Surgical Atlas of
Transcanal Endoscopic Ear Surgery
A Step by Step Guide

Video Contents

Scan QR code to access the videos

Surgical Atlas of
Transcanal Endoscopic Ear Surgery
A Step by Step Guide

Authors

Arindam Das
MS (ENT)
Consultant Otologist and Endoscopic Ear Surgeon
Assistant Professor
Institute of Otorhinolaryngology & Head and Neck Surgery (IORL & HNS)
Institute of Postgraduate Medical Education and Research (IPGMER) and SSKM Hospital
Kolkata, West Bengal, India

Sandipta Mitra
MBBS MS MRCS (London) DNB
Senior Resident (Academic)
All India Institute of Medical Sciences, New Delhi
Former Senior Resident
Institute of Otorhinolaryngology & Head and Neck Surgery (IORL & HNS)
Institute of Postgraduate Medical Education and Research (IPGMER) and SSKM Hospital
Kolkata, West Bengal, India

Sayan Hazra
MBBS MS-ENT (Gold Medal) DNB
Consultant Otologist and Endoscopic Ear Surgeon
Senior Resident (ENT)
Institute of Otorhinolaryngology & Head and Neck Surgery (IORL & HNS)
Institute of Postgraduate Medical Education and Research (IPGMER) and SSKM Hospital
Kolkata, West Bengal, India

Forewords

Mohamed MK Badr-El-Dine
Nirmal Patel

JAYPEE

JAYPEE BROTHERS MEDICAL PUBLISHERS
The Health Sciences Publisher
New Delhi | London

JAYPEE Jaypee Brothers Medical Publishers (P) Ltd

Headquarters
EMCA House
23/23-B, Ansari Road, Daryaganj
New Delhi 110 002, India
Landline: +91-11-23272143, +91-11-23272703
+91-11-23282021, +91-11-23245672
E-mail: jaypee@jaypeebrothers.com

Corporate Office
Jaypee Brothers Medical Publishers (P) Ltd.
4838/24, Ansari Road, Daryaganj
New Delhi 110 002, India
Phone: +91-11-43574357
Fax: +91-11-43574314
E-mail: jaypee@jaypeebrothers.com

Overseas Office
JP Medical Ltd.
83, Victoria Street, London
SW1H 0HW (UK)
Phone: +44-20 3170 8910
E-mail: info@jpmedpub.com

EU GPSR Authorised Representative
Logos Europe, 9 rue Nicolas Poussin
17000, La Rochelle, France
Phone: +33 (0) 6 67 93 73 78
E-mail: Contact@logoseurope.eu

Website: www.jaypeebrothers.com
Website: www.jaypeedigital.com

Surgical Atlas of Transcanal Endoscopic Ear Surgery: A Step by Step Guide

First Edition: **2023**

Reprint 2026

ISBN 978-93-5465-888-4

Printed at Replika Press Pvt. Ltd.

Dedicated to

Our teacher
Prof. (Dr) Arunabha Sengupta
who inspires us to
believe that everything is possible and leaves no stone
unturned in making anything possible.

Foreword

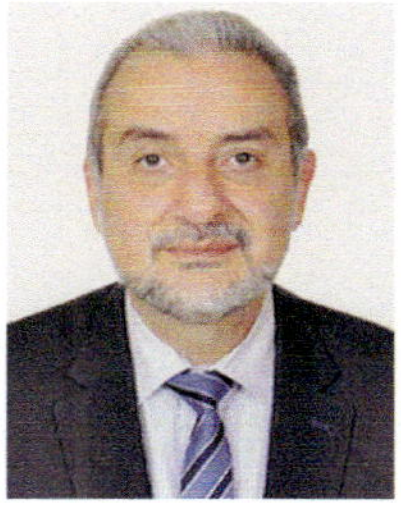

Over the last two decades, it was evident that endoscopic ear surgery would dramatically change our techniques in performing otologic surgery. The sheer introduction of transcanal endoscopic procedures rediscovered the complex anatomy of the ear and enabled better visualization of all hidden recesses otherwise not visible by microscopic techniques. Progress in endoscopic instrumentations, along with the experience gained over the years extended our indications for endoscopic ear surgery to cover most of the otologic procedures. Based on the vast technical progress in the field of otology in the past few decades, the rational to accept trends towards less-invasive procedures and embrace a better quality of life will proceed. In all likelihood, the concept of functional endoscopic ear surgery will prevail in the near future.

I am very appreciative to Dr Arindam Das and his team, for asking me to write a foreword for this comprehensive and fascinating book on endoscopic ear surgery titled *Surgical Atlas of Transcanal Endoscopic Ear Surgery: A Step by Step Guide*. I was very impressed by the idea and content of this atlas discussing the importance of endoscopic ear surgery and describing in an easy instructive way the different surgical procedures used.

The book not only reflects an impressive amount of work, but also great teaching capabilities. The elaborate illustrations facilitated the understanding of surgical anatomy in a straightforward manner. The surgical pearls presented reflect deep experience and provide practical tips important for practitioners in the field of otology and endoscopic ear surgery.

I am certain that this book will be used as a reference to both junior ENT surgeons as well as senior otologists. Residents using this book will have a useful practical guide before and after each surgery during their training program.

My sincere congratulations and deep appreciation goes to Dr Arindam Das and his team for this excellent contribution to the literature that will promote endoscopic ear surgery not only in India but all over the world.

Mohamed MK Badr-El-Dine MD PhD
Professor (Otolaryngology)
Faculty of Medicine
Alexandria University
Alexandria, Egypt
Consultant (Otology, Neurotology and
Skull Base Surgery)
Sultan Qaboos University Hospital
Muscat, Oman
President
International Working Group on
Endoscopic Ear Surgery (IWGEES)

Foreword

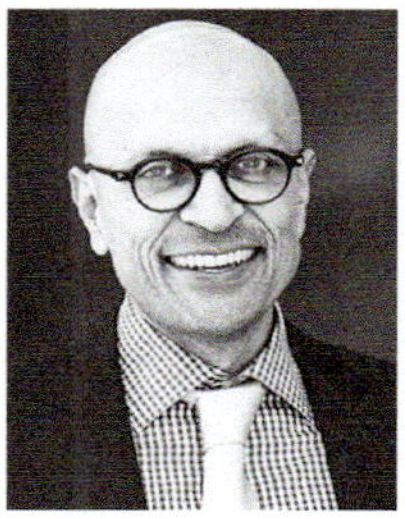

Endoscopic ear surgery has gone from an esoteric discipline to mainstream surgery in the last 10 years. Following the same historical path as endoscopic sinus surgery, the method was initially scorned as dangerous and illogical single-handed application of something which could easily be performed with two hands. There were doubters but now, all our trainees and recent graduates will agree that the endoscope delivers superior views and surgical techniques to the middle ear when compared to the microscope. By bringing the surgeons eye into the ear, contextual anatomy is better understood and surgical education is enhanced as the teacher sees the same as the learner.

Indeed, now we find that the majority of tympanoplasties and middle ear cholesteatoma can be performed transcanal saving the incisions and destruction of normal tissue to access the pathological site. This has become especially noticeable in my own pediatric practice where now most children are saved an incision for these surgeries. A huge relief for parents. Robust evidence now points to better surgical education, better quality of life outcomes and similar if not superior results with tympanoplasty and middle ear cholesteatoma surgery when comparing the endoscope to the microscope.

As with all adoption of newer surgical techniques clear concise visual explanations serve to enhance the understanding of the learner. Drs Arindam Das, Sandipta Mitra and Sayan Hazra have created a beautiful surgical atlas of the method. Beginning with the anatomy, OR setup and then progressing through basic and more complex methods the book walks the readers through the technique with high quality photography and illustrations to enhance the text. The readers will gain an in-depth understanding of all the endoscopic steps for all major pathologies of the middle ear.

This book will be an important addition to the library of all trainees and junior consultants. All senior microscopic surgeons looking to introduce the technique of endoscopic ear surgery to their practice will gain benefit from the detailed descriptions and pearls presented in the book. I congratulate Arindam Das, Sandipta Mitra and Sayan Hazra on this major effort!

Nirmal Patel MBBS (Hons) FRACS (OHNS) MS (Research UNSW)
General Secretary
International Working Group on Endoscopic Ear Surgery
Clinical Professor (Surgery)
Macquarie University, Sydney
Clinical Associate Professor (Surgery)
University of Sydney
Head (Surgical Training)
Department of Otolaryngology: Head and Neck Surgery
Royal North Shore Hospital
Sydney, Australia
Fellowship Director: SEES Group

Preface

Why is endoscopic ear surgery gaining enormous popularity amongst otologists in the last few years? We believe it is a very relevant question in recent times. At present, endoscopic ear surgery can address majority of the otological procedures that were done in the conventional manner, since inception. Interestingly, conventional microscopic ear surgical techniques got a whole new perspective after introduction of endoscopy in otology. Pathophysiology of a disease rarely changes, but we, as surgeons, are constantly evolving our surgical approaches in order to improve the result of the surgery. Endoscopic ear surgery provides a panoramic view of the surgical field and gives a close and magnified view of the vital structures. Once exposed to such a perspective, it is difficult for otologists and endoscopic ear surgeons alike, not to get addicted to this brilliant visualization. But before embarking upon this surgery, it is imperative to know the endoscopic middle ear anatomy thoroughly and understand the new principles of endoscopic ear surgery. At this opportunity, we would like to introduce our atlas which is aimed to give the readers a virtual tour into the realm of endoscopic ear surgery. It is a manual of this newly evolving surgical technique, meticulously described, to make it possible to perform, even for beginners.

In the era of minimally invasive surgery, it is a treat for every otologist to learn this highly specialized skill. We have observed that the newer generation of otologist, especially the residents, are keen to learn endoscopic techniques of ear surgery. Every aspiring surgeon searches for a surgical manual, which shall give them the insight into the surgical technique by narrating every minute detail of the surgery, make them aware of the difficulties of the technique and guide them to overcome them. This was exactly the idea behind this endeavor.

The atlas covers minor OPD procedures, such as myringotomy and grommet insertion to extremely complicated endoscopic surgery like facial nerve decompression. Endoscopic ear anatomy includes the fine micro-details of the tympanic cavity. Retrotympanum, epitympanum and protympanum have been vividly described in the atlas to make the young aspiring surgeons familiar with these new anatomical landmarks. We have tried to describe the anatomy of chorda tympani nerve in unique way, adapting to the endoscopic perspective. Starting from operation theater setup to special instruments and their use have been documented here. We have recorded all surgeries in best quality in high definition and provided crisp and clear surgical pictures, as far as possible. To make learning lucid and interesting we have included digital art diagrams to describe the anatomical landmarks and the latest anatomical concepts. "Surgical importance", "Pearls" and "Tips" have also been included to make it more relevant for practicing otologic surgeons. We have included new concepts and grading system which we have formulated, that have been published in peer reviewed, PubMed indexed, world-renowned journals. As per authors' knowledge, endoscopic facial nerve decompression has never been documented in such extensive manner.

A few lessons from our journey into the world of endoscopic ear surgery: At the start of endoscopic ear surgery, owing to its intricacies, one will encounter many difficulties, often leading to disappointment. But one needs to continue the surgical endeavor slowly and patiently. With the correct approach and practice, one will surely overcome the obstacles eventually. Single handed surgery is the most challenging factor of endoscopic ear surgery. But the trick is to learn the alternative techniques to overcome its hindrances. We believe it is a mere thought-block that keeps a surgeon from achieving his true potential. Bleeding is another limitation that needs to be controlled using proper measures, to improve visualization of the surgical field. Every such minute detail of endoscopic surgical technique and its complications have been dealt with in this atlas.

We should always remember that there is no tussle between endoscopic and microscopic ear surgery. Both are pillars in the foundation of otologic surgery, having their own advantages and disadvantages. Most importantly, every endoscopic ear surgeon should understand the limitations and contraindications of this new technique.

Arindam Das
Sandipta Mitra
Sayan Hazra

Acknowledgments

It gives us immense pleasure in introducing the first edition of our book. We would like to express our earnest indebtedness to eminent professors and teachers for their relentless support and invaluable suggestions. We would like to specially thank Drs Mohamed MK Badr-El-Dine and Nirmal Patel for penning the valuable forewords of our book.

We owe a debt of gratitude towards the Institute of Otorhinolaryngology & Head and Neck Surgery (IORL & HNS) for providing us with state-of-the-art facilities, including the best endoscopes, three-chip camera, facial nerve monitor, CO_2 laser and skeeter drill. We express our heartfelt gratitude to our teacher, Professor (Dr) Arunabha Sengupta for his immense support and guidance behind this book. We are thankful to Professor (Dr) Debasis Barman (Director and Head, IORL & HNS), Professor (Dr) Manimoy Bandhopadhyay (Director, IPGMER), and Professor (Dr) Piyush Kumar Roy (MSVP, IPGMER) for their unstinting backing.

Dr RN Patil, pioneer of endoscopic ear surgery in India has been instrumental in igniting the passion in us to pursue the art. Concepts taught by Professor (Dr) H Vijeyandra and Professor (Dr) KP Morwani on basics of otology have been the building blocks of our otology journey.

Endoscopic ear surgery is incomplete without the mention of Drs Joao Flavio, Muaaz Tarabichi, Livio Presutti and Daniele Marchioni, whose remarkable work in the field of endoscopic ear surgery has enlightened one and all.

We are overwhelmed to be associated with doyens in the field of otorhinolaryngology in India, Professor (Dr) Dulal Kumar Basu and Professor (Dr) Amitabha Roychoudhury, who have always guided and supported us.

We truly appreciate the valuable inputs given by our teachers Professor (Dr) Sumanta Kumar Dutta, Professor (Dr) Bijan Basak, Dr Alok Ranjan Mondal, Dr Sourav Dutta and Dr Kaustuv Das Biswas. We are thankful to our anesthesiologist colleagues, residents and staffs of Institute of Otorhinolaryngology, SSKM Hospital. We thank the Senior Residents of the Institute, Drs Pranay Agarwal, Ankit Choudhary, Soutrik Kumar, Mridul Janweja, Aryabrata Dubey and Sauravmoy Banerjee, who have helped us in various stages of preparation of this book.

A special mention goes to Drs Monish Bose, Sanjay Gupta, Deepjoy Basu and Lopamudra (Misra) Chakraborty, who have supported us in every possible way in performing and documentation of surgeries on regular basis.

We are extremely thankful to Shri Jitendar P Vij (Group Chairman), Mr Ankit Vij (Managing Director), Mr MS Mani (Group President), Ms Chetna Malhotra (Senior Director – Professional Publishing, Marketing and Business Development), Ms Pooja Bhandari (Production Head), and Dr Rajul Jain (Senior Development Editor) of M/s Jaypee Brothers Medical Publishers (P) Ltd, New Delhi, India, for making all efforts in editing the manuscript to finally bring the printed version to our readers.

It is impossible to thank our parents and family enough, who stood by us during the entire process.

Last but not the least, we are forever indebted to our patients who trusted us to perform the surgeries and document them for publication.

We hope the readers enjoy the book as much as we enjoyed writing it.

Contents

CHAPTER 1

History of Endoscopic Ear Surgery

Arindam Das, Sayan Hazra

Chapter Outline

INTRODUCTION

Developed in the 1960s, the Hopkins rod endoscope was a major improvement over the old endoscopes, with a wider field of view and much better optics. By the late 1960s, it was possible to visualize unprecedented anatomic detail in vibrant true colors. Coupled with the cold light source, the Hopkins rod endoscope allowed the emergence of endoscopic minimally-invasive surgical techniques in many surgical specialties, including otorhinolaryngology.

EARLY DAYS OF ENDOSCOPIC EAR SURGERY

It did not take long before someone put an endoscope in an ear to look around, first in cadavers and animal ears, then in living human patients. In 1967, Mer et al. reported on the use of endoscopes to examine the middle ears of human cadavers and ears of living animals through iatrogenic myringotomies. In 1975, Marquet introduced an endoscope of 1.7 mm diameter through a tympanic perforation to observe the tympanic cavity. He already foresaw the great possibilities of the technique and wrote: "The retrotympanic regions, such as the sinus tympani, can be observed in a precise manner". In 1982, Nomura described endoscopic explorations of middle ears of living patients through a myringotomy and using an angled endoscope known as needle otoscope. His focus was on middle ear photography. Kansaki, in 1983, was the first to anticipate the importance of endoscopy in postoperative surveillance of the posterior cavities of the middle ear in patients operated for cholesteatoma by a closed technique. Under local anesthesia, he introduced an endoscope via a retroauricular incision and reported a series of 26 cases.

Endoscopic Ear Surgery in the 1990s

Thomassin et al. started investigating the advantages of this mode of endoscopic visualizations in ear surgery. The first publications on the application of endoscopy in ear surgery were seen in the 1990s. Otologists started using endoscopic approaches not only for inspection but also to guide intervention. McKennan used it as "transcutaneous mastoidoscope" for second look mastoidectomies to avoid another postauricular incision during second look surgery for cholesteatoma. EL-Guindy from Egypt investigated the utility of endoscope to perform a myringoplasty with fat graft material in 1992.

Muaaz Tarabichi embraced endoscope as a sole mode of visualization for ear surgery and by late 1990s published an important series on "endoscopic management of acquired cholesteatoma[1]" in 1997 in which 38 cases underwent a transcanal endoscopic tympanotomy and extended atticotomy for removal of cholesteatoma. In 1999, he published another series "endoscopic middle ear surgery[2]" in 165 patients enumerating the advantages and disadvantages of transcanal operative endoscopy as the primary approach to the management of middle ear disease.

Endoscopic Ear Surgery in the 2000s

During this century, more investigators and otologic surgeons explored the potential benefits of endoscopic techniques in middle ear cavities and in cerebellopontine angle (CPA). From 1967 to 1990, there were no reports on TEES in the literature. This compares with more than 300 publications on TEES from 2010 to present day. In adjunct to this, surgeons such as Livio Presutti, Daniele Marchioni, and Natasha Pollak have gifted us with books titled "Endoscopic Ear Surgery" (EES) in 2014, exploring the role of endoscopy in the evolution of otologic surgery, and to introduce surgeons to basic and advanced EES. Rich with color images, the books also serve as an atlas of temporal bone anatomy and pathologic processes as seen through an endoscope which have aided in better understanding of EES and encouraged surgeons worldwide to use endoscopes as a primary tool or as an adjunct to microscope for various middle ear surgeries. In 2016, Muaaz Tarabichi and Joao Flavio Nogueira brought out another landmark paper in an issue of OCNA on "Endoscopic ear and Eustachian tube".

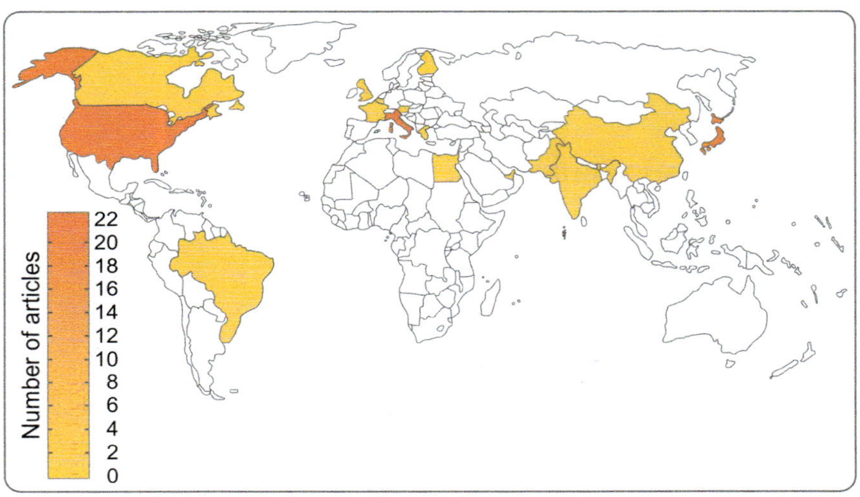

Fig. 1: Publication of articles on endoscopic ear surgery across the globe.

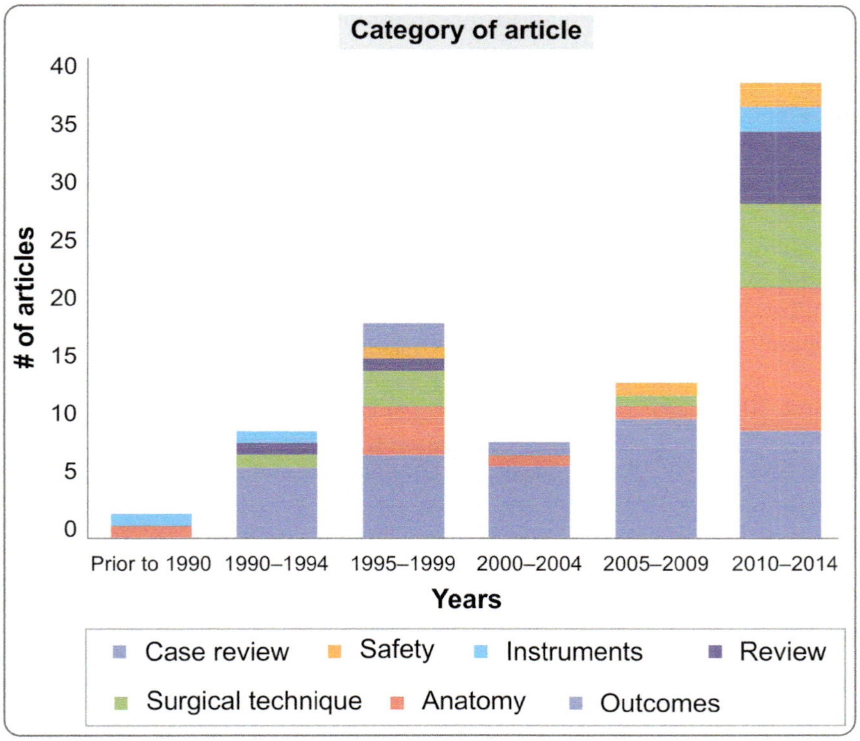

Fig. 2: Category and volume of articles on endoscopic ear surgery being published.

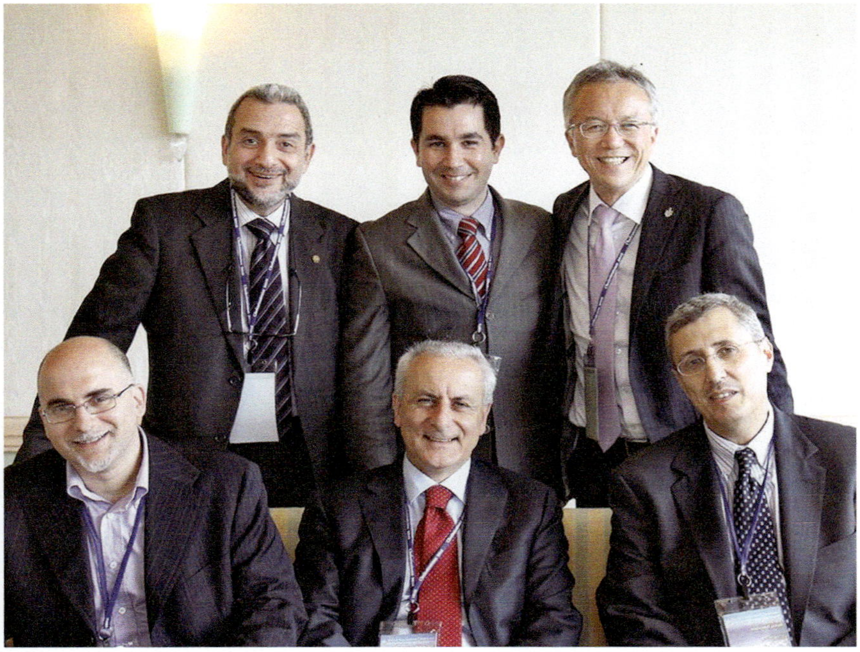

Fig. 3: Founding Members of International Working Group on Endoscopic Ear Surgery (IWGEES).
1st row (left to right sitting): Daniele Marchioni; Livio Presutti; Muaaz Tarabichi
2nd row (left to right standing): Mohamed Badr-El-Dine; Joao Flavio Nogueira; Seiji Kakehata

Badr-El-Dine in 2002 published a series of 82 canal-wall-up (CWU) surgeries and 10 canal-wall-down (CWD) surgeries for cholesteatoma. After microscopic excision, endoscope detected residual disease in 23% of cases. Common sites of residual disease were the sinus tympani, facial recess and undersurface of the scutum.

Endoscopic Ear Surgery: Present Day

Recent development of modern video-endoscopy with high-definition 4K, and 3-dimensional imaging along with high-definition recording devices have aided in sharing of knowledge further on this ever-evolving field. Surgeons are exploring areas beyond middle ear cleft onto the cochlea, CP angle, posterior fossa, etc. with better understanding of the endoscopic anatomy, angled endoscopes, and instruments with curvature and multifunctionality. Minimally invasive endoscope assisted retrosigmoid approach (MIRA) or key-hole brain surgery is one such approach that allows access to the internal auditory canal and CP angle through 2-cm^2 craniotomy performed posterior to the sigmoid sinus.

Vestibular nerve section, microvascular decompression, surgery for vestibular schwannomas, nonacoustic tumors, or insertion of auditory brainstem implants are being done almost exclusively with endoscopes. It gives a better view of the CPA and allows early identification of various neurovascular structures, more complete removal of lesions, lesser morbidity and better functional results in terms of hearing and facial nerve preservation. Giuseppe Panetti is one of the forerunners of EES and his major contributions to ENT has been through designing bespoke equipment since 2009 to assist in some of the challenges of operating endoscopically.

In 2007, Stephane Ayache (France) proposed "the creation of an International Society of Otoendoscopy" [later to be renamed the International Working Group on Endoscopic Ear Surgery (IWGEES)] to advocate and collaborate for further development of this approach to ear surgery. The founding members included Muaaz Tarabichi (UAE), Daniele Marchioni (Italy), Livio Presutti (Italy), Dave Pothier (Canada), Mohamed Badr-El-Dine (Egypt), and Seiji Kakehata (Japan). The IWGEES has grown to a membership of 205 members from 55 countries and has been instrumental in standardizing, teaching, and spreading of the technique.

REFERENCES

1. Tarabichi M. Endoscopic management of acquired cholesteatoma. Am J Otol. 1997;18(5):544-9.
2. Tarabichi M. Endoscopic middle ear surgery. Ann Otol Rhinol Laryngol. 1999;108(1):39-46.
3. Tarabichi M, Noguerira JF. Endoscopic Ear and Eustachian Tube Surgery. Otolaryngol Clin North Am. 2016;49(5):1097-132.

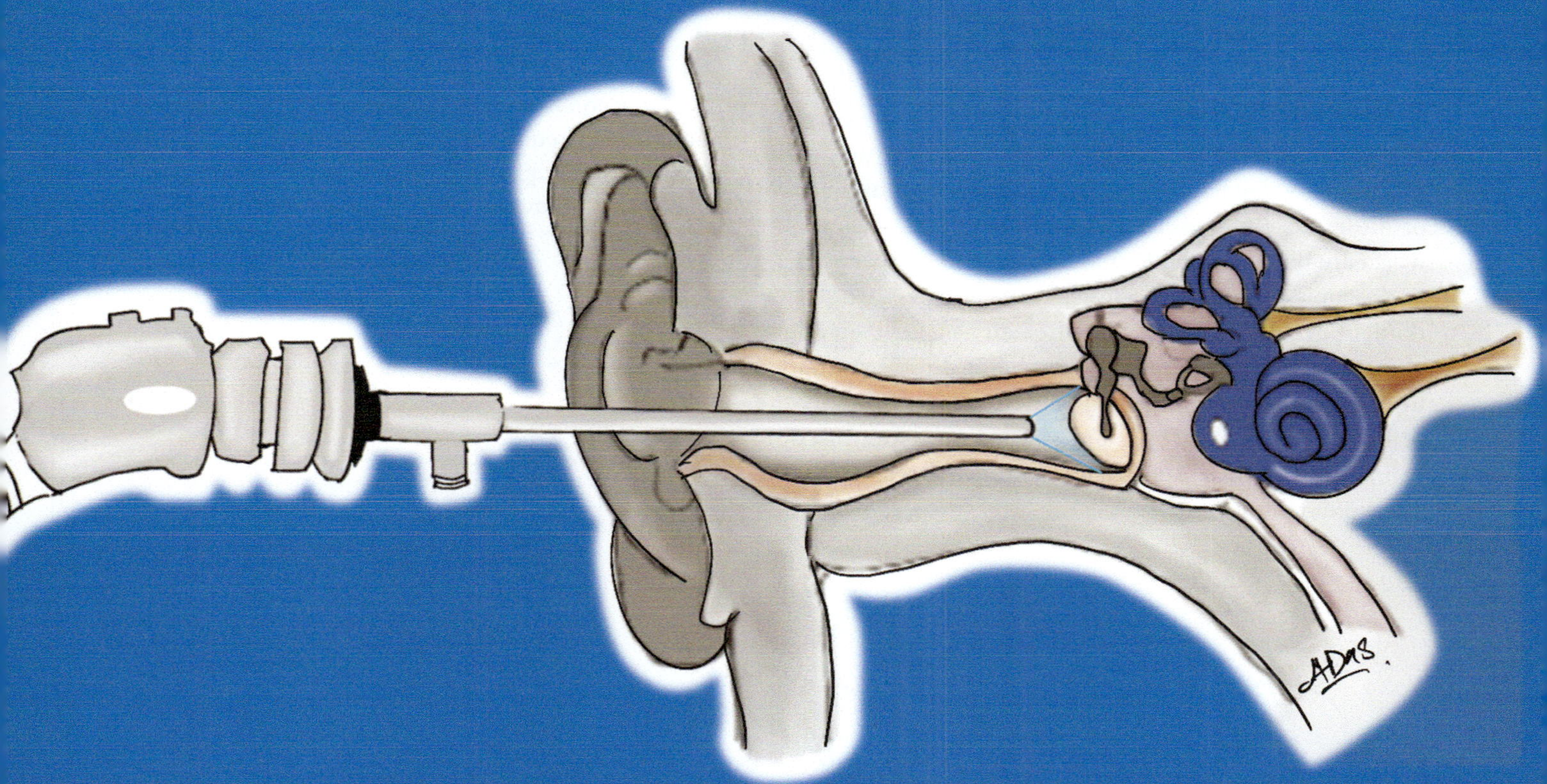

CHAPTER **2**

Principles of Endoscopic Ear Surgery

Arindam Das, Sandipta Mitra

Chapter Outline

INTRODUCTION

The basic training in otologic surgery, all over the world, traditionally has been using microscope. With the advent of the endoscope, more and more surgeons all over the world are being trained to undergo endoscopic ear surgery. Endoscopic ear surgery, technically speaking, is a whole new domain in itself and should be treated as a new technique altogether. However, most surgeons being previously trained in microscopic ear surgery, instinctively try to apply the principles of microscopic ear surgery to its endoscopic counterpart. In this respect, it is imperative to realize that the principles guiding endoscopic ear surgery are very different from the conventional microscopic ear surgery that has been propagated for decades. The spectrum of endoscopic ear surgery for chronic otitis media (COM) may be broadly classified as follows:

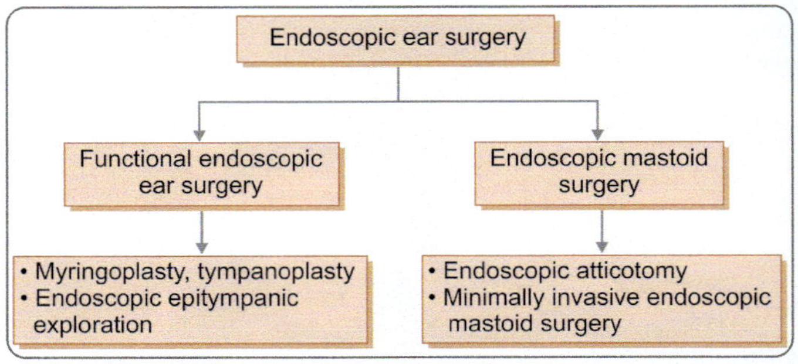

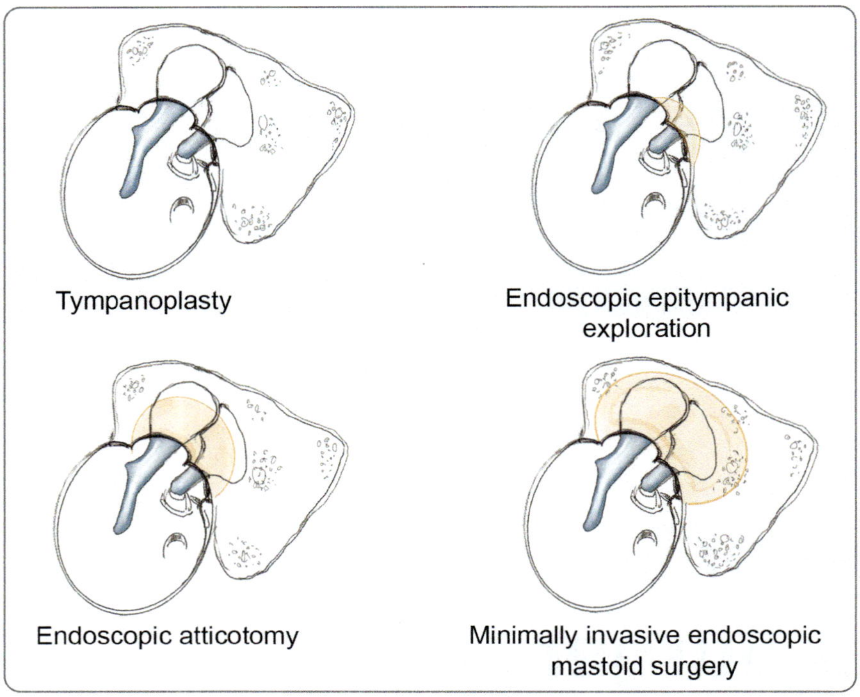

Fig. 1: Types of endoscopic ear surgery.

CLINICOPATHOLOGICAL BASIS

Endoscopic ear surgery, as a treatment modality, encompasses a wide spectrum. At one end of it, lies the *functional* endoscopic ear surgeries, that includes myringoplasty, tympanoplasty, and endoscopic epitympanic exploration. This is mainly reserved for managing the mucosal variety of chronic otitis media (both active and inactive) in which the key principle is maximal tissue preservation. Minimal bone removal, maximal soft tissue preservation with minimally invasive techniques to restore the normal physiology of ventilation pathways are the cornerstones. Whereas, on the other hand, lies endoscopic mastoid surgery that may be an atticotomy or more extensive mastoidectomy, depending on the disease extent. However, endoscopic ear surgery is not limited to surgical management of chronic otitis media. It spans to include other functional surgeries as well such as endoscopic stapes surgery (stapedotomy/stapedectomy) and facial nerve decompression surgery. Furthermore, it is also being utilised to explore diseases and tumors of lateral skull base as well as performing cochlear implant.

MICROSCOPIC TO ENDOSCOPIC EAR SURGERY: A PARADIGM SHIFT

There are a number of reasons as to why endoscopic ear surgery has gained immense popularity among otologic surgeons worldwide. To list a few, endoscopes offer the following advantages which are not available to us while performing the same surgery using the conventional microscope:[1,2]

- Wide panoramic view
- Better illumination

- Close-up view of intricate details of each anatomical structure
- Angled endoscopes (30, 45, and 70°) allow visualization of remote nooks and corners inside the middle ear cleft obviating the need for extra bone and soft tissue removal.
- Preservation of soft tissues, bone and minimal mucosal disruption lead to faster healing, early, and better hearing outcomes
- Less complications associated with bone drilling or curettage

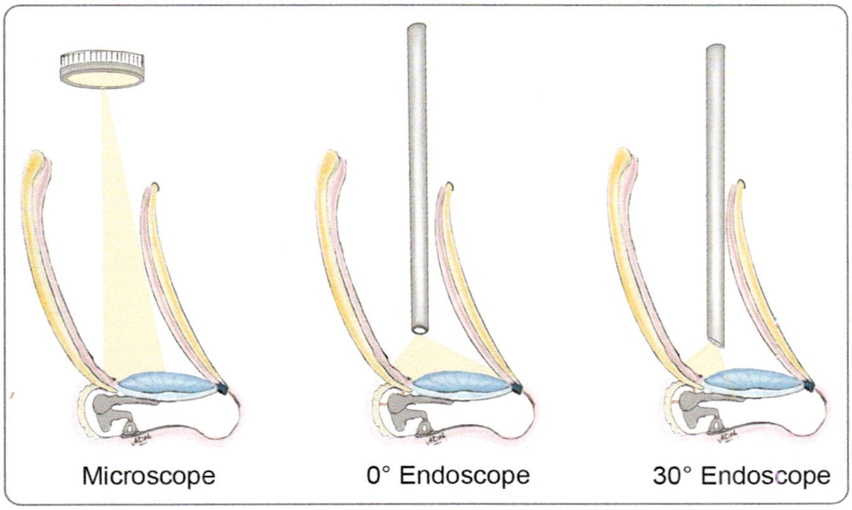

Fig. 2: Difference in angulation and field of visualization between a microscope, 0° endoscope and 30° endoscope.

INSTRUMENTATION IN ENDOSCOPIC EAR SURGERY

Endoscopes

Zero-degree endoscopes: We recommend use of 0° endoscope of 4 mm diameter and 18 cm length for majority of the operative work. The main reason for this is superior visualization, which is the key to any surgery.

Zero-degree scopes of lesser diameter such as 3 mm or 2.7 mm are not preferred as there is a decline in the quality of resolution with downsizing of scopes.

- Additionally, the shorter length of otoendoscope causes the two working hands to come in close proximity while maneuvering and frequent crossover, which is against the principles of endoscopic surgery

Angled endoscopes: In contrary, angled scopes such as 30°, 45°, 70°, etc. should be preferably of 3 mm or 2.7 mm diameter. This is because while working around a corner, the angled scope needs to be placed in the diametrically opposite position and at the same time the working instrument needs to operate in the same limited space.

Let us say the operating instrument needs to work in the area of sinus tympani. Hence, scope needs to be stationed near the protympanum or over the promontory. Now, it will be difficult to fit in scope of a larger diameter in the limited space along with another working instrument. Moreover, the tip of the angled scope being in a blind spot for the surgeon, it may cause inadvertent injury to middle ear structures, especially in beginners.

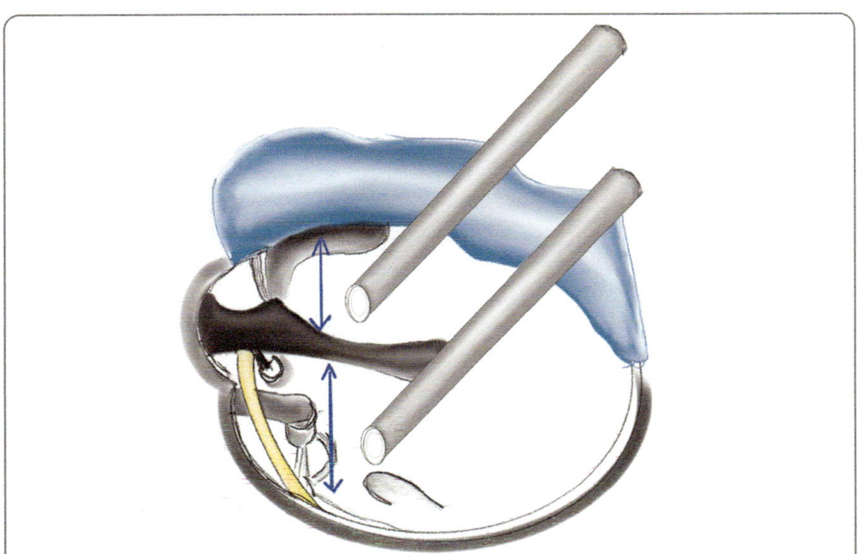

Fig. 3A: Rationale for use of 3 mm or 2.7 mm angled scope: The anteroposterior diameter of mesotympanum is roughly 10 mm which may be divided into two halves by the handle of malleus. Angled scopes are usually lodged in one of these halves (either anterior or posterior to the handle of malleus), which is roughly 4–5 mm in diameter each. Angled scopes of wider diameter such as 4 mm are difficult to negotiate in such limited spaces and hence not preferred.

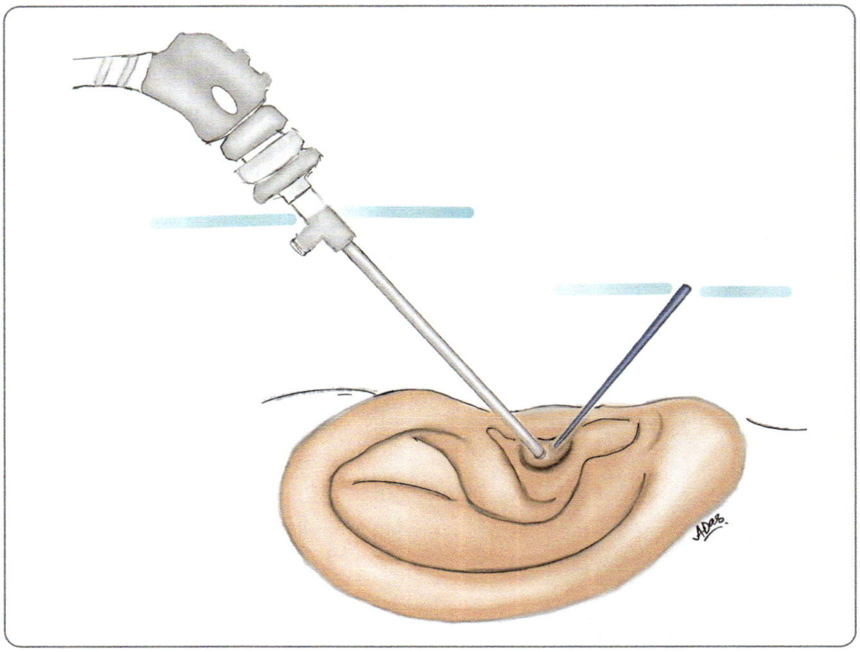

Fig. 3B: Endoscope shaft and working instrument should be of different lengths to prevent close proximity of the surgeon's hands.

Angled Microinstruments

Maximum tissue preservation by working around the corners is one of the key principles of endoscopic ear surgery. For that purpose, use of angled endoscopes requires concomitant use of specialized angled instruments for ease of operability. It is prudent to have in one's set, 45° and 90° angled microinstruments such as microscissors, alligator, and cup forceps (analogous to a Rhinologist's set for functional endoscopic sinus surgery).

Suction Instruments

Endoscopic ear surgery being practically single-handed surgery, role of suction instruments is paramount. Apart from its obvious role of keeping the surgical field clear, suction also plays the crucial function of providing *counter traction* to tissues, for example, during dissection of cholesteatoma sac in endoscopic mastoidectomy.

Complete specialized set of endoscopic ear surgery instruments have been developed by Prof Giuseppe Panetti. Each microinstrument has a suction control port on the handpiece. This enables the surgeon to perform dissection as well as suction simultaneously.

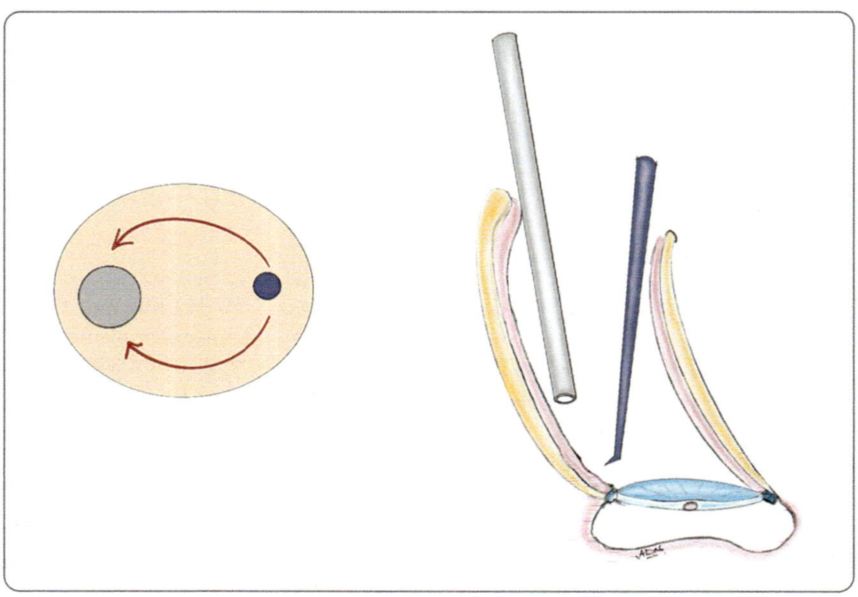

Fig. 4: Position of instrument with respect to the endoscope: Endoscope is kept stable, resting over the canal, while the instrument navigates according to the step being performed.

ROLE OF PREOPERATIVE OTOENDOSCOPY IN ENDOSCOPIC EAR SURGERY

We recommend preoperative otoendoscopy before every case planned to undergo endoscopic ear surgery. The major benefits of this simple procedure before the surgery are:

- Real-time assessment of external auditory canal architecture, its curvature, slope, dimension, any major anatomical hindrances, if any (which may have to be addressed and hence planned accordingly)
- Confirmation of the disease (e.g., small retraction pockets or ossicular erosion)
- Extent of the disease (e.g., extension of a retraction pocket, whether it has extended beyond the lateral semicircular canal)

As every case of endoscopic ear surgery is performed permeatally, a preoperative otoendoscopy may be imagined as a practice simulation prior to the actual surgery, which gives the surgeon valuable clues regarding the anatomy and the pathology itself so that he/she may be well equipped and have a ready plan on the day of the surgery.

ANATOMICAL CONSIDERATIONS IN ENDOSCOPIC EAR SURGERY

Endoscopes have opened up a new horizon in the domain of otology, facilitating visualization of structures which was poorly understood before. This has dramatically shaped new concepts and helped to understand the pathophysiology of some of the most common ear pathologies dealt with, since centuries.

As endoscopic ear surgeons, we need to orient ourselves accordingly and imbibe the recent concepts that have been put forward.[4,5] The anatomy of key areas that one needs to have a clear concept about before embarking on any endoscopic otological surgery are:

- *Retrotympanum*: Recesses around the facial nerve
- Protympanum and the anatomy of tympanic part of Eustachian tube
- Middle ear mucosal folds and anatomy of the ventilation pathways
- Three-dimensional concept of the layout of vital structures encountered from attic to the antrum when viewed from mesotympanum (since this is the natural course/path an endoscope follows in contrary to a posterior to anterior approach in microscopic canal wall-up mastoidectomy)

It is important to understand that in routine endoscopic ear surgery, all the vital structures are encountered first. This means:

- The structures are clearly viewed directly right in front of us
- Such a direct visualization carries lesser chances of iatrogenic injury (which may often occur due to lack of proper visualization)
- Not only normal anatomical landmarks, better visualization of the pathology also means a more complete disease clearance
- Better reconstruction (incudostapedial complex area being clearly visualized with better magnification)

SAFETY CONCERNS IN ENDOSCOPIC EAR SURGERY

Thermal Injury

The outer hair cells of cochlea are delicate structures which are susceptible to external stimuli such as temperature changes.[6] Temperature rise in middle ear endoscopy can cause a rise in temperature in the lateral semicircular canal, similar to a warm caloric stimulation, which is responsible for the vestibular symptoms such as vertigo and vomiting. Longer duration of thermal exposure in endoscopic ear surgery has been found to be associated with significant rise in the middle ear temperature with Xenon light source. Furthermore, a high-frequency sensorineural hearing loss has been noted in the higher frequencies such as 4, 6, and 8 kHz with Xenon light source and at 8 kHz with LED light source. This study was performed in vivo and hence represents actual temperature changes that might not be evident in studies conducted in cadaveric or simulation models due to the "heat sink" effect of circulating blood and inner ear fluids.

In the light of the above-mentioned evidence, *certain precautions* need to be adopted to avoid adverse outcomes:

- Proper surgical time management to avoid unnecessary exposure
- Use of cooler light sources such as LED
- Intensity to be kept at 50% for optimal illumination and minimal heat generation
- Intermittent cold saline irrigation of the surgical field
- Ambient operating room temperature to be kept on the cooler side of the normal range.

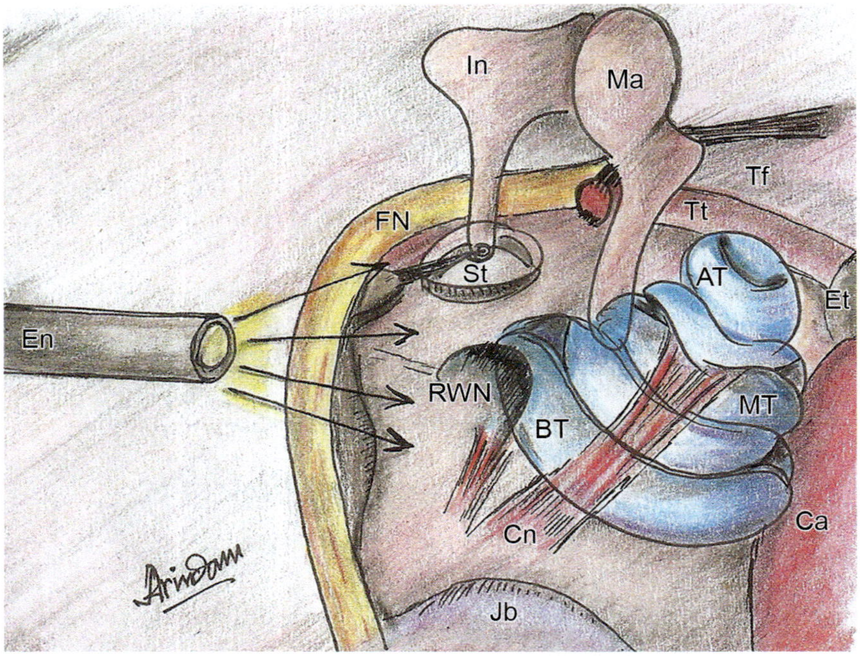

Fig. 5: Middle ear and inner ear structures exposed to heat from a light source during endoscopic ear surgery. Note the relative proximity of the basal turn of cochlea to the light source.
(AT: apical turn; BT: basal turn; Ca: carotid artery; Cn: cochlear nerve; En: endoscope; Et: Eustachian tube; FN: facial nerve; In: incus; Jb: jugular bulb; Ma: malleus; MT: middle turn; RWN: round window niche; St: stapes; Tf: tensor fold; Tt: tensor tympani)

Direct Mechanical Injury

Inadvertent injury with the tip of the scope is common in beginners. This is because endoscopic ear surgery requires finer movements with precise hand-eye coordination that is more challenging than a fixed microscopic set-up with the advantage of ambidexterity.

Controlled movements, coordination between the scope and instruments, spatial awareness of instruments especially the sharp, cutting ones should be nurtured with regular practice in cadaveric and simulator models. One may say that he/she has achieved the skill when he/she shall be able to move a particular instrument freely at any desired anatomical position at any point of time.

HEMOSTASIS IN ENDOSCOPIC EAR SURGERY

One of the major concerns of an endoscopic surgeon is bleeding and soiling of the scope during surgery. In order to avoid such a situation, the preparation of the patient must begin even before the surgery. The important checklist in this respect includes:

- Detailed *patient history* and addressing *comorbidities* like hematological and cardiovascular disorders
- *Active local infection must be controlled prior to posting for surgery:*
  - We prefer to administer one course of systemic antibiotics in all patients undergoing endoscopic ear surgery except stapes surgery
- *Steroid-containing ear drops* are avoided immediately prior to surgery and must be stopped at least 1 week before surgery.
  - This is because topical steroids have known to cause thinning of skin which makes the flap friable during surgery and increases the chances of bleeding.[7]
- *Role of middle ear packing:*
  - Cotton balls soaked in 4% lignocaine with adrenaline (1:1,000) are used to pack the external auditory canal and middle ear following four quadrant infiltrations.
  - This serves three purposes:
    1. Surface anesthesia
    2. Canal skin decongestion (similar to nasal packing just prior to endoscopic sinus surgery)
    3. Avoidance of canal wall bleb formation following local infiltration due to tamponade effect
- *Tranexamic acid protocol:*
  - Tranexamic acid has been found to play a role in hemostasis in endoscopic ear surgery. Though, it is never a substitute of a good local infiltration, it is administered in the following protocol for better intraoperative hemostasis[8]:
  - *Slow intravenous tranexamic acid bolus (10 mg/kg) half an hour before the start of surgery followed by infusion (5 mg/kg/hour). The infusion is prepared in normal saline.*
- Meticulous *local anesthetic infiltration* of *adequate amount* and *concentration* in the *right plane*

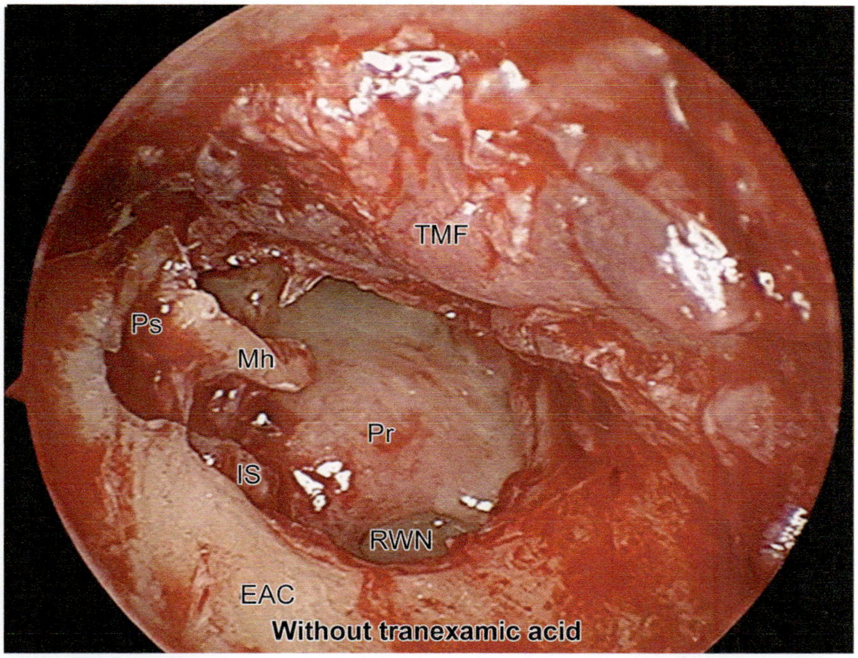

Fig. 6A: Intraoperative field in endoscopic ear surgery without tranexamic acid.
TMF: tympanomeatal flap; Ps: Prussak's space; Mh: handle of Malleus; Pr: promontory; IS: incudostapedial joint; RWN: Round window niche; EAC: external auditory canal)

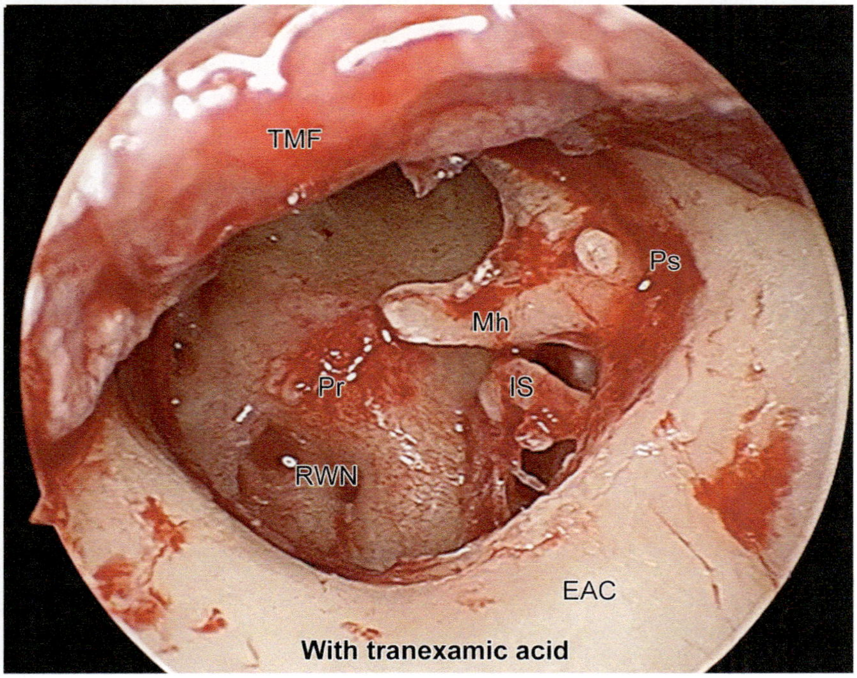

Fig. 6B: Intraoperative field in endoscopic ear surgery with tranexamic acid.
TMF: tympanomeatal flap; Ps: Prussak's space; Mh: handle of Malleus; Pr: promontory; IS: incudostapedial joint; RWN: Round window niche; EAC: external auditory canal)

Das and Mitra EES Bleeding and Field Visibility Score (D&M EES score):

Grade	*Amount of bleeding*	*Description*	*Quality of field visibility*
0	None	Suctioning not required	Excellent
1	Minimal	Suctioning rarely required	Very good
2	Slight	Intermittent suctioning required	Good
3	Moderate	Adrenaline soaked cotton balls + intermittent suctioning	Fair
4	Moderately severe	Adrenaline soaked cotton balls + suction instrument required to maintain visibility	Poor
5	Severe	Procedure converted to microscopic approach/abandoned	Visualization not possible

A stepwise approach to achieving hemostasis in endoscopic ear surgery can be summarized as follows:

Cotton pledgets soaked in undiluted adrenaline

↓

Packing with hemostats like gelfoam

↓

Cauterization with ball point probe with monopolar diathermy at low current setting (only applicable in external auditory canal)

ROLE OF ENDOSCOPE HOLDER IN ENDOSCOPIC EAR SURGERY

Holders for stabilizing the endoscope have been used in different surgical specialties including neurosurgery.[9] Endoscope holders have been developed for otologic surgery as well. It allows the surgeon to fix the endoscope to an operating microscope. This allows both hands of the surgeon to be utilized for instrumentation.

However, use of endoscope holder has its own disadvantages:

- Dynamic component of endoscopic ear surgery is one of its key strengths as compared to the fixed system of microscope.
- Simultaneous synchronous movements of the scope along with the instrument are very crucial for proper visualization of the desired area and maneuvering.
- Ability to move the endoscope in centimeters, manually, helps the surgeon to attain that perfect position from where the entire working field can be visualized.
- In a fixed endoscope, sudden jerky movement by the patient under local anesthesia can cause damage to the patient as well the endoscope

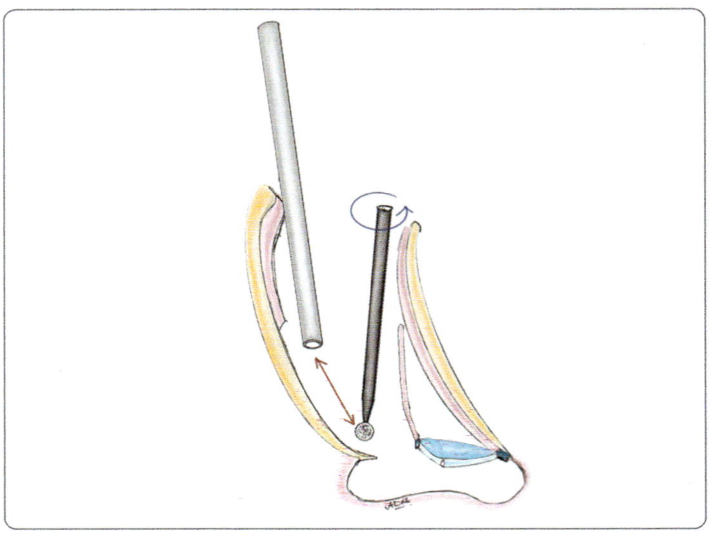

ENDOSCOPIC BONE DRILLING: THE ART

Single-handed bone drilling using the endoscope happens to be one of the biggest challenges of endoscopic ear surgery. This is true for beginners as well as surgeons classically trained in microscopic ear surgery, who always had the luxury of ambidexterity.

However, with sustained practice and strict adherence to certain basic principles, it is possible to perform single-handed endoscopic bone drilling safely and efficiently. The basic principles of endoscopic bone drilling are:

- *Safe distance:*
  - One should always maintain a safe distance between the tip of the endoscope and the rotating burr.
  - Simultaneous synchronous movement of the two makes it a dynamic process
  - "Brushless motor" in which the burr comes to an immediate halt as soon as the foot pedal is stopped, it is very useful and should be used for endoscopic bone drilling.
- *Mind the shaft:*
  - The rotating shaft of the burr may cause inadvertent injury to the canal soft tissue.
  - To avoid it, an aluminum foil of a suture pack such as catgut may be laid to protect the canal soft tissues during drilling.
- *Coarse diamond burr:* Coarse diamond burr should be used for bone drilling as it is less tissue destructive, lest there is a slip of the hand.
- *Wilson bone punch:*
  - The major bulk of the outer attic wall may be easily punched out using a Wilson bone punch while performing endoscopic atticotomy.
  - Having removed the major bulk of the bone, the remaining bone is then carefully drilled using an appropriately sized burr tip.
- *Angled curettes:* High quality angled curettes are useful for endoscopic bone removal and should be an integral part of an endoscopic ear surgeon's instrument set.

Fig. 7: The safe distance between the rotating tip of the burr and the tip of the endoscope.

EXPOSURE IN ENDOSCOPIC EAR SURGERY

- Exposure is the key to a successful surgical procedure.
- Middle Ear Structural Visibility Index (MESVI) is a 10-point grading system based on certain critical anatomical landmarks devised by the authors to specify the extent of exposure of surgical field in mastoid surgery.
- In a study conducted by the authors, when this MESVI score was correlated with the area of optimal exposure required for disease clearance, it was found that for an approximately equal area of exposure, endoscopic approach offered a superior median MESVI when compared to microscopic approach.

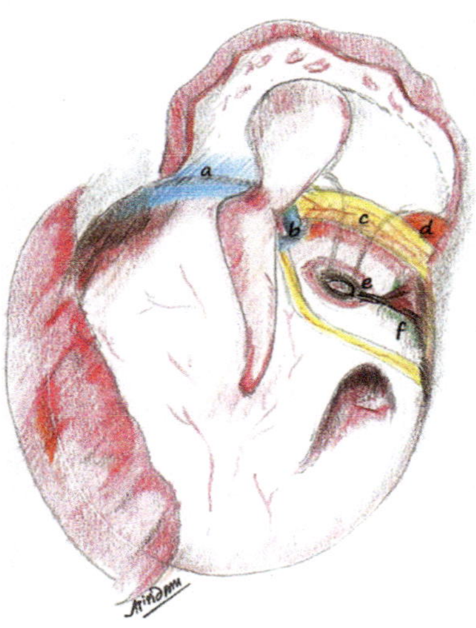

Anatomical landmarks	Score
a. Tensor fold	2
b. Processus cochleariformis	1
c. Facial nerve (Horizontal segment)	1
b. Lateral semicircular canal (Ampullary end)	2
e. Footplate of stapes	2
f. Sinus tympani	2
Total score	**10**

1	2	3	4	5	6	7	8	9	10

Poor (1–3) Good (4–7) Excellent (>7)

Fig. 8: Middle ear structural visibility index (MESVI).

ENDOSCOPIC EAR SURGERY AS A TEACHING TOOL

Endoscopic ear surgery serves as an extremely useful teaching tool for budding otologists. Intricate anatomical details, hand movements, and surgical step demonstration which were otherwise difficult to comprehend in the microscopic era can be readily illustrated.

ENDOSCOPIC EAR SURGERY: THE SHORTCOMINGS

Depth Perception

The lack of binocular vision makes endoscopic ear surgery essentially two-dimensional. This makes it a major reason for this surgery to have a steep learning curve. However, the way to overcome this limitation is to develop the sense of *"tactile feedback"*. Developing the sense of *surgical proprioception* by touching the nearest safe landmark in the surgical field is the key to overcoming this limitation, apart from regular endoscopic temporal bone dissection. Recently, 3D camera has been introduced to overcome this shortcoming.[10]

Lack of Stability due to Single-handedness

Single-handedness has always been a limiting factor in endoscopic ear surgery, more so in case of beginners. The lack of support by the second instrument in the nondominant hand needs to be tackled by devising instruments such as combined suction-dissectors and improvising new surgical techniques in order to fill in the deficit.

Severe Hemorrhage Soiling the Scope

Severe hemorrhage (Grade 5 of Das and Mitra EES Bleeding and Field Visibility Score) soiling the scope and completely obscuring the vision is one the rare instances where the surgeon may have to abandon the procedure endoscopically and shift to the microscope.

CONCLUSION

Endoscopic ear surgery is a highly specialized surgery of finesse and precision. With clear understanding of the endoscopic anatomy, strict adherence to the basic principles and sustained practice, one can surely master the skills to perform this surgery. However, one should remember that the endoscope and the microscope are both tools for otologic surgery. Each has its own merits and demerits. The decision to choose the appropriate tool or a combination of tools should be customized according to the patient's disease as well as the surgeon's own capability.

SPECIAL POINTS

- Endoscopic ear surgery is an entirely different entity in itself and should not be compared with microscopic ear surgery in that sense.
- One should imbibe the anatomical concepts and surgical principles relevant to endoscopic ear surgery.
- Dedicated specialized instruments must be available with the surgeon embarking on any endoscopic ear surgery.
- One should never compromise on the quality of the camera as visualization is the key.
- Learning curve of endoscopic ear surgery largely depends in ability to pick up the precise movements, hand-eye coordination, and sense of depth.
- A surgeon should never be biased and at any point of time should be ready to convert it into a microscopic approach, if the need arises.
- Lastly, otologists must step out of the rigid conventional institution of microscopic ear surgery, embrace endoscopic ear surgery as a highly specialized branch and explore its possibilities in future.

REFERENCES

1. Tarabichi M. Endoscopic management of limited attic cholesteatoma. Laryngoscope. 2004;114(7):1157-62.
2. Bennett ML, Zhang D, Labadie RF, Noble JH. Comparison of middle ear visualization with endoscopy and microscopy. Otol Neurotol. 2016;37:362-6.
3. Marchioni D, Mattioli F, Alicandri-Ciufelli M, Presutti L. Transcanal endoscopic approach to the sinus tympani: a clinical report. Otol Neurotol. 2009;30(6):758-65.
4. Bonali M, Anschuetz L, Fermi M, Villari D, Mariani GA, Manzoli L, et al. The variants of the retro- and hypotympanum: an endoscopic anatomical study. Eur Arch Otorhinolaryngol. 2017;274(5):2141-48.
5. Alicandri-Ciufelli M, Marchioni D, Kakehata S, Presutti L, Villari D. Endoscopic management of attic cholesteatoma: long-term results. Otolaryngol Clin North Am. 2016;49(5):1265-70.
6. Das A, Mitra S, Agarwal P, Sengupta A. Prolonged intra-operative thermal exposure in endoscopic ear surgery: is it really safe? J Laryngol Otol. 2020;134(8):727-31.
7. Das A, Mitra S, Ghosh D, Kumar S, Sengupta A. Does tranexamic acid improve intra-operative visualisation in endoscopic ear surgery? A double-blind, randomised, controlled trial. J Laryngol Otol. 2019;133(12): 1033-7.
8. Coondoo A, Phiske M, Verma S, Lahiri K. Side-effects of topical steroids: a long overdue revisit. Indian Dermatol Online J. 2014;5(4):416-25.
9. Morita A, Okada Y, Kitano M, Hori T, Taneda M, Kirino T. Development of hybrid integrated endoscope-holder system for endoscopic microneurosurgery. Neurosurgery. 2004;55(4):926-32.
10. Bernardeschi D, Lahlou G, De Seta D, Russo FY, Mosnier I, Sterkers O. 3D endoscopic ear surgery: a clinical pilot study. Eur Arch Otorhinolaryngol. 2018;275(2):379-84.

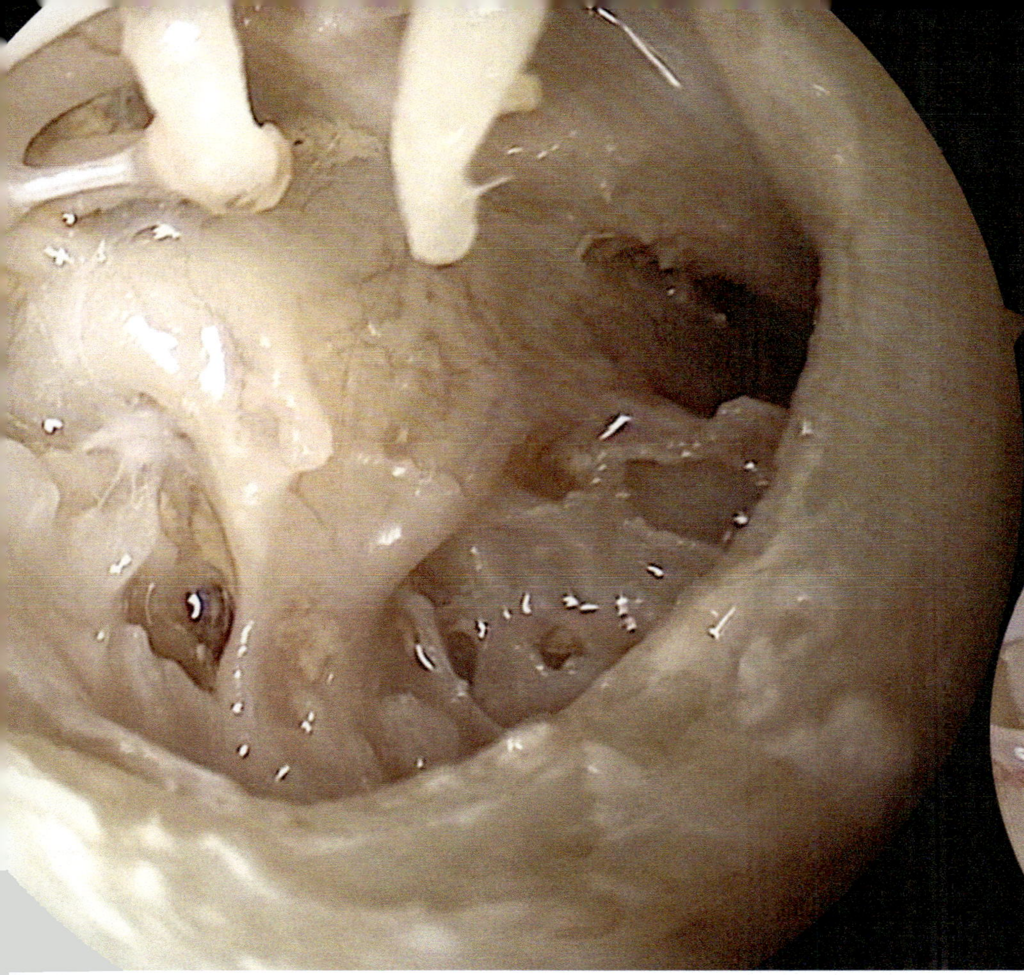

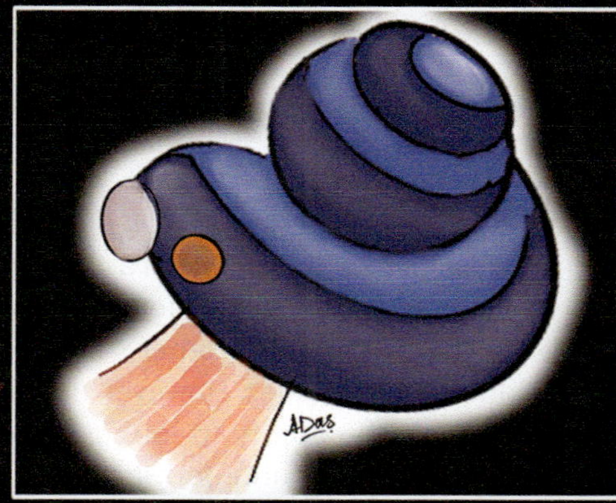

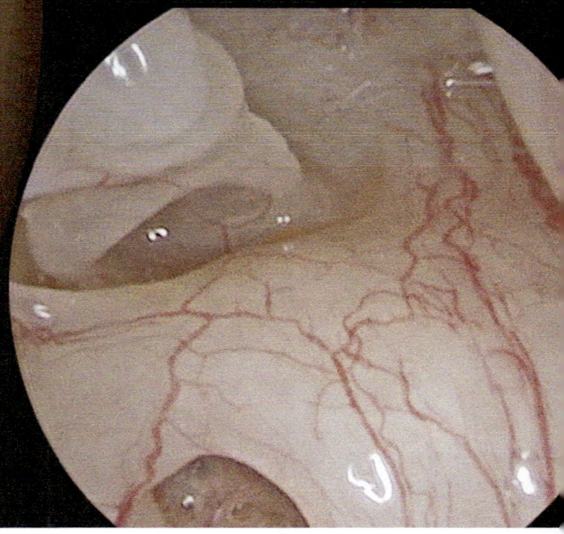

CHAPTER **3**

Endoscopic Anatomy of Middle Ear: A Surgeon's Perspective

Arindam Das, Sandipta Mitra

Chapter Outline

INTRODUCTION

Endoscopes have introduced a new perspective of looking at the middle ear and its contents. The anatomy of the middle ear and its relations to other structures has been known to otologists for decades. However, the magnified, wide-angled view, with the ability to look around bends and corners have made it possible for otologists to better understand the anatomy and physiological principles of this extremely complex region of the human body.

There is excellent documentation of minute detail of every anatomical structure present in each compartment of the middle ear, in world literature, owing to the impeccable visualization that endoscopes have made possible. The aim of this chapter is to summarize them region-wise, from the surgical point of view.

Anatomically, the middle ear has been compartmentalized into **Figures 1 and 2**.

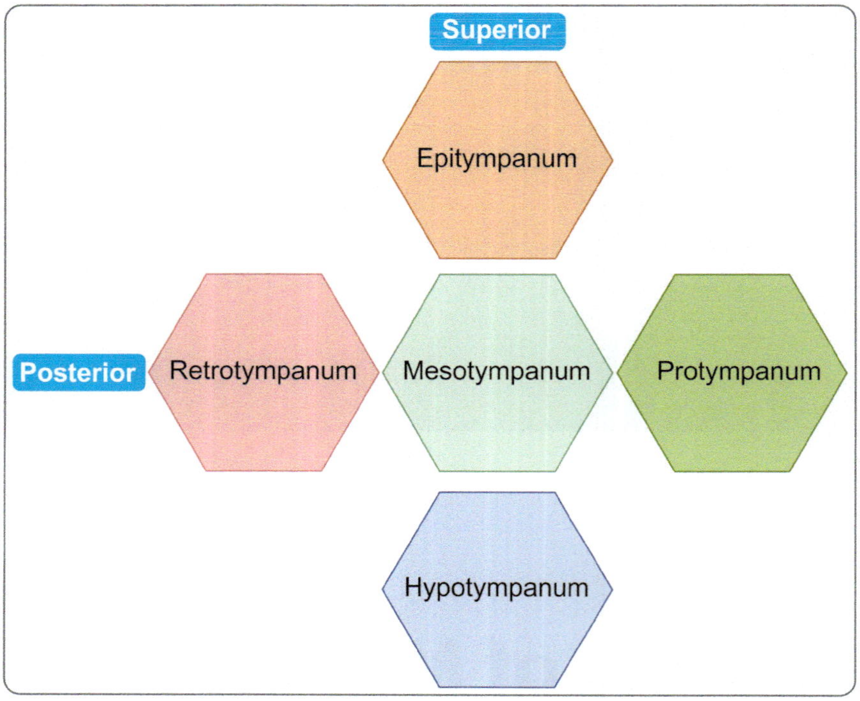

Fig. 1: Schematic diagram depicting right middle ear compartments as visualized endoscopically.

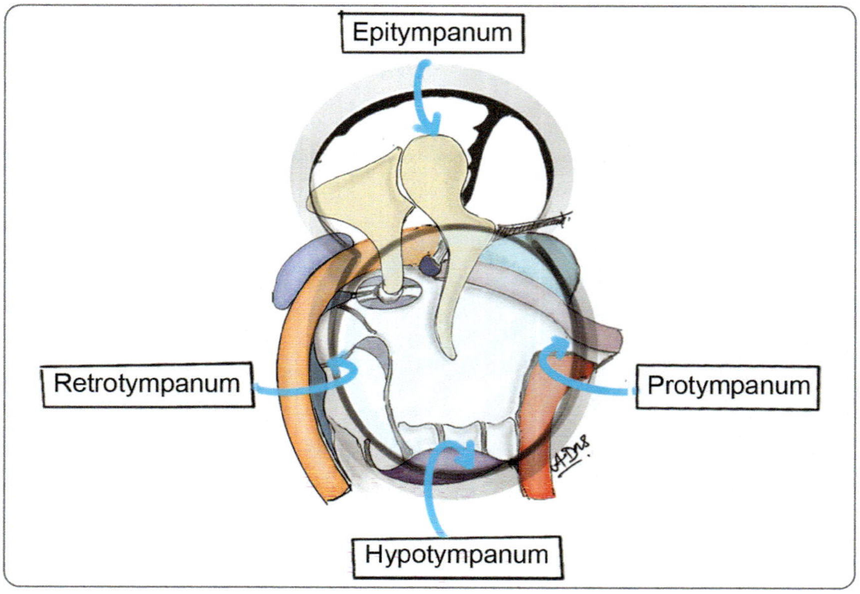

Fig. 2A: Compartments of right middle ear (Pictorial depiction).

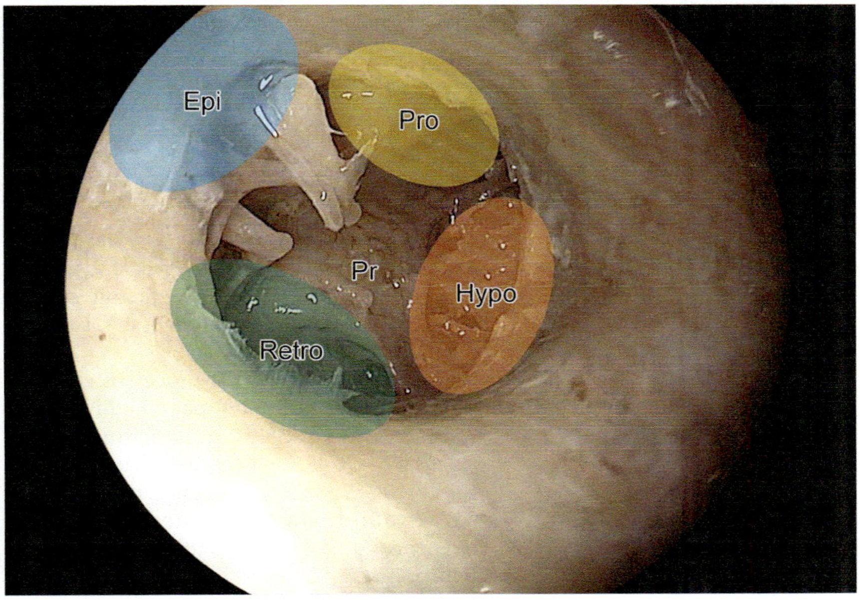

Figs. 2B: Compartments of right middle ear. (Pr: promontory)

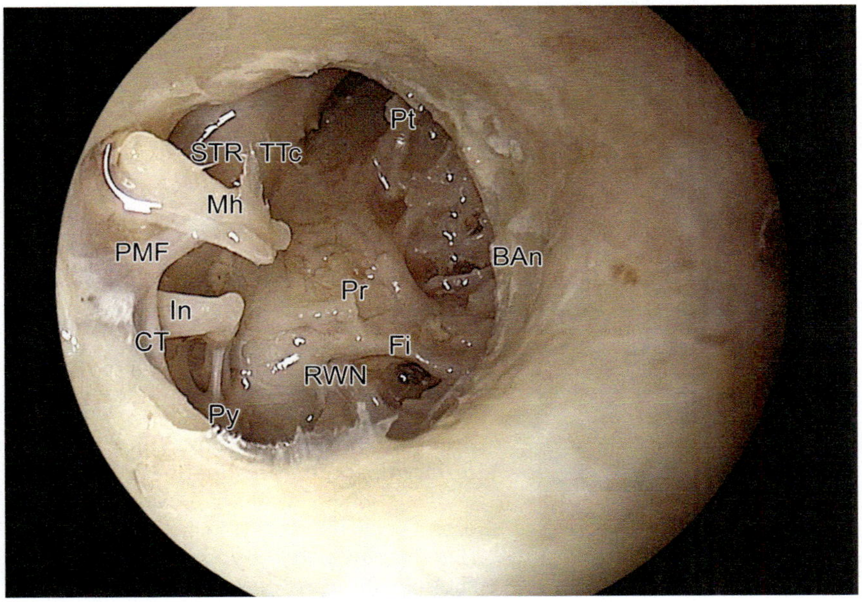

Figs. 2C: Critical landmarks of right middle ear. (CT: chorda tympani; Fi: finiculus; In: incus; Mh: malleus handle; PMF: posterior malleolar fold; Pr: promontory; Pt: protiniculum; Py: processus pyramidalis; RWN: round window niche; STR: supratubal recess; TTc: canal for tensor tympani)

SURGICAL ANATOMY OF RETROTYMPANUM

Retrotympanum is part of the middle ear which lies posterior to the mesotympanum. It houses a number of subspaces which are in close relation to important structures that are routinely dealt with in cholesteatoma surgery.

The retrotympanum is further divided into *superior* retrotympaum and *inferior* retrotympanum by *subiculum*. *Subiculum* is a bony ridge extending from styloid eminence to the posterior lip of the round window niche.

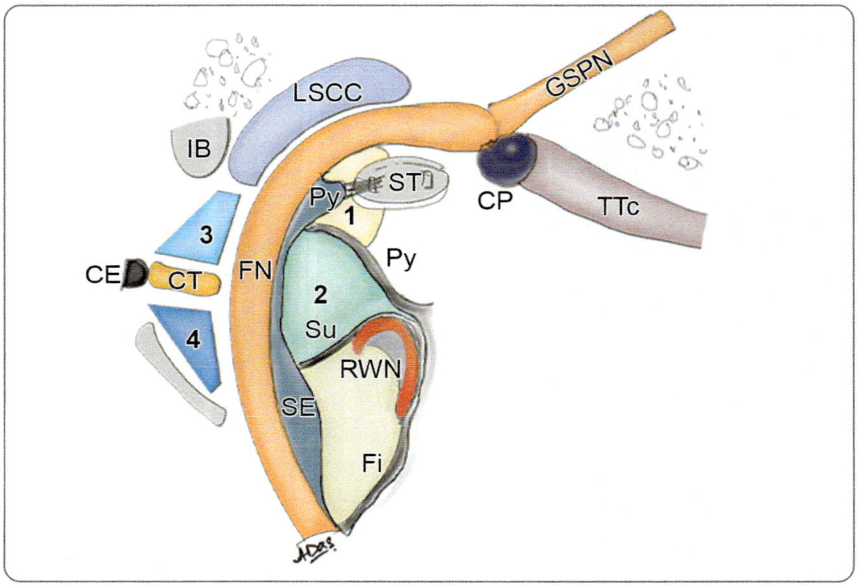

Fig. 3A: Anatomy of retrotympanum (right ear) (spaces in relation to the vertical segment of facial nerve: 1. Posterior tympanic sinus; 2. Sinus tympani; 3. Facial recess; 4. Lateral tympanic sinus).
(CE: chordal eminence; CP: processus cochleariformis; CT: chorda tympani; Fi: finiculus; FN: facial nerve; GSPN: greater superficial petrosal nerve; IB: incus buttress; LSCC: lateral semicircular canal; Py: processus pyramidalis; RWN: round window niche; SE: styloid eminence; Su: subiculum; TTc: canal for tensor tympani)

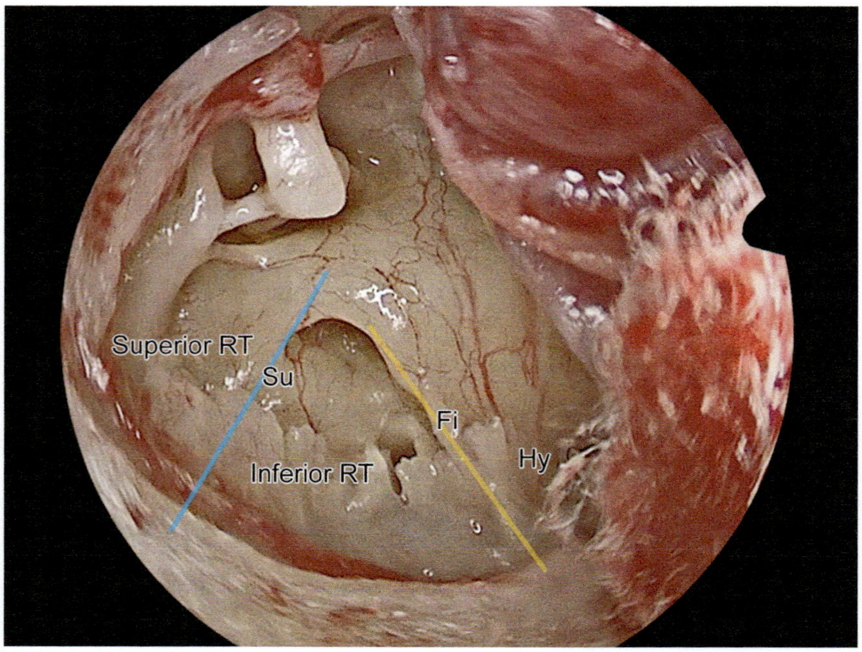

Fig. 3B: Subiculum (blue line) divides retrotympanum into superior and inferior divisions, while finiculus (Fi) marks the lower extent of inferior retrotympanum (right ear).
(Fi: finiculus; Hy: hypotympanum; Su: subiculum)

Superior Retrotympanum

Superior retrotymapnum has four important sinuses in relation to the vertical segment of the facial nerve and the pyramidal eminence.

- Two spaces located *medially and anteriorly* are:
  1. Posterior tympanic sinus (superiorly)
  2. Sinus tympani (inferiorly)

Separated by ponticulus: A ridge of bone from *processus Pyramidalis to promontory*

- Two spaces located *laterally and posteriorly* are:
  1. Facial recess (superiorly)
  2. Lateral tympanic sinus (inferiorly)

Separated by chordal ridge: A ridge of bone extending from posterior aspect of *pyramidal eminence*

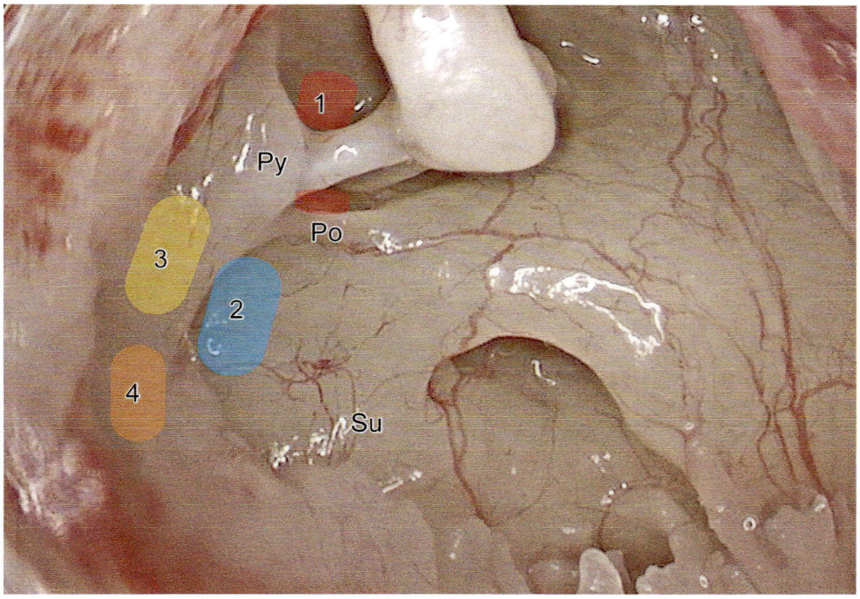

Fig. 4A: Spaces of superior retrotympanum (right ear); (1. Posterior tympanic sinus; 2. Sinus tympani; 3. Facial recess; 4. Lateral tympanic sinus).

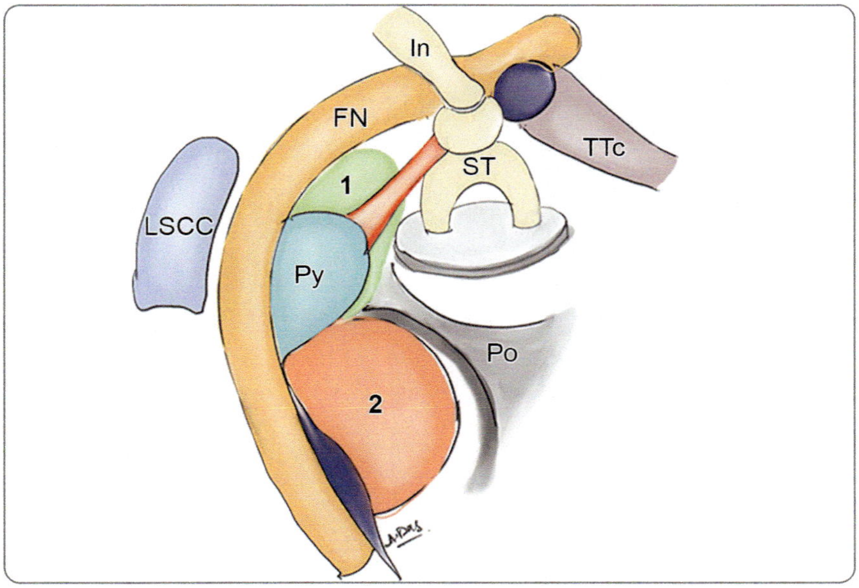

Fig. 4B: Pictorial depiction of sinuses medial to vertical segment of facial nerve (right ear) (1. Posterior tympanic sinus; 2. Sinus tympani).

Sinus tympani (ST) is a space in superior retrotympanum bounded superiorly by ponticulus and inferiorly by subiculum. Sinus tympani been classified based on its depth into[1]:

- *Type A:* The medial limit of the vertical part of the facial nerve corresponds to the depth of the sinus. In these cases, the ST is small and does not extend medial and posterior to facial nerve.
- *Type B:* The medial boundary of the ST lies medially with respect to the vertical segment of the facial nerve; however, it does not present a posterior extension to the facial nerve.
- *Type C:* ST is deep with posterior extension. The medial boundary of the ST lies medial and posterior to the third portion of the facial nerve. In these cases, ST is very large and deep, and all these patients have a well-developed mastoid.

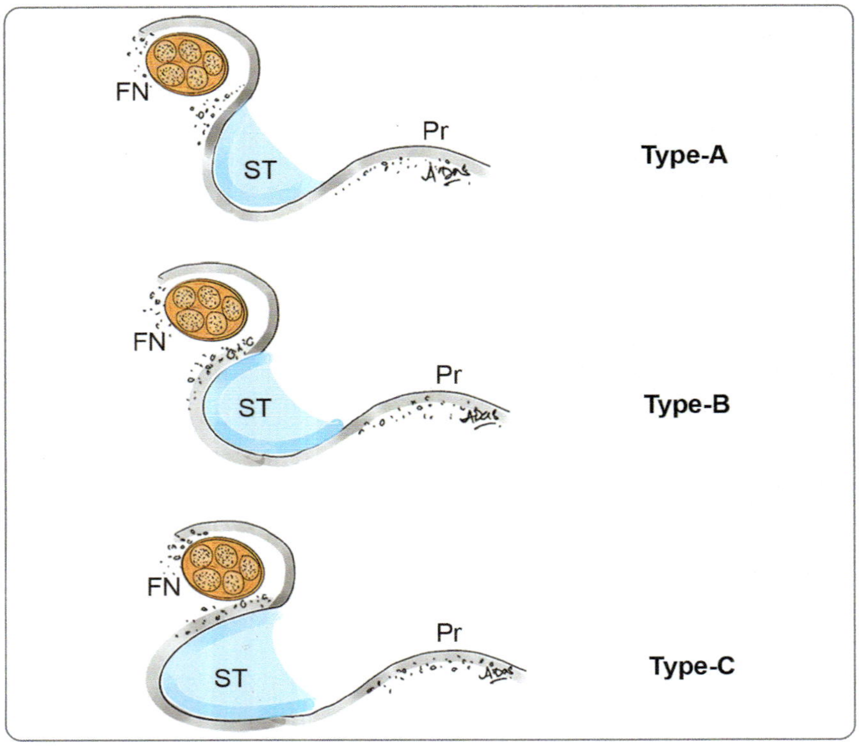

Fig. 5: Pictorial depiction of the classification of the depth of sinus tympani with respect to the facial nerve.
(FN: facial nerve; Pr: promontory; ST: sinus tympani)

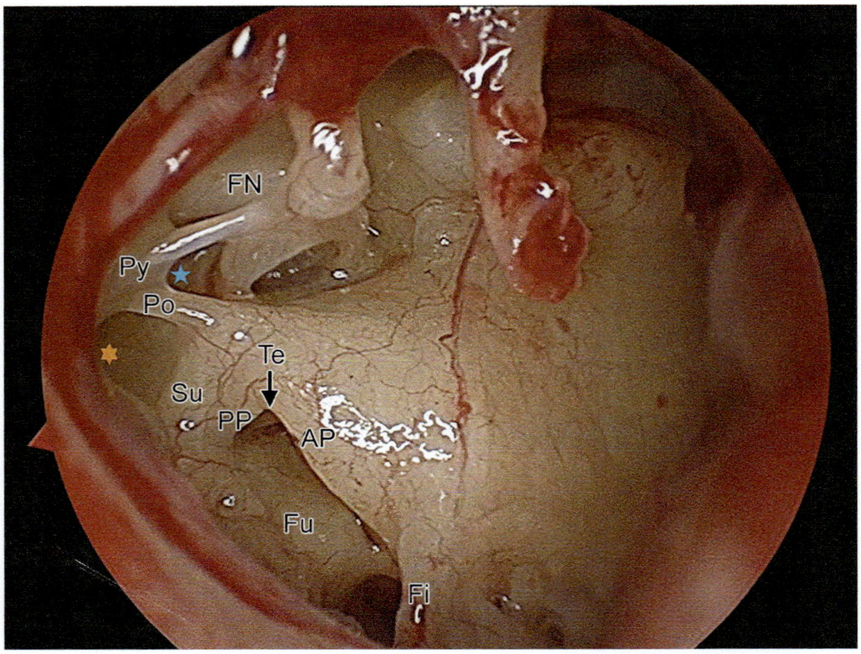

Fig. 6: Endoscopic view of posterior tympanic sinus (right ear) (blue star) and sinus tympani (yellow star).

Clinical Significance

- *Sinus tympani is notorious for residual cholesteatoma since it is a hidden recess, not easily accessible by routine surgical approaches.*[2]
- *Cholesteatoma extending deep into the depths of ST (especially Type C) is often difficult to clear by transcanal microscopic (visualization done using the reflective surface of a round knife) or straight endoscopic approach.*
- *In such cases, even angled endoscopes (45° and 70°) may not be sufficient to clear the disease entirely if it extends posterior to the nerve.*
- *A microscopic postauricular facial recess approach should be performed in such cases.*
- *Retraction pocket in inactive squamosal variety of chronic otitis media may invade into the depths of ST. Endoscopic approach using curved picks are useful for dissection.*

Sinus subpyramidalis or subpyramidal space (SS) is the recess extending under the pyramidal eminence. Depending on the extent of pneumatization, an excessively pneumatized SS may be another hidden area of extensive cholesteatoma and hence a potential site of disease recurrence.[3,4]

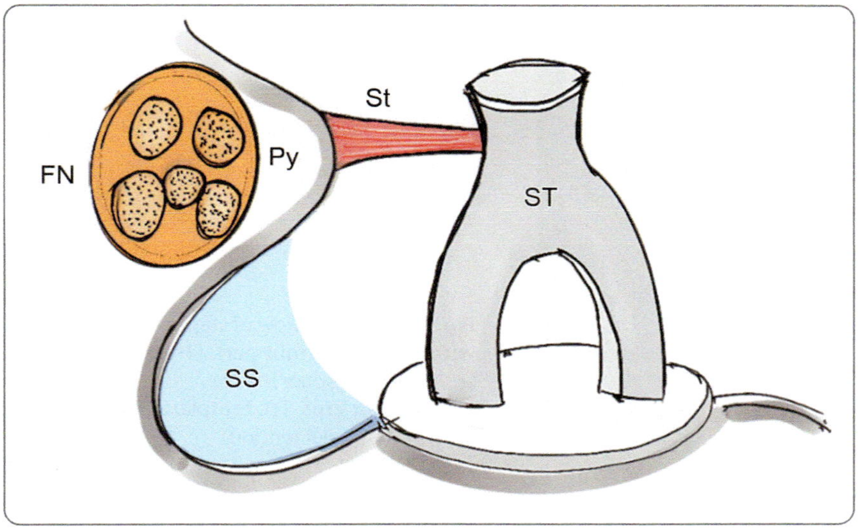

Fig. 7: Anatomy of the subpyramidal space (SS) (right ear)
(FN: facial nerve; Py: pyramidal eminence; St: stapedial tendon; ST: stapes).

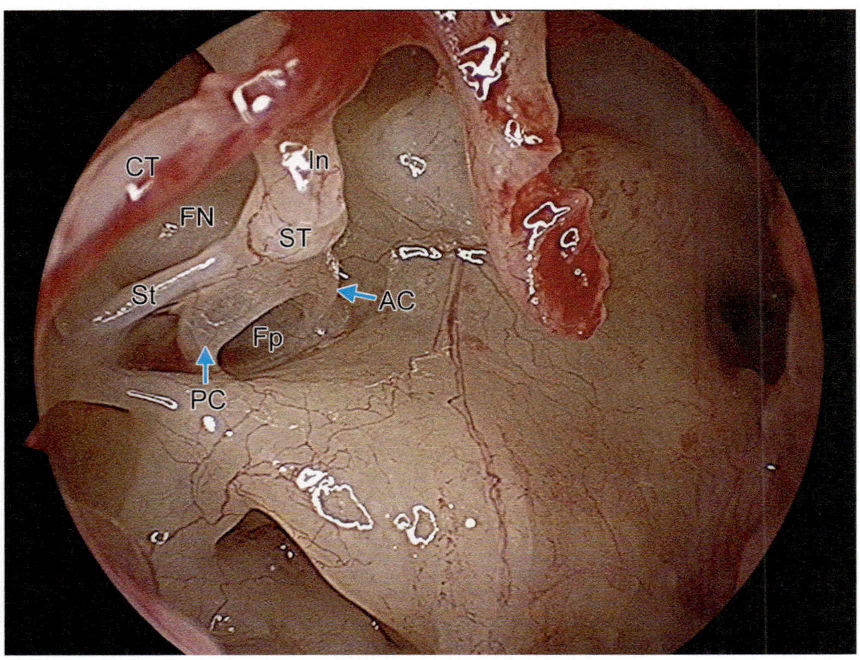

Fig. 8A: Endoscopic view of incudostapedial complex (right ear).
(Ac: anterior crus; CT: chorda tympani; FN: facial nerve; Fp: footplate; In: incus; PC: posterior crus; ST: stapes; St: stapedial tendon)

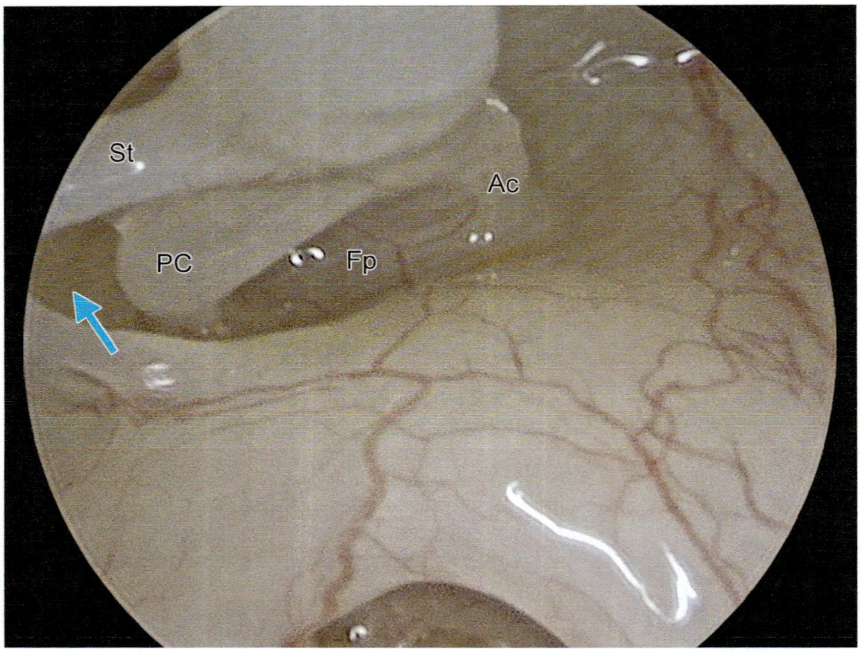

Fig. 8B: Close-up view of stapes suprastructure with footplate (right ear). (Thick blue arrow: subpyramidal space).
(Ac: anterior crus; Fp: footplate; PC: posterior crus; St: stapedial tendon)

Inferior Retrotympanum

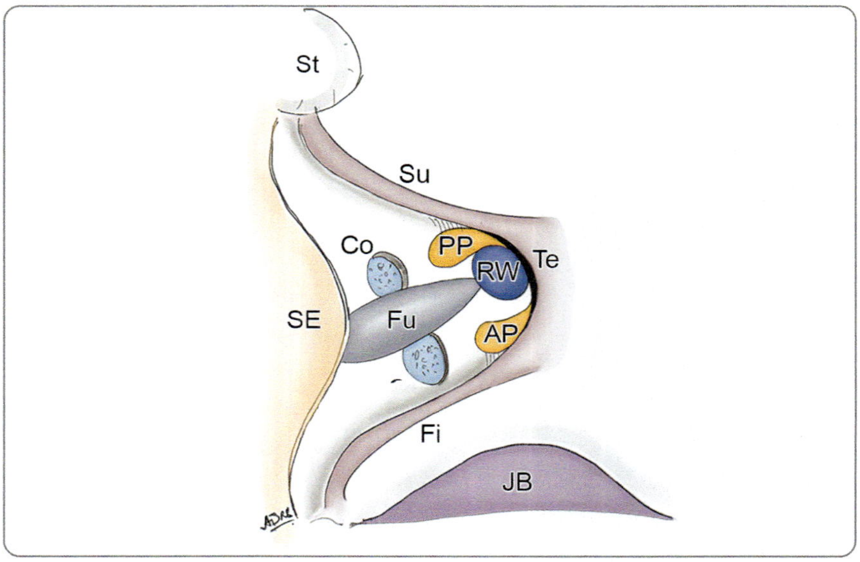

Fig. 9: Anatomy of sinus subtympanicus (right ear).
(AP: anterior pillar; Co: cochlea; Fi: finiculus; Fu: fustis; JB: jugular bulb; PP: posterior pillar; RW: round window; SE: styloid eminence; Su: subiculum; Te: tegmen)

- *Sinus subtympanicus:* Marchioni et al. described a sinus lying inferior to the ST. It is a well-defined recess lying between subiculum superiorly and posteriorly, finiculus inferiorly and anteriorly, limited posteriorly and laterally by styloid eminence and posteriorly and medially by otic capsule and open anteriorly and medially to the round window niche.[5]
- *Sustentaculum promontorii:* Proctor and colleagues have identified a relatively constant ridge of bone connecting the basal turn of cochlea to the inferior wall of the tympanum. This ridge of bone lies in relation to the anterior pillar of the round window niche and was named sustentaculum promontorii. The word "sustentaculum" originated in Latin meaning "support". It was named so because it was believed that it sustained the inferior tympanic artery, covering it during the developmental process.[6]
- *Finiculus:* Marchioni et al. renamed "sustentaculum promontorii" to "finiculus" as "fin" in Latin meant "borderline". This was done to define a clear demarcation

between the retrotympanum and hypotympanum.[1,5] Moreover, they found that the inferior tympanic artery was not always found in this constant anatomical position as proposed by Proctor.

- *Area concamerata:* Proctor described "area concamerata" as the floor of the retrotympanum.
- *Fustis:* "Fustis" is a smooth bony column leading into the round window niche that is found in the "area concamerata".

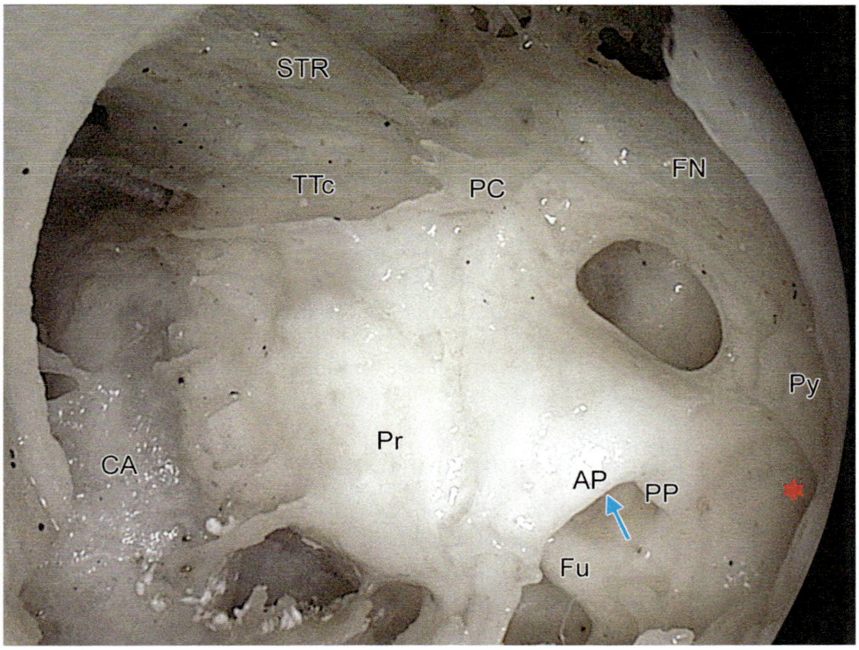

Fig. 10A: Dry left temporal bone dissection showing round window niche. (Blue arrow: leads to round window membrane; orange star: sinus tympani).
(AP: anterior pillar; CA: carotid artery; FN: facial nerve; Fu: fustis; PC: processus cochleariformis; PP: posterior pillar; Pr: promontory; STR: supratubal recess; TTc: canal for tensor tympani); Py: Pyramidal eminence)

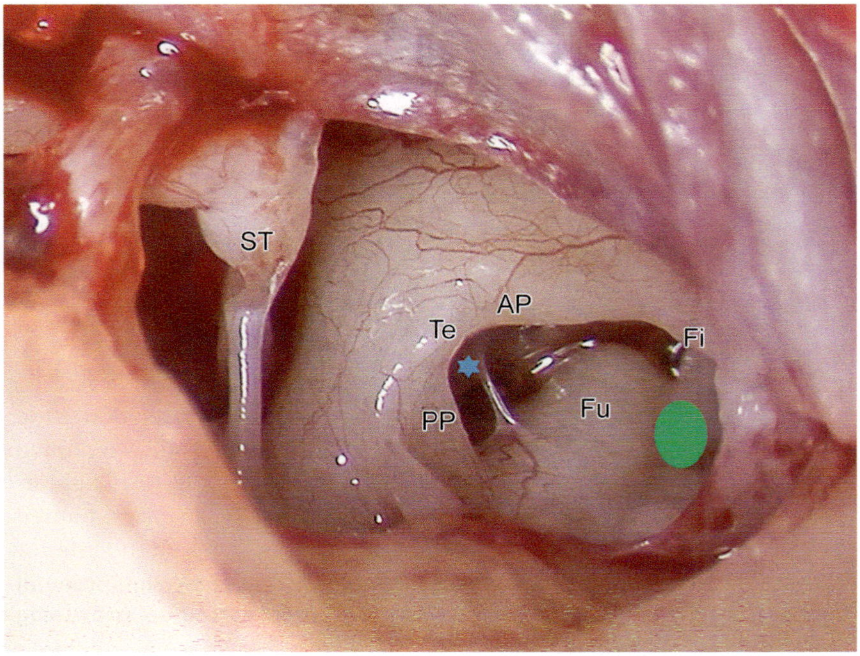

Fig. 10B: Endoscopic view of round window anatomy (right ear). (Blue star: round window membrane; green circle: "area concamerata").
(AP: anterior pillar; Fu: fustis; PP: posterior pillar; Te: tegmen)

SURGICAL ANATOMY OF EPITYMPANUM

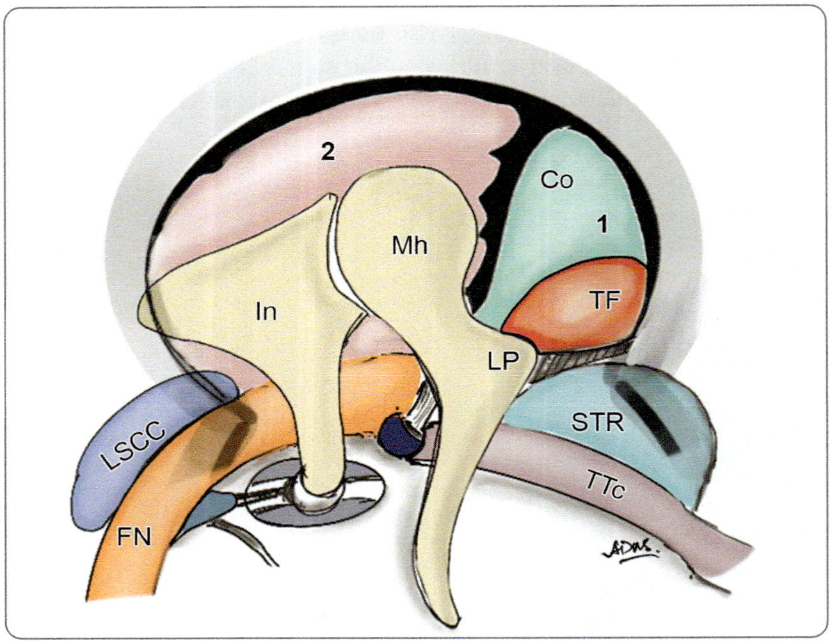

Fig. 11: Anatomy of epitympanum (right ear) (1. Anterior epitympanic space, 2. Posterior epitympanic space).
(Co: cog; FN: facial nerve; In: incus; LP: lateral process of malleus; LSCC: lateral semicircular canal; Mh: malleus handle; STR: supratubal recess; TF: tensor fold; TTc: canal for tensor tympani)

Epitympanum is the pneumatized compartment of the middle ear lying superior to mesotympanum.

Epitympanum is being divided into two subspaces by a bony anatomical structure called "cog" (described later):

1. Anterior epitympanic space
2. Posterior epitympanic space

Posterior Epitympanic Space

Posterior epitympanic space is a part of the epitympanum lying posterior to the cog. The larger and posterior of the two spaces, it houses the head of the malleus and the body and short process of incus.

The posterior epitympanic space communicates and is ventilated by the tympanic isthmus (anterior and posterior).

Anterior Epitympanic Space

Anterior epitympanic space is the space located anterior to bony cog. Located far anteriorly, this space often harbors residual squamosal disease that causes cholesteatoma recurrence. It is separated from the supratubal recess (part of protympanum) by tensor fold.

The ventilation of the anterior epitympanic space depends on the configuration and completeness of the tensor fold. If the tensor fold is complete, the AES becomes a closed recess which depends on the tympanic isthmus (anterior and posterior), for its ventilation via mesotympanum.[7] In case of an incomplete tensor fold, the ventilation occurs via the protympanum and then into the Eustachian tube.

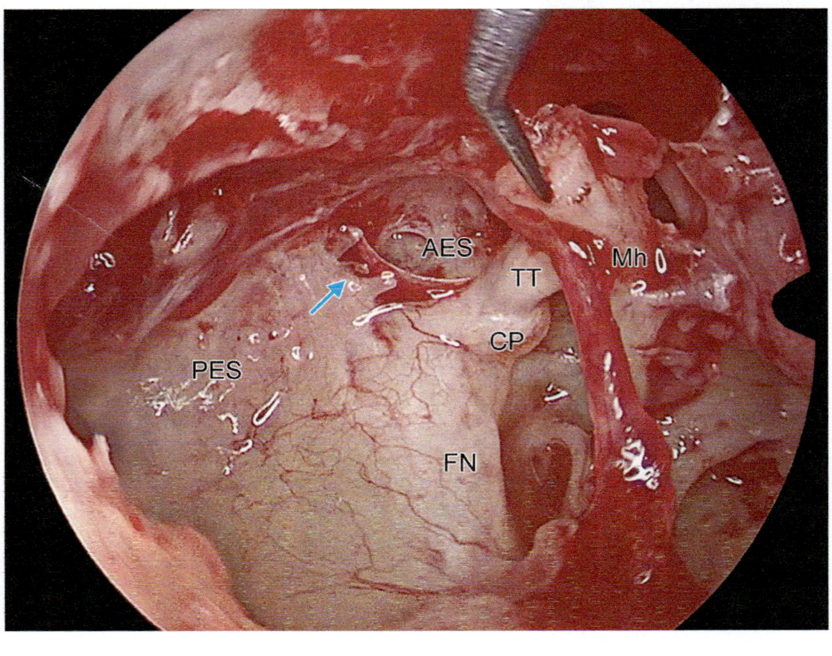

Fig. 12: Intraoperative endoscopic view of epitympanum (right ear). Blue arrow: cog separating AES from PES.
(AES: anterior epitympanic space; CP: processus cochleariformis; FN: facial nerve; Mh: malleus handle; PES: posterior epitympanic space; TT: tensor tympani tendon)

Cog

- The cog is a bony septum extending from tegmen tympani superiorly, vertically downward toward the cochleariform process, in front of the malleus head.
- It represents the embryologic remnant of the fusion plane between saccus anticus and medius
- It separates the anterior epitympanic space from the posterior epitympanic space
- From the viewpoint of microscopic ear surgery, the cog was thought to be a structure located far anteriorly, that would often be difficult to identify in ears with extensive disease, either due to the disease bulk or erosion of the landmark itself.
- However, it is routinely identified in endoscopic ear surgery and serves as a valuable landmark.
- The perspective of cog has changed with the advent of endoscopes. It is now thought to be central landmark of the middle ear cleft, lying approximately at the midpoint, pointing toward the processus cochleariformis.

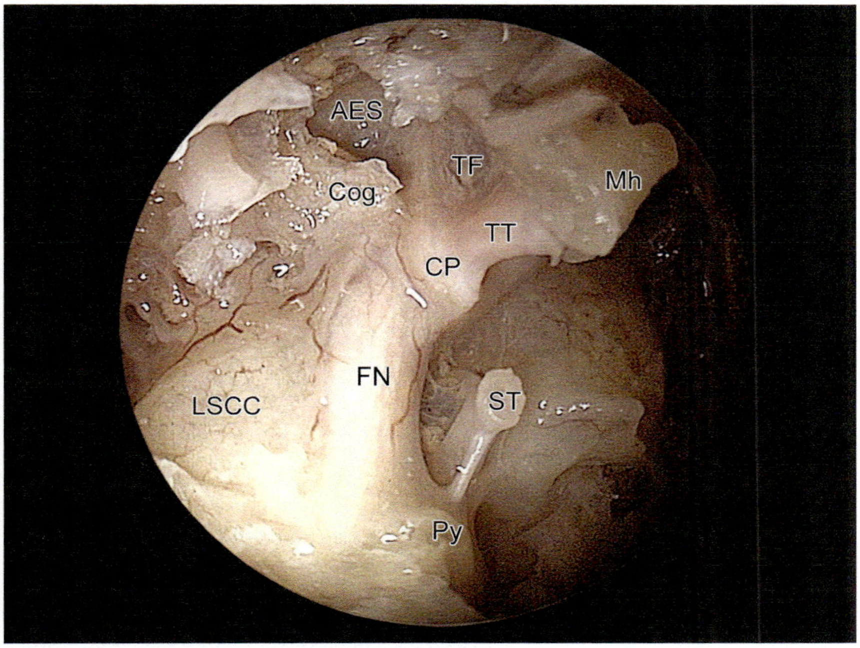

Fig. 13A: Temporal bone dissection showing anatomy of cog (right ear).
(AES: anterior epitympanic space; FN: facial nerve; Mh: malleus handle; Py: processus pyramidalis; TT: tensor tympani tendon; ST: stapes)

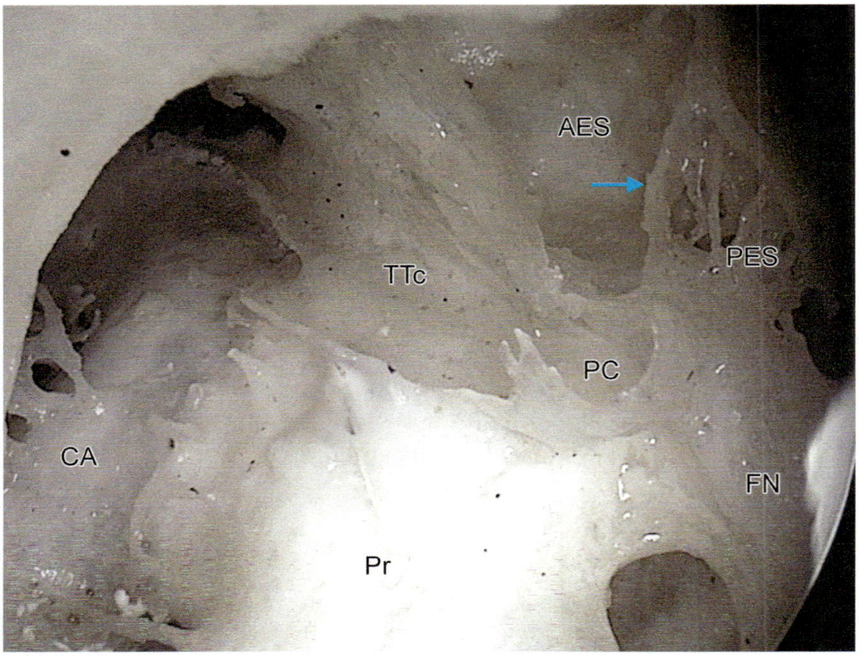

Fig. 13B: Temporal bone dissection showing anatomy of cog (left ear). (Blue arrow: cog separating AES from PES)
(AES: anterior epitympanic space; FN: facial nerve; PC: processus cochleariformis; PES: posterior epitympanic space)

Tensor Fold

Tensor fold is one of the mucosal folds forming the epitympanic diaphragm. It is located between the tensor tympani tendon and the lateral bony attic wall.[8]

Tensor fold may show variations. The types and their clinical significance are:[9]

- *Complete tensor fold:* The tensor fold separates the AES from supratubal recess. The ventilation of AES solely depends on the tympanic isthmus (anticus and posticus)
- *Incomplete tensor fold*: The tensor fold is incomplete, thus creating an additional anterior ventilation pathway apart from the tympanic isthmus.

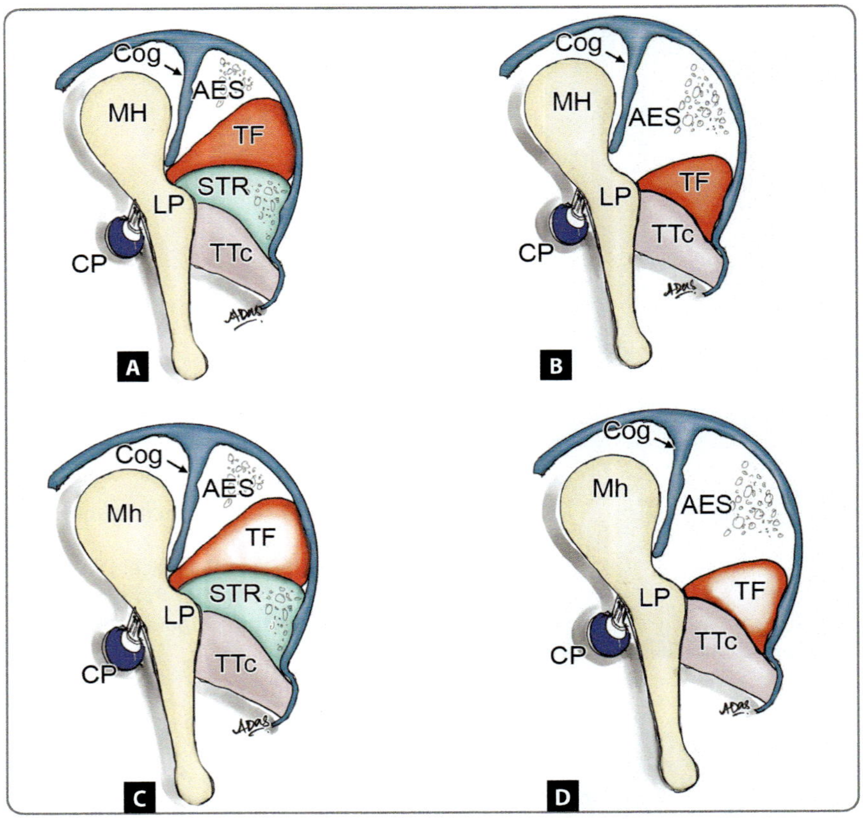

Figs. 14A to D: Anatomy of tensor fold. (A) Vertical disposition of complete tensor fold (note the resultant area of supratubal recess); (B) Complete horizontal tensor fold (note the resultant area of anterior epitympanic space); (C) Incomplete vertical tensor fold; and (D) Incomplete horizontal tensor fold. (AES: anterior epitympanic space; CP: processus cochleariformis; LP: lateral process of malleus; Mh: malleus handle; TF: tensor fold; TTc: canal for tensor tympani)

Clinical Significance

- In case of blockage of the tympanic isthmus with a complete tensor fold, there is practically no ventilation of the epitympanum. This subsequently leads to retraction pocket formation.
- Endoscopic epitympanic exploration (EEE) is a minimally invasive approach to clear hypertrophied mucosal folds blocking the tympanic isthmus and the anterior pathway.[10]
- Angled endoscopes with appropriately curved picks allow dissection of the mucosal folds blocking the ventilation pathways without the need to remove the ossicles or excess bone drilling.

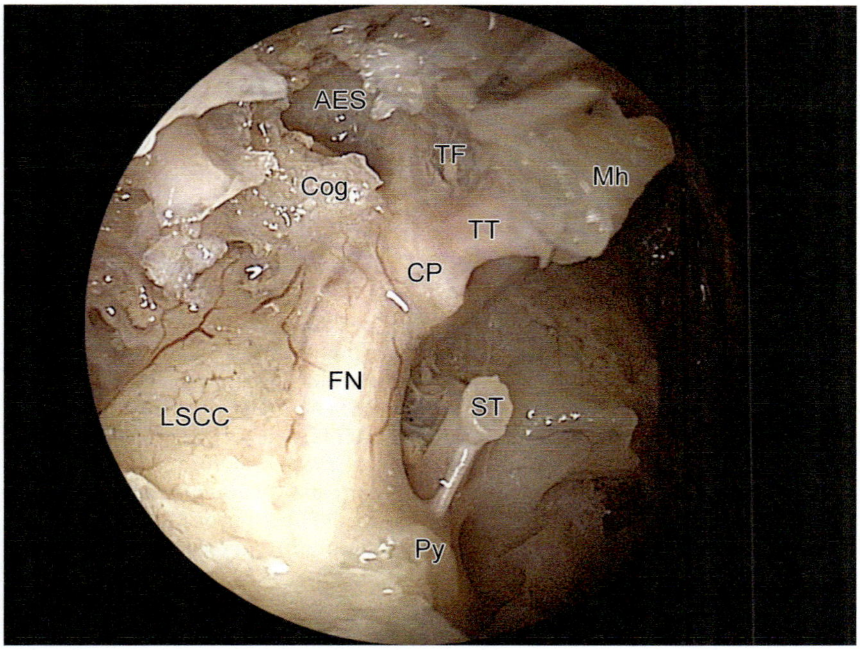

Fig. 15A: Wet right temporal bone dissection specimen showing complete tensor folds. (AES: anterior epitympanic space; CP: processus cochleariformis; FN: facial nerve; Mh: malleus handle; Py: processus pyramidalis; TT: tensor tympani tendon; ST: stapes; TF: tensor fold)

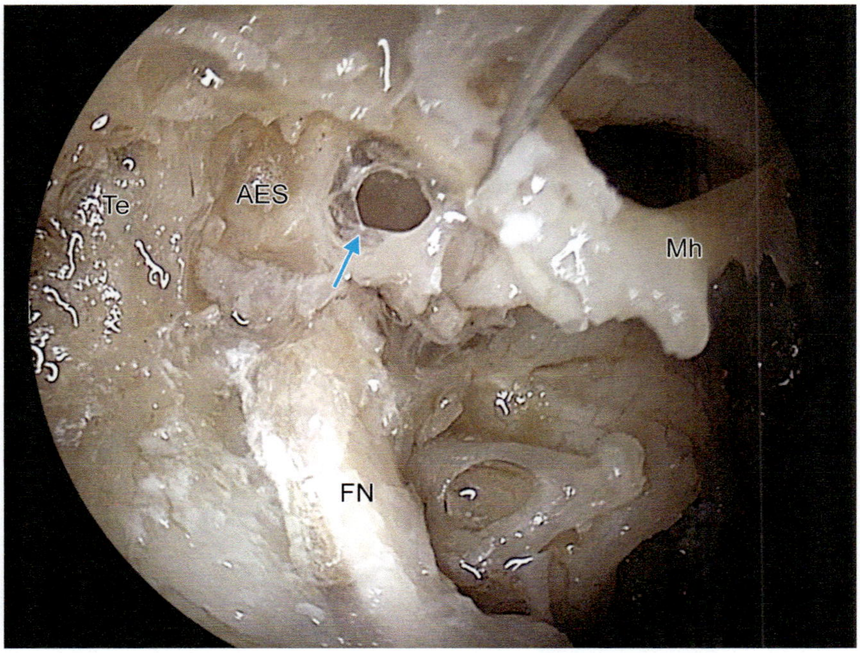

Fig. 15B: Wet right temporal bone dissection specimen showing incomplete tensor folds. (Blue arrow: incomplete tensor fold leading to communication between anterior epitympanic space and supratubal recess)
(AES: anterior epitympanic space; FN: facial nerve; Mh: malleus handle; Te: tegmen)

Epitympanic Diaphragm

Epitympanic diaphragm is a collection of mucosal folds and ligaments that separate epitympanum from the mesotympanum. First described by Chatellier and Lemoine as "attico-tympanic diaphragm" and further explored by Palva et al. who named it "epitympanic diaphragm", the diaphragm is composed of three malleal ligamental folds (anterior, lateral, and posterior), posterior incudal ligamental fold and two purely membranous folds (tensor fold and lateral incudomalleal fold) along with malleus and incus.[11,12]

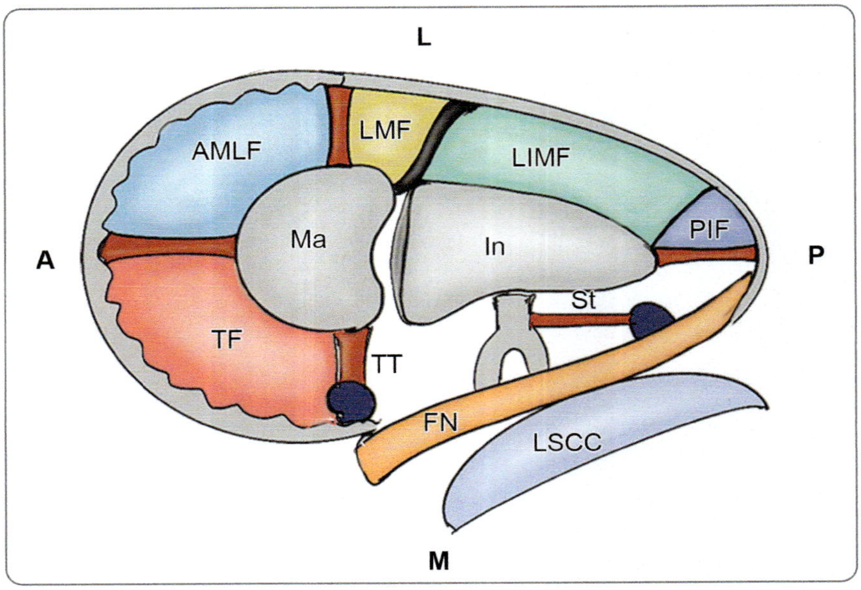

Fig. 16: Epitympanic diaphragm as viewed from above (right ear).
(A: anterior; AMLF: anterior malleolar ligamental fold; FN: facial nerve; In: incus; L: lateral; LIMF: lateral incudomalleolar fold; LMF: lateral malleolar fold; LSCC: lateral semicircular canal; M: medial; Ma: malleus; P: posterior; PIF: posterior incudal fold; St: stapedial tendon; TF: tensor fold; TT: tensor tympani)

The intricate folds and ligaments that are strategically arranged in this limited space are fascinating and have been explored over the years by otologists by meticulous temporal bone dissections. However, in clinical practice, individual folds are rarely discernible in every case, especially in diseased ears, where the mucosa is inflamed.

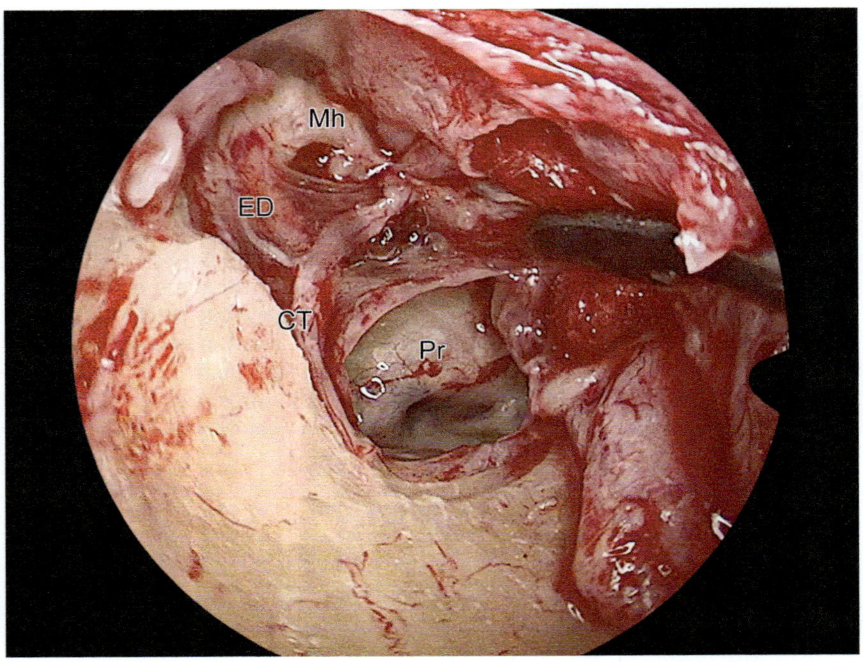

Fig. 17A: Intraoperative pictures showing epitympanic diaphragm (ED), (right ear).
(CT: chorda tympani; ED: epitympanic diaphragm; Mh: malleus handle; Pr: promontory)

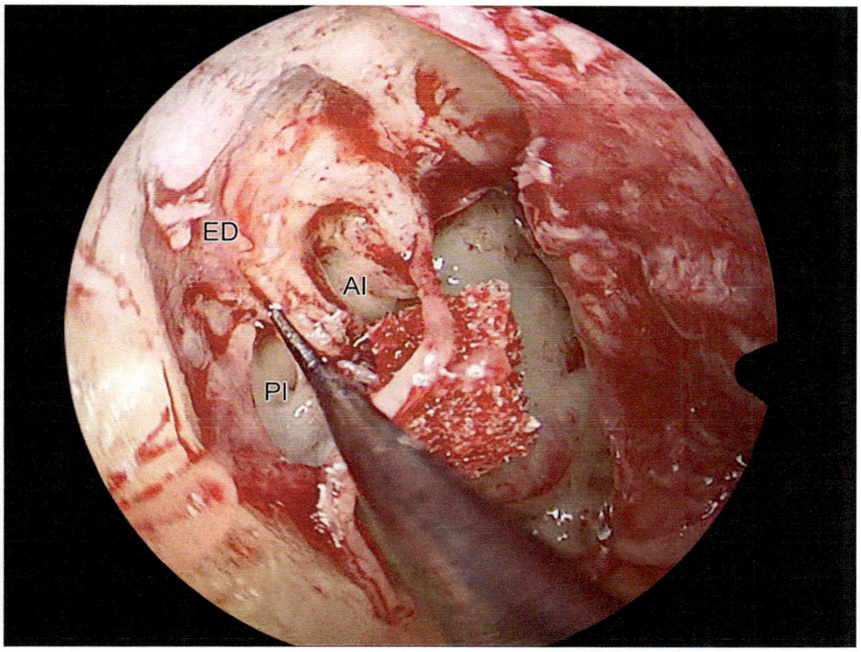

Fig. 17B: Intraoperative pictures showing epitympanic diaphragm (ED), isthmus anticus (AI), and posticus (PI) (right ear).

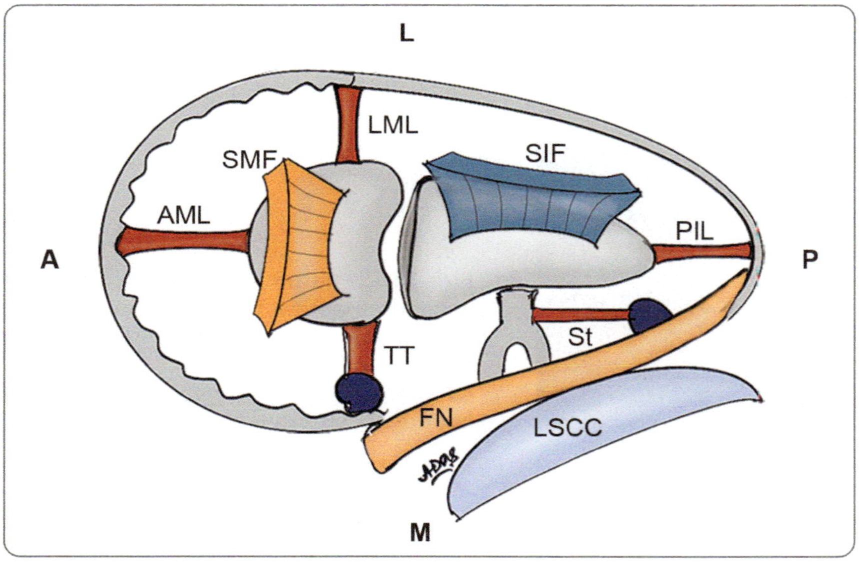

Fig. 18: Vertical folds of epitympanum.
(A: anterior; AML: anterior malleolar ligament FN: facial nerve; L: lateral; LML: lateral malleolar ligament; LSCC: lateral semicircular canal; M: medial; P: posterior; PIL: posterior incudal ligament; SIF: superior incudal fold; SMF: superior malleolar fold; St: stapedial tendon; TT: tensor tympani)

Ventilation Pathways

The epitympanum is ventilated by the following pathways:

- *Tympanic isthmus*:
    - *Isthmus anticus/anterior isthmus*: Proctor described it as the space between the incudostapedial joint and cochleariform process with the tensor tympani tendon
    - *Isthmus posticus/posterior isthmus*: Space between the pyramidal process and the short process of the incus
- *Additional anterior pathway*: An incomplete tensor fold physiologically or a surgically created opening by dissection of a complete tensor fold gives rise to an additional path of ventilation of the anterior epitympanic space, communicating directly into the protympanum.

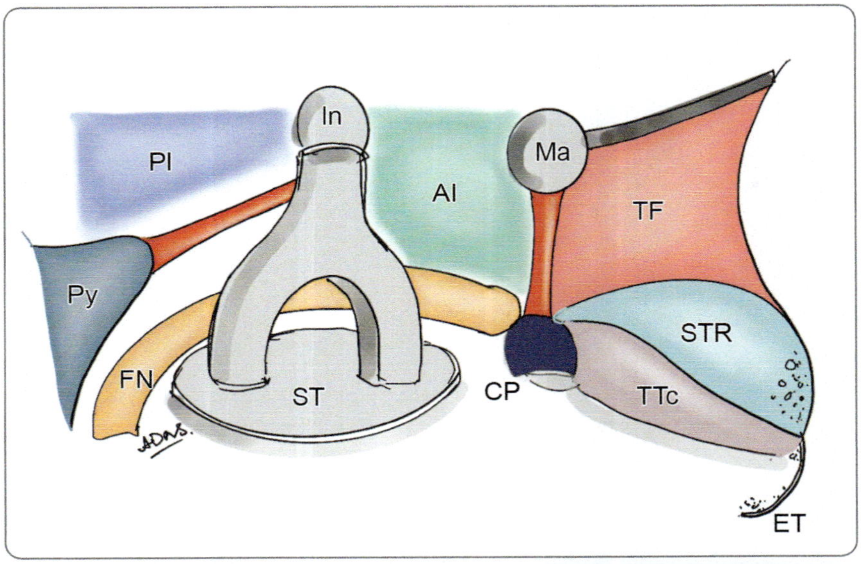

Fig. 19A: Anatomy of middle ear ventilation pathways.
(AI: isthmus anticus; PI: isthmus posticus; CP: processus cochleariformis; FN: facial nerve; In: incus; Ma: malleus; Py: processus pyramidalis; ST: stapes; STR: supratubal recess; TF: tensor fold; TTc: canal for tensor tympani)

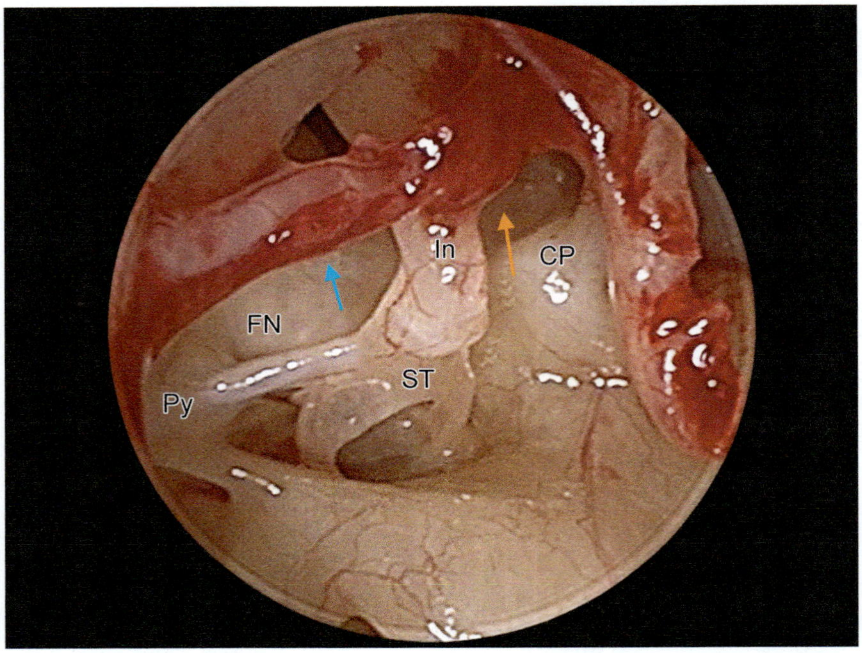

Fig. 19B: Anatomy of right middle ear ventilation pathways. AI: isthmus anticus (orange arrow); PI: isthmus posticus (blue arrow).
(CP: processus cochleariformis; FN: facial nerve; In: incus; Py: processus pyramidalis; ST: stapes)

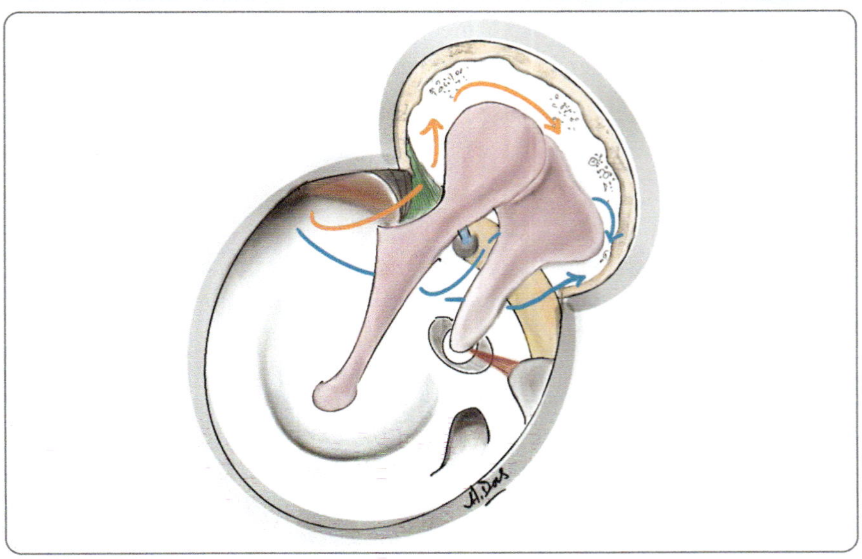

Fig. 20: Pathways of left middle ear ventilation. (Blue arrow: epitympanum is ventilated via two major ventilation routes anterior isthmus and posterior isthmus; orange arrow: additional anterior pathway via an incomplete or surgically opened complete tensor fold).

Prussak's Space

- Prussak's space is a subcomponent of the lateral epitympanic space.
- It is bounded by:
  - *Lateral:* Pars flaccida of the tympanic membrane
  - *Medial:* Neck of the malleus
  - *Superior:* Lateral malleal ligament fold
  - *Inferior:* Lateral (short) process of the malleus
- From the endoscopic viewpoint, it has been described as the space located inferior to the epitympanic diaphragm.
- It is separated from the epitympanic compartments by the lateral malleolar ligament fold which forms the roof of Prussak's space.
- The posterior wall of Prussak's space contains an opening called the posterior pocket of von Tröltsch, which forms the main route of ventilation of this space.

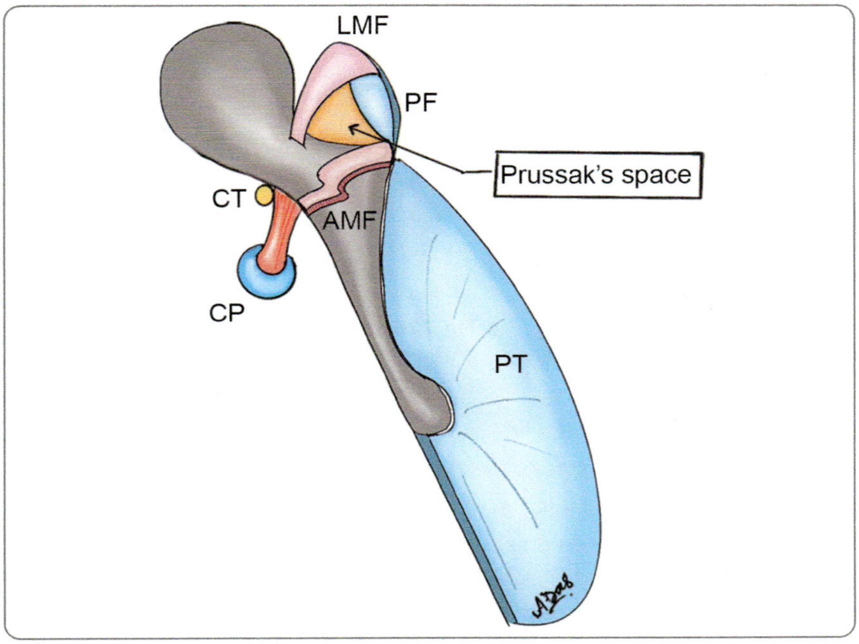

Fig. 21: Boundaries of Prussak's space. (AMF: anterior malleolar fold; CP: processus cochleariformis; CT: chorda tympani; LMF: lateral malleolar fold; PF: pars flaccida; PT: pars tensa)

Clinical Significance

- Prussak's space is believed to be the site of origin of epitympanic cholesteatoma
- The probable reason is that the ventilation of Prussak's space through the posterior pocket of von Tröltsch is narrow.[13]
- Hence, granulations or thick viscid secretions may block the ventilation and cause retraction of the pars flaccida, forming its lateral boundary, eventually progressing into cholesteatoma.
- From the Prussak's space, the cholesteatoma assumes the pathways of least resistance for its spread

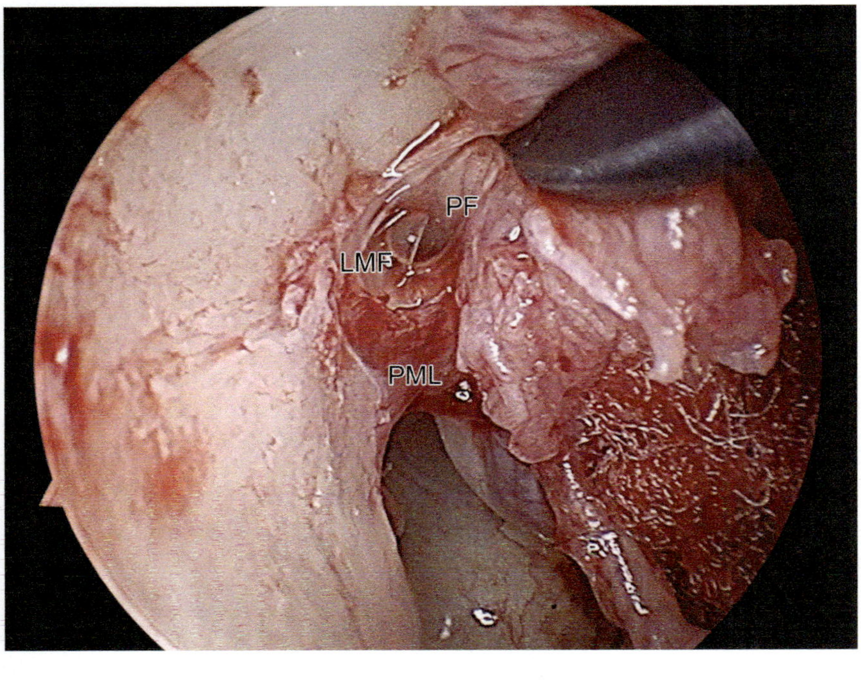

Fig. 22A: Intraoperative pictures showing Prussak's space (right ear). (LMF: lateral malleolar fold; PF: pars flaccida; PML: posterior malleolar ligament)

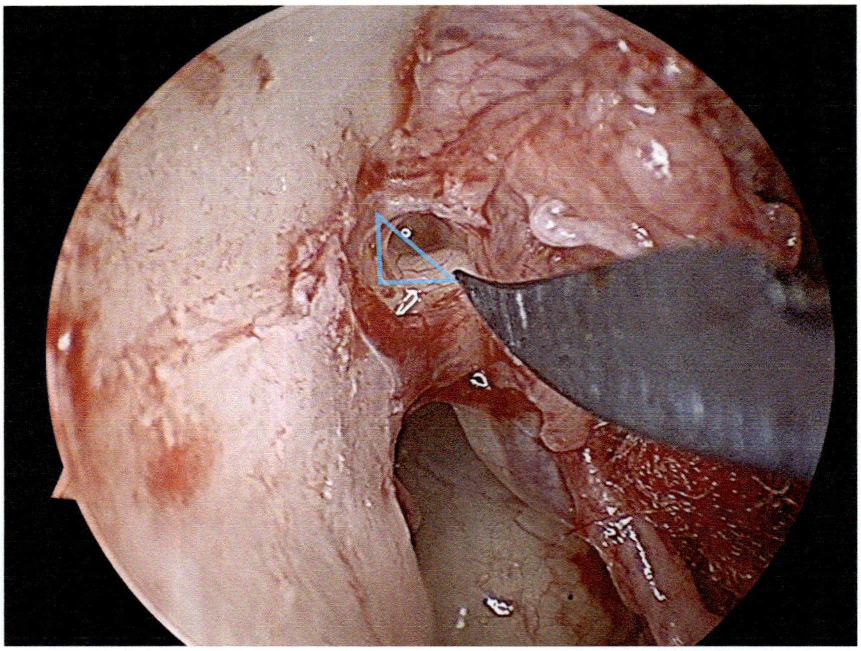

Fig. 22B: Intra-operative picture showing Prussak's space (right ear) (blue triangle).

SURGICAL ANATOMY OF PROTYMPANUM

The protympanum is a part of the middle ear lying anterior to the mesotympanum.

- Protympanum communicates with cartilaginous Eustachian tube anteriorly, mesotympanum posteriorly, epitympanum superiorly, and hypotympanum inferiorly.
- Protympanum has been described as the final common pathway of ventilation between tympanic cavity and the external environment.[14]

Changes in Anatomical Concept with Advent of Endoscopes

- The protympanum, tympanic cavity, and the bony Eustachian tube have been classically described as distinct anatomical entities.
- Endoscopic observation has made this distinction obsolete and established that the protympanum is actually a continuation of the bony Eustachian tube.[15]
- Eustachian tube as such is redefined as a fibrocartilaginous structure that extends from the most anterior part of the tympanic cavity (that is protympanum with anterior bony tube) to the nasopharynx.
- The interventions are actually directed toward the cartilaginous Eustachian tube (the malleable segment).

Boundaries of Protympanum

- Classically, the boundaries of protympanum have been described as the vertical and horizontal tangents to the boundaries of the bony tympanic ring.[16]
- With the advent of endoscopes, especially angled scopes, the boundaries of this space have been defined more clearly:
  - *Superior*: Tegmen tympani and entire tensor tympani canal, merging posteriorly with and including the supratubal recess if present
  - *Inferior:* From the protiniculum (described later) posteriorly to protympanic air cells anteriorly which are an anterior extension of the hypotympanic cell complex
  - *Anterior:* Confluent with the junctional and cartilaginous portion of the Eustachian tube
  - *Posterior:* Communicates with mesotympanum
  - *Medial:* Lateral wall of the carotid canal, extending from the caroticocochlear recess anteriorly, with caroticotympanic vessels, and nerves including anterior branches from Jacobson's (tympanic branch of glossopharyngeal) nerve.
  - *Lateral*: Bony wall separating the space from the mandibular fossa extending to the anterior annulus, from the level of the protiniculum inferiorly to the anterior limit of the notch of Rivinus at the anterior tympanic spine.

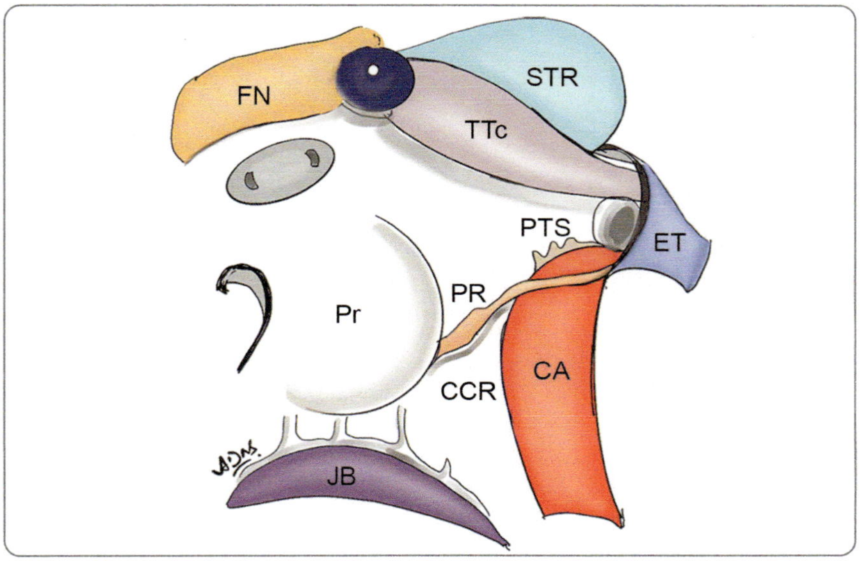

Fig. 23: Anatomy of protympanum (right ear). (CA: carotid artery; CCR: cochleo-carotid recess; ET: Eustachian tube; FN: facial nerve; JB: jugular bulb; Pr: promontory; PR: protiniculum; PTS: protympanic spine; STR: supratubal recess; TTc: canal for tensor tympani)

Supratubal Recess

Supratubal recess is a superomedial extension of protympanum and anterior mesotympanum, located anterior to the tensor fold.[17]

- The tensor fold separates the anterior epitympanic space from the supratubal recess
- The size of the supratubal recess depends on the anatomical orientation of the tensor fold
- In case of a vertically oriented, tensor fold, the supratubal recess is present as a large space; the opposite being the case in horizontally placed tensor fold.
- The supratubal recess is a smooth-walled cavity, whereas, the anterior epitympanic space has numerous sharp bony excrescences.[18]

Subtensor Recess

Subtensor recess is an area of pneumatization located inferomedial to the tensor tympani canal.

- Its conformation depends on the morphology of the tensor canal
- Based on the above, the subtensor recess can be of three types[1]:
  1. *Type A*: Flat tensor canal with absent subtensor recess
  2. *Type B*: Raised tensor canal and shallow subtensor recess with fundus of recess easily visible
  3. *Type C*: Raised tensor canal and deep subtensor recess. Limits of fundus of the recess difficult to visualize
- Demarcation between a type B and type C subtensor recess is when the fundus of the recess extends superior to the midpoint of the tensor tympani canal.

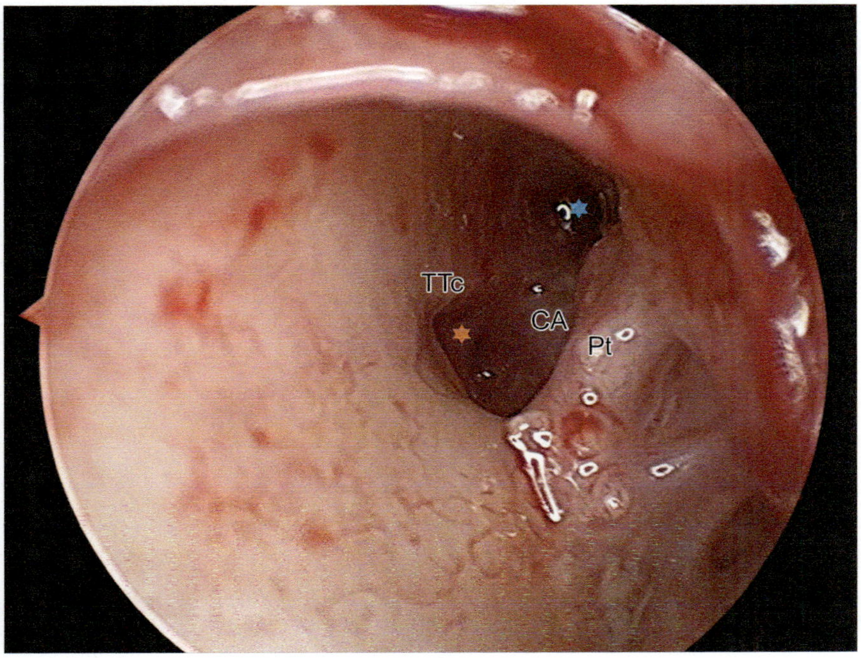

Fig. 24A: Endoscopic anatomy of protympanum [orange star: subtensor recess; blue star: Eustachian tube (ET)]
(CA: Carotid artery; Pt: protiniculum; TTc: canal for tensor tympani)

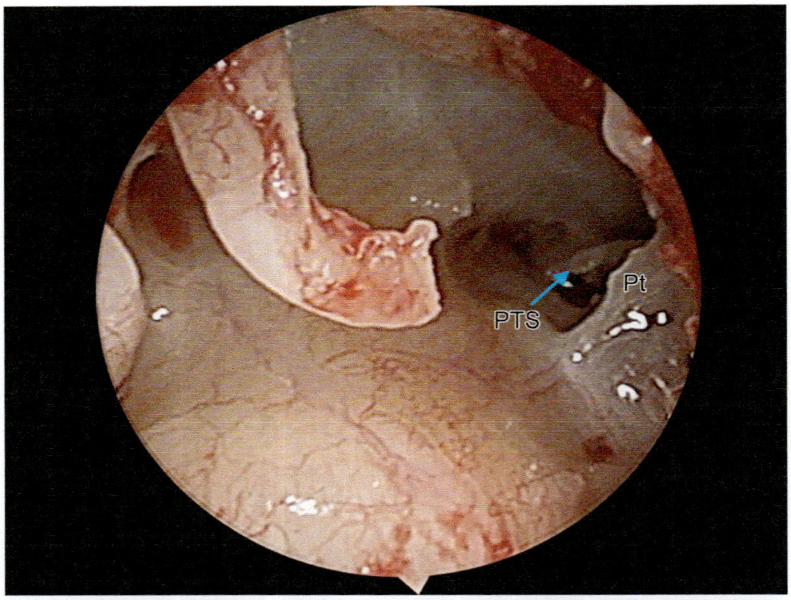

Fig. 24B: Endoscopic anatomy of protympanum (right ear)
(Pt: protiniculum; PTS: protympanic spine)

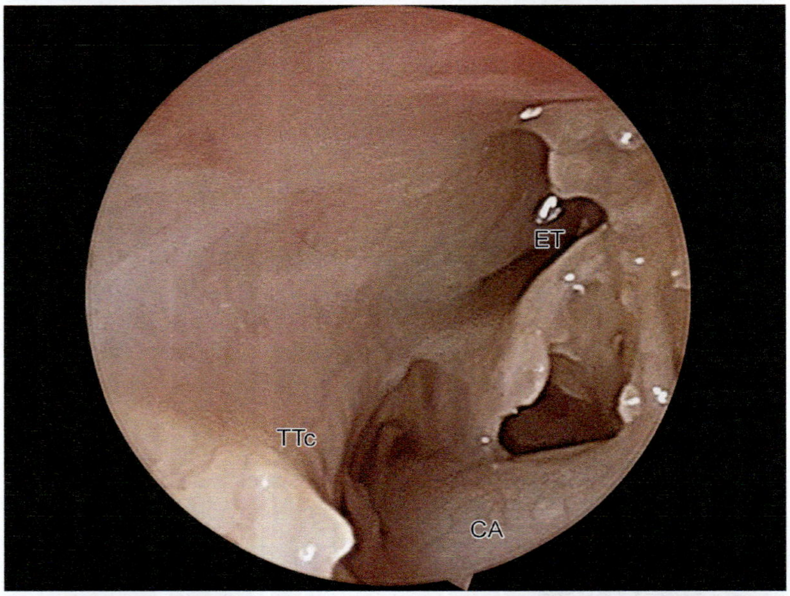

Fig. 24C: Endoscopic anatomy of protympanum.
(CA: Carotid artery; ET: Eustachian tube; TTc: canal for tensor tympani)

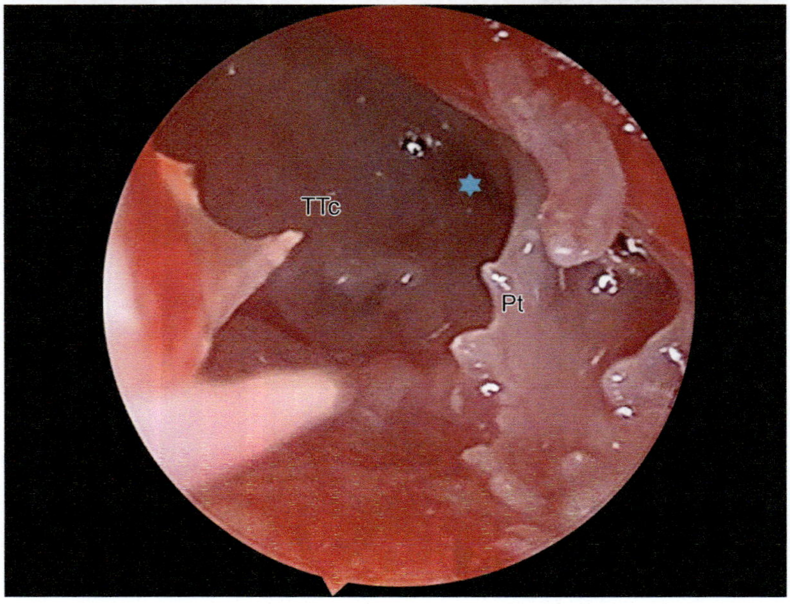

Fig. 24D: Endoscopic anatomy of protympanum [Blue star: Eustachian tube (ET)]
(Pt: protiniculum; TTc: canal for tensor tympani)

Protiniculum

Protiniculum is a bony ridge extending from the promontory medially, across the inferior wall and merging with the lateral wall of the tympanic cavity.

- It marks the demarcation between hypotympanum and protympanum
- The protiniculum has three conformations:[5]
  1. *Type A*: Ridge, with no air cells passing medially
  2. *Type B*: Bridge, with hypotympanic air cells extending inferiorly into protympanum
  3. *Type C*: Absent, no discernible protiniculum, hypotympanum fusing with protympanum

Protympanic Spine

Protympanic spine is a rough spine composed of either bony ridges or spicules is seen over the carotid artery prominence

- It has been hypothesized to be related to fusion of the two laminae (superior and inferior) of the carotid canal during embryologic development
- Its presence indicates less chances of carotid canal dehiscence in the protympanum

Caroticocochlear Recess

Caroticocochlear recess is the space between the anterior border of the promontory and carotid canal

- It is traversed by caroticotympanic nerves carrying postganglionic sympathetic efferent.

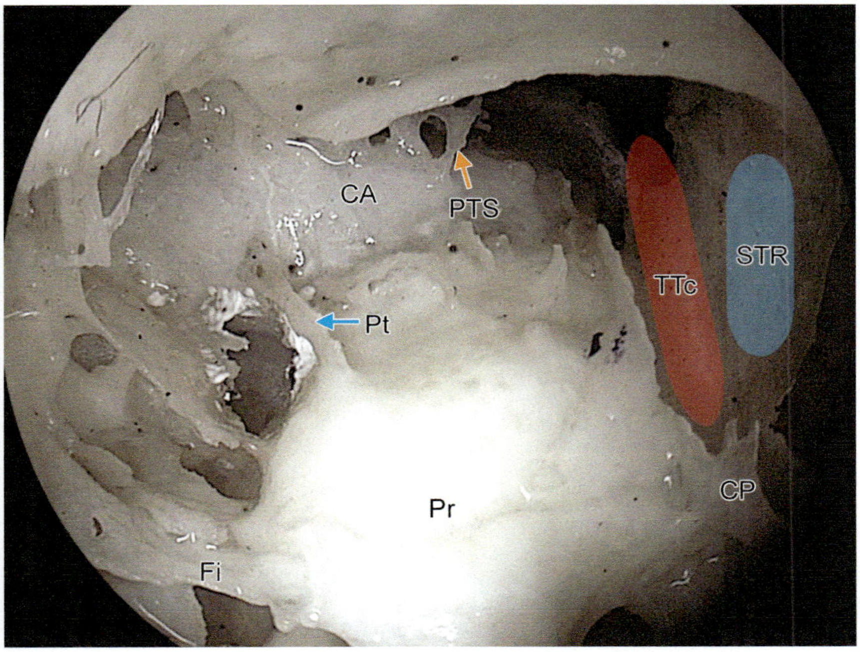

Fig. 25: Dry temporal bone specimen (left ear) showing important landmarks of protympanum.
(CA: carotid artery; CP: processus cochleariformis; Fi: finiculus; Pt: protiniculum; PTS: protympanic spine; Pr: promontory; STR: supratubal recess; TTc: canal for tensor tympani)

Morphological Significance of Protympanum

- Protympanum is lined by *pseudostratified ciliated columnar* epithelium bearing numerous *cilia* that beat and propel secretions toward the Eustachian tube
- The epithelium also bears *goblet cells* that secrete *mucus*
- Any pathology involving this region affects both the functions, causing stagnation of secretions leading to otitis media and subsequent perforation or negative pressure and tympanic membrane retraction.[19]
- *Biofilms* causing resistant middle ear infection are also likely to be located in this region.

Surgical Importance of Protympanum[20]

Final common pathway of ventilation:

- *Cholesteatoma in the protympanum*: A hidden area and a cause of residual and recurrence of disease
- *Surgical access to the Eustachian tube*
- *Otic neuralgia and tympanic neurectomy:* Branches of Jacobson's nerve in the protympanum need to be addressed as well; better visualized with angled endoscopes.
- *Cerebrospinal fluid leak:* Visualization with an angled endoscope can help the surgeon to identify the true

Eustachian tube for safely packing the region to control transnasal leak in recalcitrant cases.

SURGICAL ANATOMY OF HYPOTYMPANUM

Hypotympanum is the part of the middle ear lying below the level of lower border of external auditory canal.

- Contains numerous air cells
- Anteriorly, it is separated from the protympanum by protiniculum.
- The floor of the hypotympanum separates the tympanic cavity from the jugular bulb

Clinical Importance

- The jugular bulb may extend high up into the tympanic cavity in 25.3% of the population.[21]
- High jugular bulb is defined as jugular bulb extending up to or beyond inferior bony annulus.
- The bone over the jugular bulb may be dehiscent.
- The surgical importance of it lies during the elevation of the annulus in the inferior quadrant. Inadvertent injury to the jugular bulb may cause devastating bleeding.
- Acts as a corridor for the transcanal infracochlear approach to the petrous apex[22]

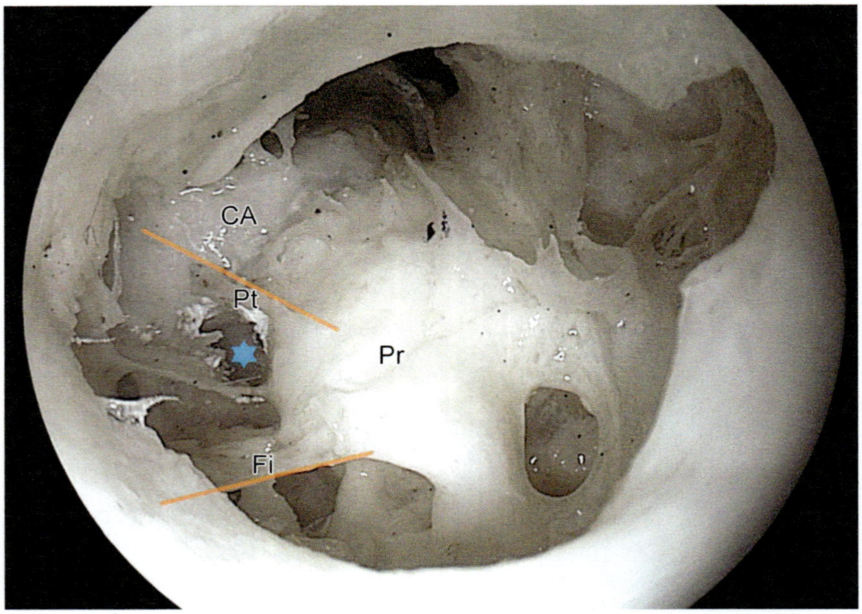

Fig. 26A: Anatomical extent of hypotympanum from protiniculum anteriorly to finiculus posteriorly (left ear).
(CA: carotid artery; Fi: finiculus; Pr: promontory; Pt: protiniculum)

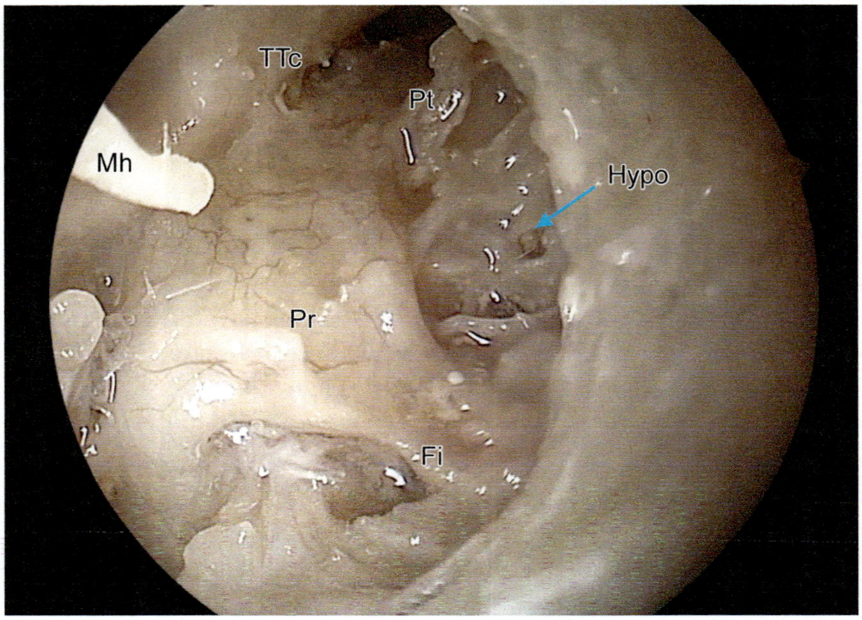

Fig. 26B: Bony landmarks of hypotympanum (right ear).
(Fi: finiculus; Mh: malleus handle; Pr: promontory; Pt: protiniculum; TTc: canal for tensor tympani)

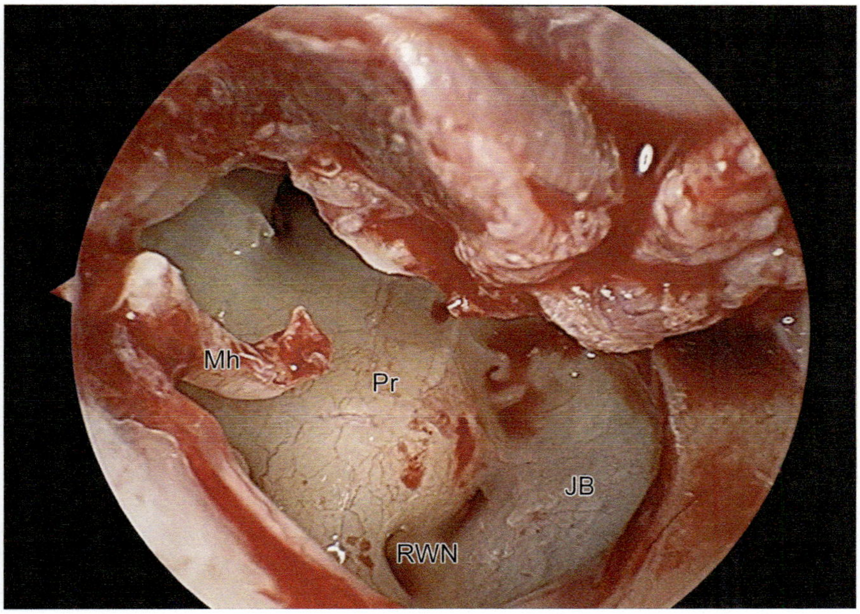

Fig. 26C: Landmarks of hypotympanum (right ear).
(JB: jugular bulb; Mh: malleus handle; Pr: promontory; RWN: round window niche)

SURGICAL ANATOMY OF CHORDA TYMPANI

Chorda tympani is the largest branch of facial nerve in its intratemporal segment.

- It carries two types of fibers:
  1. *Special sensory fibers*: Taste sensation from anterior two-thirds of tongue
  2. *Presynaptic parasympathetic fibers*:
     i. Secretomotor fibers to submandibular and sublingual glands
     ii. Blood vessel of tongue and causes dilatation of these vessels
- Chorda tympani exits from the facial nerve distal to the nerve to stapedius and proximal to the stylomastoid foramen
- *Mean angle:* Chord tympani forms a mean angle of 22° with the trunk of the facial nerve, where it arises from the facial nerve
- *Anatomical variations: Branching of the nerve may occur anywhere at the mastoid segment of the facial nerve*
  - Mid-third of mastoid segment (70%)
  - Proximal third (20%)
  - Distal third (10%)
- *Course of chorda tympani:*
  - After arising from facial nerve, chorda tympani traverses anterosuperiorly in a posterior canaliculus, usually accompanied by posterior tympanic branch of stylomastoid artery
  - The opening of the posterior canaliculus lies just medial to the tympanic annulus
  - Length of the posterior canaliculus is highly variable (3–14 mm) and average diameter is 0.5 mm.
  - In 10%, the posterior canaliculus is a sulcus on the posterior wall of external auditory canal, rather than a canaliculus.
  - Chorda tympani then arches upward and passes medial to the upper part of handle or neck of malleus, above the insertion of tensor tympani
  - The nerve exits the middle ear through the anterior canaliculus, which is a separate canal, also known as "canal of Huguier"
  - The canal of Huguier runs in the medial part of the petrotympanic fissure
  - The nerve is accompanied by anterior tympanic branch of the maxillary artery in the canal of Huguier.

Clinical Importance

- Chorda tympani is a structure which has been relatively less explored in literature.
- However, from the surgical point of view, one has to deal with the nerve in almost every case of endoscopic ear surgery during access into middle ear
- Chorda tympani has strong *inhibitory* action on other taste fibers.
- *Taste constancy:* This is a phenomenon in which if the chorda tympani is *denervated*, this *inhibitory* action is *lost*. Subsequently, it is *"neuroplasticity"* that can *compensate* for the *partial* loss of taste sensation that may occur due to damage of chorda tympani from disease or surgery.

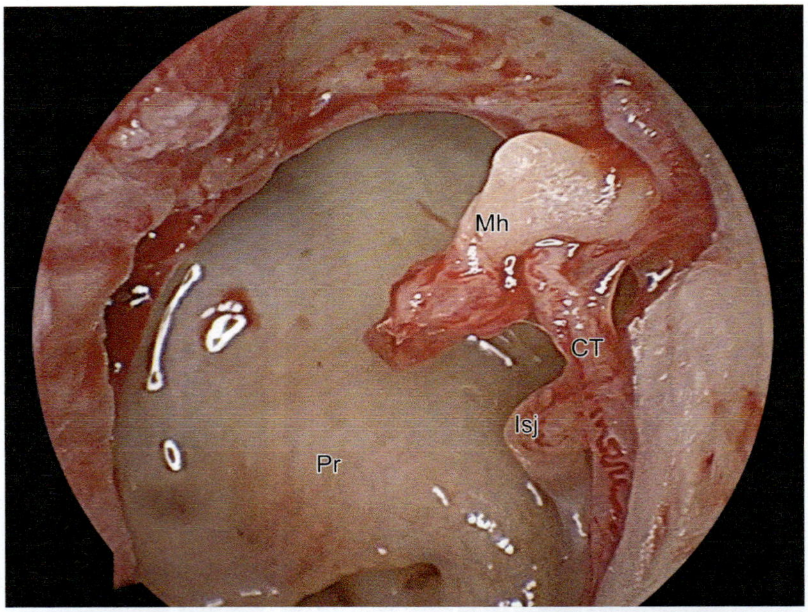

Fig. 27A: Endoscopic view of chorda tympani.
(CT: chorda tympani; Isj: incudostapedial joint; Mh: malleus handle; Pr: promontory)

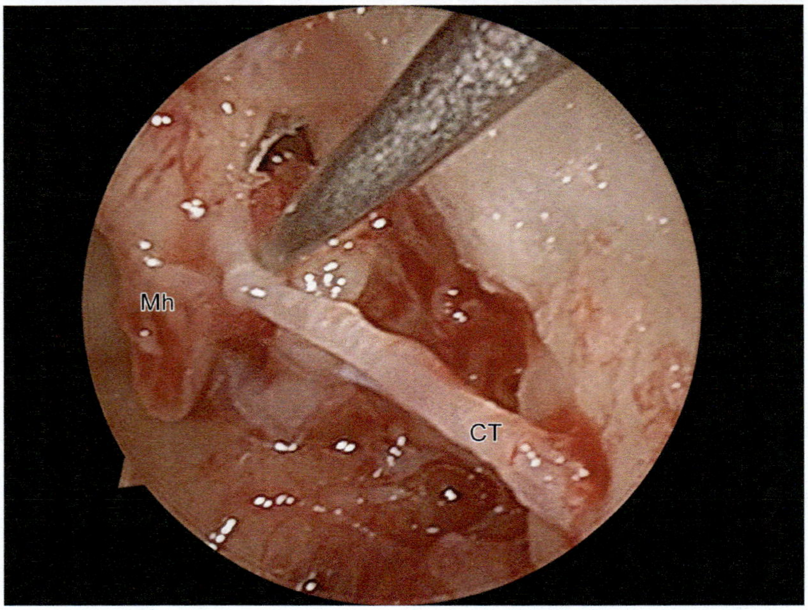

Fig. 27B: Course of chorda tympani.
(CT: chorda tympani; Mh: malleus handle)

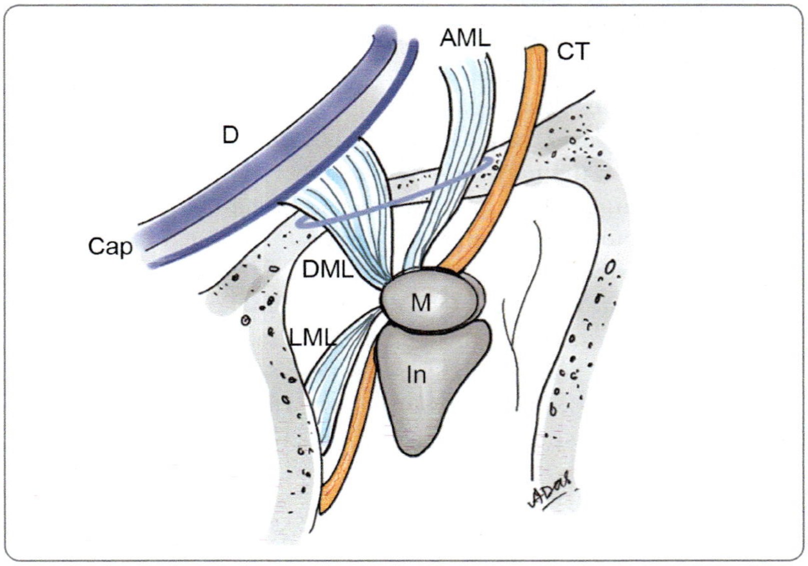

Fig. 27C: Anatomy of chorda tympani.
(AML: anterior malleolar ligament; Cap: capsule of temporomandibular joint; CT: chorda tympani; D: disk of temporomandibular joint; DML: discomalleolar ligament; In: incus; LML: lateral malleolar ligament; M: malleus)

ENDOSCOPIC ANATOMY OF COCHLEA AND ITS NEIGHBORING STRUCTURES

Cochlea, the sense organ of hearing, is housed within the temporal bone. Shaped like a snail's shell, it comprises of 2¾ turns around a bony pyramid, known as the *modiolus*. The cochlea houses three chambers inside it, namely:

1. *Scala media (filled with endolymph)*: Houses the organ of corti
2. *Scala vestibuli (filled with perilymph)*: Lying superior to scala media and abuts the oval window
3. *Scala tympani (filled with perilymph)*: Lying inferior to scala media and opens into the round window

The scala vestibuli and tympani communicate with each other at the apex via the *helicotrema*.

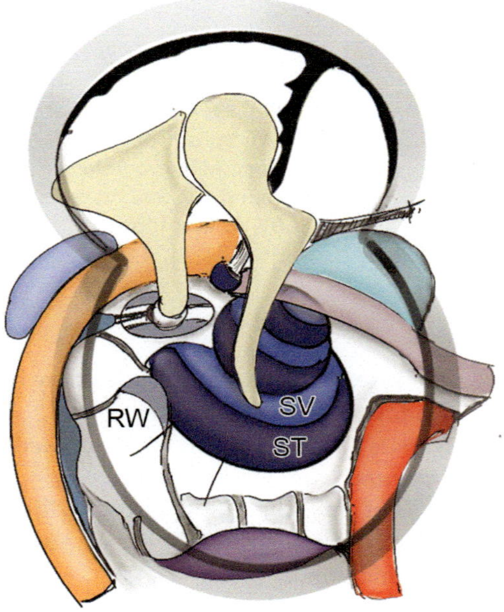

Fig 28: Anatomical disposition of cochlea with respect to right middle ear structures. (RW: round window; ST: scala tympani; SV: scala vestibuli)

Promontory

The most profound bulge seen at the medial wall of the middle ear is called the promontory which is formed by the basal turn of cochlea.

Jacobson's Nerve

The tympanic branch of the glossopharyngeal nerve (also known as the Jacobson's nerve) is the most prominent structure seen traversing the surface of promontory. It unites with the sympathetic plexus around carotid artery to form the tympanic plexus over the promontory. The nerve divides into two branches. An anterior branch travels toward the Eustachian tube and a posterior branch arches around the bony margin of the round window.[23,24]

Round Window

The opening of scala tympani to middle ear covered by secondary tympanic membrane.

Round Window Niche

The bony overhang that overlies the true round window membrane is called round window niche. It is formed by *anterior pillar* (postis anterior), *posterior pillar* (postis posterior) and tegmen, connecting the two pillars.[25] Composed of the above-mentioned landmarks, the niche is a tunnel-like structure that leads to the round window membrane. Several anatomical variations of the round window niche have been described such as- "cylindrical-type", "j-type" and "truncated cone-type", which all have implications in round window membrane visibility during surgery.[26]

Round Window Membrane

- The true round window membrane is also known as the secondary tympanic membrane.
- It separates the middle ear from the scala tympani
- It is a three-layered structure comprising an outer squamous epithelium, a middle connective tissue and an inner layer of mesothelial cells.[27]
- Often a false membrane is mistaken for the true round window membrane, which is usually a draping of the mucosal folds of the middle ear over the true membrane.
- This confusion can be sorted out by testing the round window reflex- gentle palpation of the ossicles shall cause the true round window membrane to move outward, causing the shining.

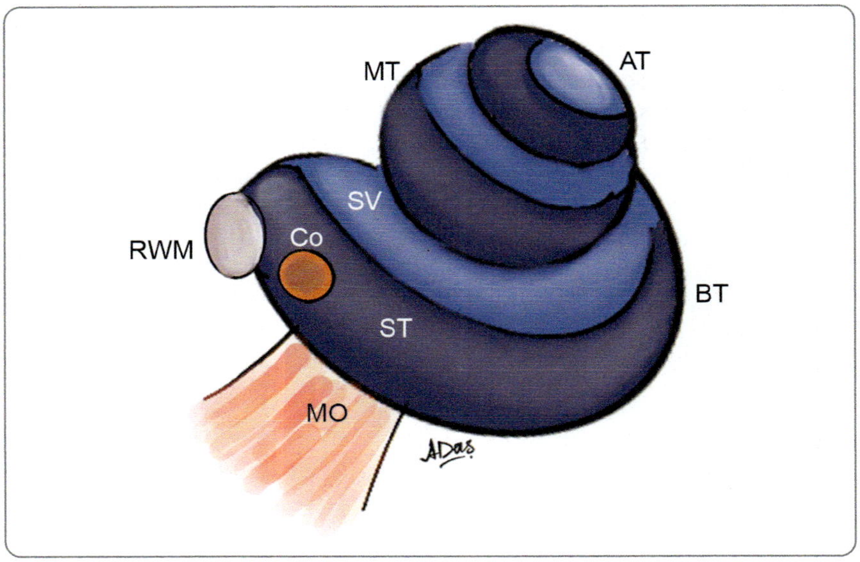

Fig. 29: Anatomy of cochlea (right)
(AT: apical turn; BT: basal turn; Co: cochlear duct; MO: modiolus; MT: middle turn; RWM: round window membrane; ST: scala tympani; SV: scala vestibuli)

- Reflection of a small amount of water placed in the hypotympanum to move
- However, in presence of a mucosal fold over it, that is, a false membrane, the reflex will be absent.

Surgical Importance of Round Window Membrane

- The portal of entry of the electrodes of cochlear implant into the cochlea is via the round window.
- The insertion of the electrodes may be done by round window insertion or cochleostomy.
- The site of cochleostomy is determined by the position of the *round window membrane.*
- A slight miscalculation of this critical landmark may cause insertion into a wrong place and render the implant nonfunctional.

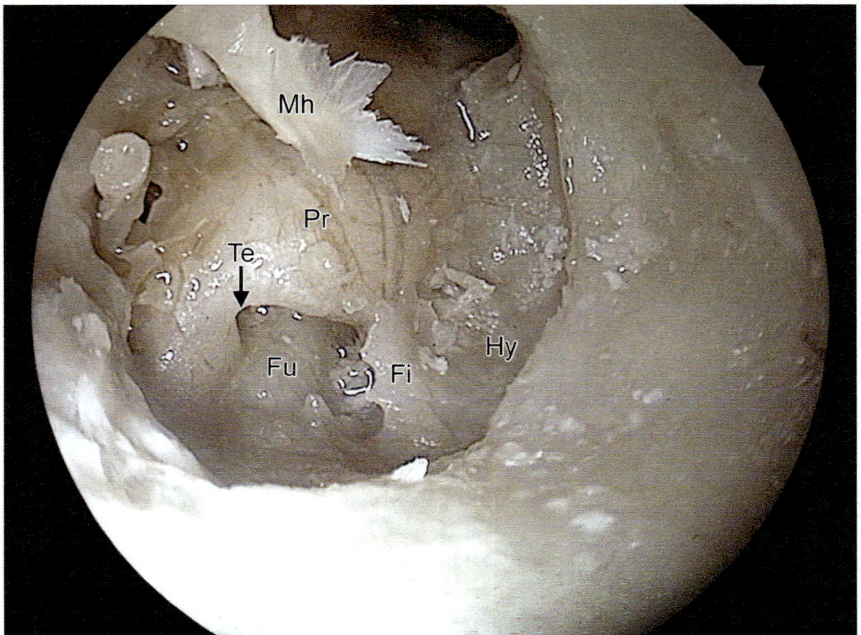

Fig. 30A: Steps of exposure of round window membrane: Round window niche (arrow) (right ear).
(Fi: finiculus; Fu: fustis; Hy: hypotympanum; Mh: malleus handle; Pr: promontory)

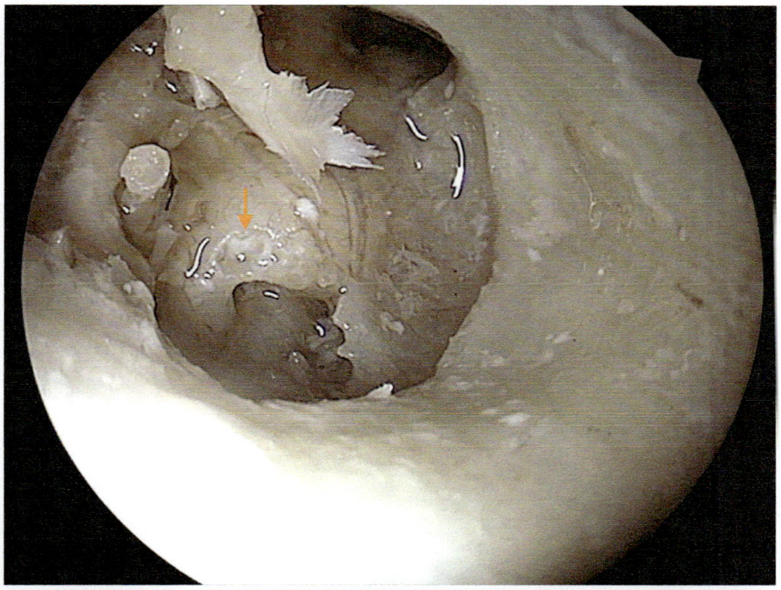

Fig. 30B: Steps of exposure of round window membrane: Site of drilling of round window niche for exposure of round window membrane (right ear) (orange arrow).

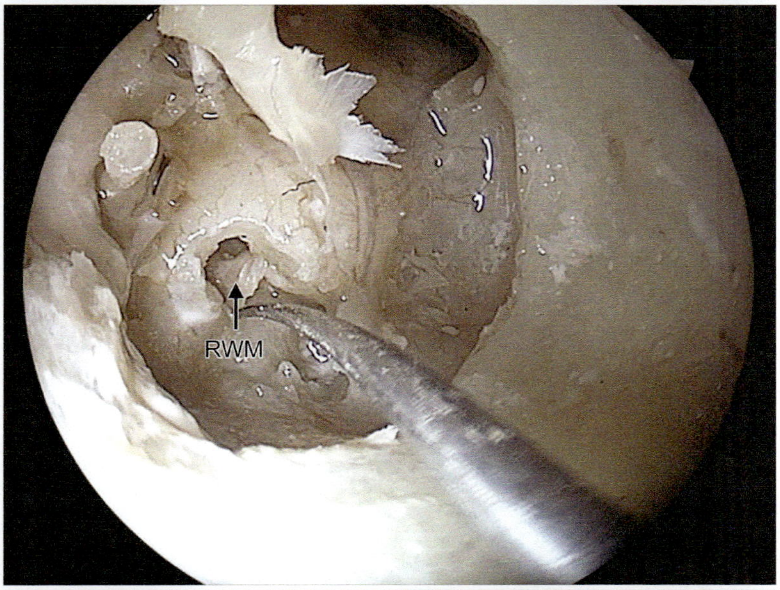

Fig. 30C: Steps of exposure of round window membrane: Exposure and reflection of round window membrane (right ear).
(RWM: round window membrane)

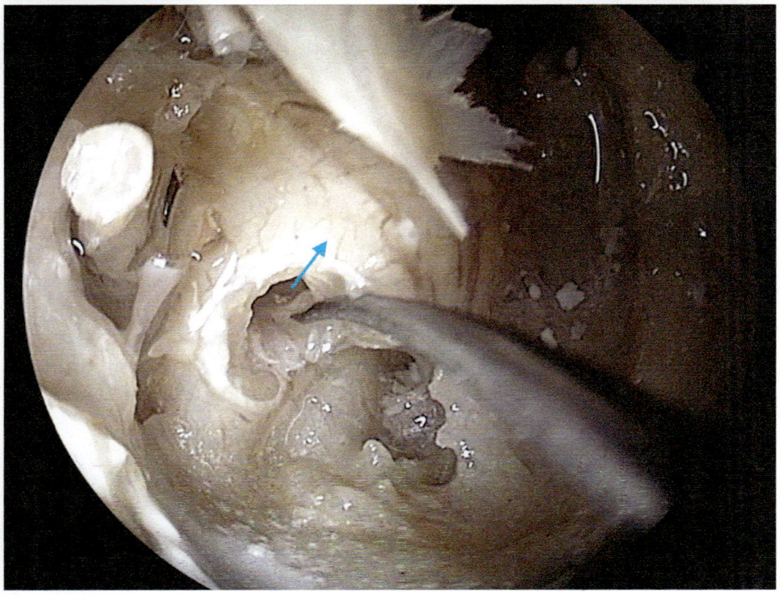

Fig. 30D: Steps of exposure of round window membrane: Direction of scala tympani of the basal turn of cochlea— site of cochlear implant insertion (right ear).

Crista Fenestra

It is a sharp bony ridge located at the anteroinferior aspect of the round window, forming the narrowest portion of round window, called the *hook region.*

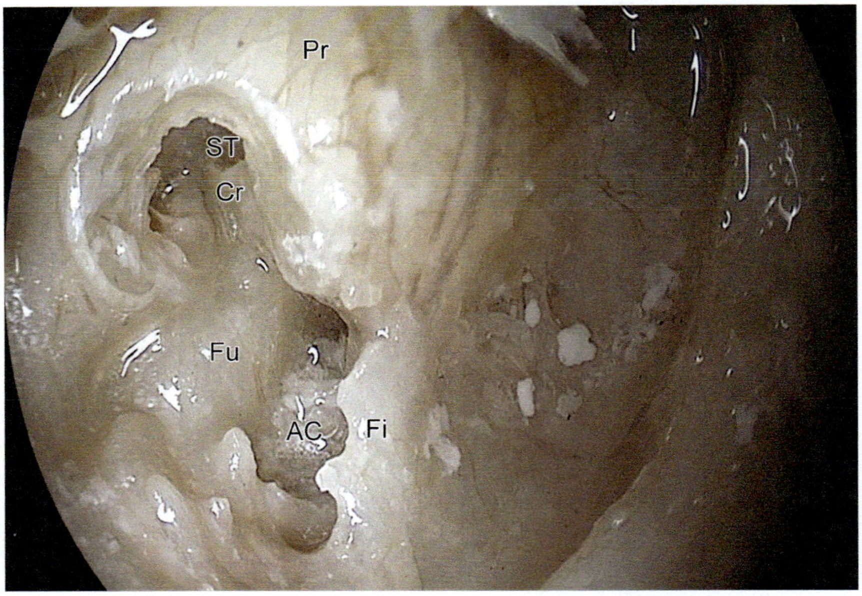

Fig. 31A: Wet temporal bone dissection specimen showing important landmarks around the round window (right ear).
(AC: area conchamerata; Cr: crista; Fi: finiculus; Fu: fustis; Pr: promontory; ST: scala tympani)

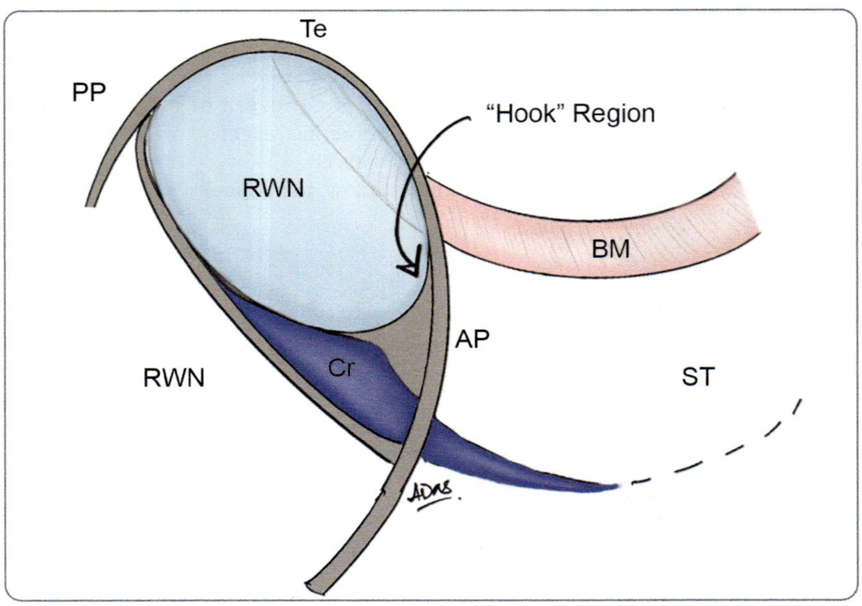

Fig. 31B: Pictorial depiction of hook region anatomy (right ear).
(AP: anterior pillar; BM: basilar membrane; Cr: crista; PP: posterior pillar; RWN: round window niche; ST: scala tympani; Te: tegmen)

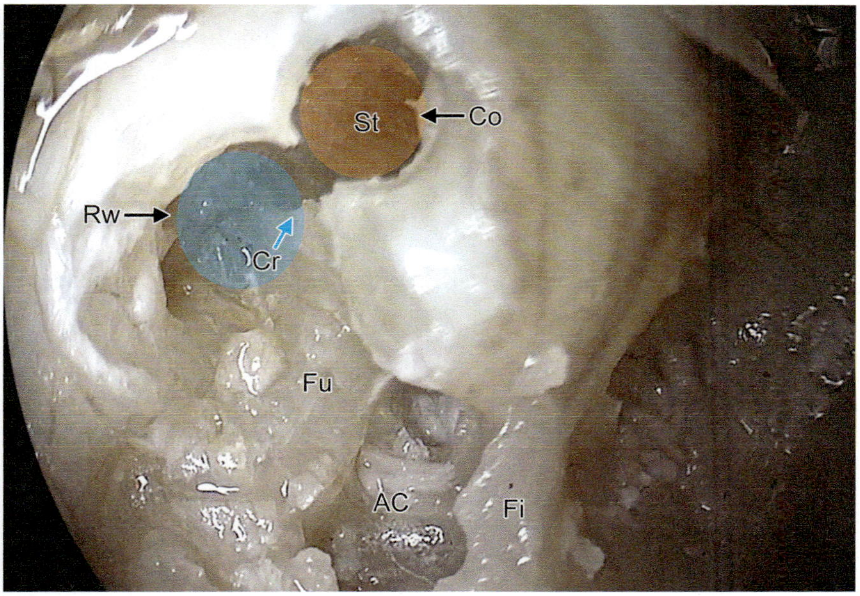

Fig. 32: Magnified endoscopic view of hook region (right ear).
(AC: area conchamerata; Co: cochlear duct; Cr: crista; Fi: finiculus; Fu: fustis; Rw: round window; St: scala tympani)

Surgical Importance of Crista Fenestra

- Crista fenestra poses a surgical challenge in relation to cochlear implant electrode insertion as it causes narrowing of the natural opening of the round window, in case of round window insertion
- This results in an acute angulation while directing the electrodes into scala tympani
- In case of cochleostomy, this anatomical bottleneck is bypassed and a direct access into scala tympani is attained.
- However, this requires meticulous surgical anatomical precision, as a wrong cochleostomy can misdirect the electrodes into scala vestibuli superiorly or carotid canal anteriorly or hypotympanic air cell inferiorly.

Osseous Spiral Lamina

It is a shelf of bone arising from the modiolus, projecting into the cochlea, taking the winding contour of the turns of cochlea.

Basilar Membrane

The basilar membrane runs from the tympanic lip of the osseous spiral lamina to the spiral ligament's basilar crest. It forms the floor of the scala media and the base of organ of Corti.

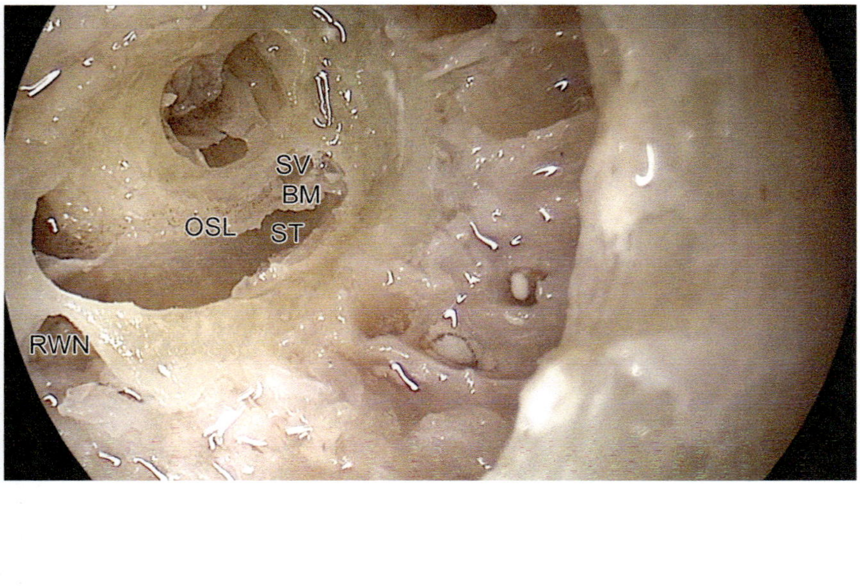

Fig. 33: Wet temporal bone dissection specimen showing internal anatomy of cochlea (right ear).
(BM: basilar membrane; OSL: osseous spiral lamina; RWN: round window niche; ST: scala tympani; SV: scala vestibuli)

REFERENCES

1. Marchioni D, Mattioli F, Alicandri-Ciufelli M, Presutti L. Transcanal endoscopic approach to the sinus tympani: a clinical report. Otol Neurotol. 2009;30(6):758-65.
2. Weiss MH, Parisier SC, Han JC, Edelstein DR. Surgery for recurrent and residual cholesteatoma. Laryngoscope. 1992;102:145-51.
3. Presutti L, Marchioni D, Mattioli F, Villari D, Alicandri-Ciufelli M. Endoscopic management of acquired cholesteatoma: our experience. J Otolaryngol Head Neck Surg. 2008;37:481-7.
4. Tarabichi M. Endoscopic management of acquired cholesteatoma. Am J Otol. 1997;18:544-9.
5. Marchioni D, Alicandri-Ciufelli M, Piccinini A, Genovese E, Presutti L. Inferior retrotympanum revisited: an endoscopic anatomic study. Laryngoscope. 2010;120(9):1880-6.
6. Proctor B. The development of the middle ear spaces and their surgical significance. J Laryngol Otol. 1964;78:631-48.
7. Marchioni D, Alicandri-Ciufelli M, Molteni G, Artioli FL, Genovese E, Presutti L. Selective epitympanic dysventilation syndrome. Laryngoscope. 2010;120(5):1028-33.
8. Palva T, Ramsay H, Böhling T. Tensor fold and anterior epitympanum. Am J Otol. 1997;18(3):307-16.
9. Marchioni D, Molteni G, Presutti L. Endoscopic anatomy of the middle ear. Indian J Otolaryngol Head Neck Surg. 2011;63(2):101-13.
10. Das A, Mitra S, Hazra S, Sengupta A. Endoscopic epitympanic exploration in mucosal chronic otitis media: is canal wall up mastoidectomy really needed?. J Laryngol Otol. 2021;135(1):39-44.
11. Chatellier HP, Lemoine J. Le diaphragme interatticotympanique du nouveau-ne. Ann Otolaryngol Chir Cervicofac. 1946;13:534-66.
12. Palva T, Johnsson L. Epitympanic compartment surgical considerations: reevaluation. Am J Otol. 1995;16:505-13.
13. Marchioni D, Alicandri-Ciufelli M, Grammatica A, Mattioli F, Genovese E, Presutti L. Lateral endoscopic approach to epitympanic diaphragm and Prussak's space: a dissection study. Surg Radiol Anat. 2010;32(9):843-52.
14. Bluestone CD, Bluestone MB. Eustachian tube. Structure, function, role in otitis media. Shelton (CT): PMPH-USA; 2005. p. 62.
15. Kapadia M, Arsiwala Z, Tarabichi M. Endoscopic transtympanic Eustachian tube dilatation: an overview of evaluation methods and dilatation technique. World J Otorhinolaryngol Head Neck Surg. 2019;5(3):152-9.
16. Nadol JB, McKenna MJ. Surgery of the ear and temporal bone. Philadelphia (PA): Lippincott Williams & Wilkins; 2005. p. 125.
17. Palva T (Ed). Color Atlas of the Anatomy and Pathology of the Epitympanum. Basel: Karger; 2001. pp. 45-52.
18. Tarabichi M, Marchioni D, Kapadia M. The epitympanum revisited: endoscopic anatomy. Indian J Otolaryngol Head Neck Surg. 2016;68(4):490-5.
19. Ars B, Ars-Piret NM. Morphofunctional partition of the middle ear cleft. Mediterr J Otol. 2007;3:31-9.
20. Jufas N, Marchioni D, Tarabichi M, Patel N. Endoscopic anatomy of the protympanum. Otolaryngol Clin North Am. 2016;49(5):1107-19.
21. Savic D, Djeric D. Surgical anatomy of the hypotympanum. J Laryngol Otol. 1987;101(5):419-25.
22. Li KL, Agarwal V, Moskowitz HS, Abuzeid WM. Surgical approaches to the petrous apex. World J Otorhinolaryngol Head Neck Surg. 2020;6(2):106-14.
23. Townsend GL, Morimoto AM, Kralemann H. Management of sialorrhea in mentally retarded patients by transtympanic neurectomy. Mayo Clin Proc. 1973;48:776-9.
24. Sinha P. Successful treatment of parotid fistula with tympanic neurectomy. Indian J Otolaryngol Head Neck Surg. 2008;60:227-30.
25. Mehanna AM, Abdelnaby MM, Eid M. The Anatomy and Anatomical Variations of the Round Window Prechamber and Their Implications on Cochlear Implantation: An Anatomical, Imaging, and Surgical Study. Int Arch Otorhinolaryngol. 2020;24(3):e288-e298.
26. Canzi P, Avato I, Manfrin M, Simoncelli AM, Magnetto M, Rebecchi E, et al. Anatomic variations of the round window niche: radiological study and related endoscopic anatomy. Surg Radiol Anat. 2019;41(7):853-7.
27. Schachern PA, Paparella MM, Duvall AJ 3rd, Choo YB. The human round window membrane. An electron microscopic study. Arch Otolaryngol. 1984;110(1):15-21.

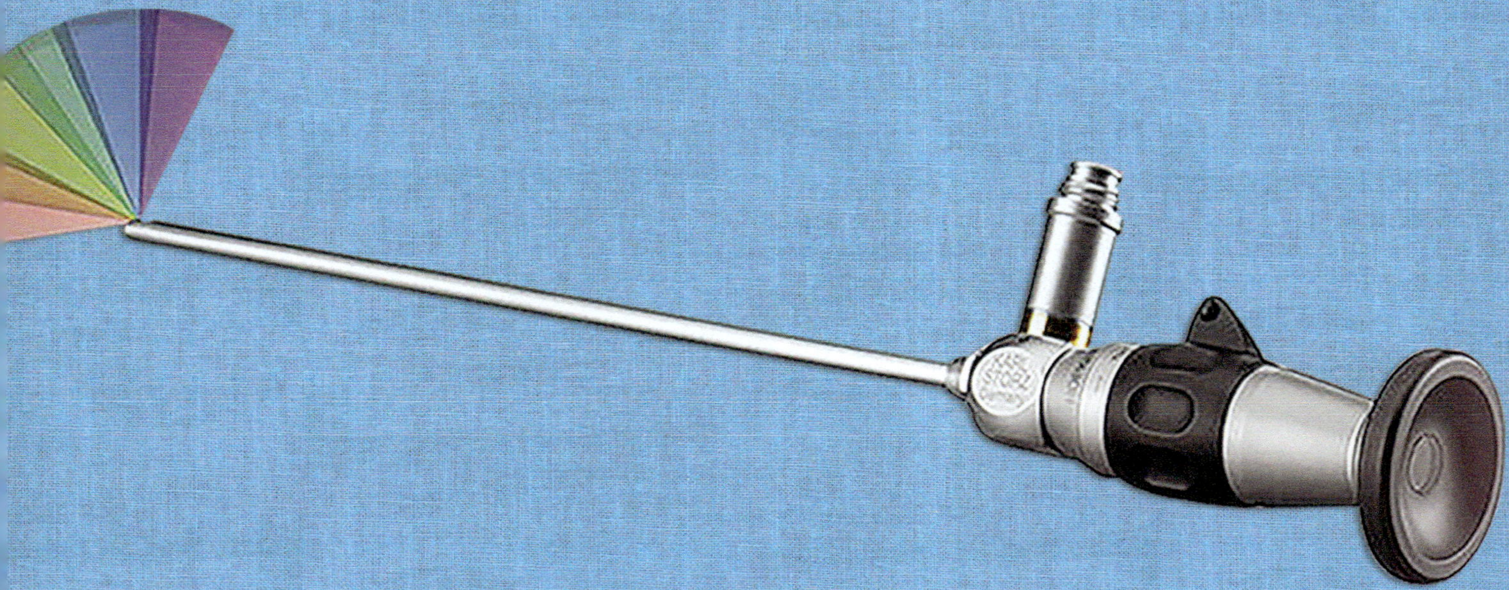

CHAPTER 4

Operation Theater Setup and Instruments

Arindam Das, Sayan Hazra

Chapter Outline

INTRODUCTION

Surgical principles employed for endoscopic and microscopic ear surgery are quite different and accordingly the basic instruments required for either technique is also different. Some special curved instruments like certain dissectors, forceps, suction apparatus, etc. need to be adapted so as to take advantage of the endoscope's ability to "see around corners." Here we give you an overview of the instrument armamentarium and operation theater (OT) set-up. Further details pertaining to each surgical procedure will be dealt with in its respective section.

ENDOSCOPE

Endoscopes vary in lengths, diameters, and angulations, each having its own advantages and disadvantages. Endoscope with larger diameter provides better field of view, better illumination delivered by the light bundles carried within the lens and thus superior clarity of image delivered. 18-cm 4 mm 0° Hopkins rod and scope is our workhorse for most of the regular otologic procedures. Longer endoscope ensures that the surgeon's two hands are at different distances from the ear canal and thus be less likely to interfere with one another during surgery. However, scopes of 3 mm diameter and 14 cm length are also used for surgical otoendoscopy. Angled scopes (30°, 45°, and 70°) of 2.7 mm diameter are kept in hand to visualize the so-called hidden areas like the tympanic sinus, facial recess, anterior epitympanic recess, orifice of Eustachian tube, etc. Slimmer scopes are preferred since an angled scope needs to be placed in diametrically opposite position while working around corners and the working instrument needs to operate in the same narrow space. 3 mm and 1.9 mm scopes of 18 cm length are beneficial in pediatric cases and in adults with very narrow canals.

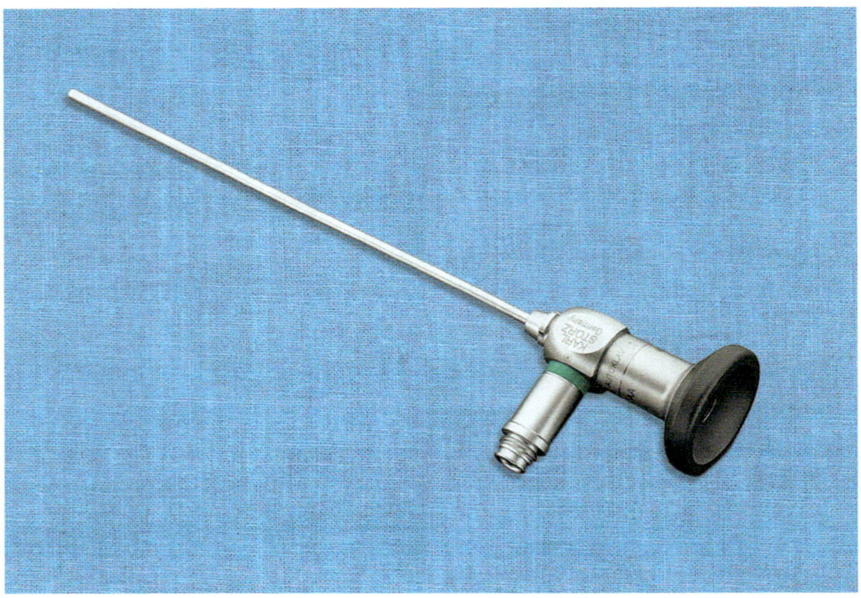

Fig. 1: A 4-mm 0° endoscope; regarded as the "workhorse" for endoscopic ear surgery (EES).

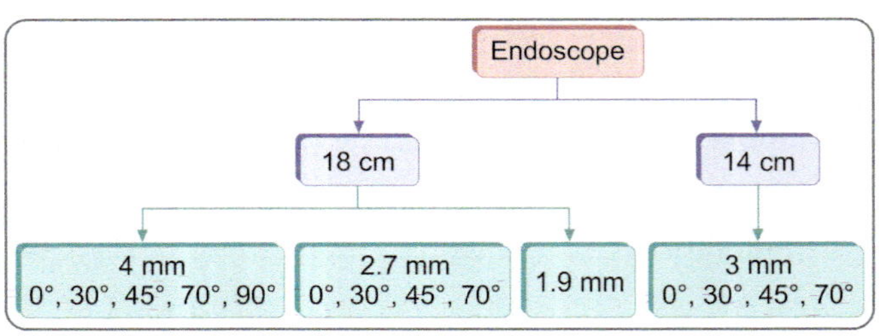

EndoCAMeleon of 4 mm 18 cm long by Karl Storz provides adjustable direction of view, ranging from 15° to 90° which has the light cable connector facing upward.

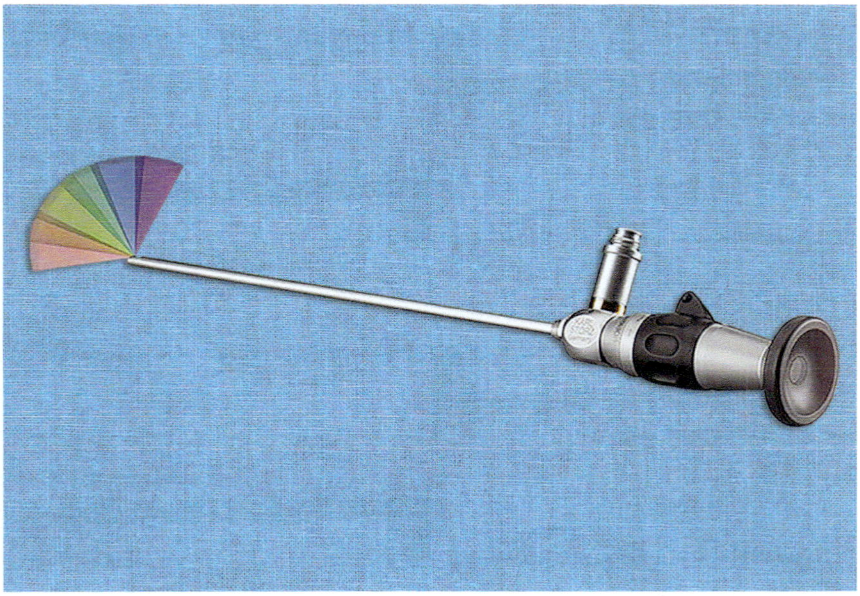

Fig. 2: EndoCAMeleon by Karl Storz.

CAMERA AND MONITOR

One of the main reasons for revolution of endoscopic ear surgery (EES) has been the technological advancement of the camera which facilitates better visualization of the complex anatomy and makes the job of the surgeon easier. Three-chip cameras, and more recently the high-definition fully digital cameras, deliver images of excellent quality and provide automatic controls over color, brightness, white balance, and digital contrast enhancement.

There are two main types of camera sensors: (1) charge-coupled device (CCD) and (2) complementary metal-oxide-semiconductor (CMOS). CCD was the better of these technologies in terms of picture quality, color reproduction and performance in low light. The technology behind CMOS is now being used in professional digital still and movie cameras. However, medical technology still predominantly employs CCD, which can either be 1-chip or 3-chip. 1-chip uses a Bayer filter, which means that a dominant color in the red-green-blue spectrum can wash-out the others, leading to a phenomenon called "redout" if bleeding is present. 3-chip devices have prisms which split the red-green-blue inputs into three separate chips, preventing this phenomenon from occurring. Thus 3-chip CCD camera is preferred in EES where small amounts of bleeding in a confined space can make a big difference. Weight and size of the camera head is also a factor to consider in terms of holding fatigability.

Some cameras have a manual focusing ring, while others rely on digital zoom. As with all digital photography, manual zoom provides a crisper/clearer image.

High-definition (HD) and ultra-high definition (4K): The video mode relates to the number of pixels that fit in each image frame, as it is linked to the size of the screen's frame (i.e., width × height). High-definition means at least 720 pixels in height per frame. 720p, 1080p, and 1440p are HD. Ultra-high definition or 4K technology displays at 2160p, while 8K technology displays at 4320p mode. A 720p screen will have a frame size of 1280 × 720 pixels, while a 1080p will have a 1920 × 1080 pixels frame size. Ultra HD will have a 3840 × 2160 size or 4096 × 2160.

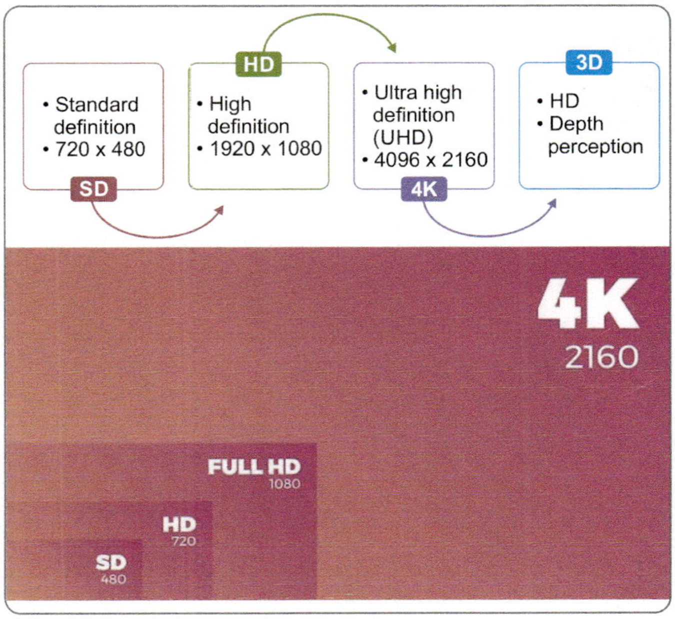

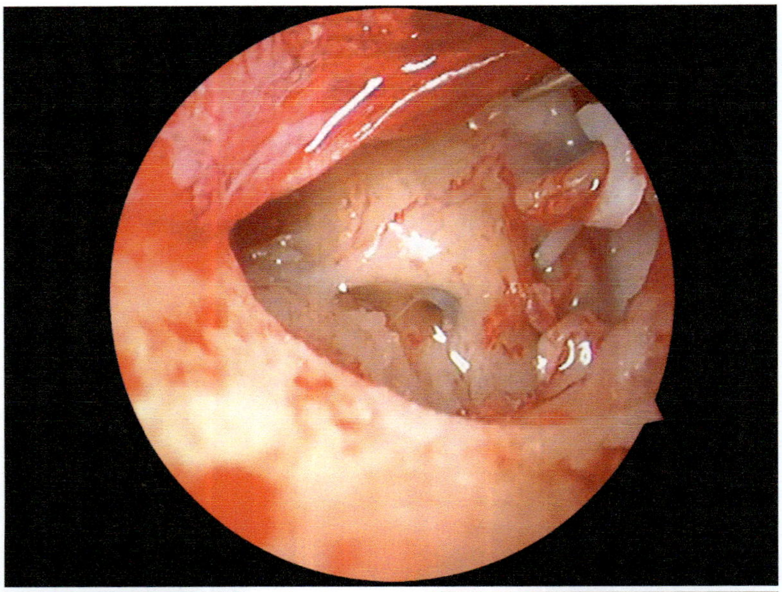

Fig. 3: Standard definition (SD) image.

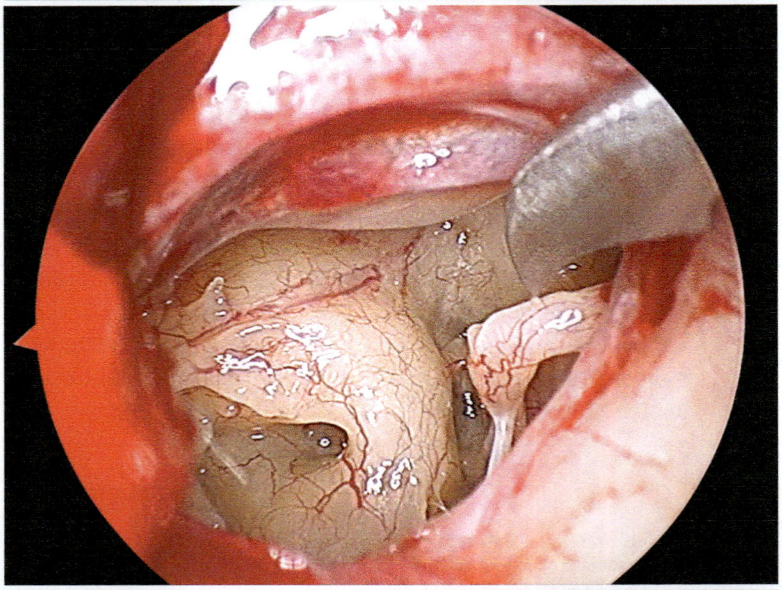

Fig. 4: High definition (HD) image.

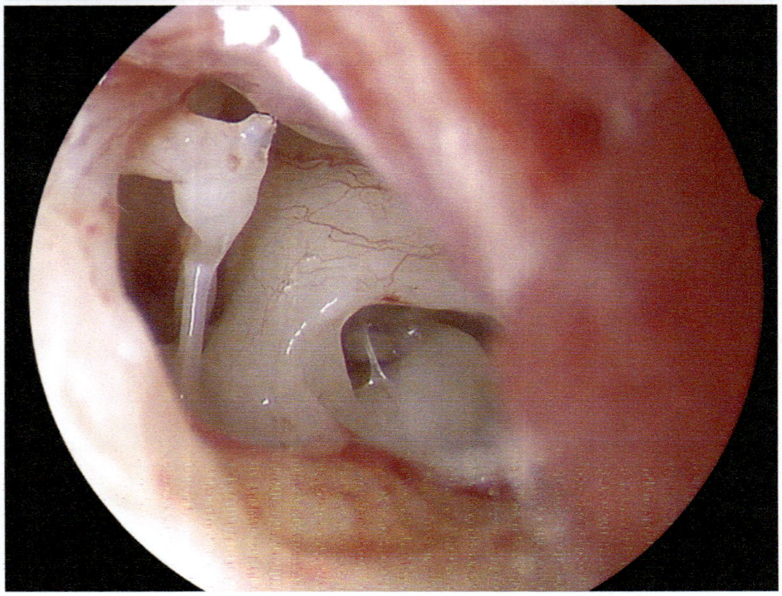

Fig. 5: 4K image.

- The image 1 system by Karl Storz instantly converts optical images to digital format with improved imaging on all digital recording and display devices. It offers 3-chip CCD fully digital high-definition camera head, having maximum resolution 1920 × 1080 pixels, with integrated image processing module, thus providing the resolution and light sensitivity necessary for the highest digital image quality.
  Image 1 S RUBINA™ and three-dimensional (3D) endoscopes are further advancement provided by Karl Storz, details of which have been described later.
- Wolf-Endocam Logic 4K camera head provides pin-sharp images using HD technology using either of CCD or CMOS sensors while its Endocam Performance HD has CCD sensors.
- Olympus CH-S400 4K camera head with high sensitivity CMOS sensor gives sharp images along with one-touch autofocus function and electronic zoom to see fine details of tissue/structures even when enlarged.

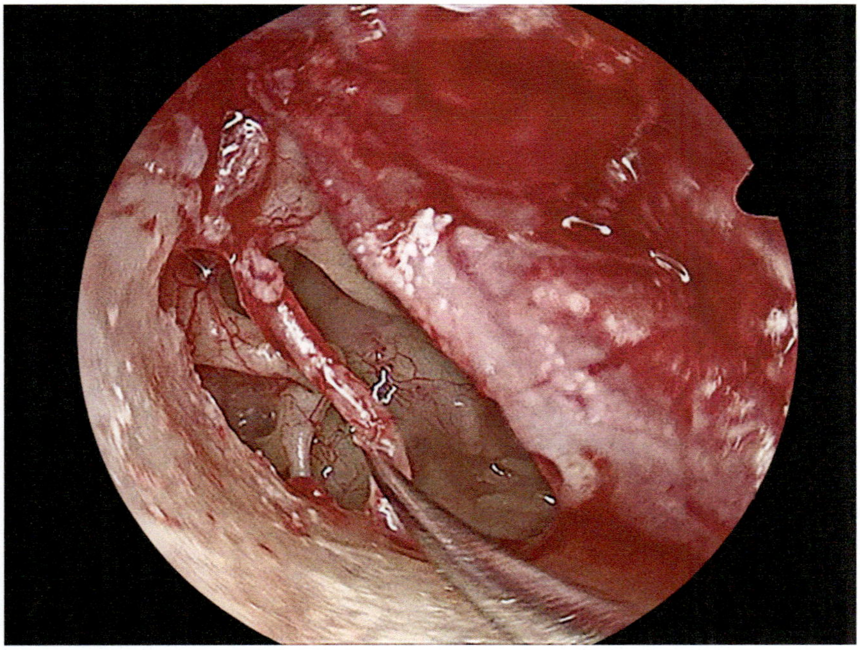

Fig. 6: Image from Storz SPIES.

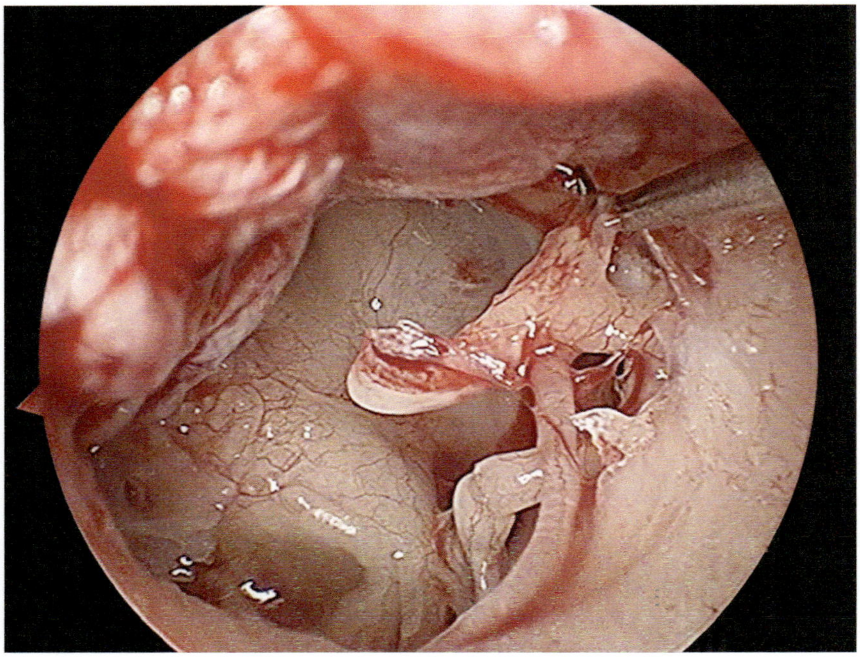

Fig. 7: Image from Stryker HD camera.

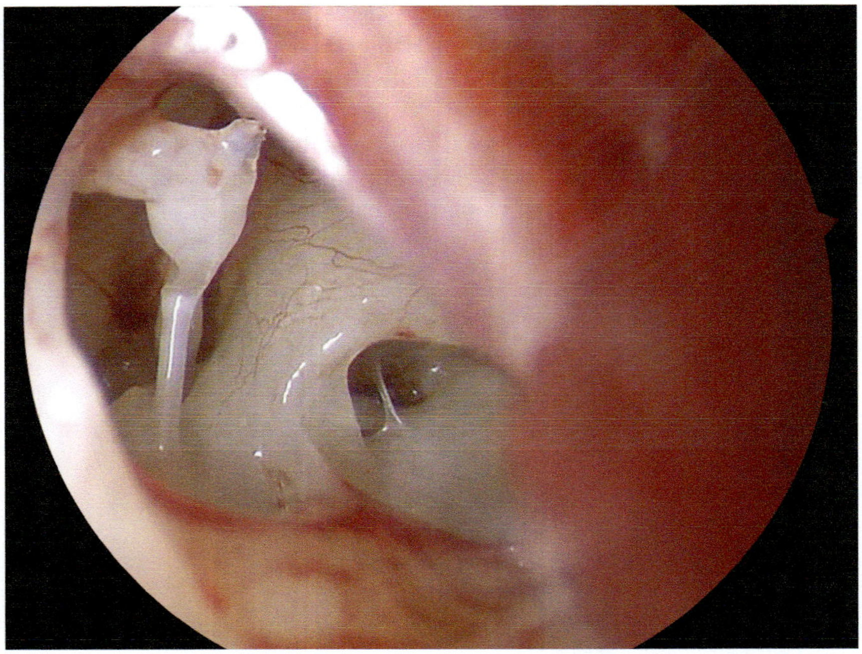

Fig. 8: Image from Wolf 4K camera.

Illumination is generated by a powerful cold-light source and transmitted to the endoscope via a 180-cm-long fiberoptic light cable. Different types of light sources (Xenon, LED, Halogen) offer light of varying brightness. Though Xenon light source provides excellent illumination, it also results in thermal injury. In this regard, a cooler source such as LED at 50% illumination is sufficient for visualization in EES as well as safe vis-à-vis its thermal effects on middle ear and inner ear.[1]

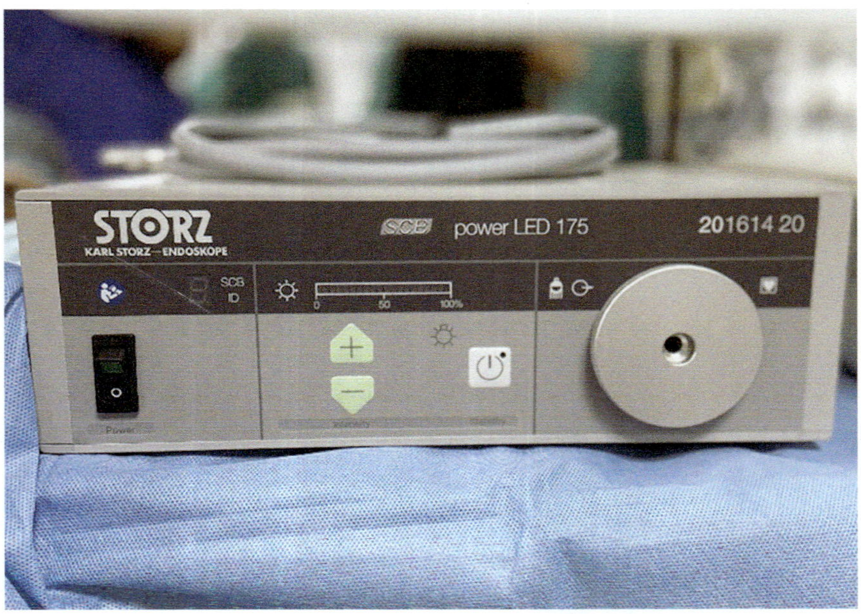

Fig. 9: LED light source with cable.

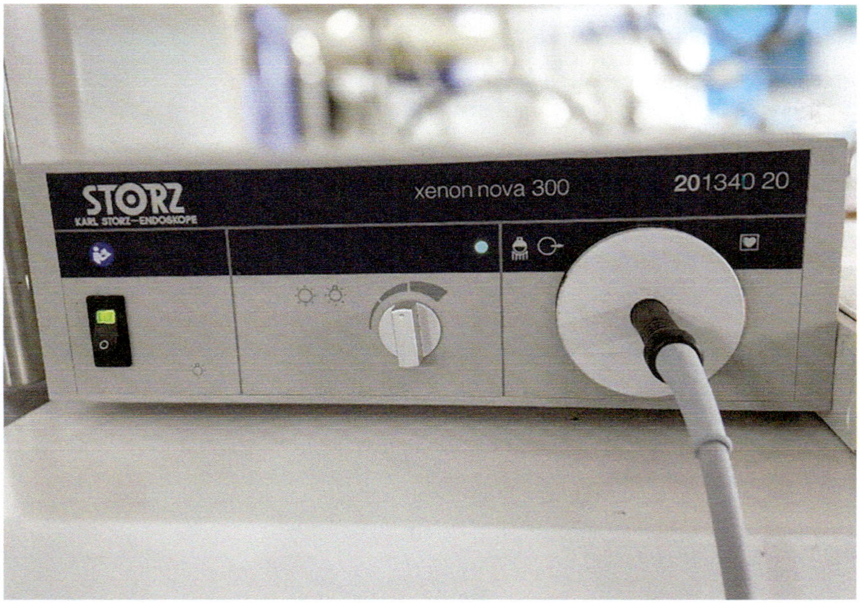

Fig. 10: Xenon light source with light cable attached.

Monitor: Modern monitors have a thin film transistor liquid crystal display (TFT-LCD or LCD) with a LED (light-emitting diode) backlight. These are connected via digital visual interface (DVI) or high-definition multimedia interface (HDMI) to the aforesaid camera head. High-definition medical grade monitors display the camera image throughout the endoscopic procedure which should be placed in direct line of view of the surgeon. It is advisable to use a bigger screen for proper enlarged visualization. Another characteristic of a monitor is the aspect ratio which refers to the ratio between width and height. The screen aspect ratio of a traditional television screen is 4:3. High-definition monitors use an aspect ratio of 16:9. Pixel shapes correspond to the shape of the aspect ratio. In simple terms, pixels for the 4:3 format are thin, while that of 16:9 format are wide.

27" HD monitor is used in the Image 1 system while OEV262H 26" LCD monitor by Olympus having advanced display technology makes it possible to realize the full potential of its endoscopy system. Wolf has medical LCD 4K monitors starting from 21.5" and going up to 55".

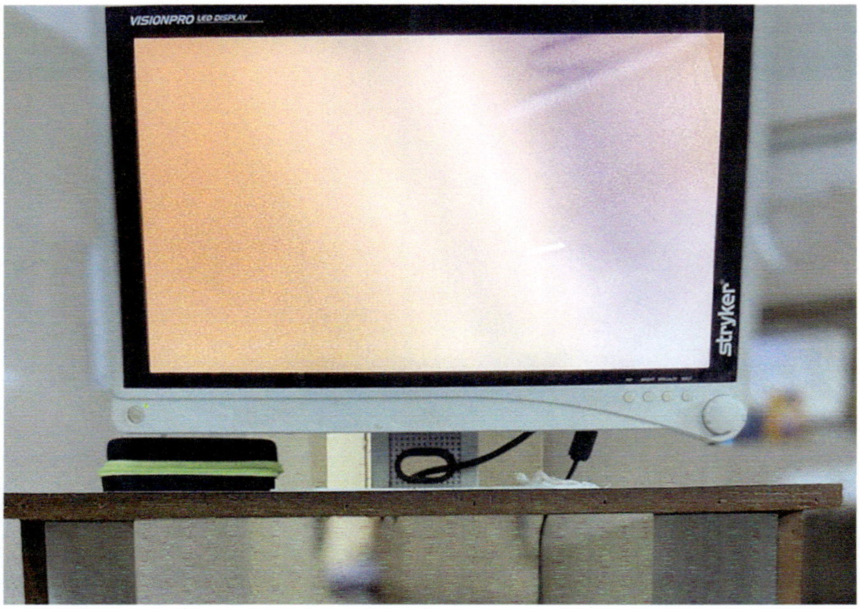

Fig. 11: Medical grade monitor by Stryker.

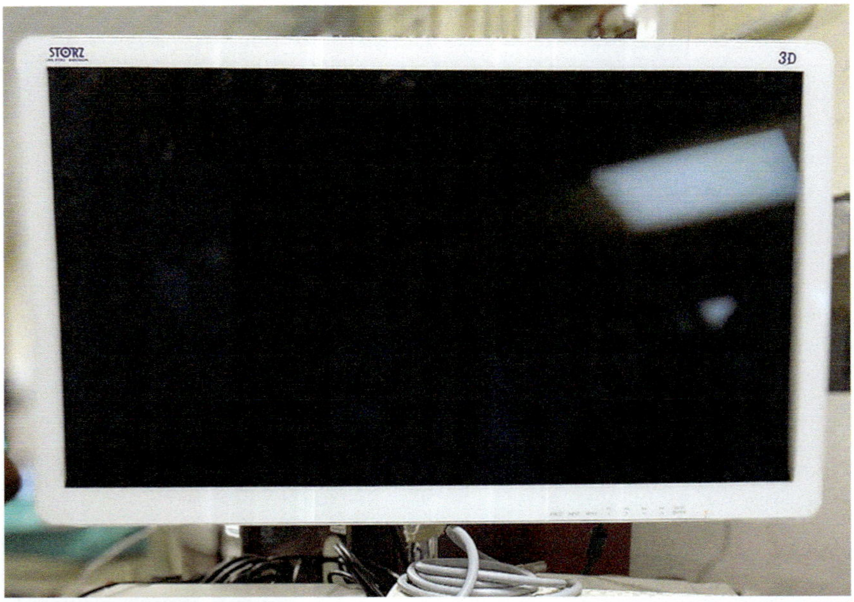

Fig. 12: 3D monitor.

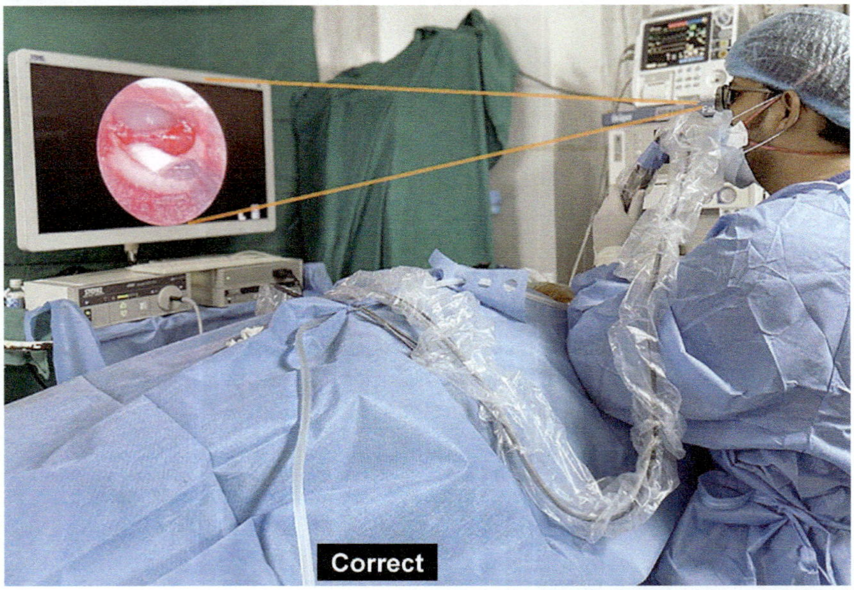

Fig. 13A: Depiction of correct eye level of surgeon with respect to the monitor.

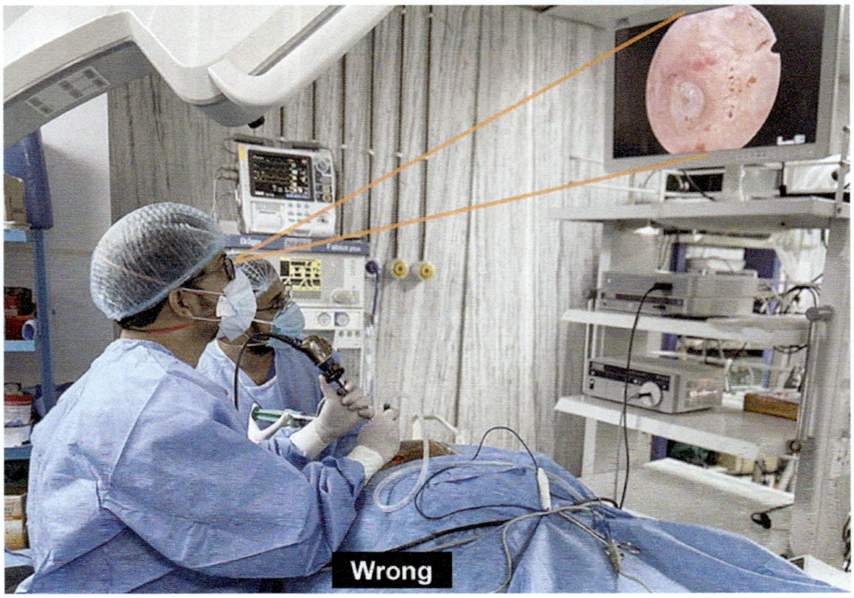

Fig. 13B: Depiction of incorrect eye level of surgeon with respect to the monitor.

Data archiving and recording: The AIDA compact HD (Advanced Image and Data Archiving) digital documentation system provides convenient image, video, and audio archiving of important stages and results of a procedure. This ensures a continuous information flow from the operating table to the patient files and also captures high-quality images for self-audit of surgical steps, as well as a master teaching tool. There's provision for direct recording from the recently developed Image 1 system. However, in case such systems are not available due to financial and other constraints, one can look for external recording devices having capacity to record images in the same output quality as in the capturing system.

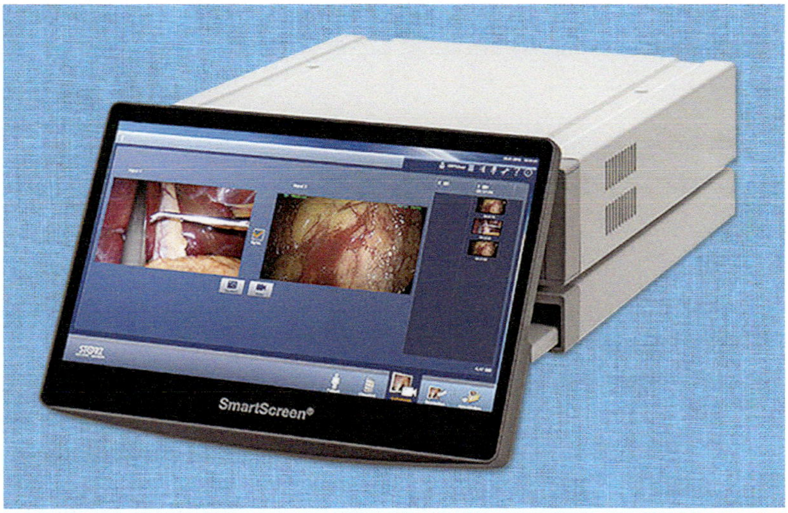

Fig. 14A: Recording device: Advanced Image and Data Archiving (AIDA) compact HD video recorder.

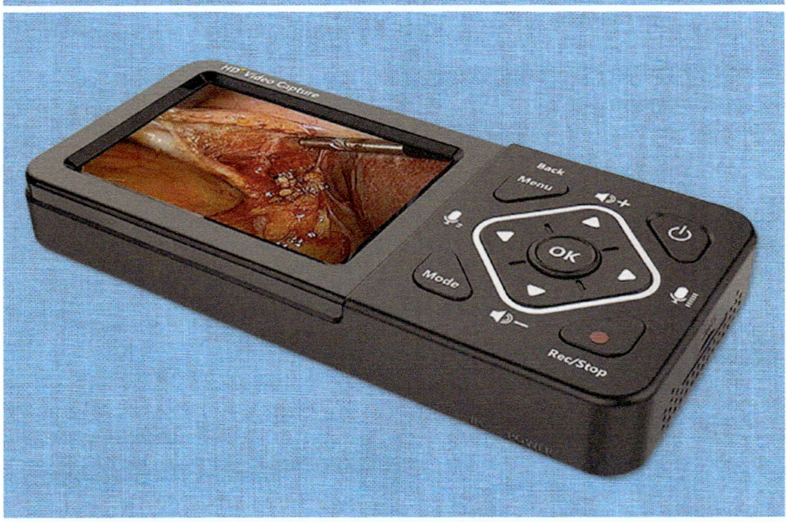

Fig. 14B: Recording device: HD video recorder.

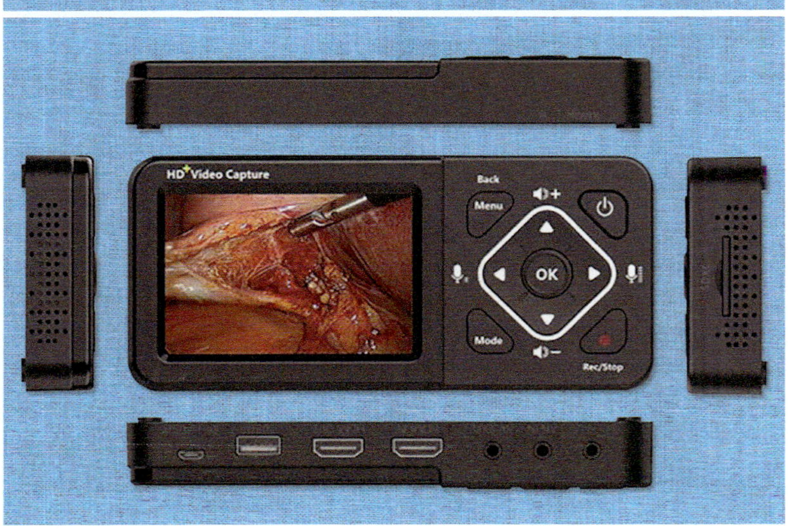

Fig. 14C: Recording device: HD video recorder.

OPERATION THEATER SETUP

- *Endoscope console* placed diametrically opposite to surgeon and at his/her eye level
- *Scrub nurse/assistant and instrument trolley* at head-end of OT table. This enables proper assistance, particularly regarding the size of the burr ends, the choice of the proper instruments, and the rate of supply of the irrigating water.
- *Operating microscope* kept as a "standby" beside the endoscope console
- *Diathermy, suction apparatus, and anesthetic workstation* kept at/around foot-end of OT table.
- *Ambient illumination* of the theater should be kept at a minimum level to avoid reflection on the monitor.

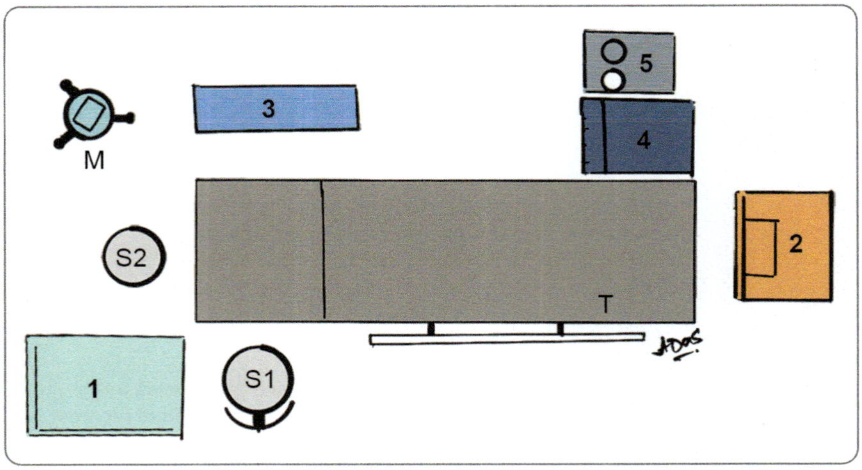

Fig. 15A: Schematic diagram of OT room set-up for endoscopic ear surgery (EES): For right ear.
(1: instrument trolley; 2: anesthesia workstation; 3: camera and monitor; 4: diathermy; 5: suction machine; M: microscope; T: OT table; S1: surgeon; S2: assistant)

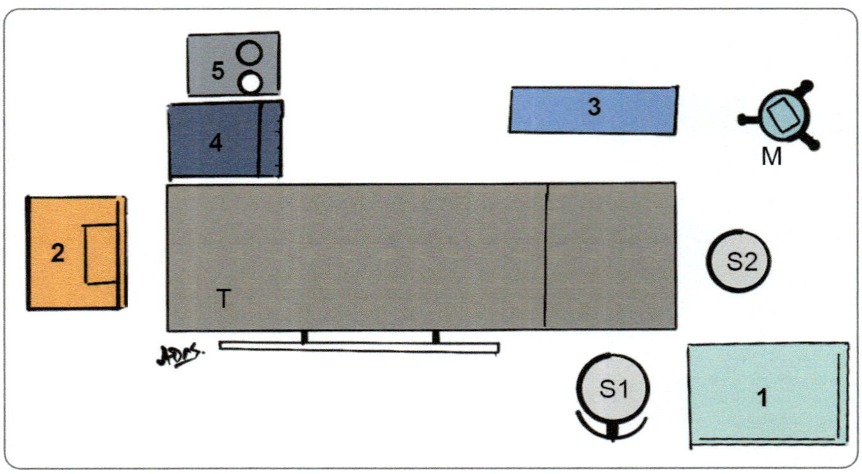

Fig. 15B: Schematic diagram of OT room set-up for endoscopic ear surgery (EES): For left ear.
(1: instrument trolley; 2: anesthesia workstation; 3: camera and monitor; 4: diathermy; 5: suction machine; M: microscope; T: OT table; S1: surgeon; S2: assistant)

INSTRUMENT SETS

Bulk of the surgical steps are carried out with classic microscopic ear surgery instruments having straight or mildly curved shafts, but because EES necessitates working with the angled 30° or 45° endoscopes, instruments ought to be fashioned accordingly with single-bent or double-bent shafts or even significantly curved shafts. This facilitates reaching into the hidden recesses of the middle ear without the need for any extra drilling purely for the sake visualization and instrument handling. Of late, instruments incorporating suction into the shaft are in vogue, thereby facilitating dissection with a single hand while the surgeon's other hand is holding the endoscope.

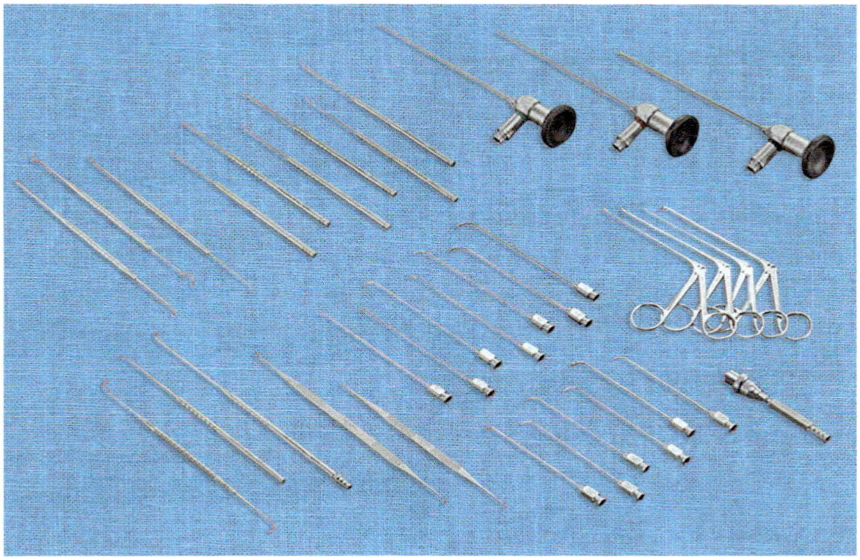

Fig. 16A: Storz endoscopic ear surgery instrument set.

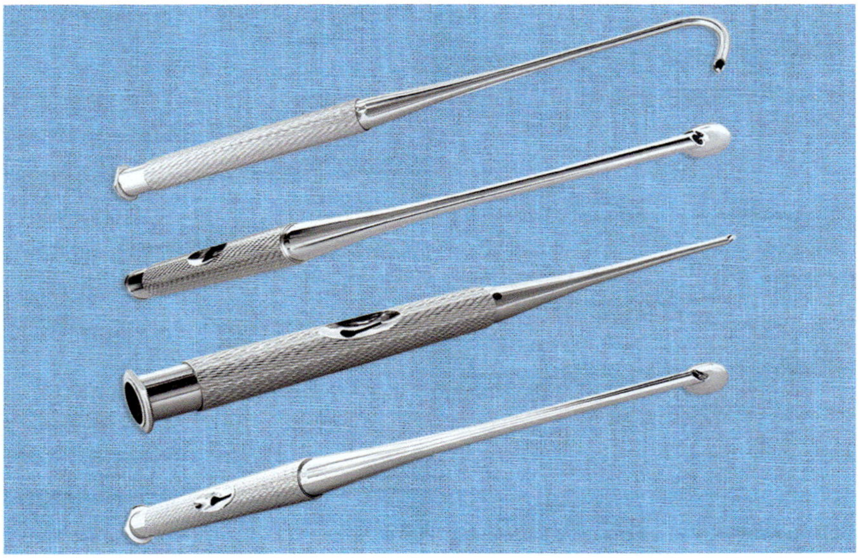

Fig. 16B: Panetti suction instruments set.

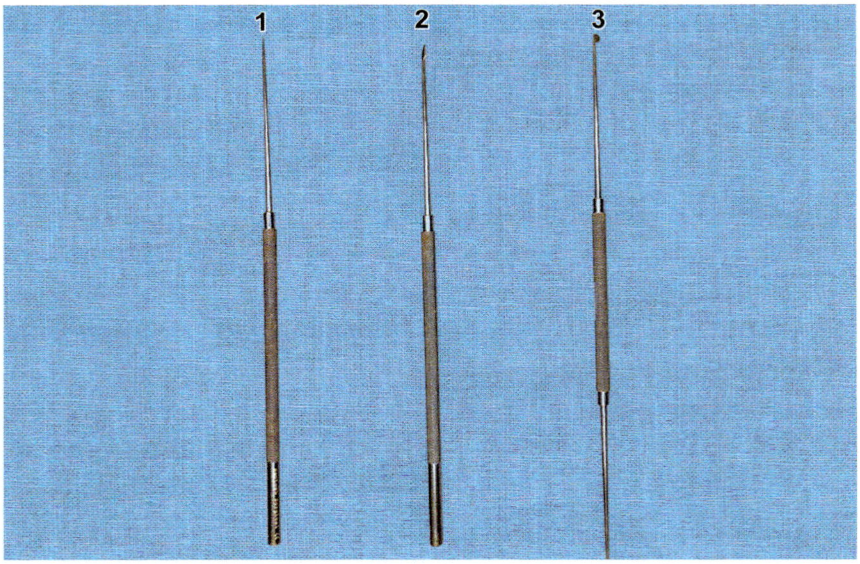

Fig. 17: Titanium instruments. 1: curved pick, 2: sickle, 3: double-ended round and side knife.

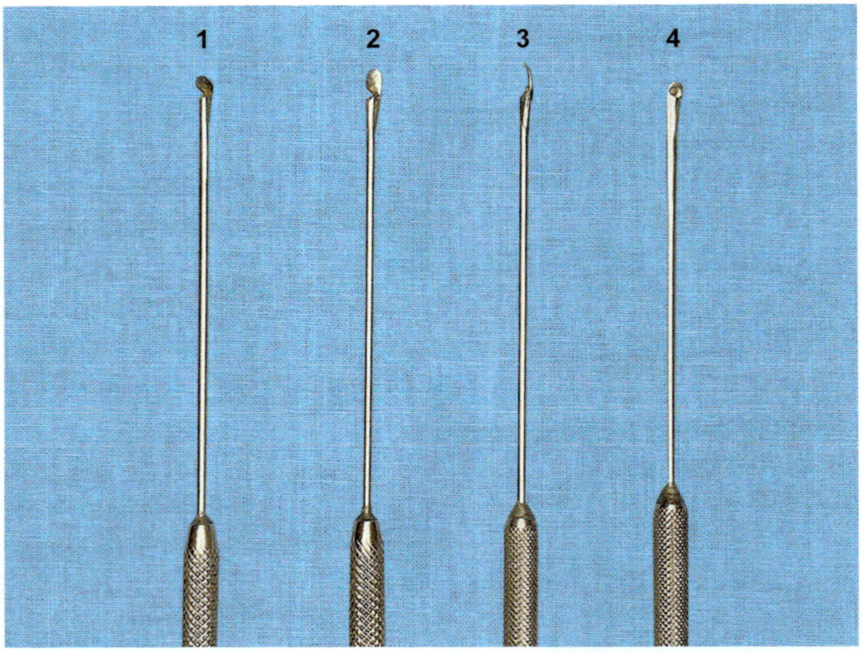

Fig. 18: Integrated suction instruments. 1: round knife, 2: side knife, 3: sickle knife, 4: middle ear dissector.

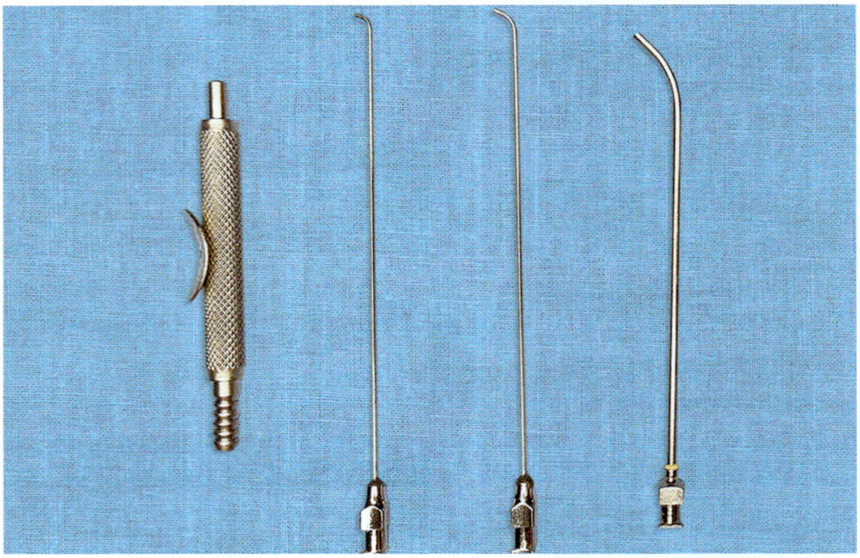

Fig. 19: Suction set with adapter.

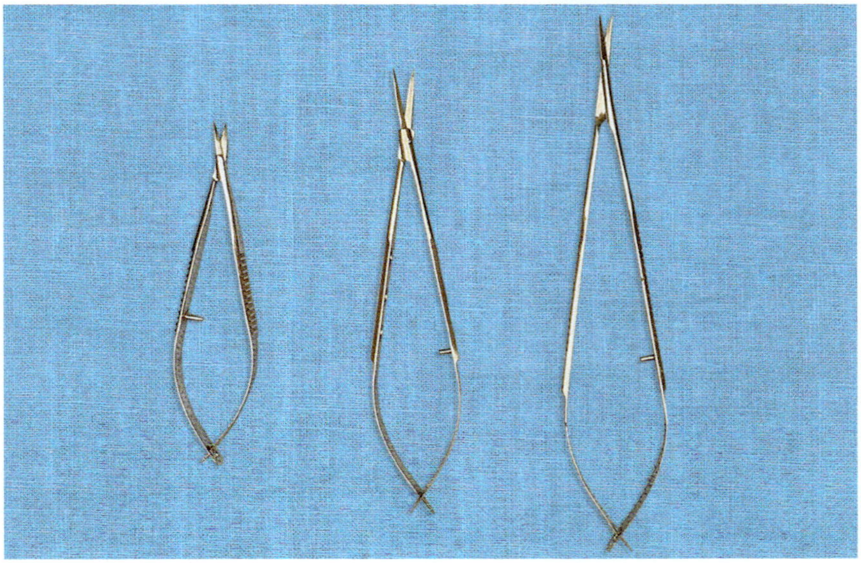

Fig. 20: Iris scissors of various sizes (curved).

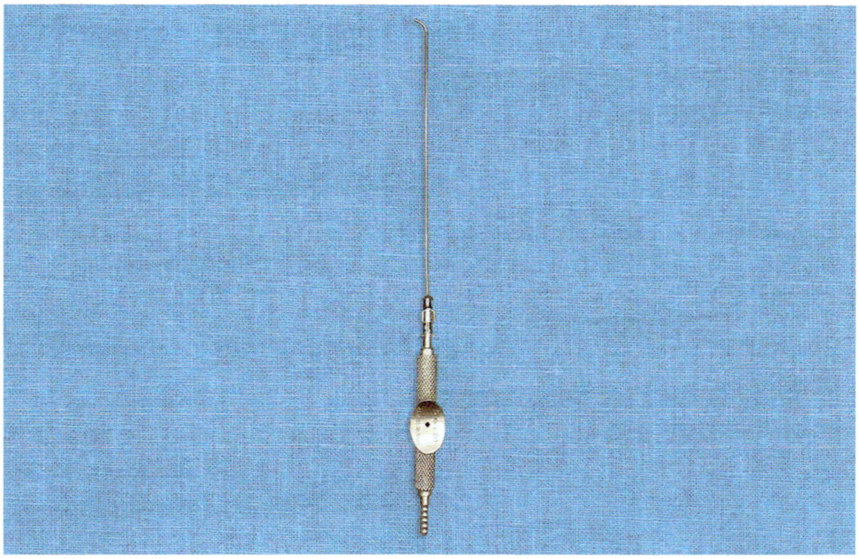

Fig. 21: Long curved suction cannula with adapter.

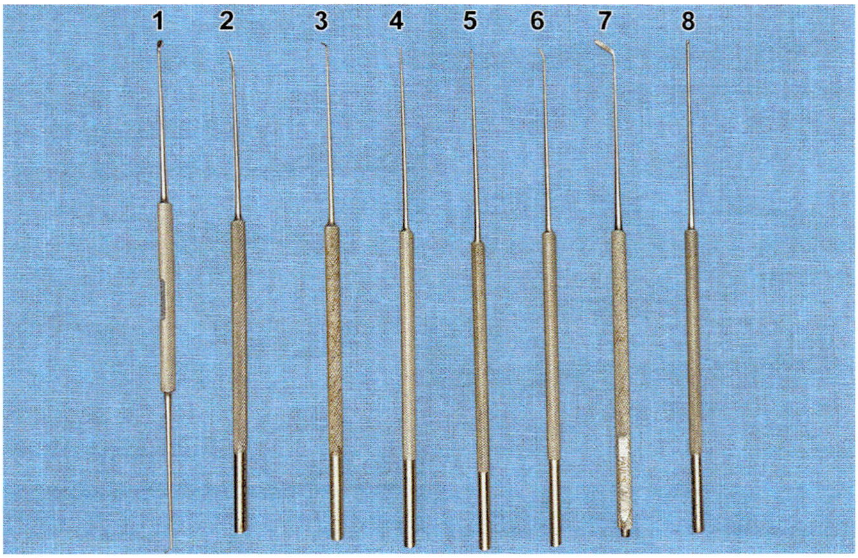

Fig. 22: Endoscopic ear surgery set.
1: double-ended round and side knife, 2: sickle knife, 3: ballpoint probe, 4: 90° pick, 5: 45° pick, 6: smooth curved pick, 7: middle ear gauge, 8: 0.9 mm trephine.

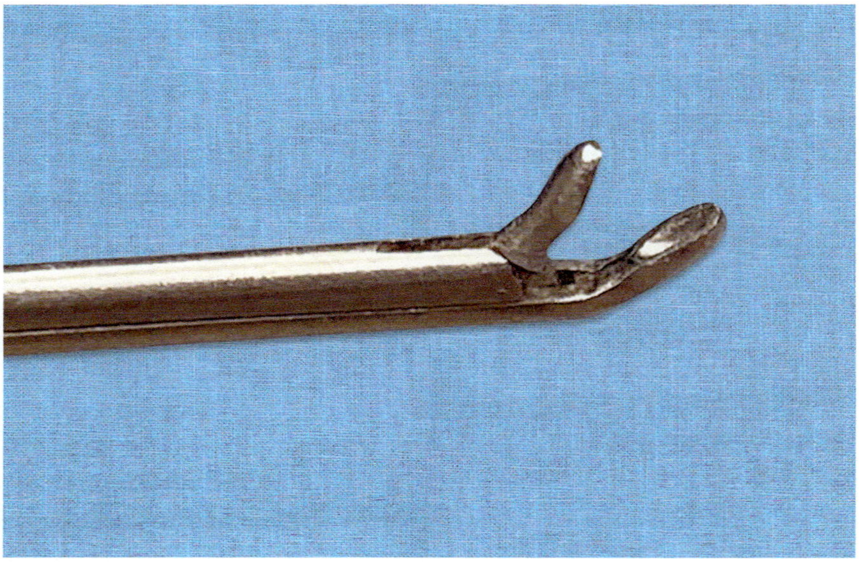

Fig. 23: Upturned micro-cup forceps.

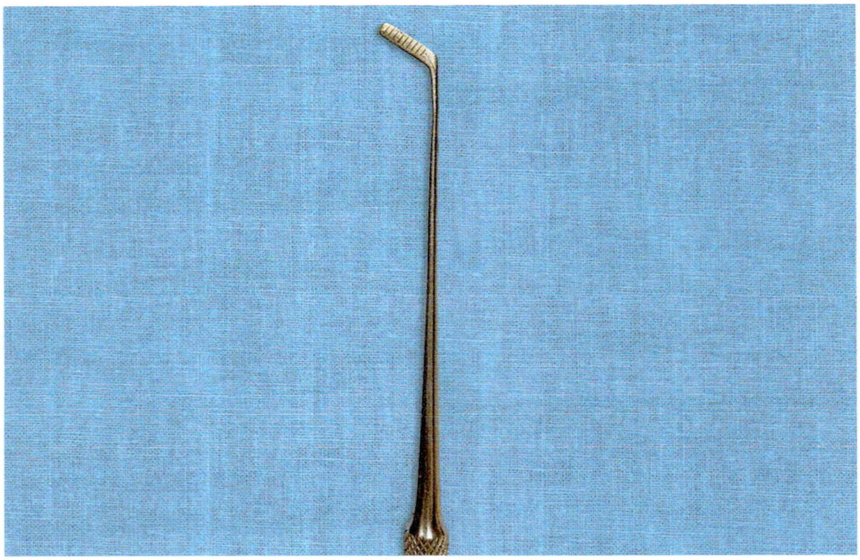

Fig. 24: Middle ear gauge.

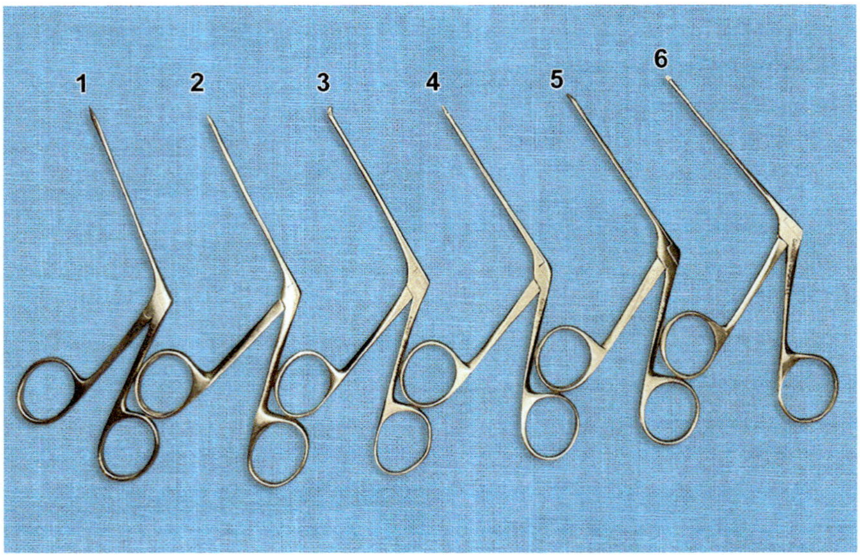

Fig. 25: Micro-forceps set.
1: micro scissors, 2: micro alligator forceps, 3: upturned micro-cup forceps, 4: left-turned micro alligator forceps, 5: right-turned micro alligator forceps, 6: malleus nipper.

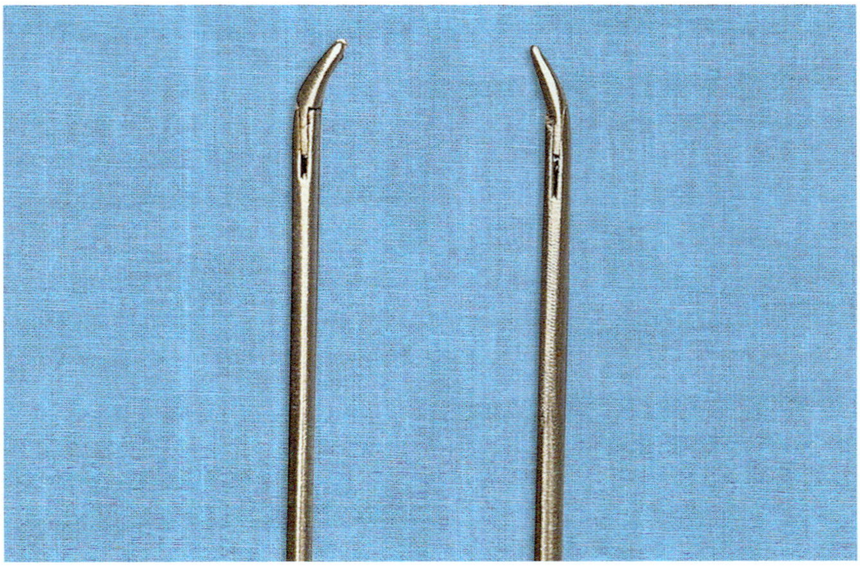

Fig. 26: Right and left-turned micro alligator forceps.

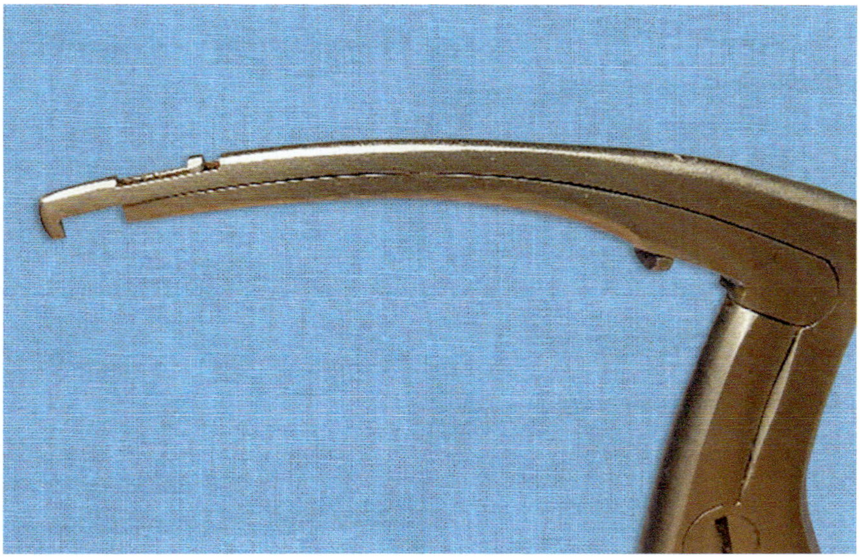

Fig. 27: Wilson's down-biting bone punch.

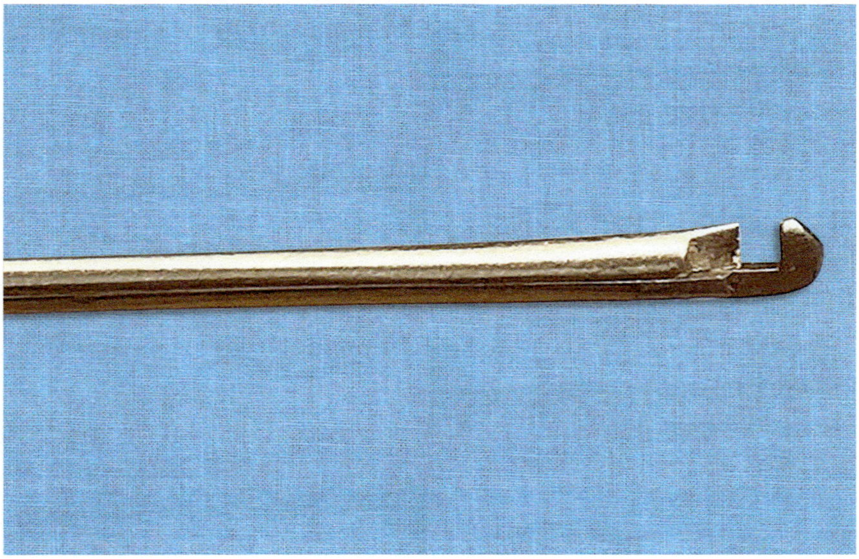

Fig. 28: Malleus nipper.

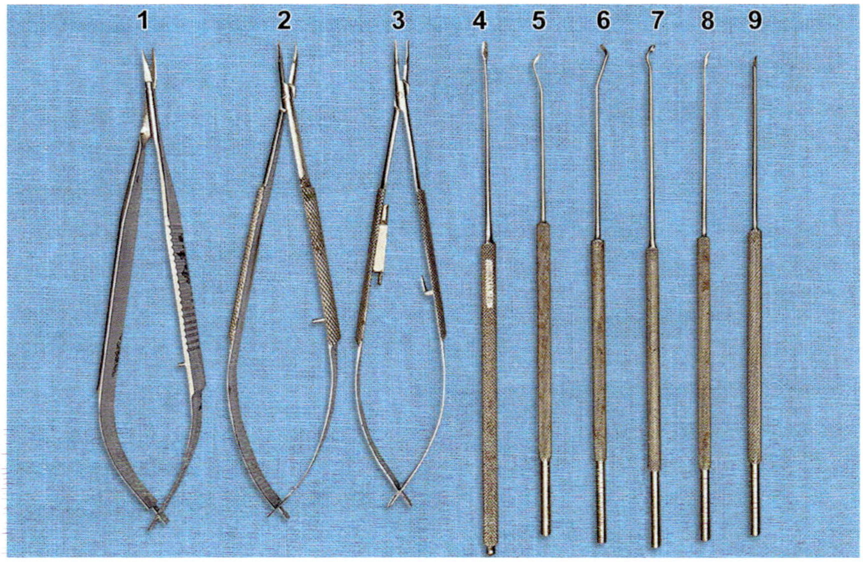

Fig. 29: Facial nerve decompression set. 1: iris scissors, 2: nerve holding forceps, 3: micro-needle holder, 4: Duckbill elevator, 5 and 6: double-curved Bill's elevator, 7: curette, 8: sickle knife, 9: tenotome.

Cartilage Slicer

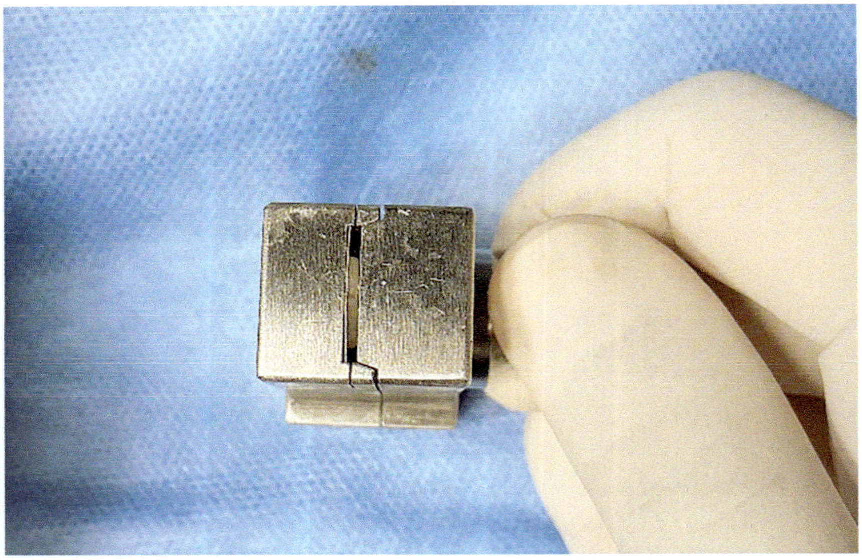

Fig. 30A: Use of cartilage slicer: Cartilage piece kept within recess of cutting block with thickness of 0.7 mm.

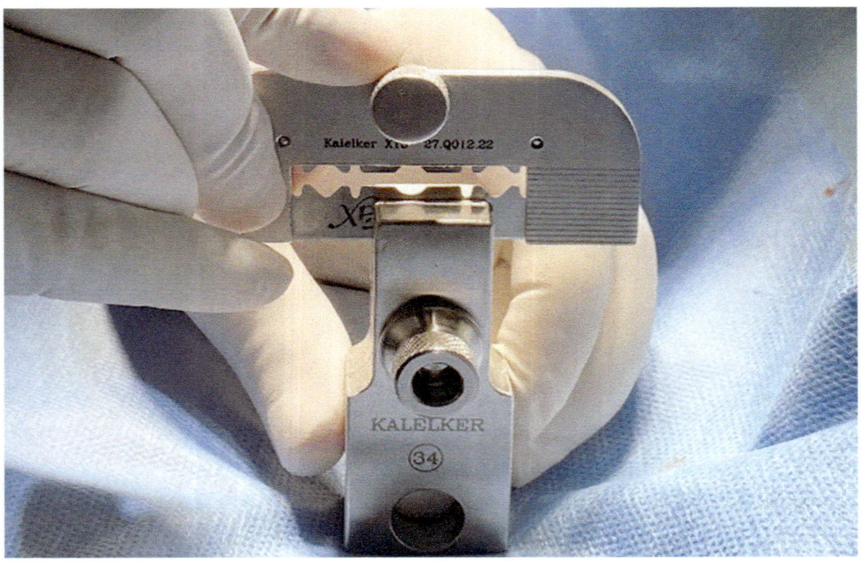

Fig. 30B: Use of cartilage slicer: With sawing movements blade is gently lowered onto the slot of the recess (front view).

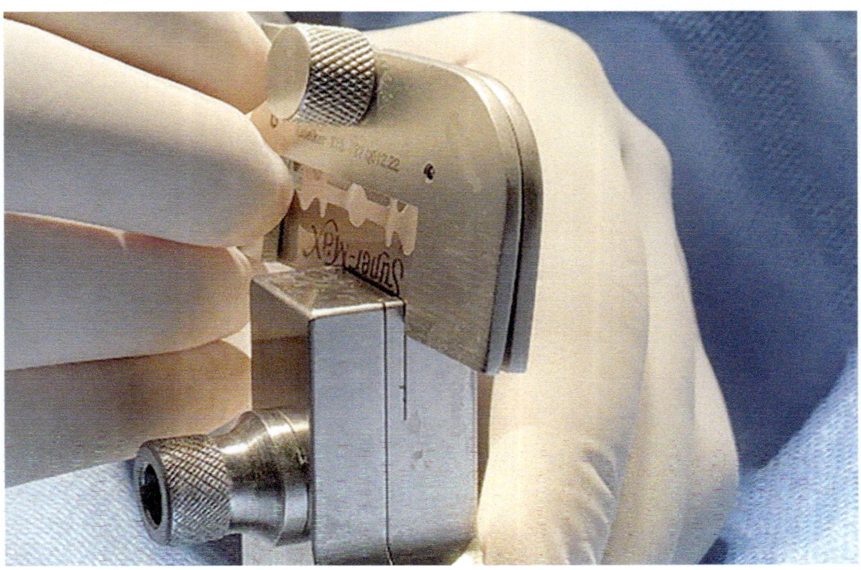

Fig. 30C: Use of cartilage slicer: With sawing movements blade is gently lowered onto the slot of the recess (side view).

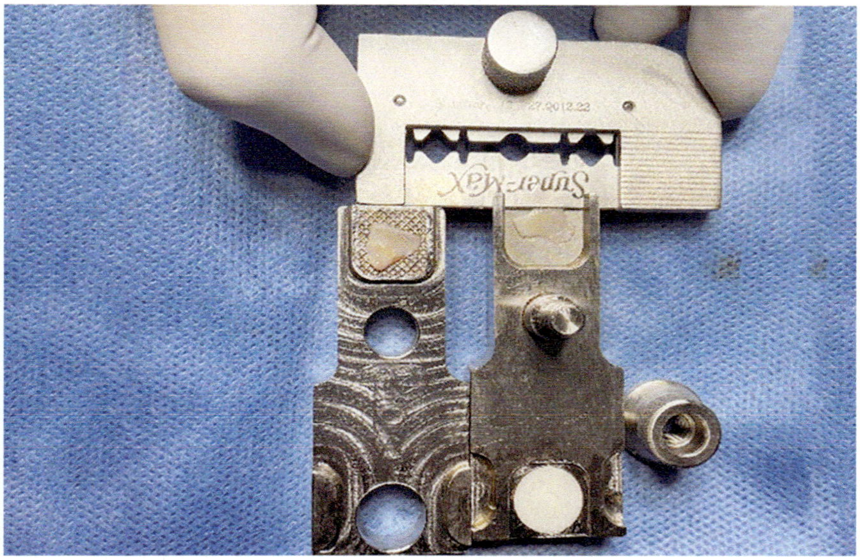

Fig. 30D: Use of cartilage slicer: Cutting block is opened by unscrewing, [thickness of desired cartilage is calculated as: (0.7 mm—thickness of metal plate used within the recess)], metal plates of 0.1, 0.2, and 0.3 mm are available for the same.

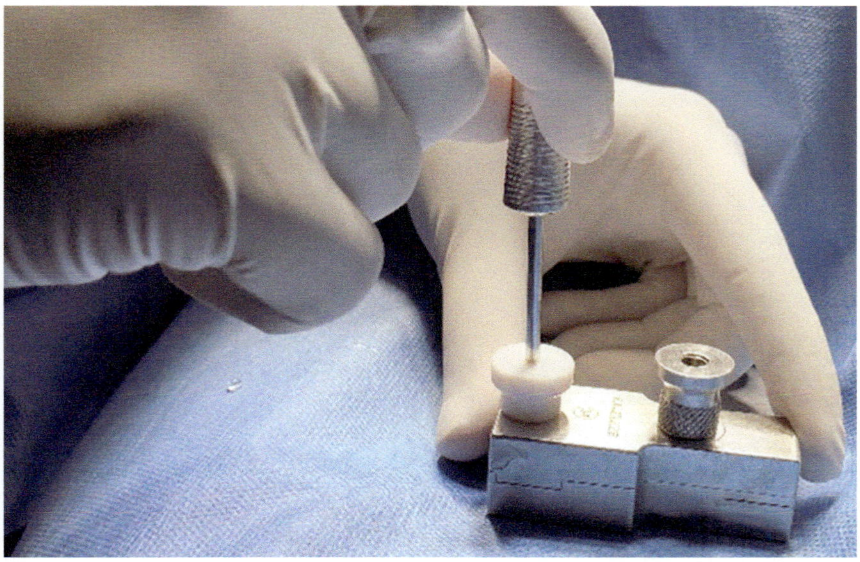

Fig. 30E: Use of cartilage slicer: Trephine being done for cartilage to be placed onto footplate area.

Microdrill and handpiece: High speed drill with foot control; brushless motor is advised. Straight and contra-angled handpiece is used as per requirement. Few otologic micromotor drills in vogue are:

- NSK system
- Medtronic Indigo drill system
- Storz unidrive
- Skeeter slow-speed drill by Medtronic

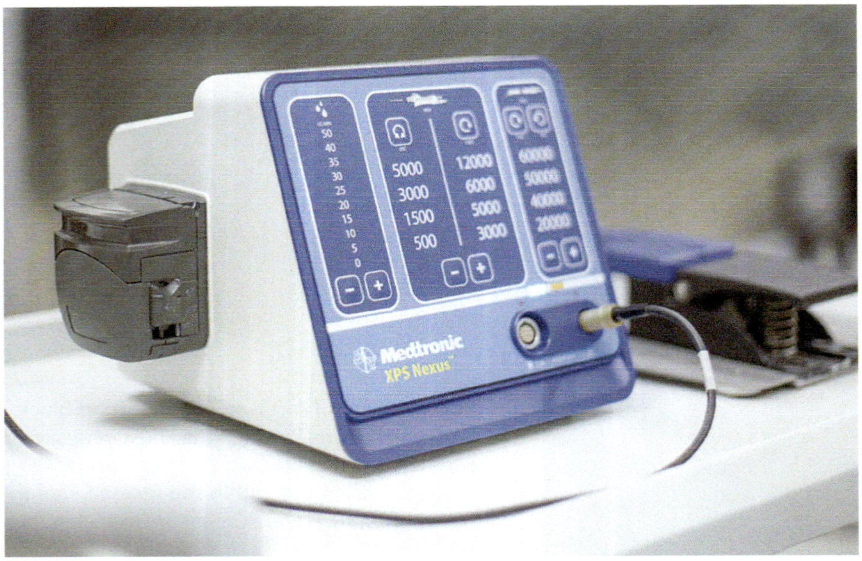

Fig. 31A: Medtronic Indigo drill system with console.

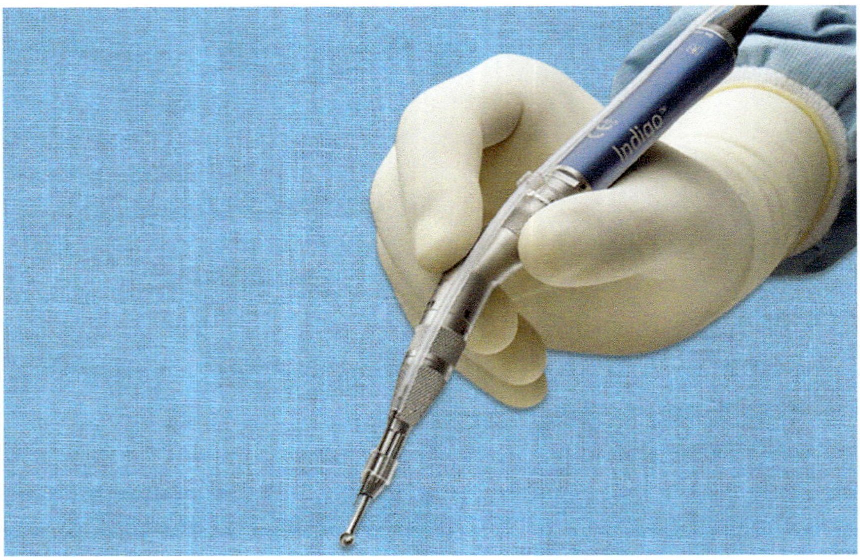

Fig. 31B: Medtronic Indigo drill with contra-angle handpiece.

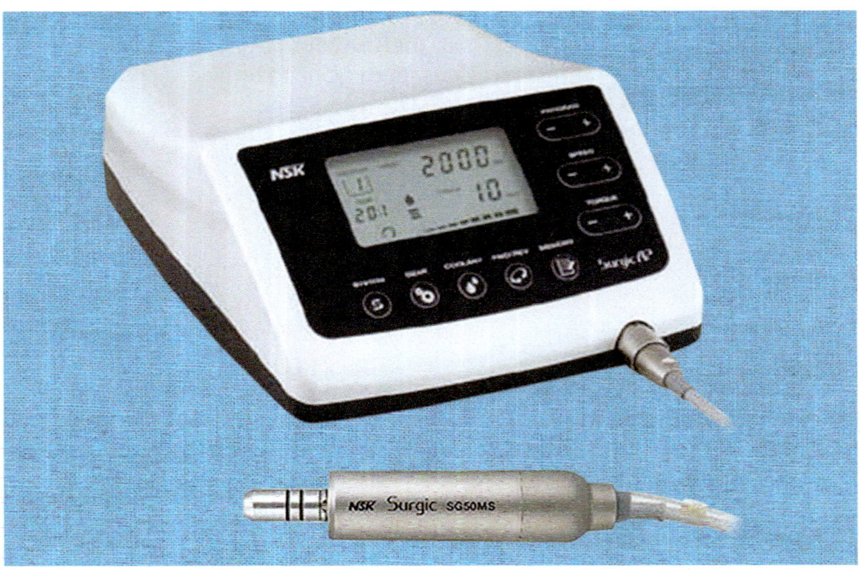

Fig. 32: NSK brushless motor.

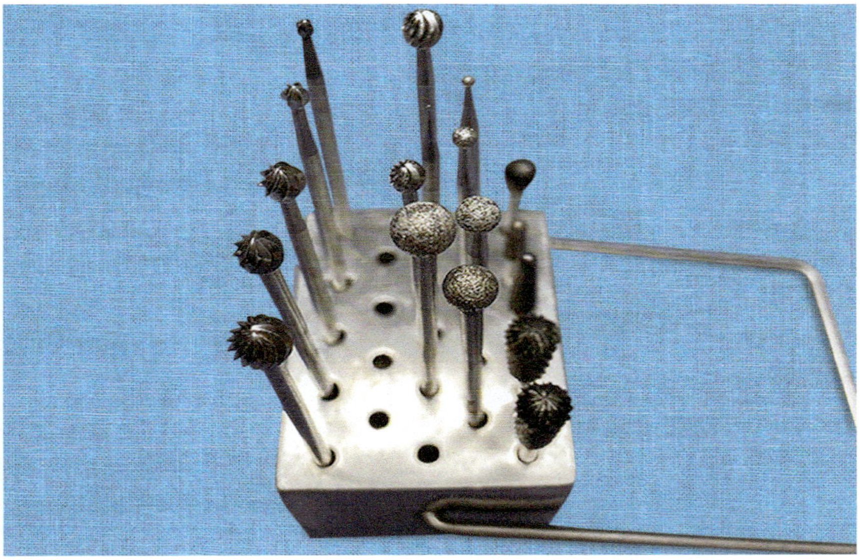

Fig. 33: Various burrs on holder.

- *Diathermy*: Valleylab^{TM} monopolar and bipolar diathermy is used for control of soft tissue bleed as in any otologic procedure. Specially designed insulated ball-point probe is used mostly during tympanomeatal flap elevation at low current setting.

PATIENT PREPARATION

Preoperative Medication

- *Antibiotics*: Third-generation cephalosporin (ceftriaxone) 1 g IV for adults and 30 mg/kg for children after proper skin sensitivity test is given 30–60 minutes prior to incision.
- *Analgesics*:
    - Injection pentazocine is given IM at 30 mg/mL—single dose 15–20 minutes prior to surgery, except for patients having coronary ischemia or history of myocardial infarction.
    - *Injection diazepam (10 mg/2 mL)*: 1 mL each IM and charged into IV fluid for slow infusion over 1 hour.
- *Antiemetics*: Injection ondansetron (2 mg/mL)—4 mg is given IV 1 hour prior to surgery to prevent postoperative nausea and vomiting.
- *Tranexamic acid injection and infusion*: Slow intravenous tranexamic acid bolus (10 mg/kg) half an hour before the start of surgery followed by infusion (5 mg/kg/hour). The infusion is prepared in normal saline.[2]

Anesthesia

Local anesthesia is preferred as far as possible using 2% xylocaine mixed with 1:2 lac to 1:40,000 adrenaline along with topical solution of 4% xylocaine and adrenaline as when needed. This has certain benefits like:

- Suitable for day-care surgery
- Better hemostasis
- Subjective assessment of hearing gain intraoperative
- Continuous assessment of facial nerve weakness, if any

General anesthesia is preserved for children and apprehensive adult patients. However, it is imperative to follow certain principles for better outcomes:

- Hypotensive anesthesia to reduce oozing and thus neater operative field
- Low mean arterial pressure of around 60–70 mm Hg
- Heart rate to be kept on the lower side to reduce cardiac output
- Premature reversal from anesthesia to be avoided

Shaving/ear preparation: Male patients are encouraged to cut their hair short prior to admission and females are asked to tie their hair neatly and place nonmetallic clips for the same. Hairs on the pinna and tragus are clipped. Patients are asked to apply shampoo on the day before surgery and prohibited from applying any oil on the hair/scalp. 1 inch of hair-bearing scalp behind the postauricular groove is shaved on the day of surgery with 7.5% povidone-iodine scrub. For myringotomy/grommet insertion and stapes surgery we do not advice hair shaving. Hair from the EAC is trimmed to prevent frequent soiling of the scope which is done during surgical procedure using curved iris scissor.

Skin preparation: Operative field is smeared with 70% isopropyl alcohol (surgical spirit), followed by 10% povidone-iodine in aqueous solution and again with surgical spirit. Field is allowed to dry before placing adhesive drape sheet.

Drape sheet: Three-layered standard draping is followed as in any otologic procedure.

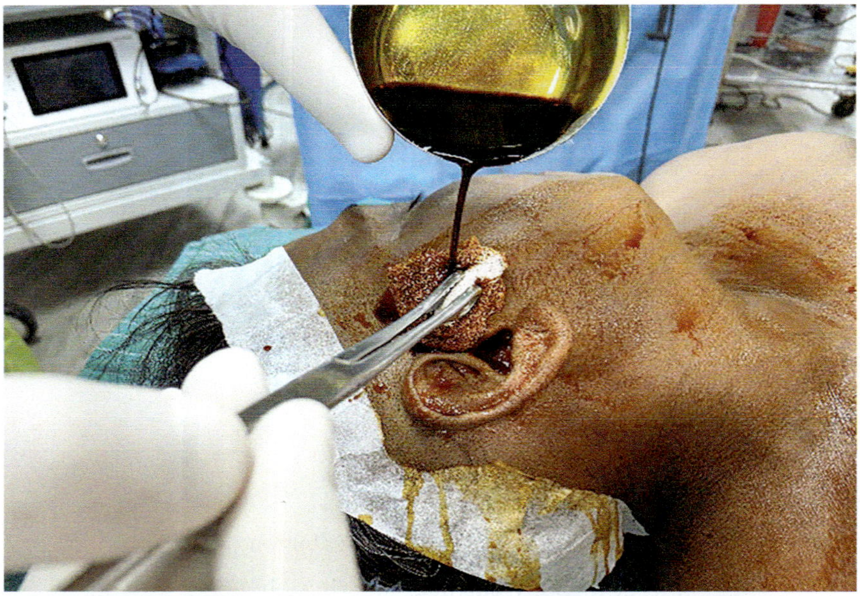

Fig. 34A: Scrubbing with povidone-iodine.

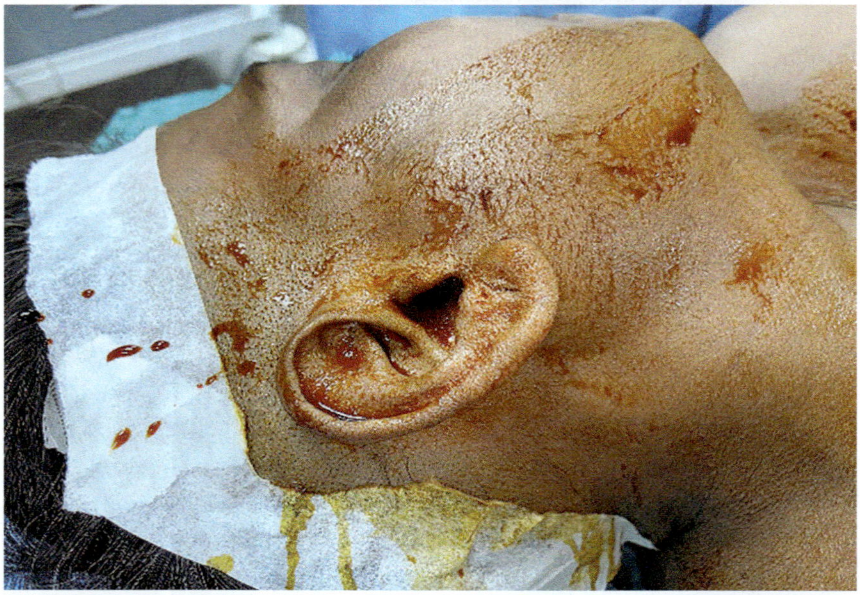

Fig. 34B: Scrubbing with povidone-iodine.

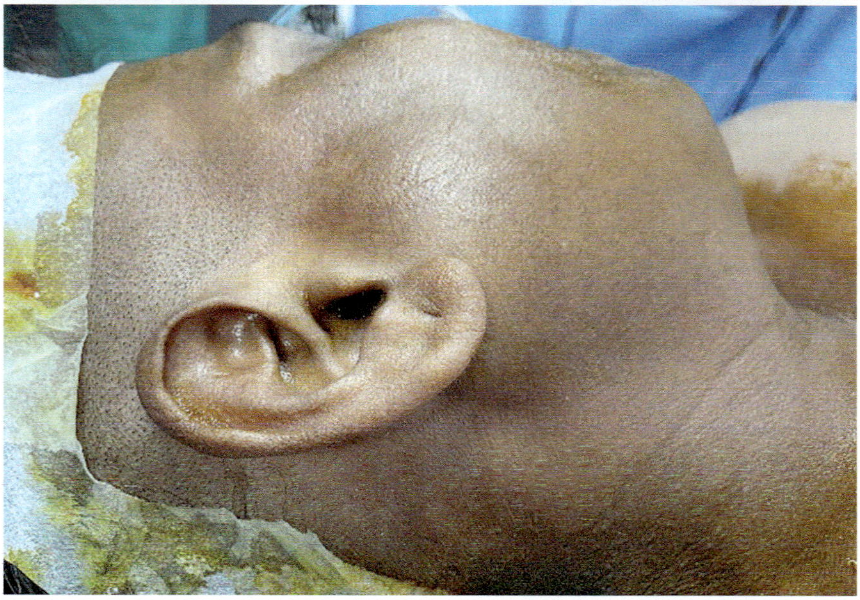

Fig. 34C: Surgical site dried prior to application of Steri-Drape sheet.

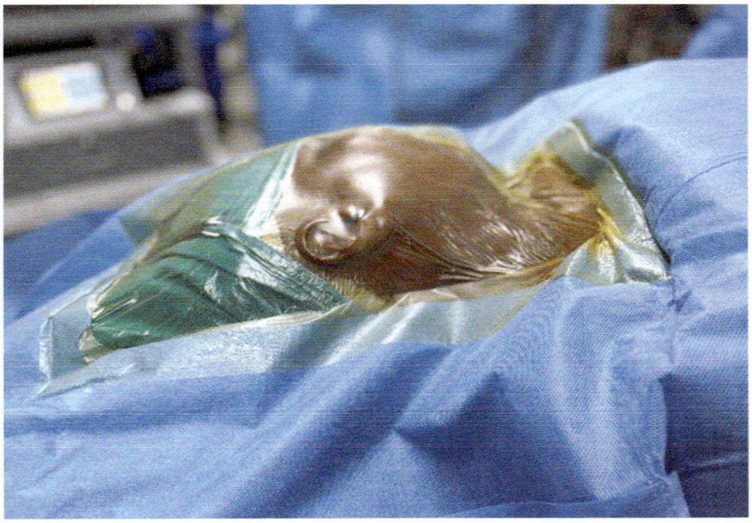

Fig. 34D: Draping of surgical site on right ear.

Stay suture: The cartilaginous and bony portions of the EAC need to be aligned to insert the endoscope. The cartilaginous portion of the EAC is often pushed posteriorly using the shaft of the endoscope. Certain techniques such as the stay suture can be used to straighten the EAC and increase the working space for the endoscope. 1-0 silk suture[3] is placed just lateral to bony-cartilaginous junction of EAC and fixed with the drape sheet to maintain traction on the conchal cartilage, thus aligning the EAC for easy insertion of the scope.

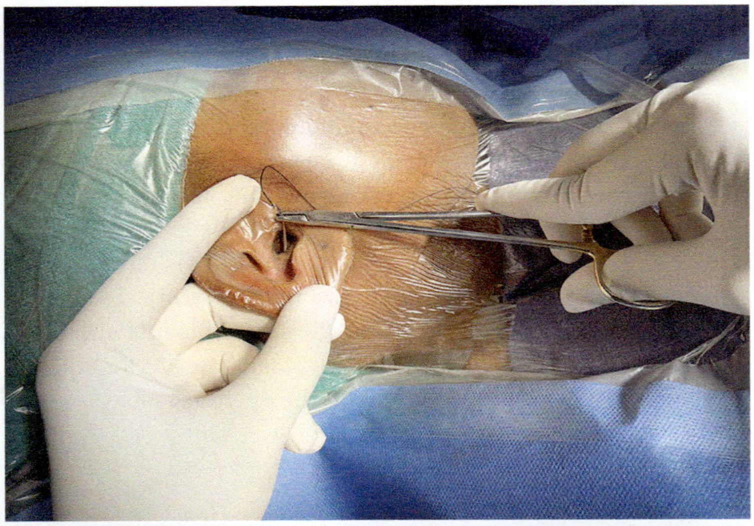

Fig. 35A: Stay suture being placed lateral to bony-cartilaginous junction.

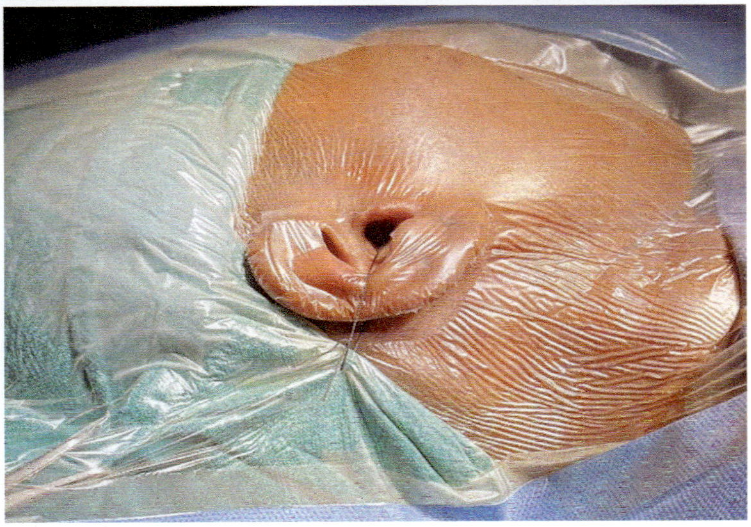

Fig. 35B: Stay suture fixed to drape sheet.

Antifog solution: Gauze pieces are taken in two metal bowls, one soaked in antifog solution like Savlon (chlorhexidine gluconate + cetrimide) and the other in normal saline to clean the tip of the scope. It is imperative to note that only adequate amount of the antifog solution is to be soaked, since excess solution at the tip of the scope will result in transfer of the same into the operative field and thus increases the chances of postoperative crusting. Whereas inadequately soaked gauze will lead to lesser antifog action and damage of the tip of the scope due to mechanical trauma.

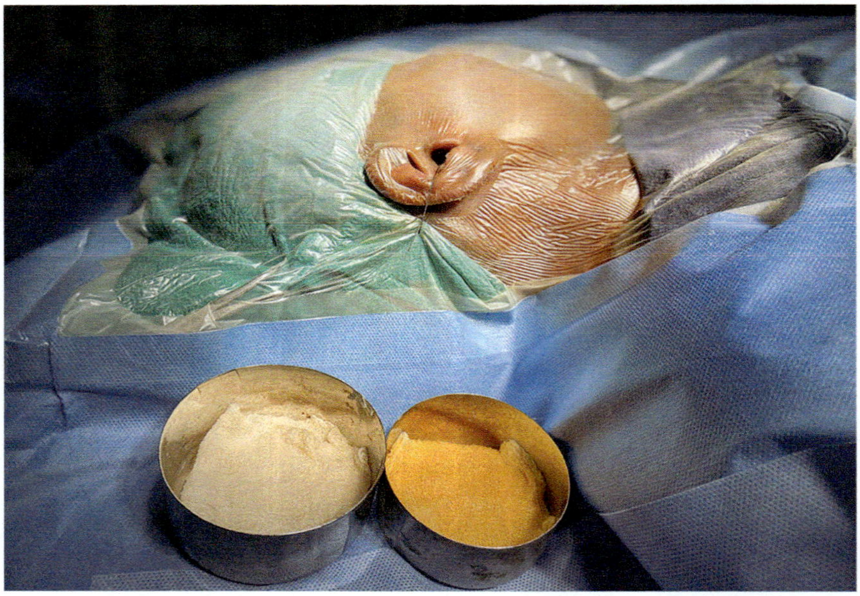

Fig. 35C: Gauze pieces soaked in antifog solution and normal saline kept in two separate metal bowls.

SURGEON AND PATIENT POSITION

Patient lies supine with head rotated to opposite side at angle 30° with the table and rested on a soft blanket for support.

Surgeon sits comfortably on a height-adjustable rotatable chair, with arm-rest preferably. One should avoid leaning onto the operating table and surgeon's back should be straight with a back-rest during the surgical procedure. The chair should have wheels to allow free movement. Most instruments are held like a pen. During fine manipulations, the surgeon's hand should be supported on the patient's head. This enables precise manipulations without tremors. It also lessens the tension on the arms and decreases fatigue.

In case arm rests are not available, for a right-hand dominant surgeon, during operative procedure on left ear, the nondominant (left) hand of the surgeon is to be placed on the operating table to stabilize the endoscope. Similarly, while operating on the right ear, the nondominant (left) hand of the surgeon is to be placed on a separate sterile trolley/ table of the same height as that of the operating table.

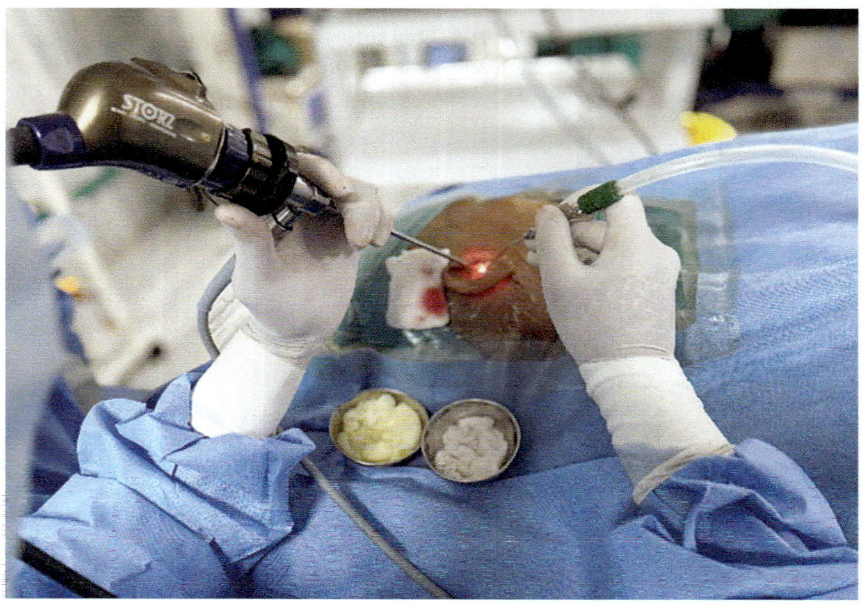

Fig. 36A: Right-handed surgeon holding endoscope on nondominant hand and both hands supported on operating table.

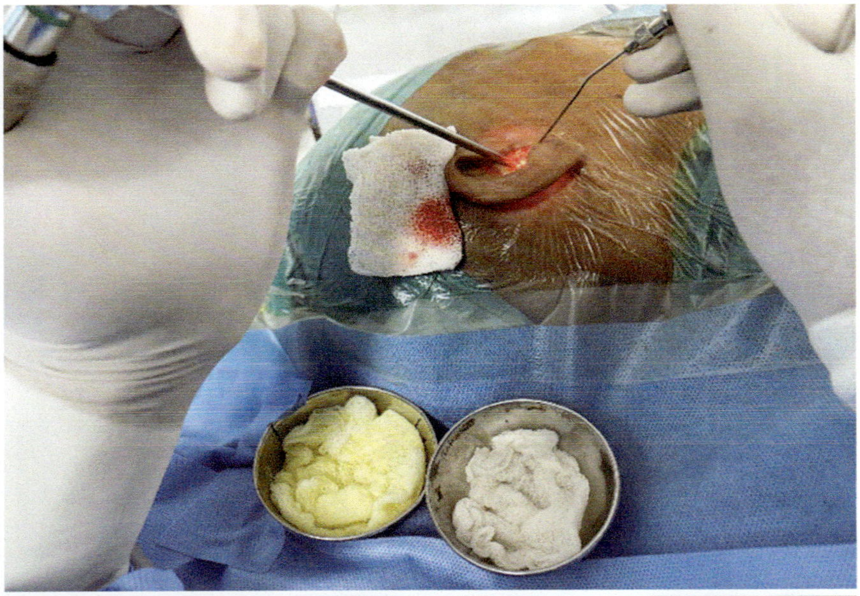

Fig. 36B: Relative hand positions. Endoscope parked on superior aspect of external auditory canal and suction cannula being introduced from inferior aspect.

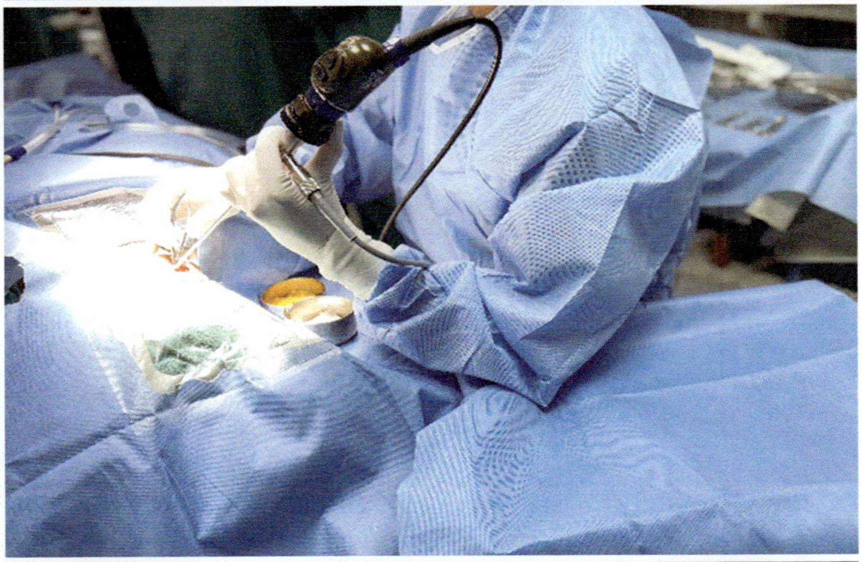

Fig. 36C: Nondominant endoscope holding hand can also be steadied by placing on separate side trolley (side view)

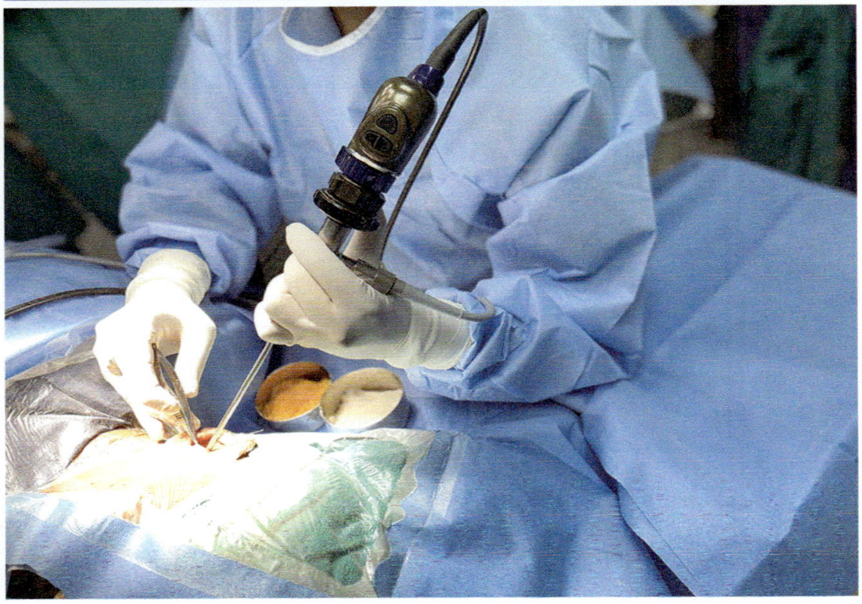

Fig. 36D: Nondominant endoscope holding hand being steadied by placing on separate side trolley (front view).

TABLE ARRANGEMENT

Stand Table Arrangement

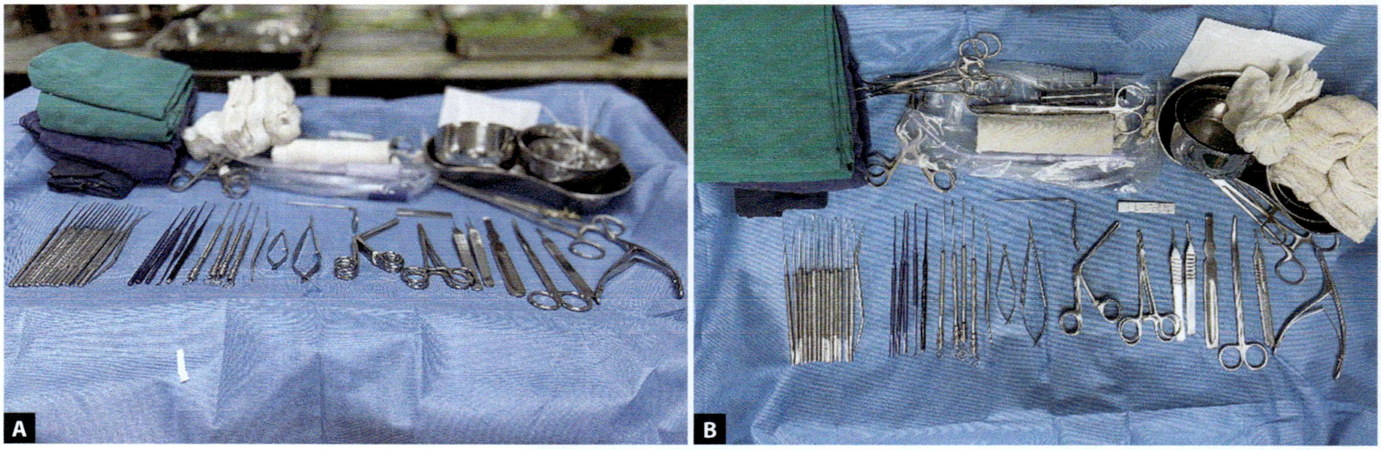

Figs. 37A and B: Stand table arrangement.

POSTOPERATIVE CARE

Standard mastoid bandage is applied for at least 24 hours and then changed to smaller dressing prior to discharge.

Third-generation cephalosporin or similar wide spectrum antibiotics, painkillers, and antiemetics are given in usual dosage to all patients in the postoperative period.

Certain special cases such as patients undergoing stapes surgery and facial nerve decompression are given intravenous steroids during hospital stay and oral steroids to be continued after discharge.

Vestibular sedatives are given to patients complaining of severe postoperative nausea/vomiting, like in stapes surgery.

REFERENCES

1. Das A, Mitra S, Agarwal P, Sengupta A. Prolonged intra-operative thermal exposure in endoscopic ear surgery: is it really safe? J Laryngol Otol. 2020;134(8):727-31.
2. Das A, Mitra S, Ghosh D, Kumar S, Sengupta A. Does tranexamic acid improve intra-operative visualisation in endoscopic ear surgery? A double-blind, randomised, controlled trial. J Laryngol Otol. 2019;133(12):1033-7.
3. Parab SR, Khan MM. Pinna stay suture in two handed endoscopic ear surgery: Our experience. Otolaryngology. 2020;41(5):102582.

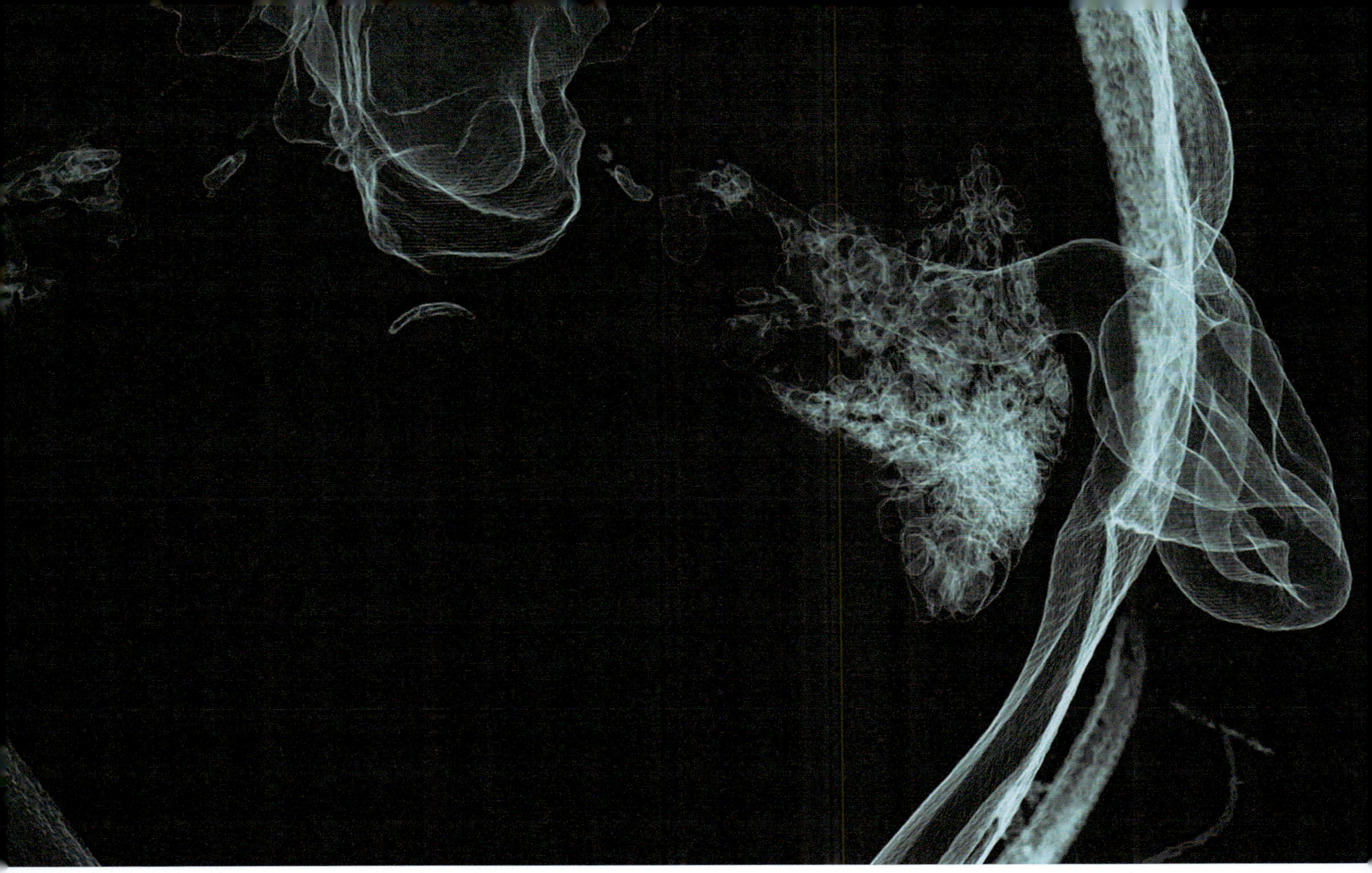

CHAPTER 5

Imaging for Endoscopic Ear Surgery

Arindam Das, Sayan Hazra

Chapter Outline

INTRODUCTION

Computed tomography (CT) and MRI provide information about anatomy of the region under study, localization of pathology (if any), its relation to adjacent structures, and expansive or infiltrative characteristics—factors that play important role in therapeutic decision making and planning of surgical intervention. Temporal bone has the maximum number of anatomical variations in the human body and thus it is important that the surgeon is well verse of the intricate details of it before any surgical procedure.

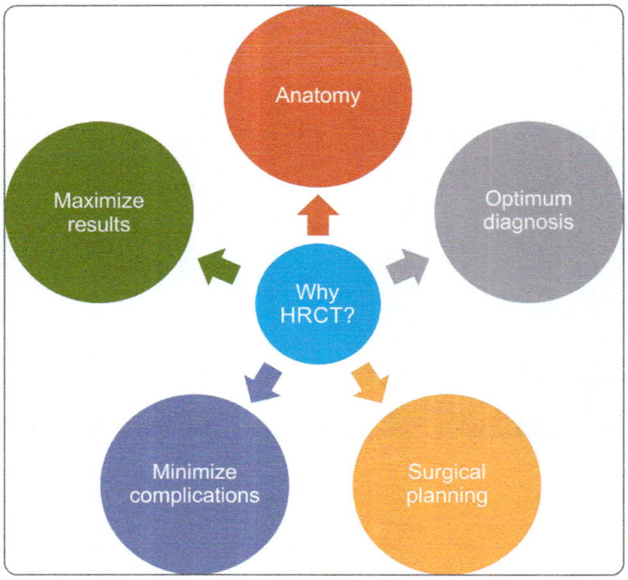

(HRCT: high-resolution computed tomography)

PREIMAGING PREPARATION: ITS ROLE AND IMPORTANCE

Before proceeding for any imaging study, one should do an endoscopic evaluation of the ear. This will give opportunity to the surgeon regarding:

- Assessment of anatomical contour and dimensions of the external auditory canal (EAC)
- Presence of any mass/lesion (like cerumen, debris, exostosis, canal cholesteatoma, fibrous dysplasia, etc.) in the EAC
- Presence of retraction of any part of the tympanic membrane
- Peek into the middle ear if there is any perforation.

ROLE OF PREOPERATIVE COMPUTED TOMOGRAPHY SCAN

Computed tomography scan is one of the basic tools nowadays for evaluation of the temporomastoid region. It is useful for:

- Evaluation of bony outlines
- Pneumatization and mineralization patterns
- Position and aspect of soft tissue like facial nerve, internal carotid artery (ICA), jugular bulb, etc.
- Status of ossicular chain.

Role of CT scan as a preoperative diagnostic tool is even more in case of endoscopic ear surgery (EES) than in any routine tympanomastoid surgery. The reason being, CT scan gives vital information regarding the dimensions and architecture of EAC which is imperative to know before taking up an endoscopic endeavor. A very narrow or tortuous canal will jeopardize the surgery. Similarly, cholesteatoma sac extending beyond the ampullary end of lateral semicircular canal (LSCC) is regarded as a relative contraindication for EES and better off dealt by microscopic approach. Though the realms of EES are increasing every day, still such cases are better taken up for endoscopic approach only in expert hands. Another such scenario is the mastoid pneumatization, where EES scores over microscope in contracted/less pneumatized temporal bones. Thus, CT scan not only provides the surgical road map but also raises the red flags for the surgeon.

A comprehensive list of evaluation points of structures to be noted while studying CT images is given below, from EES point of view:

Axial	*Coronal*	*Sagittal*
Semicircular canals with vestibular aqueduct	EAC	Dimensions and morphology of EAC
Mastoid pneumatization	Dural plate	Vertical portion of VII CN
Dural plate	Scutum	Epitympanum, mesotympanum, and hypotympanum together
EAC and IAC	Ossicles	Ossicular chain
Facial nerve (genu and tympanic segment)	Epitympanum	Tegmen integrity
Cog, AES, PES	Hypotympanum	
Cochlea with cochlear aqueduct	IAC with falciform crest	
RW niche and sinus tympani		
Ossicles with footplate area	Semicircular canals	
Skull base fracture	Facial nerve (genu, mastoid segment)	
E. tube	Cochlea	
Foramen spinosum	Skull base fracture	

(AES: anterior ectosylvian sulcus; CN: cranial nerve; EAC: external auditory canal; E. tube: Eustachian tube; IAC: internal auditory canal; PES: posterior ectosylvian sulcus; RW: round window)

HOW TO READ THE COMPUTED TOMOGRAPHY SCAN?

There are some basic rules to be followed before one indulges into studying the various cuts of the CT scan.

- Read from CT console, not from limited number of plates. Technology has opened the gates for the surgeon to go through every detail of the temporal bone using softwares available, either free of cost or at minimal expenditures, such as RadiAnt™, Horos™, Osirix™, etc.
- Identification of landmarks rather than disease process and its extent. It is almost impossible to diagnose any disease process based on the CT scan alone. Clinical findings, audiological evaluation, and multimodality imaging need to be done to reach any conclusion.
- Identification of fixed normal patterns such "stack of coin" appearance of cochlea, "ice cream cone", and "molar tooth" appearance of ossicles, and "adder head" and "bucket handle" appearance of superior semicircular canal (SCC). Only then, one can identify the abnormalities associated with such structures.
- On a given cut, focus on one landmark at a time and study its relation to neighboring fixed landmark. This gives the opportunity to systematically review that particular cut instead of searching haphazardly for structures.

Speaking of the same, it is advisable to study the various cuts of the CT scan in a systematic manner described below and form a mental outline for the surgical approach.

Conventional Cuts

Axial Cuts (Above Downward)

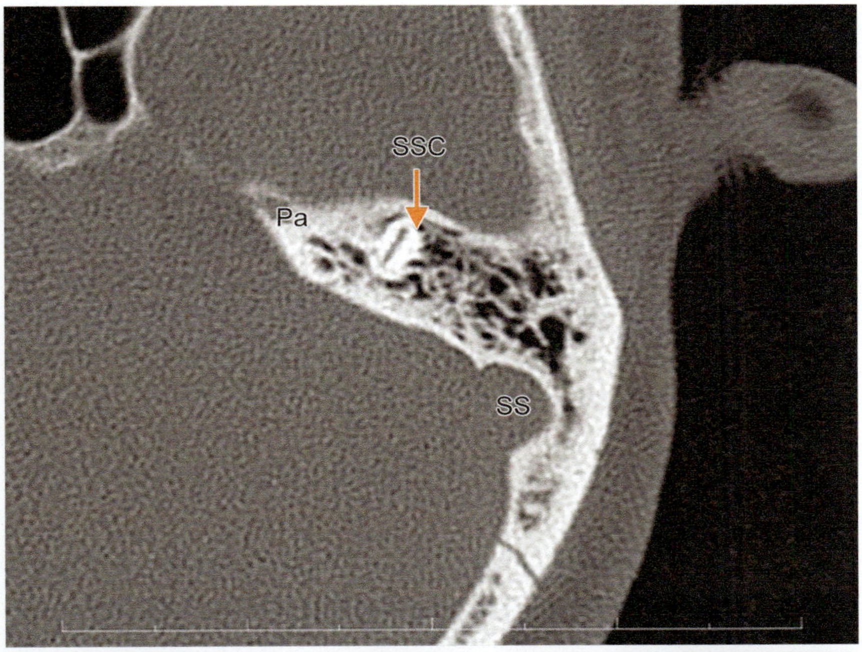

Fig. 1: At the level of SSC.
(Pa: petrous apex; SSC: superior semicircular canal; SS: sigmoid sinus)

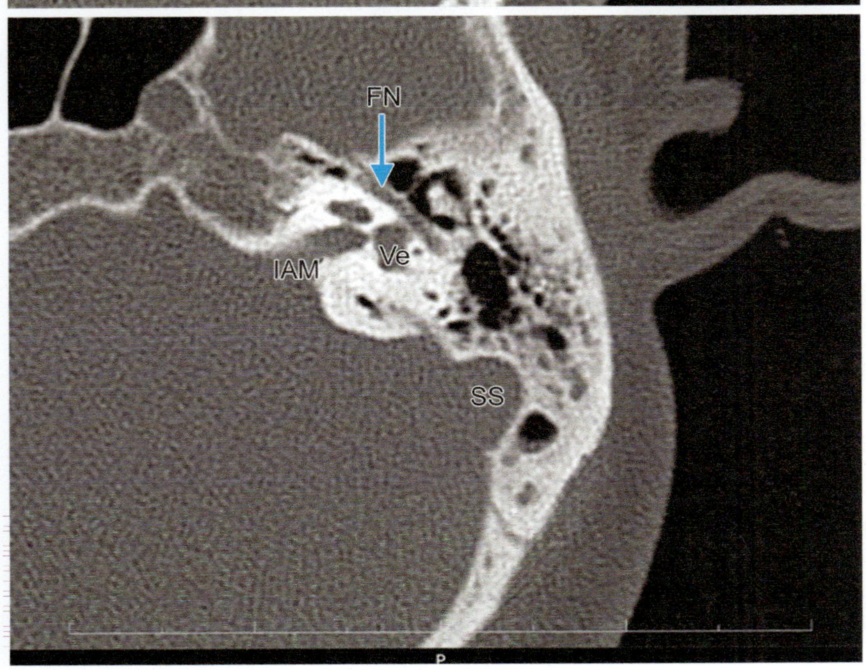

Fig. 2: Facial nerve tympanic segment.
(FN: facial nerve; IAM: internal acoustic meatus; SS: sigmoid sinus; Ve: vestibule)

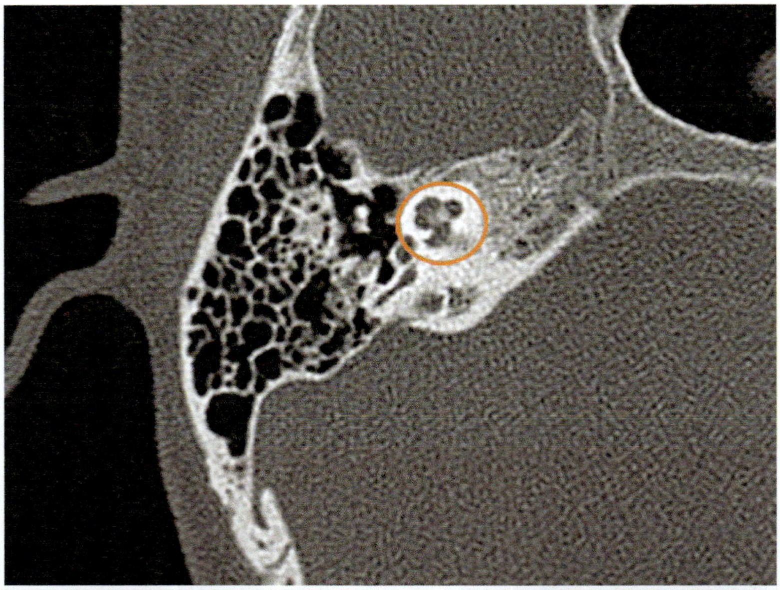

Fig. 3: Cochlea (mid-modiolus view). Clover-leaf shaped.

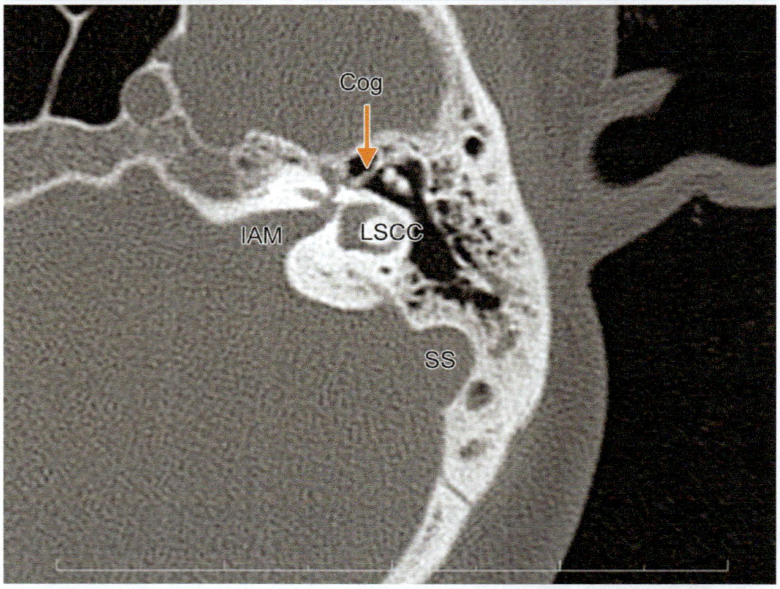

Fig. 4: Epitympanic space (Cog—orange arrow). (IAM: internal acoustic meatus; LSCC: lateral semicircular canal; SS: sigmoid sinus)

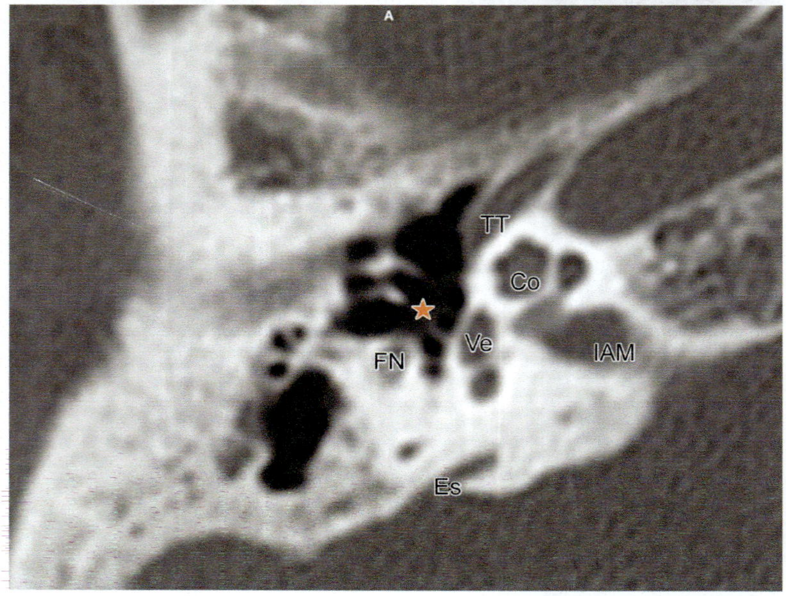

Fig. 5: Stapes (orange asterisk). (Co: cochlea, Es: endolymphatic sac; FN: facial nerve; IAM: internal acoustic meatus; TT: Tensor tympani muscle; Ve: vestibule)

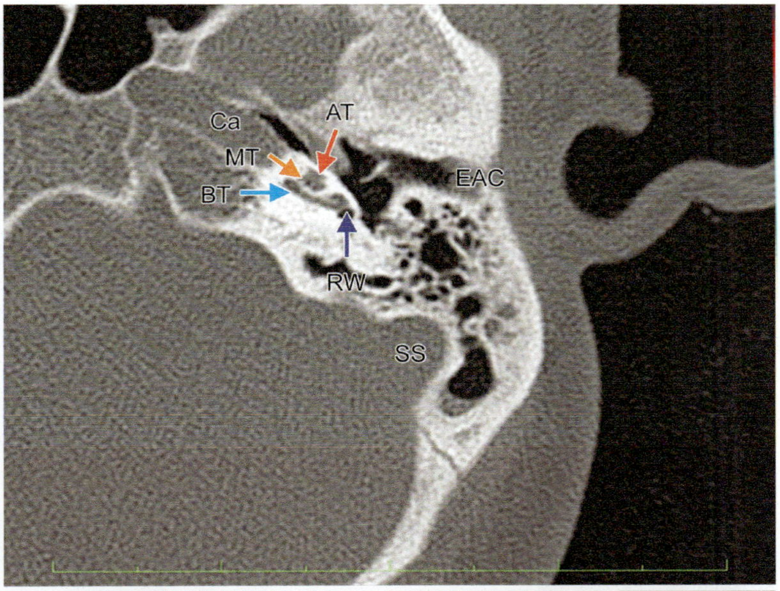

Fig. 6: Basal turn of cochlea (stack of coins appearance). (AT: apical turn, BT: basal turn; Ca: carotid artery; EAC: external auditory canal; MT: middle turn; RW: round window; SS: sigmoid sinus)

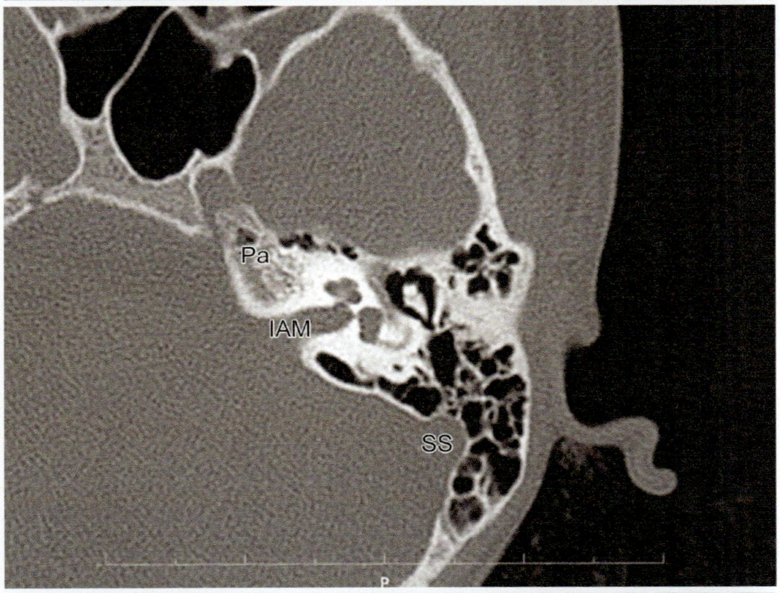

Fig. 7A: Ossicles: Ice cream cone appearance (head of malleus being the ball and body of incus being the cone of the ice cream).

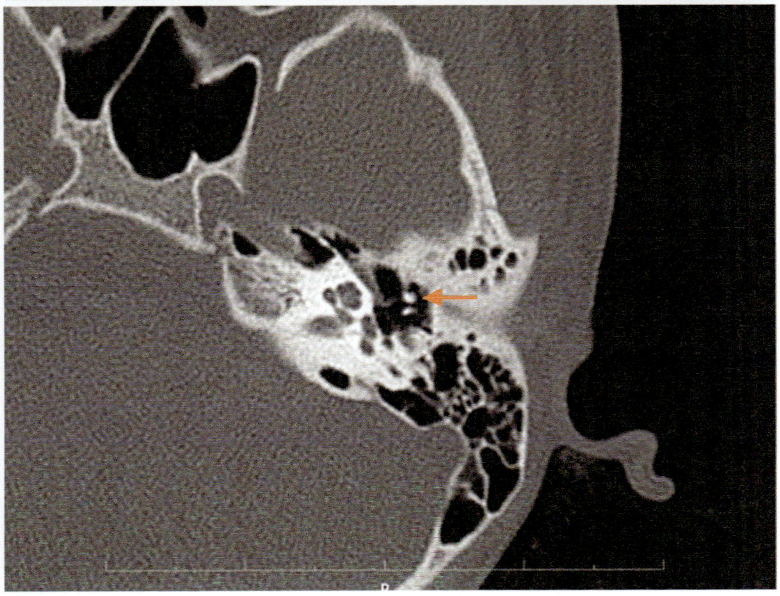

Fig. 7B: Ossicles: Double dot appearance—neck of malleus (lateral dot) and long process of incus (medial dot).

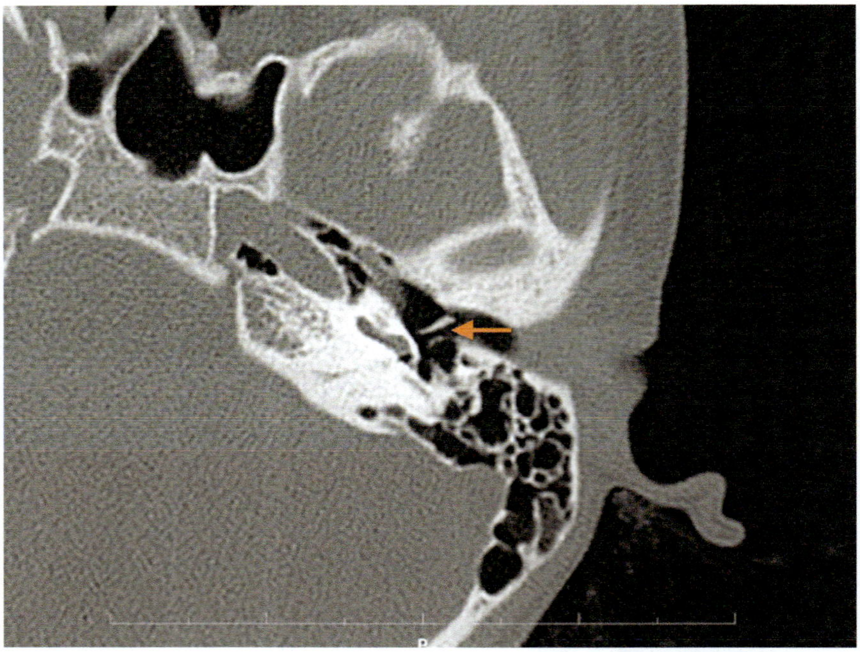

Fig. 7C: Ossicles: Double line appearance.

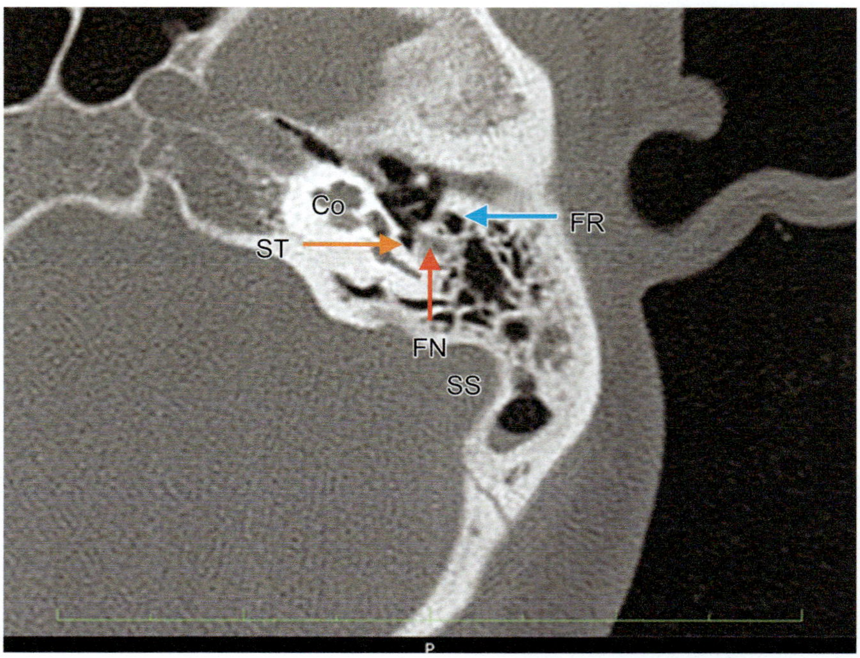

Fig. 8: Sinus tympani (ST): orange arrow and facial recess (FR): blue arrow.

Coronal Cuts (Anteroposterior)

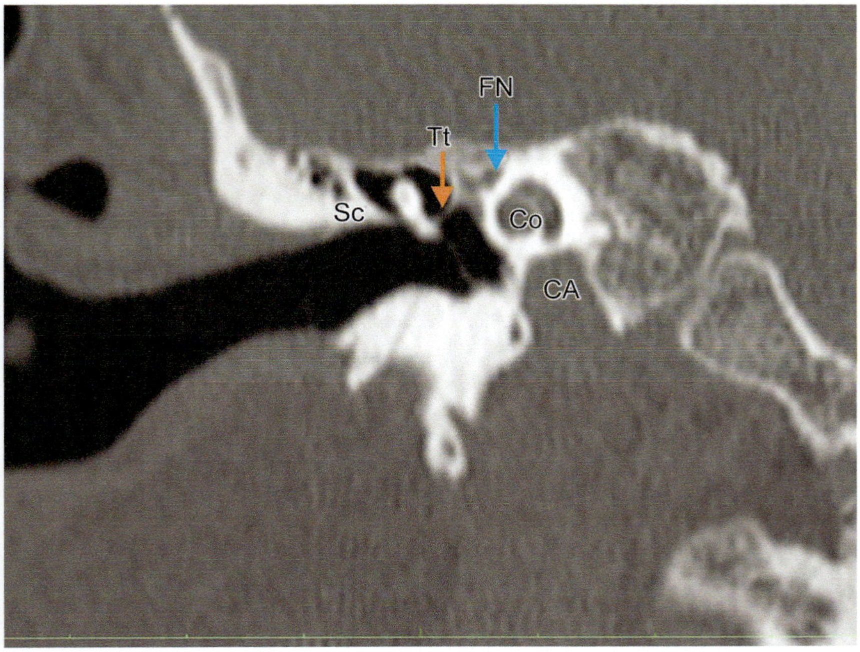

Fig. 9: Coronal cut at scutum.
(CA: carotid artery; Co: cochlea; FN: facial nerve; Sc: scutum; Tt: tensor tympani muscle)

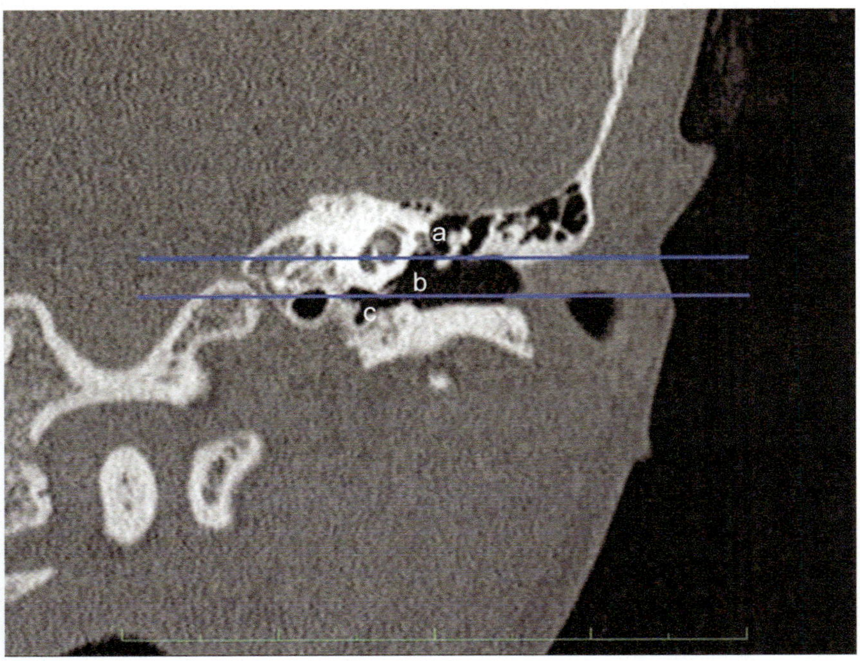

Fig. 10: Division of middle ear space.
(a) Epitympanum, (b) Mesotympanum, and
(c) Hypotympanum.

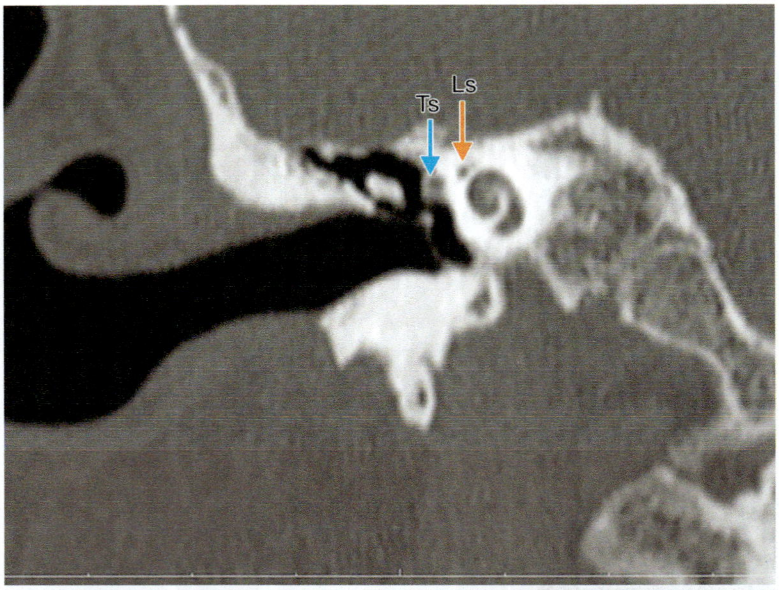

Fig. 11: Facial nerve—Ls: labyrinthine and Ts: tympanic segments.

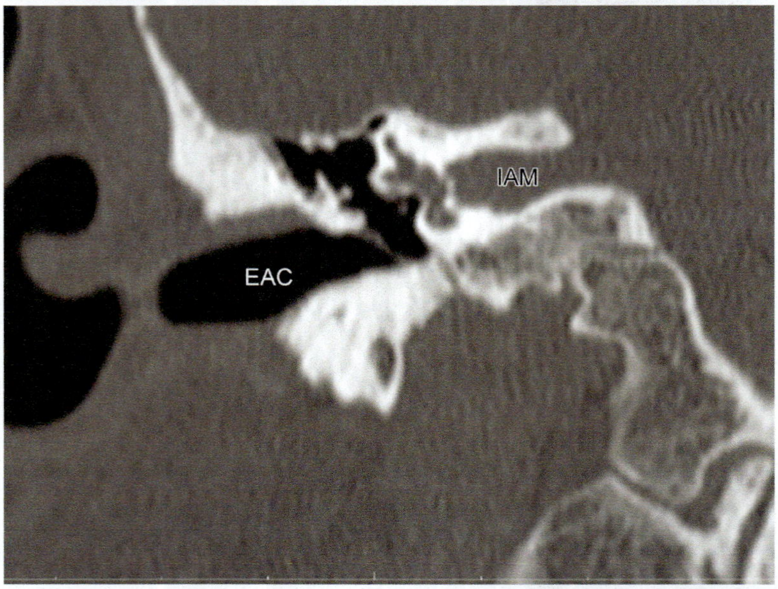

Fig. 12: Vestibule with SSC.
(EAC: external auditory canal; IAM: internal acoustic meatus; SSC: superior semicircular canal)

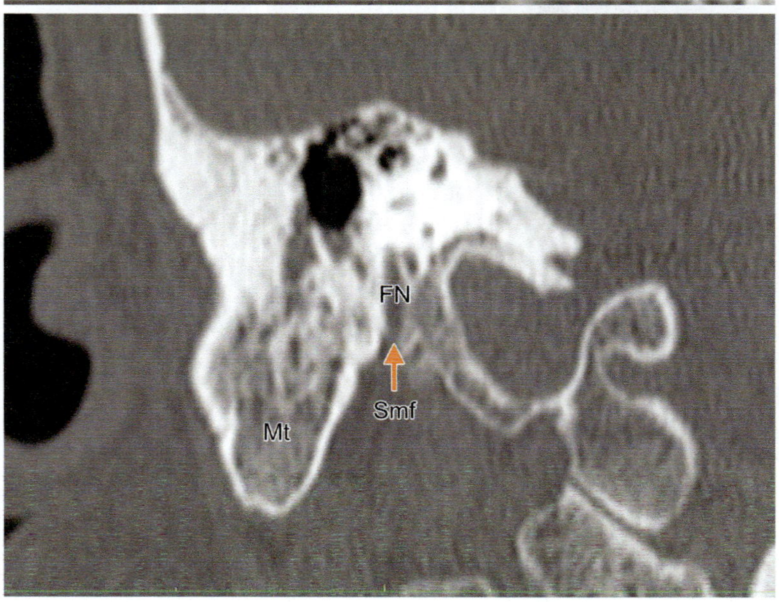

Fig. 13: Mastoid segment of facial nerve (FN).
(Mt: medial tip cell area; Smf: stylomastoid foramen)

Sagittal Cuts (Lateral to Medial)

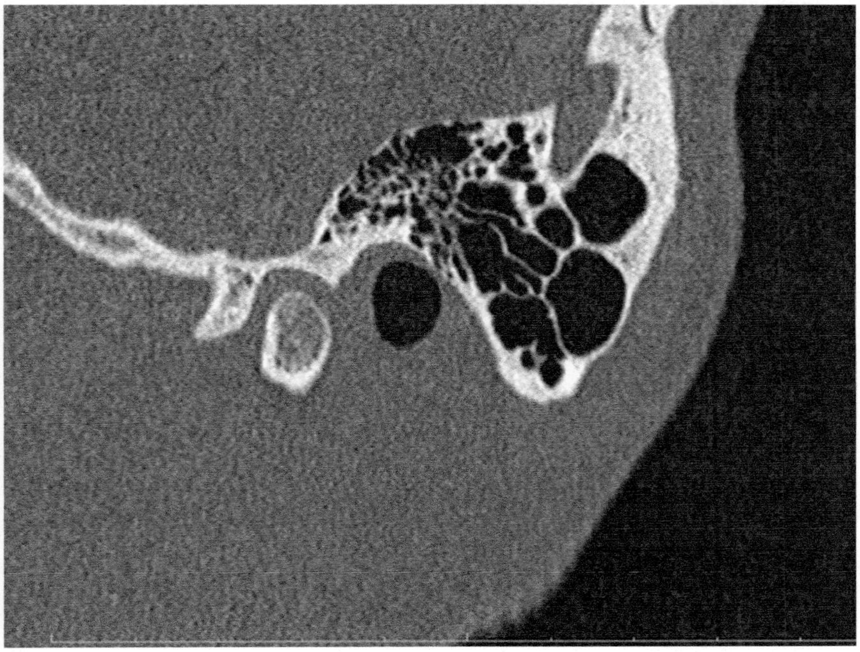

Fig. 14: Mastoid pneumatization.

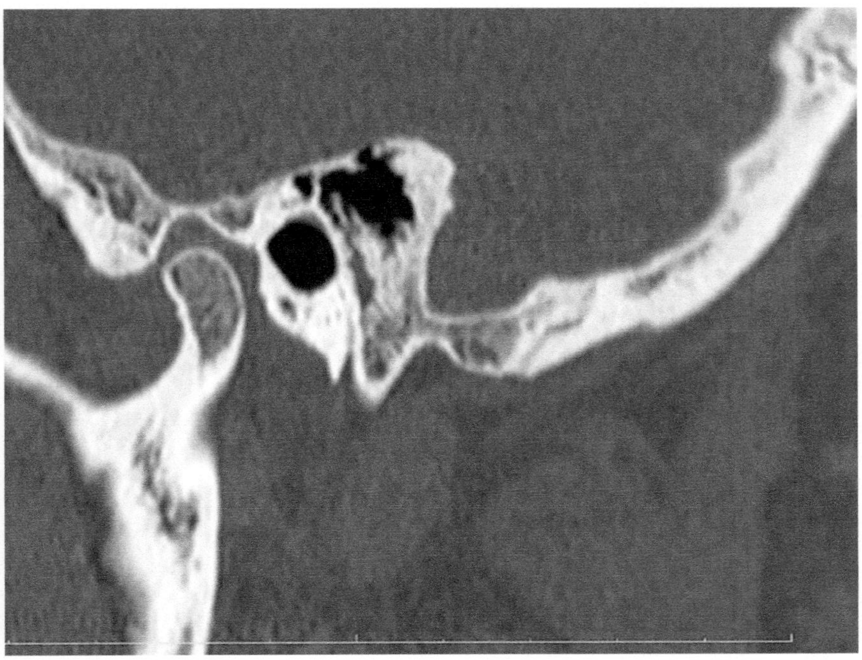

Fig. 15: External auditory canal dimensions.

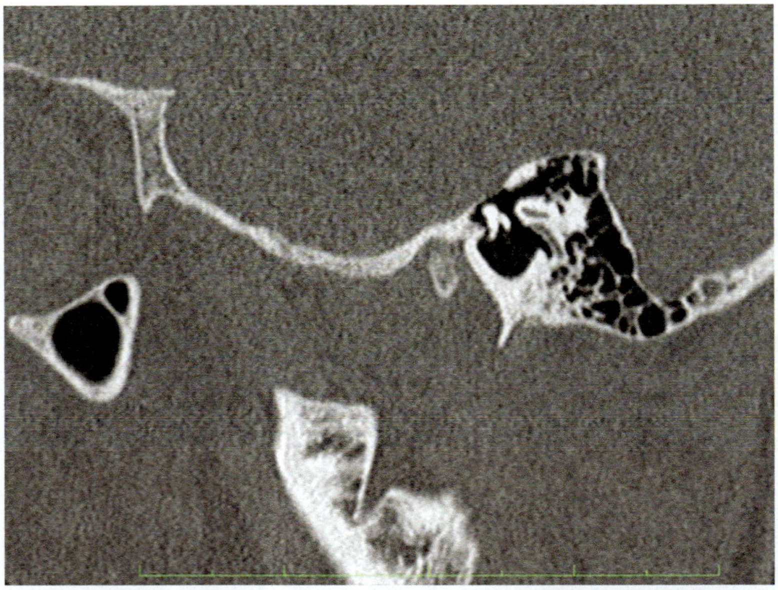

Fig. 16: Molar tooth appearance of ossicles: Handle of malleus and long process of incus.

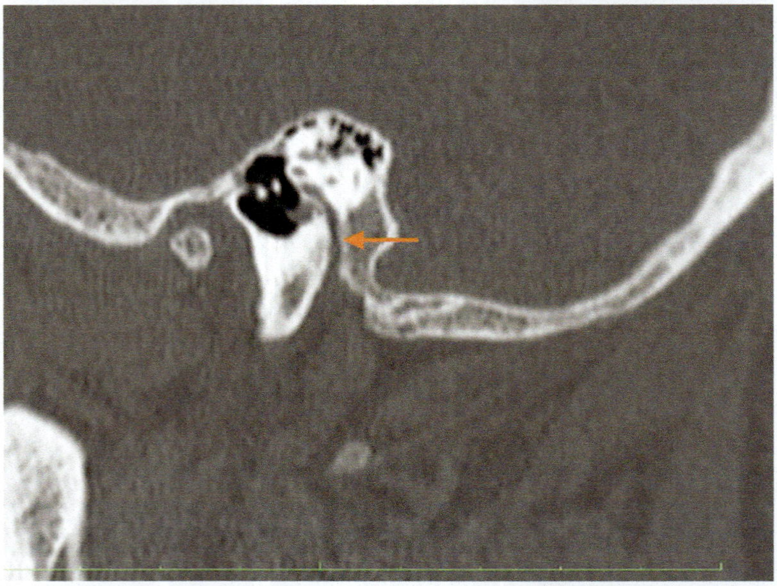

Fig. 17: Vertical segment of facial nerve (orange arrow).

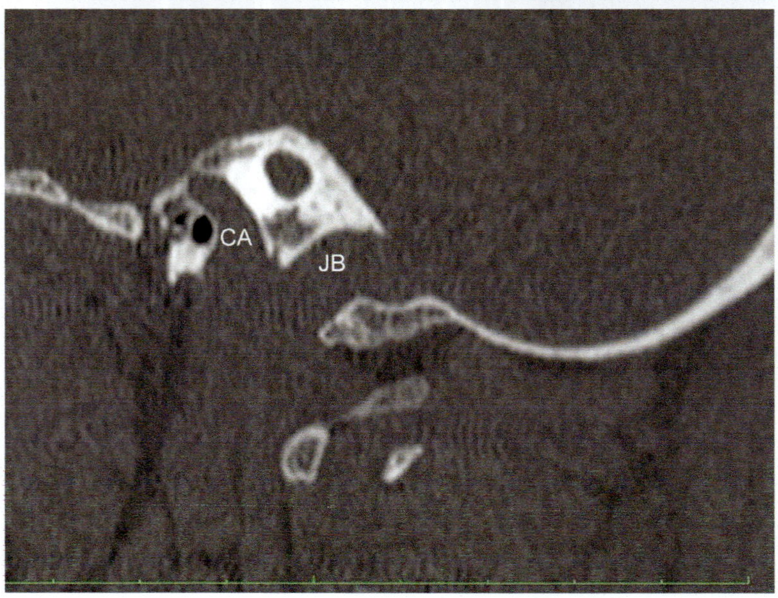

Fig. 18: Great vessels. CA: ascending internal carotid artery; JB: jugular bulb. The area between Ca and Jb is the crotch.

Special Cuts (3D Multiplanar Reconstruction Using Software)

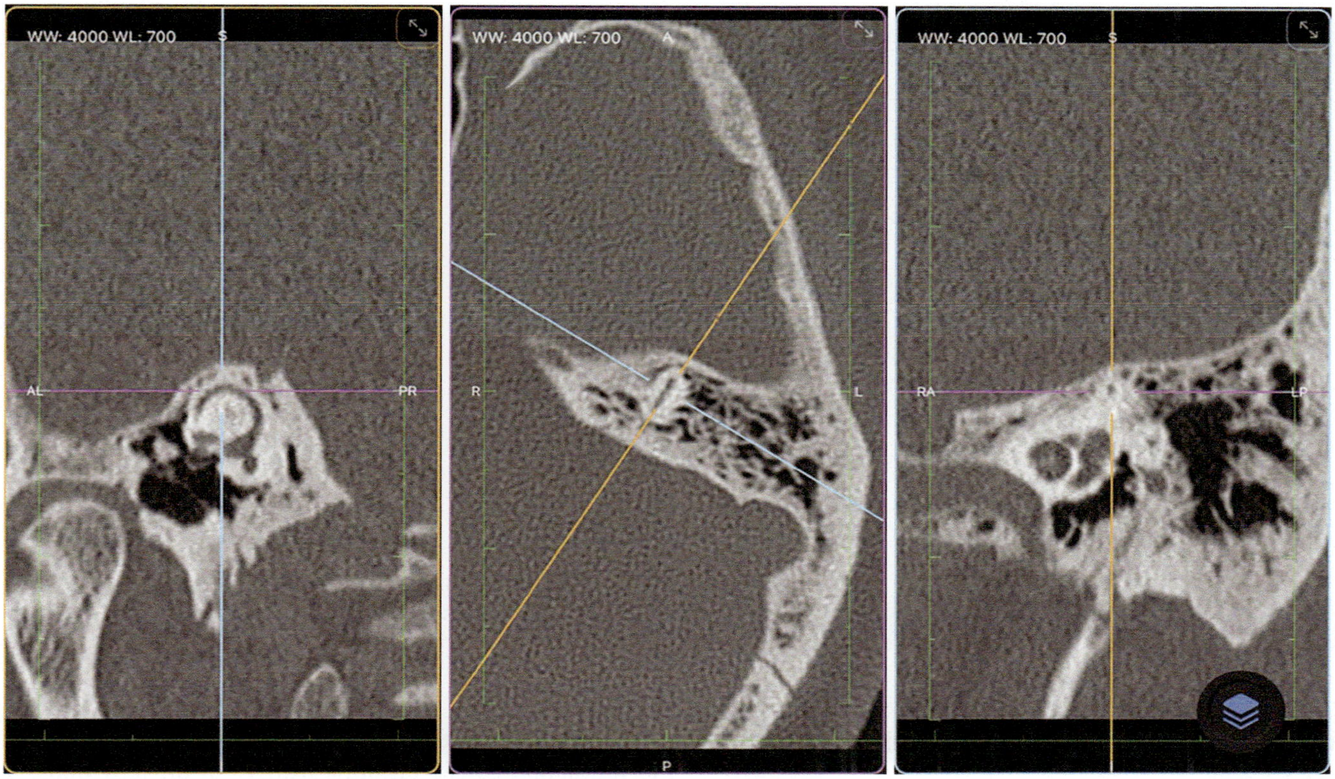

Fig. 19: Special cuts using software.

Pöschl Projection

Sagittal oblique projection of axial cut—SSC

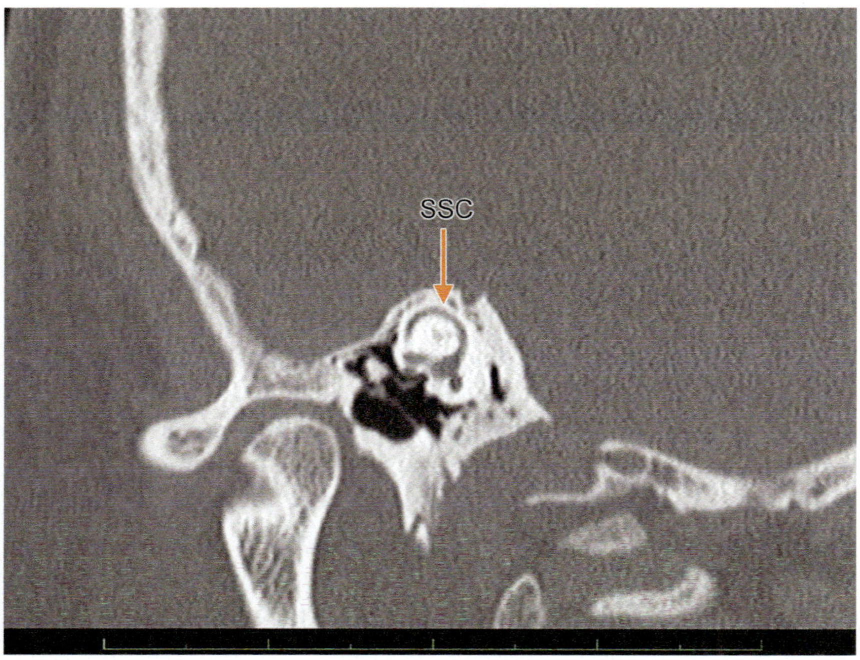

Fig. 20: Sagittal oblique projection of axial cut showing superior semicircular canal (SSC).

Stenvers View

Coronal oblique projection of axial cut—cochlea, facial nerve

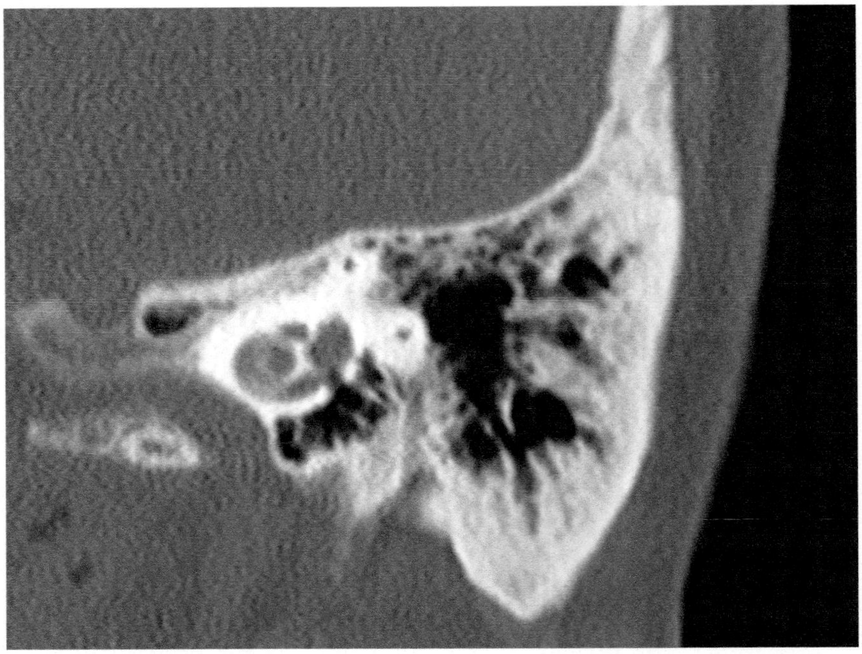

Fig. 21: Coronal oblique projection of axial cut showing entire cochlea turns along with facial nerve

CASE-BASED STUDY OF PREOPERATIVE CT SCAN

Myringoplasty/Grommet

- *EAC*:
  - Stenosis/atresia (cicatrization/developmental)
  - Debris (infection/trauma)
  - Bone malformation (exostosis/osteoma/fibrous dysplasia)
- *Middle ear*:
  - High jugular bulb
  - ICA dehiscence/aberrant
  - Mass/opacity in middle ear (glomus/congenital cholesteatoma)
  - Ossicular status (anomalous, luxation, bony ankylosis of Malleus and Incus)

Cholesteatoma

- *EAC*: Scutum erosion
- Prussak's space
- Ossicle erosion
- *Extent of sac*: Epitympanum, retrotympanum, hypotympanum, protympanum, aditus/beyond LSCC
- Fallopian canal dehiscence
- *Semicircular canals integrity*: Pöschl view and Stenver view
- Posterior cranial fossa (PCF), middle cranial fossa (MCF)

Differential diagnosis of cholesteatoma from middle ear secretion and effusion is done with diffusion-weighted MRI (DW-MRI).

Complications and intracranial extensions of cholesteatoma is assessed by MRI.

Stapes/Tympanosclerosis

- Ossicular chain
  - Fixation
  - Luxation
  - Previous surgery—dislocation/luxation/erosion
- *Demineralization*: Footplate/inner ear/retrofenestral
- Vestibular and cochlear aqueduct/inner ear malformation/gusher
- Epitympanic fixation/ossification of ligament
- Third window phenomenon/superior canal dehiscence (SCD)/carotid dehiscence
- Horizontal VII CN/prolapsing on footplate/intercrural
- Foramen spinosum and fallopian canal [persistent stapedial artery (PSA)]

Residual/Recurrence Cholesteatoma, Second Stage Ossiculoplasty

In this regard multiple imaging modalities such as CT, MRI [delayed T1 contrast-enhanced, echo-planar imaging (EPI) DWI and non-EPI DWI] and cone-beam computed tomography (CBCT) are helpful to diagnose the presence of any residual/recurrence of disease and plan for surgical intervention for the same.

INTENSITY PROJECTION IN 3D-MPR MODE

Maximum Intensity Projection

Maximum intensity projection (MIP) aims at projecting the "voxel" with high attenuation value on every view throughout the volume. Here, Z-axis represents only the pixel with highest Hounsfield number. Bone and contrast material filled structures are thus displayed preferentially. In high-resolution computed tomography (HRCT) mastoid, this mode intensifies the ossicular chain.[1]

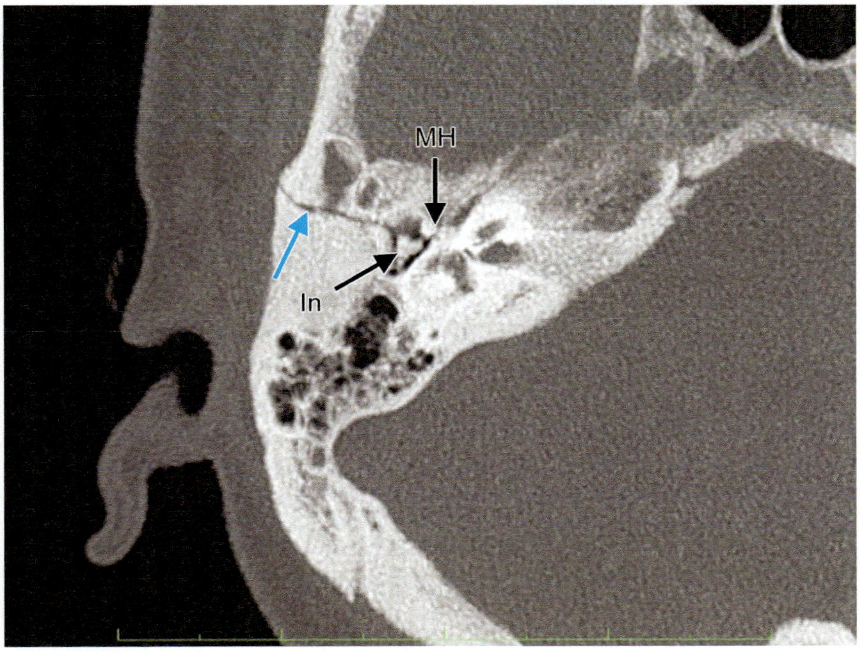

Fig. 22A: Maximum intensity projection (MIP) algorithm being used to highlight bones and ossicles. Blue arrow: fracture line. (In: incus; MH: malleus head)

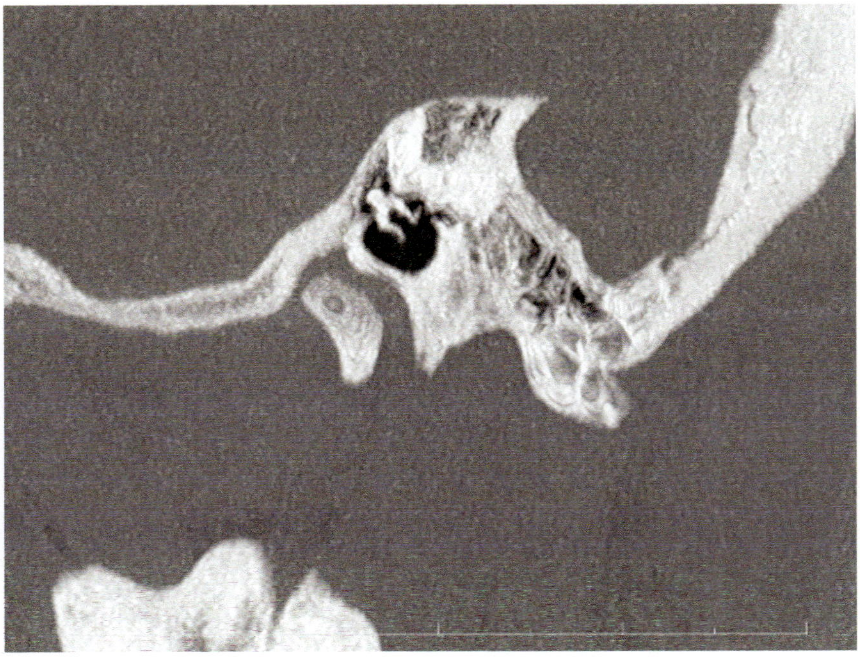

Fig. 22B: Molar tooth appearance of ossicles: Handle of malleus and long process of incus.

Minimum Intensity Projection

The minimum intensity projection (MinIP) and MIP algorithms are almost identical, with the change being, in case of MinIP, for each XY coordinate, only the lowest Hounsfield value along the Z-axis is represented. Thus, only the most hypodense structures of the volume are represented. This is helpful to augment soft tissues such as facial nerve.

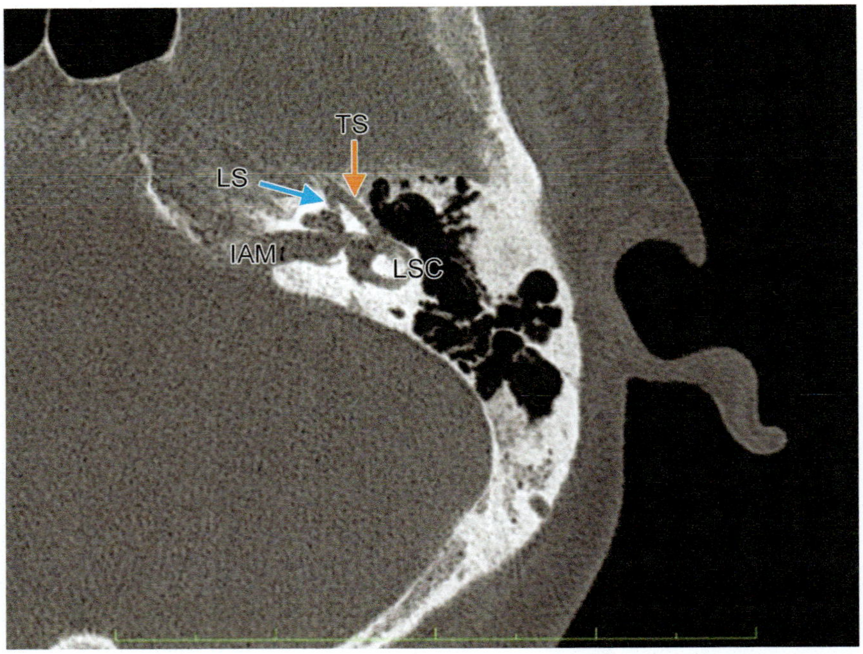

Fig. 23A: Minimum intensity projection (MinIP) algorithm being used to highlight soft tissues. TS (orange arrow): Tympanic segment and LS (blue arrow): Labyrinthine segment of facial nerve.
(IAM: internal acoustic meatus, LSC: lateral semicircular canal)

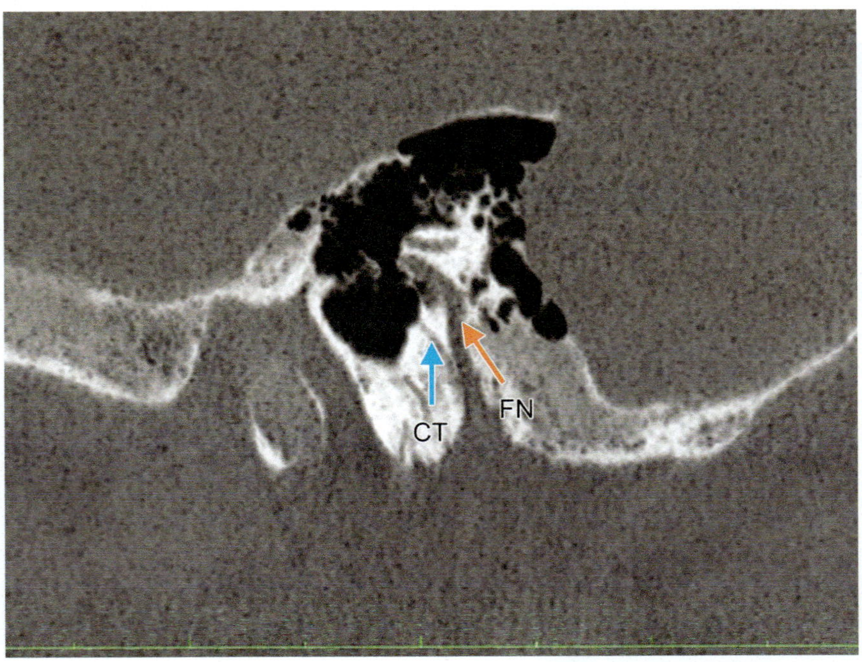

Fig. 23B: Minimum intensity projection (MinIP) algorithm being used to highlight soft tissues.
(FN: facial nerve; CT: chorda tympani)

Three-dimensional Reconstruction

This feature helps the surgeon to plan for the surgery as it provides a virtual otoendoscopy into the diseased ear based on certain aspects:

- *EAC*: Dimensions and presence of canal humps or tortuosity
- Middle ear structures
- *Ossicles*: Erosion, discontinuity, anomalies
- Fracture line in traumatic facial palsy
- Attic defects in squamosal COM or revision surgeries

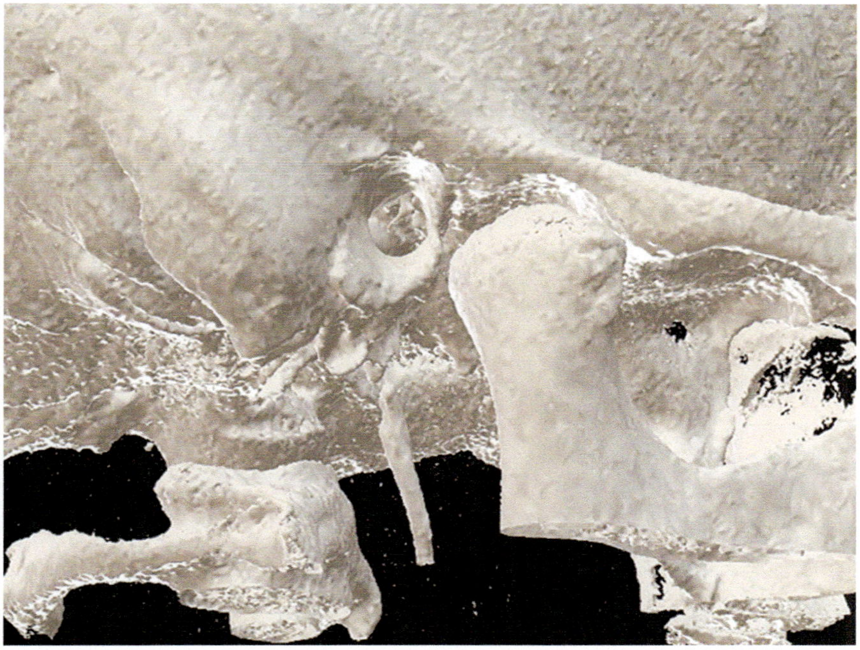

Fig. 24A: Three-dimensional (3D) reconstruction of HRCT: External auditory canal.

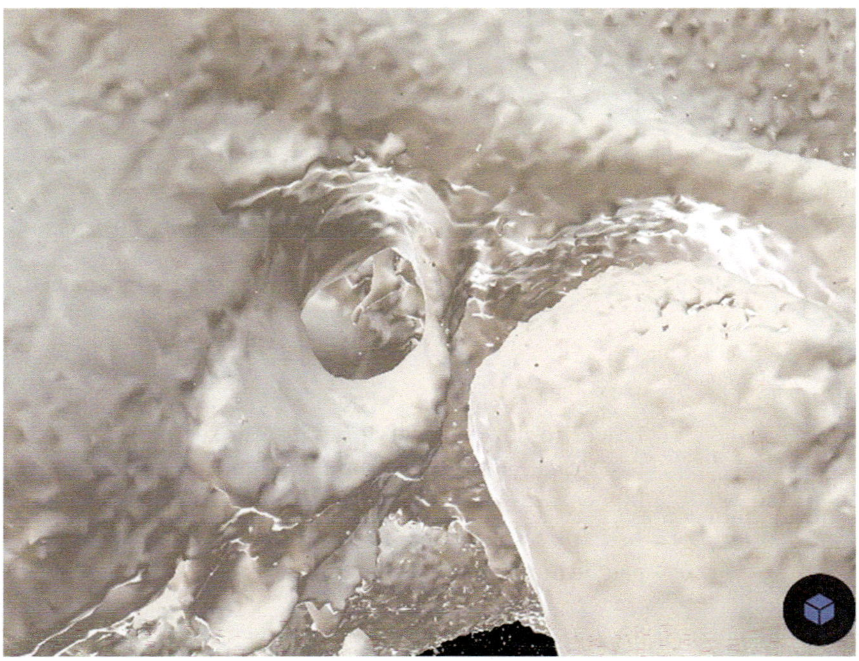

Fig. 24B: Three-dimensional (3D) reconstruction of HRCT: External auditory canal architecture.

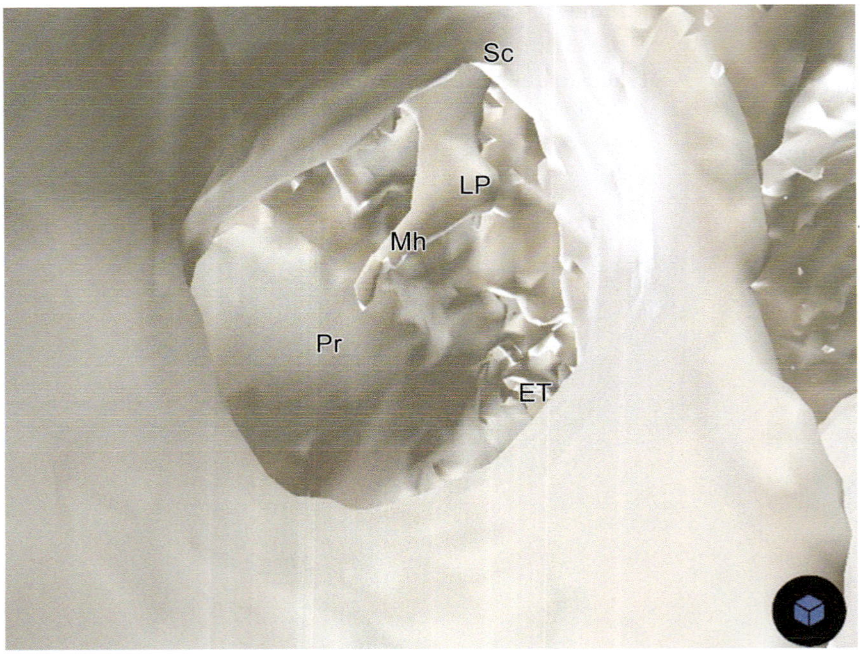

Fig. 24C: Three-dimensional (3D) reconstruction of HRCT: External auditory canal with scutum.
(Sc: scutum; LP: lateral process of malleus; Mh: malleus handle; Pr: promontory, ET: Eustachian tube)

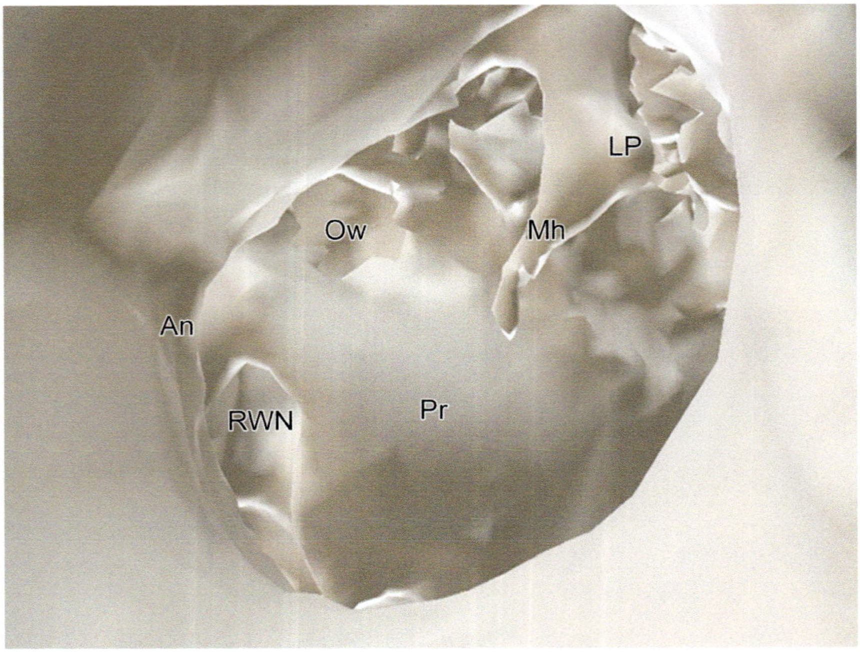

Fig. 24D: Three-dimensional (3D) reconstruction of HRCT: Middle ear landmarks.
(LP: lateral process of malleus; Mh: malleus handle; Pr: promontory, Ow: oval window; RWN: round window niche; An: annulus)

Cone-beam Computed Tomography Scan

Cone-beam imaging is a volume acquisition method introduced just before the year 2000. It was first intended for dental study of relative dimensions and preimplantation assessment, providing orthodontists and implantologists with useful images. Significant improvements and the emergence of certain intrinsic advantages have considerably changed the outlook, with respect not only to dentomaxillary imaging but also to sinus and petrosal bone exploration. Salient features of this modality include:

- Lower radiation level compared to regular CT. Thus, CBCT is ideal for repeated examination, postoperative follow-up and pediatric exploration.
- Assessment of traumatic bone lesions of the pars petrosa can be performed rapidly and easily on CBCT.

Utility of CBCT in Otology

- *Malformation and dysplasia*: CBCT is probably the most effective imaging technique for anatomic study of the ossicular chain, thanks to its excellent spatial resolution.

Ossicular chain malformation or fixation, bone dysplasia, and otospongiosis sites are clearly visible.

- ***Chronic otitis***: In chronic otitis with dense pars petrosa and middle ear opacity, cholesteatoma, and associated complications can be diagnosed on CBCT. As in CT, diagnosis is not based on specific lesion density but on the impact on neighboring bone structures (middle ear walls, ossicular chain, thin osseous labyrinthine wall, and osseous fallopian canal).
- ***Trauma***: CBCT is effective for traumatic pars petrosa bone lesions, although it must be borne in mind that associated soft-tissue and cerebral lesions will not be visualized.
- ***Postoperatively***: Follow-up of ossiculoplasty and residual air-bone gap are indications for CBCT. Postoperative follow-up of cholesteatoma is increasingly dependent on MRI, but residual surgical cavity opacity can be effectively explored by CBCT.

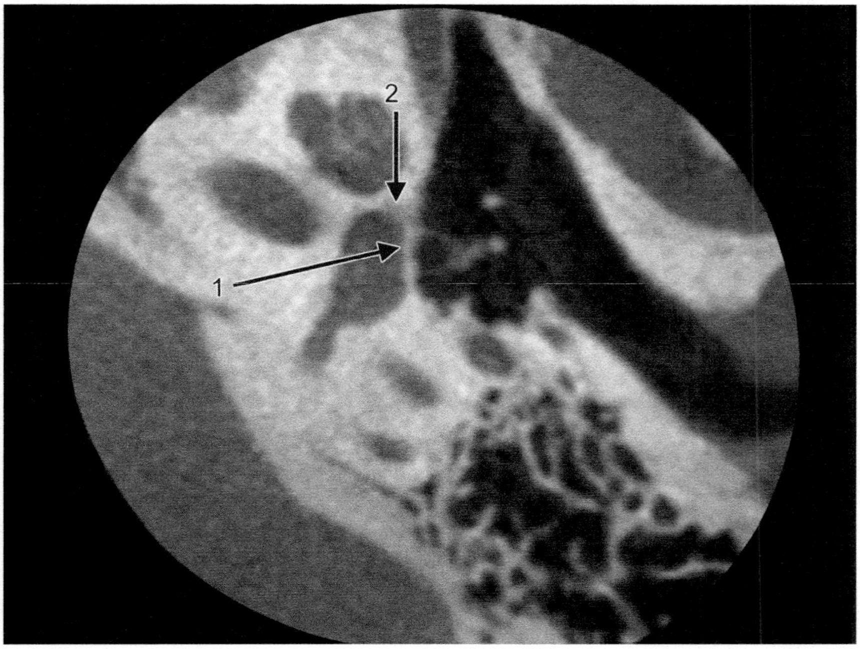

Fig. 25A: Otospongiosis: Stapediovestibular otospongiosis site.

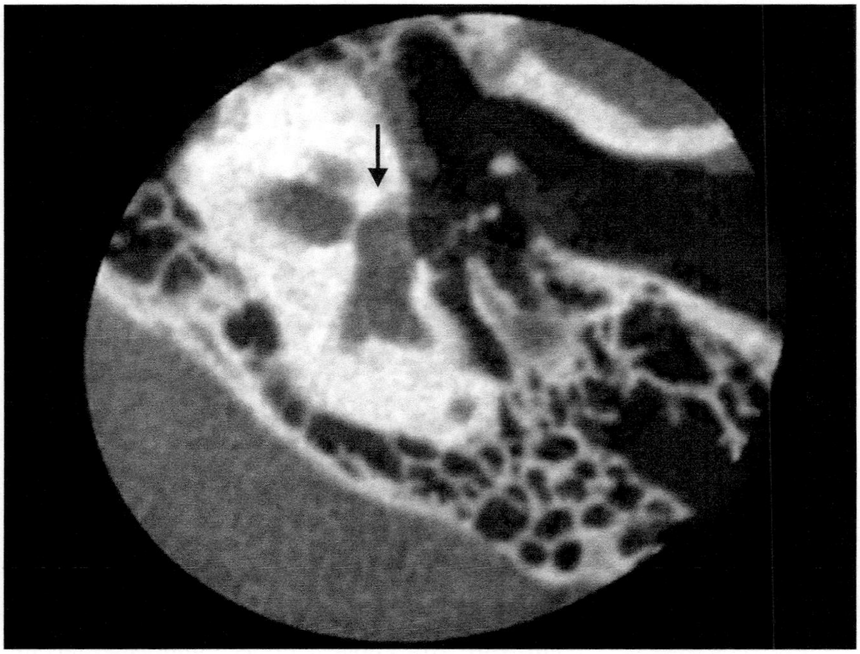

Fig. 25B: Otospongiosis: Prestapedial otospongiosis site.

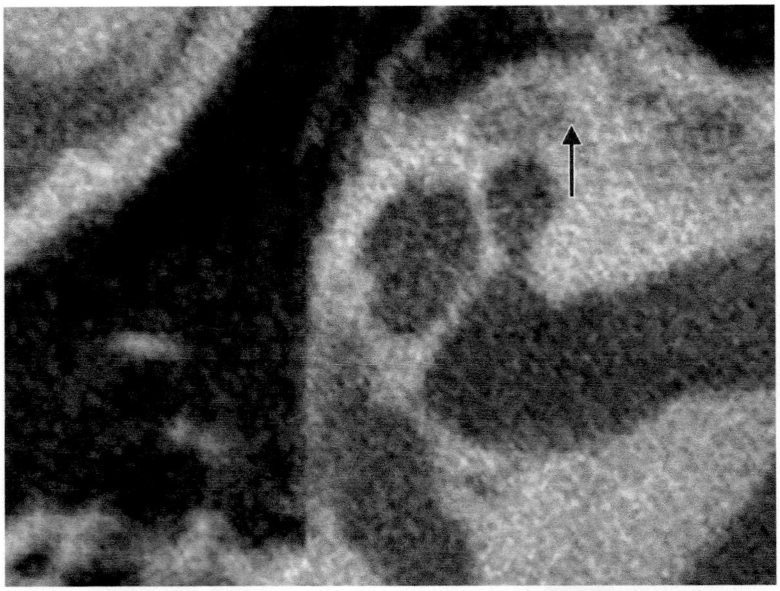

Fig. 25C: Otospongiosis: Cochlear otospongiosis site.

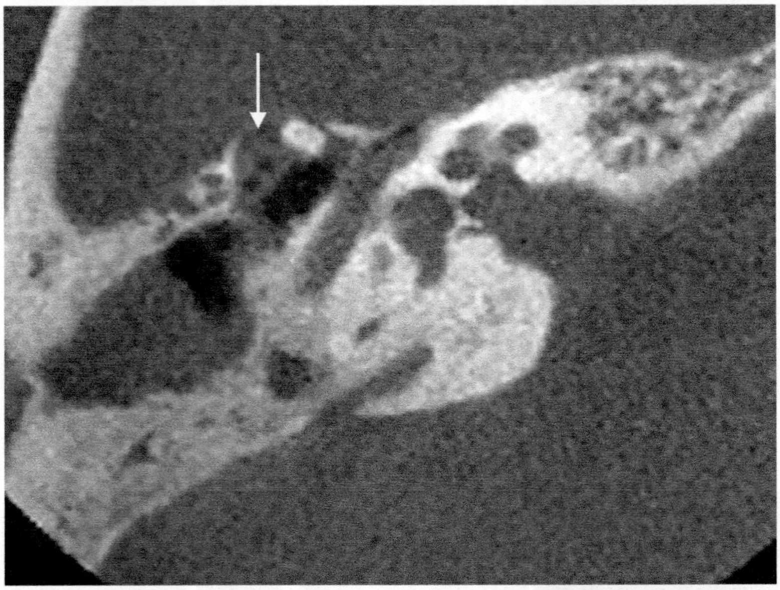

Fig. 26A: Attic cholesteatoma: multiplanar reconstructions: Axial slice.

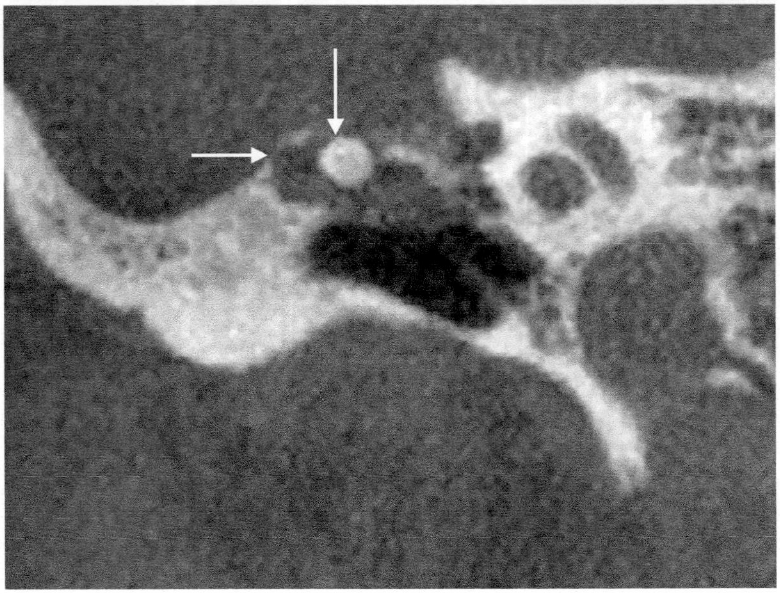

Fig. 26B: Attic cholesteatoma: multiplanar reconstructions: Coronal slices.

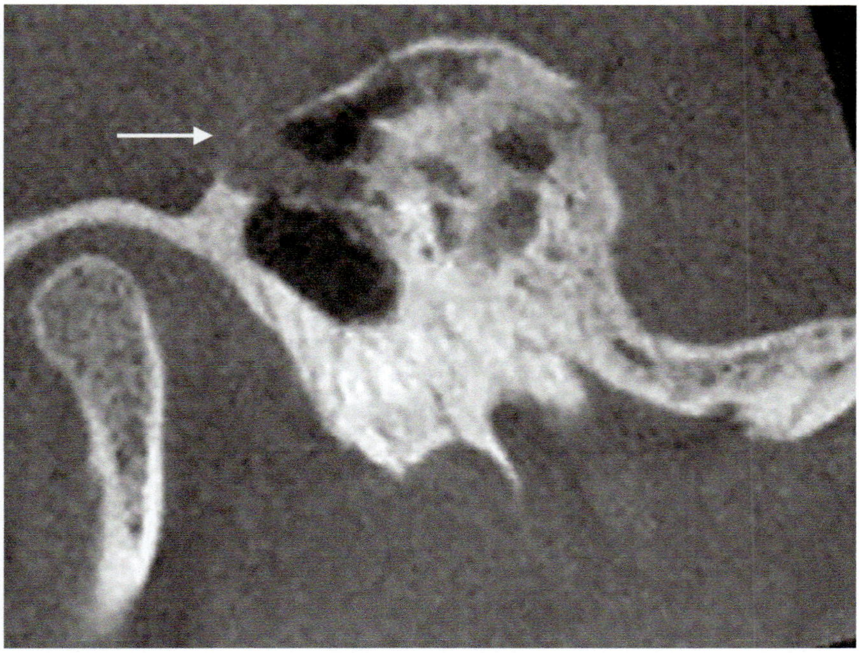

Fig. 26C: Attic cholesteatoma: multiplanar reconstructions. Sagittal slice.

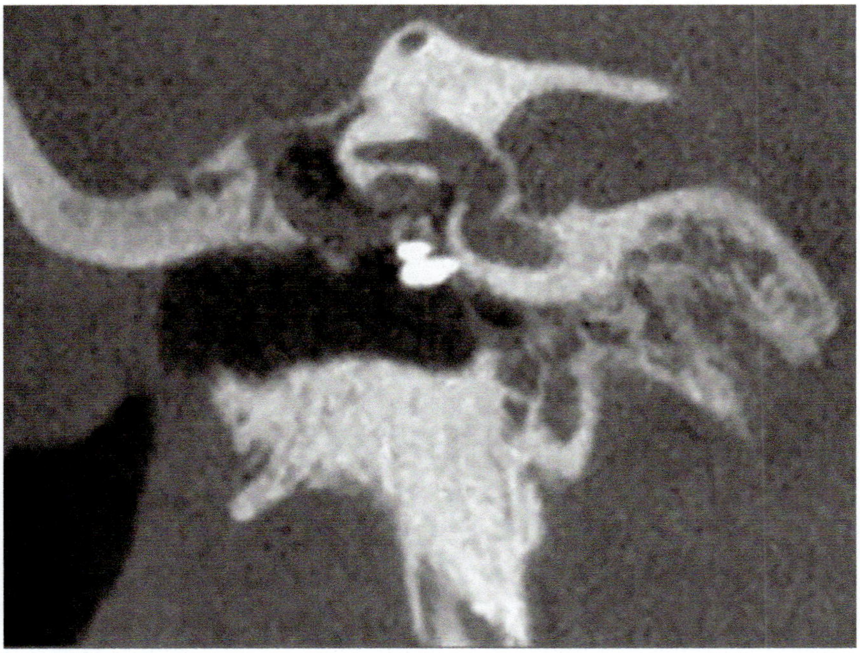

Fig. 26D: Attic cholesteatoma: multiplanar reconstructions: Partial prosthesis tilt. Good visibility of external attic opacity which, as on computed tomography (CT), appears nonspecific but which, associated with inward ossicle chain displacement and attic wall erosion, suggests cholesteatoma. Sagittal slice showing tegmen erosion.

MAGNETIC RESONANCE IMAGING FUNDAMENTALS

	T1	*T2*	*T1-Gd*
Air and bone	No signal	No signal	No signal/hypo
Water	Hypo	Hyper	Hypo
Fat	Hyper	Hyper	Hyper
Tumor	Medium (as muscle)	Hyper	Hyper
Cholesteatoma	Hypo/iso	Hypo/iso	Capsule +
Granulation	Iso	Hyper	+
Abscess	Hypo	Hyper	Capsule +

ROLE OF PREOPERATIVE MAGNETIC RESONANCE IMAGING

Magnetic resonance imaging plays an important role in the preoperative and postoperative diagnosis of specific sequences of indeterminate soft tissue abnormalities identified on HRCT of the temporal bone.

Contrast-enhanced MRI can discriminate between the nonenhancing cholesteatoma and other contrast-enhancing findings, e.g., inflammation, scar, or granulation tissue. *DWI* is more practical with a shorter examination time than delayed contrast material-enhanced imaging; there is also no need for contrast injection. The technique relies on the principles of the Brownian motion of water molecules. Cholesteatomas appear hyperintense on DWI obtained with β-factors of 800 or 1,000 s/mm^2 where the β-factor is a measure of the strength of the respective diffusion weighting. This visual characteristic is similar to a histologically identical lesion, the epidermoid cyst. Granulation tissue, fibrous tissue, cholesterol granuloma or serous fluid, on the other hand, have low signal intensity on DWI (at a b-factor of 800 s/mm^2). *Turbo spin-echo (TSE)-based DWI* is a spin-echo based multishot (MS) technique with long echo time and a high signal-to-noise ratio. The sequence is known to lack significant image distortions and it does not show the susceptibility artifacts that are observed with standard EPI DWI. Therefore, a better spatial resolution in the middle ear is possible and it permits fast multiplanar imaging. Furthermore, thinner slices can be obtained than with EPI-sequences. This so-called *non-EPI* sequence has therefore hardly any false-positive findings. False-negative findings are mostly a consequence of motion or empty retraction pockets. Primary and residual/recurrent cholesteatoma can be accurately detected on non-EPI DWI with 98% clinical and radiologic correlation.

In spite of surgical advancement of EES, there are certain constraints. Lesions <8 mm, confined to the middle ear and its extensions can be eradicated with a minimally invasive endoscopic transcanal technique. The surgeon should never be dogmatic and keep the conventional postauricular mastoidectomy approach as an alternative wherever deemed necessary depending on disease extent.[2]

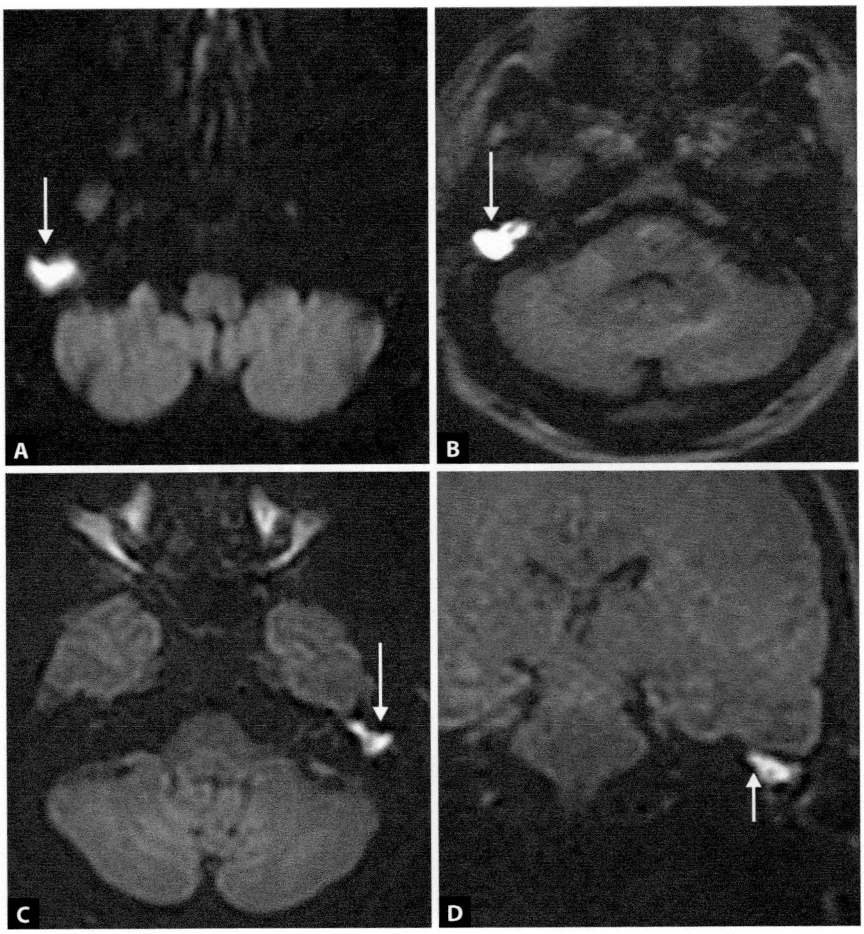

Figs. 27A to D: Comparison of different DWI techniques. (A) EPI DWI acquired in a patient undergoing evaluation for possible demyelinating disease. Abnormal DWI signal intensity in the right temporal bone (arrow) prompted further evaluation for cholesteatoma. The abnormal DWI signal intensity is clearly visible due to the large size of the lesion, but there are artifacts from the skull base; (B) SS TSE (HASTE) DWI sequences obtained in a patient with obscured visual examination due to postoperative changes. Increased diffusion signal intensity is seen in the right middle ear and mastoid defect (arrow), with cholesteatoma confirmed at surgery; (C) Multishot TSE DWI (BLADE) image in a patient with otoscopic examination obscured by cartilaginous reconstruction shows increased DWI signal intensity (arrow) in the left epitympanum, with cholesteatoma confirmed at surgery; (D) The multishot TSE DWI has the additional advantage of generating images in a coronal plane, which can be especially useful when erosion of the tegmen tympani and/or intracranial extension is suspected. Arrow indicates increased DWI in the left epitympanum.
(DWI: diffusion-weighted imaging; EPI: echo-planar imaging; SS TSE: single-shot turbo spin echo)

REFERENCES

1. Ding Y, Sun X, Li D, Zhang H, Chen Y, Xu A. [Evaluation of maximum intensity projection in HRCT in the diagnosis of the destruction of ossicular chain in chronic otitis media]. Lin Chuang Er Bi Yan Hou Ke Za Zhi. 2006;20(7): 289-92.
2. Migirov L, Wolf M, Greenberg G, Eyal A. Non-EPI DW MRI in planning the surgical approach to primary and recurrent cholesteatoma. Otol Neurotol. 2014;35(1):121-5.

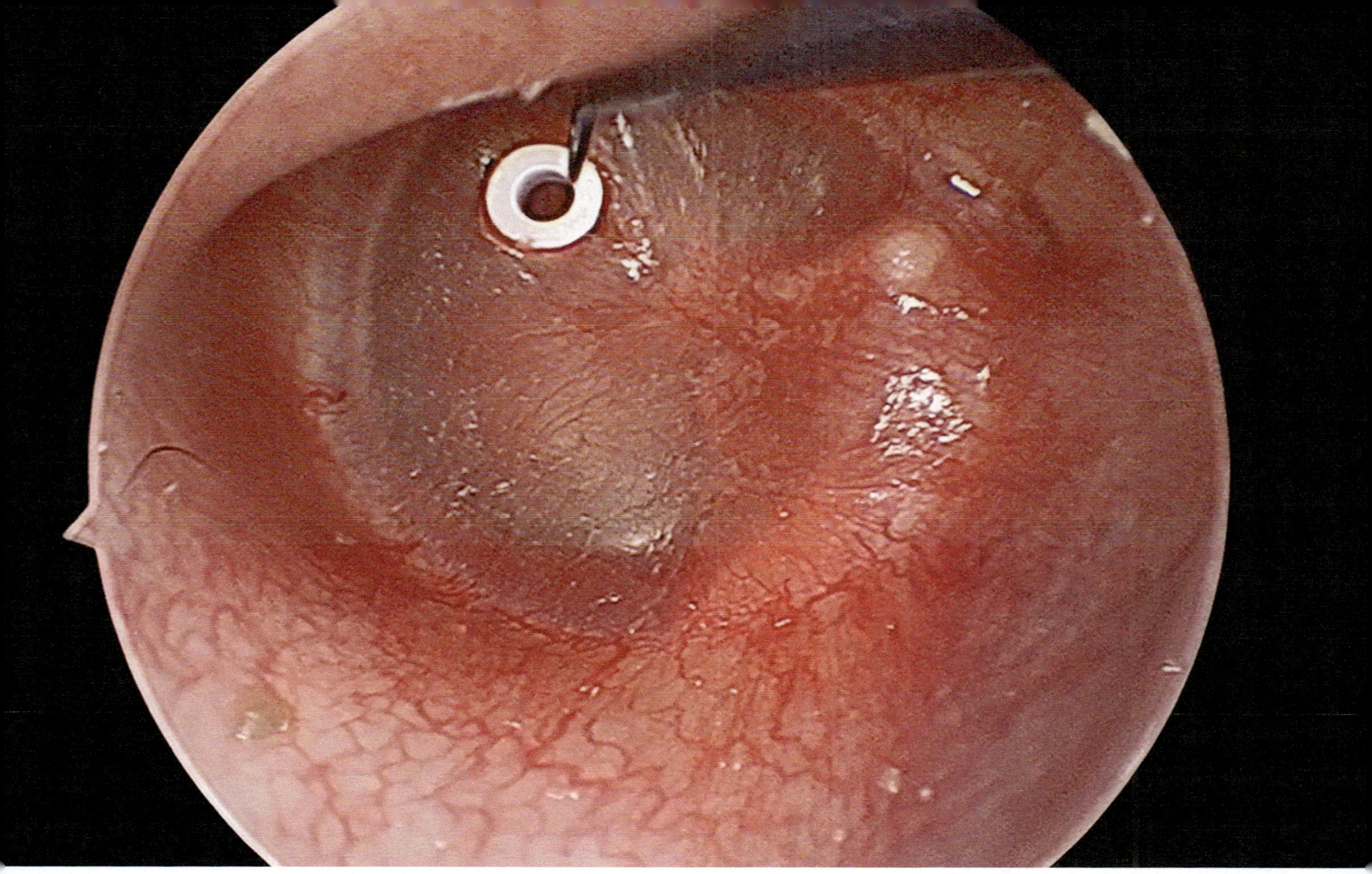

CHAPTER 6

Endoscopic Myringotomy

Arindam Das, Sayan Hazra

Chapter Outline

INTRODUCTION

Myringotomy is a surgical procedure wherein a small puncture is made on the tympanic membrane. This is done as an office procedure in adults under local anesthesia. In children and apprehensive patients, the procedure is carried under general anesthesia.

INDICATIONS

- Otitis media with effusion (OME)
- Acute otitis media
- Insertion of gentamicin-soaked microwick in Ménière's disease
- Intratympanic drug delivery in sudden sensorineural hearing loss (SNHL)
- As a prerequisite for Meniett device

PREOPERATIVE PREPARATION

Pure-tone audiometry is done to evaluate the preoperative hearing threshold and nature of hearing loss. Tympanometry using an automated impedance meter has been used widely as a method of detecting OME, which uses compliance and pressure as the numerical parameters, presented visually as a compliance curve. A type B tympanogram is frequently associated with OME; a type A is infrequently associated with OME and a type C falls in between.[1]

TYPES OF GROMMETS USED

- Shepard
- Bevel Bobbin
- Shah
- Sheehy
- T-tube

Authors prefer using the Shah variety due to presence of "shoe" which aids in easier intratympanic placement quite snuggly.

Advantages of Endoscope

- Clear, magnified, panoramic view of tympanic membrane
- Canal humps can be negotiated easily.
- Use of speculum in pediatric transcanal microscopic approach hampers visualization and decreases working space which can be easily mitigated with use of narrower 3 mm or 2.7 mm endoscopes without compromising on the exposure.
- Proper localization decreases chances of middle ear injury and thus postoperative complications such as fibrosis and permanent perforation.
- Early and accurate diagnosis of middle ear pathology and/or anomalies such as high jugular bulb, congenital cholesteatoma, prolapsed facial nerve, etc.

SURGICAL STEPS

1. *Anesthesia*: Four quadrant infiltration with 2% lidocaine with adrenaline (1:30,000)
2. *Identification of landmarks*: Critical step in deciding site to make incision

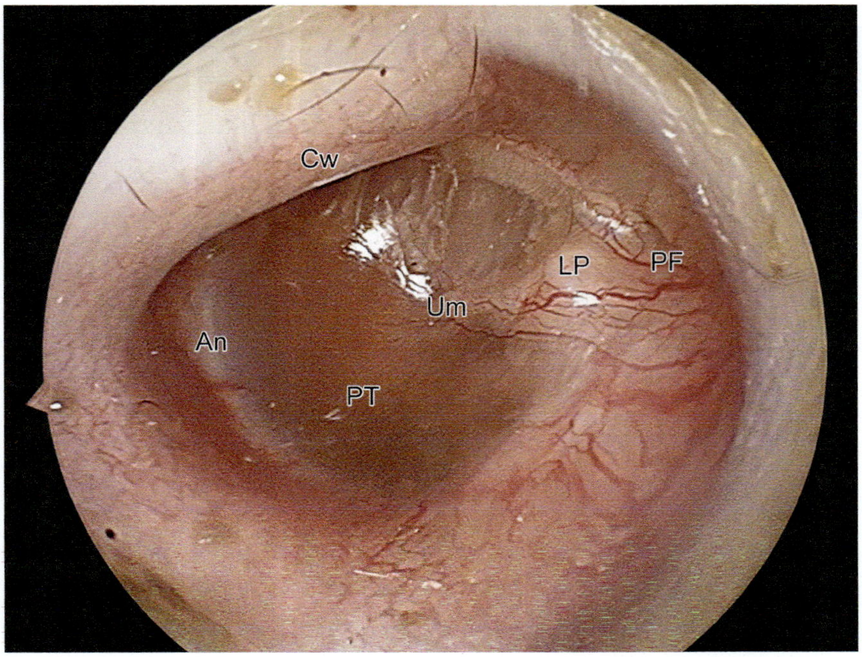

Fig. 1: Endoscopic view of left ear.
(An: annular ring; Cw: canal wall; LP: lateral process of malleus; PF: pars flaccida; PT: pars tensa; Um: umbo)

- Landmarks to be identified prior to myringotomy:
  - Lateral process of malleus (LP)
  - Tip of handle of malleus or umbo (Um)
  - Annular ring (An)

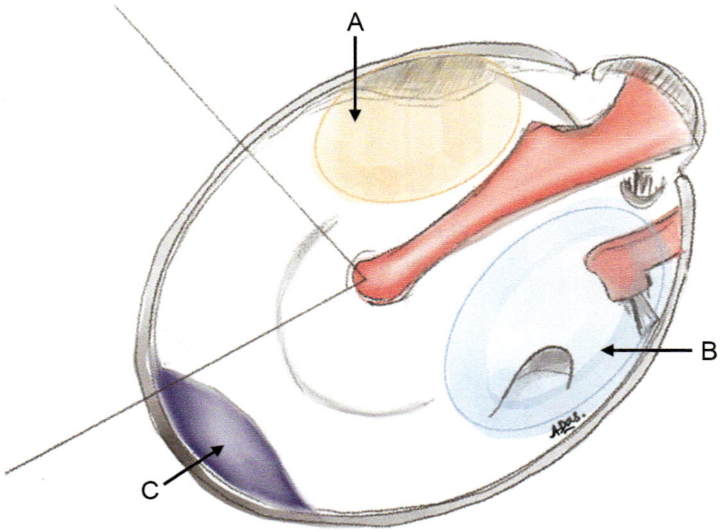

Fig. 2: Schematic depiction of landmarks for myringotomy in anteroinferior quadrant of left ear. A (Yellow zone)—Eustachian tube, B (Blue zone)—ossicular chain unit, and C (Violet zone)—jugular bulb.

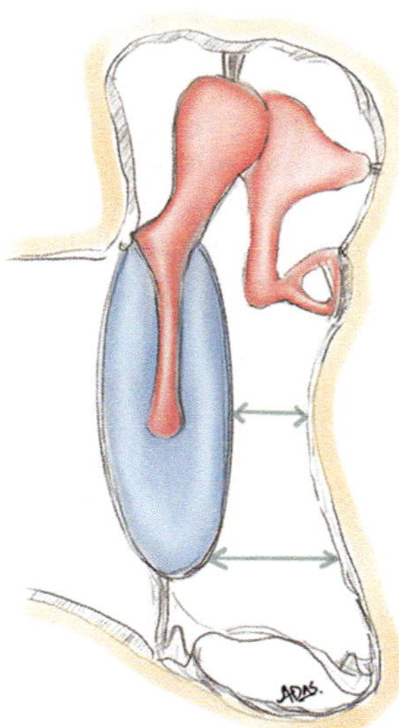

Fig. 3: Schematic depiction of coronal section of right ear as seen from front showing relative distance between tympanic membrane and medial wall.

3. *Myringotomy*: Sharp incision is placed on anteroinferior quadrant using myringotome or reasonably sharp sickle knife. Radial incision causes lesser injury on the middle fibrous layer of the drum and thus postoperative faster healing. The ventilation tube inserted via a radial or circumferential incision however does not influence the extrusion rate.[2] Anterosuperior incision can lead to unwanted injury to the medial end of Eustachian tube opening (protympanum). Posterior incision is to be avoided to prevent inadvertent injury to the ossicular chain.

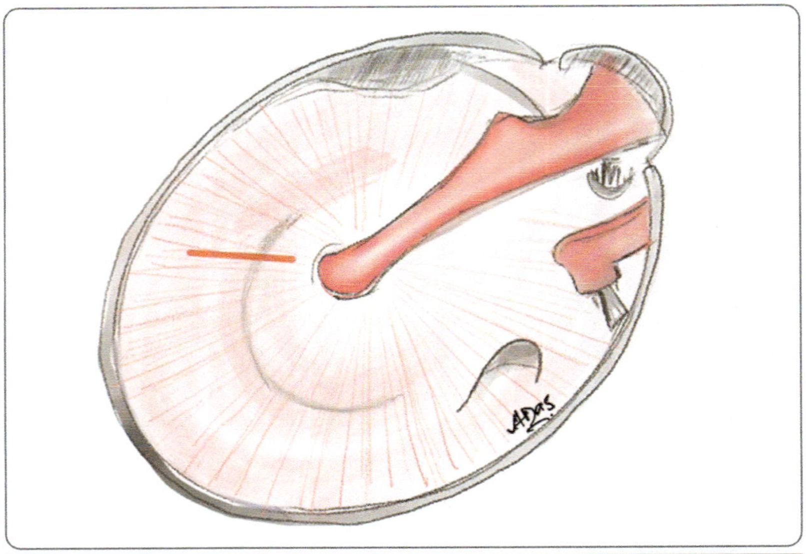

Fig. 4A: Schematic depiction of site of placing incision on left ear tympanic membrane.

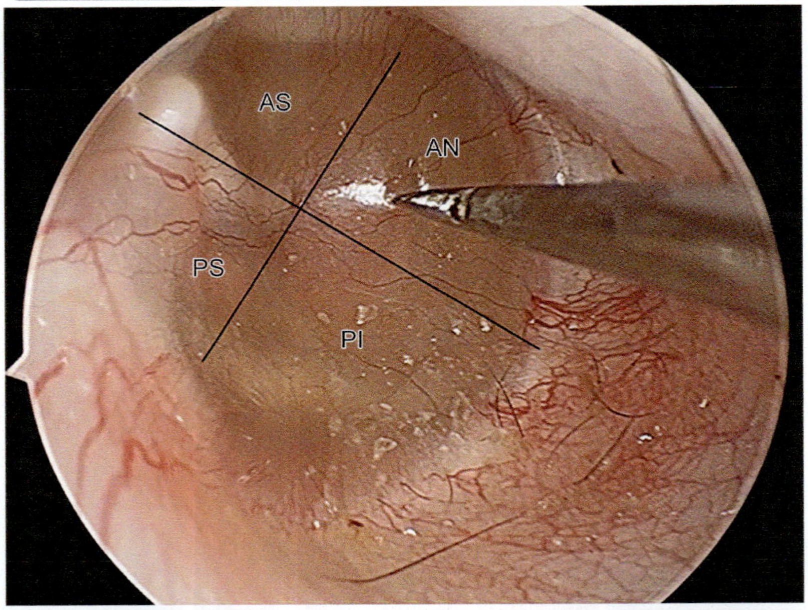

Fig. 4B: Site of placing incision being illustrated on right tympanic membrane. Quadrants—AS: anterosuperior; AN: anteroinferior; PS: posterosuperior; PI: posteroinferior.

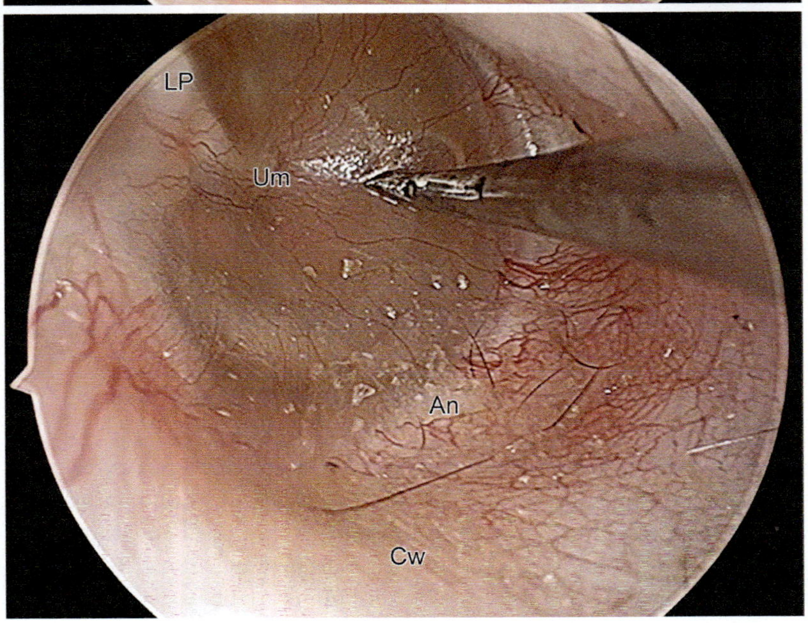

Fig. 4C: Site of placing incision being illustrated on right tympanic membrane with reference to landmarks; (An: annular ring; Cw: canal wall; LP: lateral process of malleus; Um: umbo).

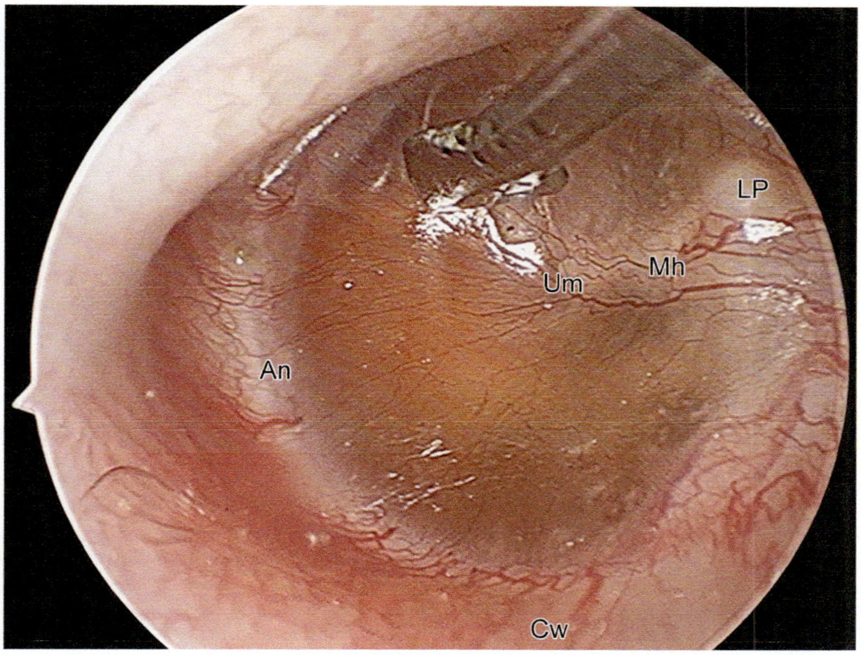

Fig. 4D: Radial incision being given on left tympanic membrane with reference to landmarks.
(An: annular ring; Cw: canal wall; LP: lateral process of malleus; Um: umbo; Mh: malleus handle).

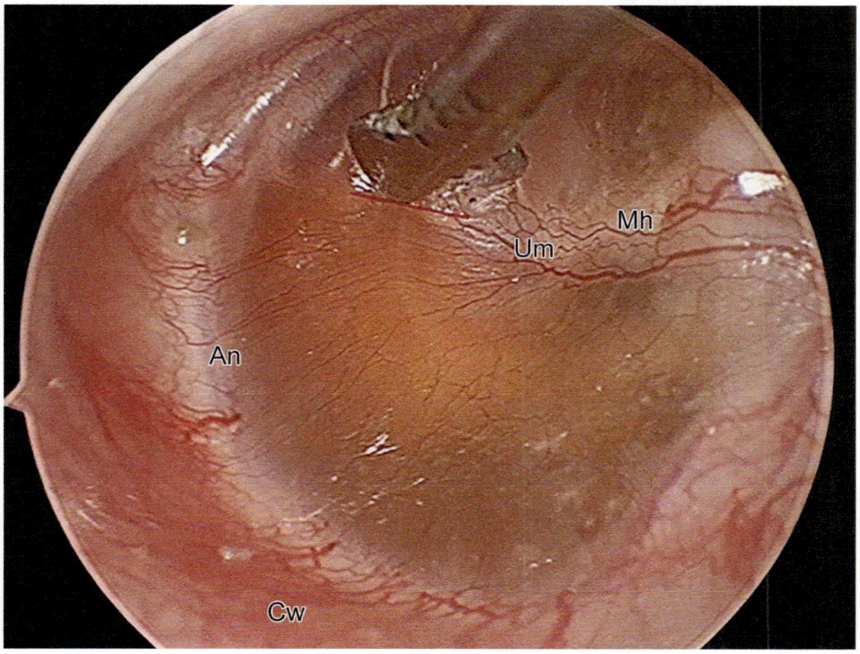

Fig. 4E: Radial incision being given on left tympanic membrane with reference to landmarks.
(An: annular ring; Cw: canal wall; LP: lateral process of malleus; Um: umbo; Mh: malleus handle).

4. *Middle ear fluid aspiration*: Using appropriate suction cannula, the middle ear fluid is aspirated. 2 mL corticosteroid (dexamethasone 4 mg/mL) is injected into the middle ear and suctioned off to prevent postoperative inflammation.[3]

TIP

- Noise from persistent aspiration may lead to permanent noise-induced hearing loss.[4]
- Suctioning to be done atraumatically to prevent injury to middle ear mucosa which can lead to bleeding and subsequent obscuring of surgical field, plugging of grommet, and long-term fibrosis.

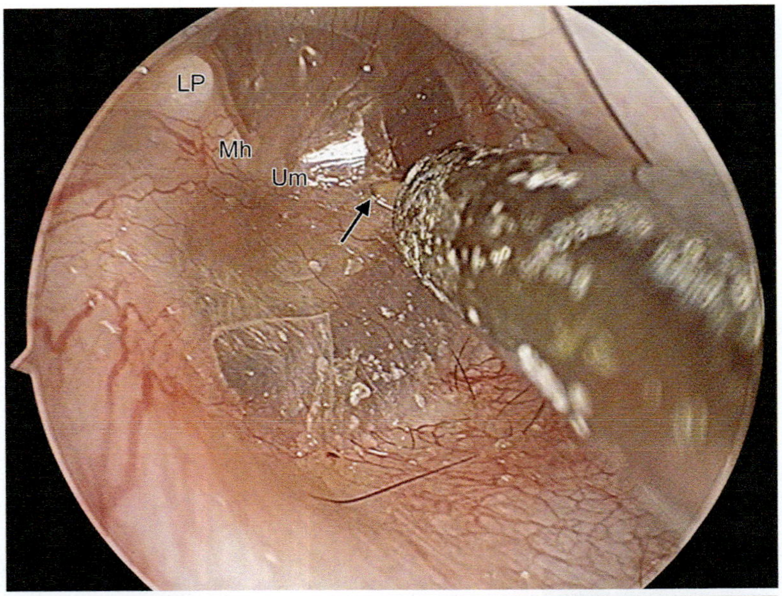

Fig. 5A: Middle ear fluid being aspirated from right ear.
(LP: lateral process of malleus; Mh: malleus handle; Um: umbo)

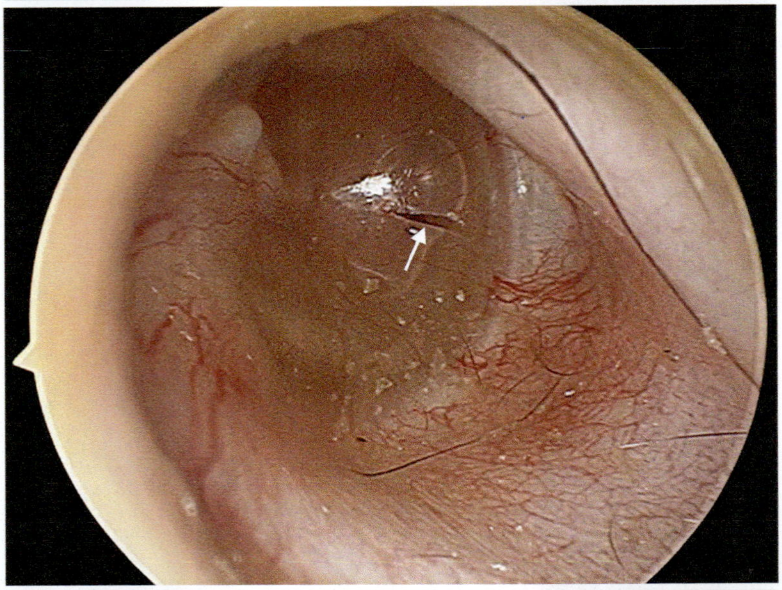

Fig. 5B: View after initial aspiration.

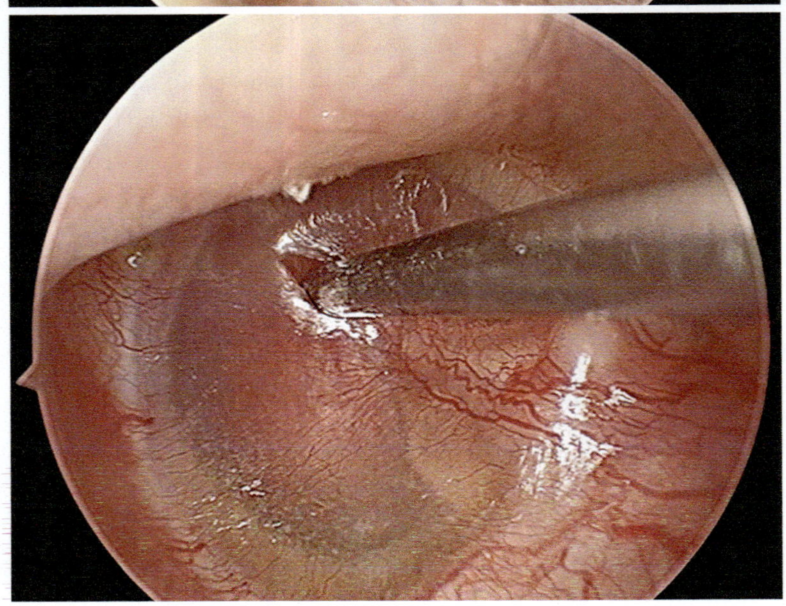

Fig. 5C: Middle ear fluid being aspirated from left ear.

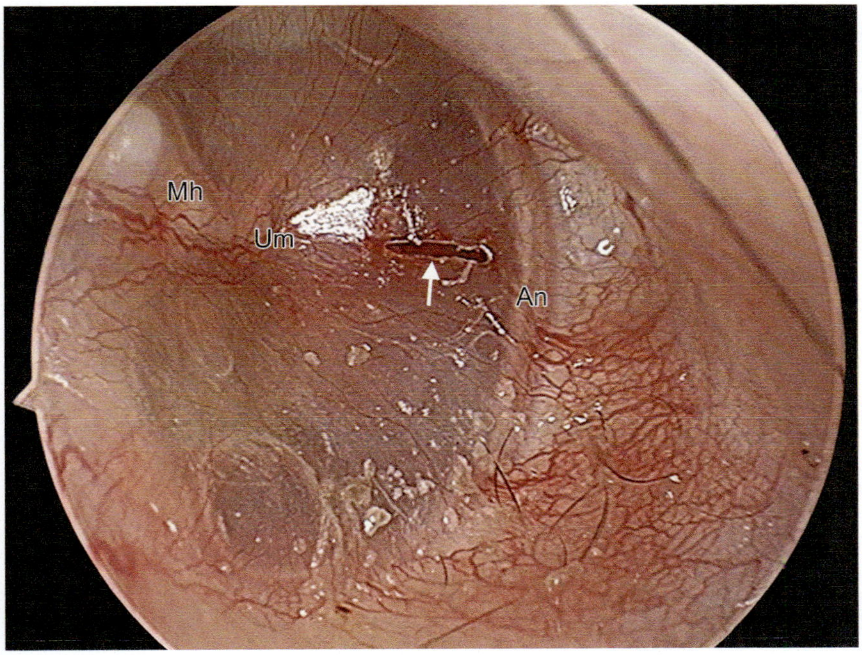

Fig. 5D: Final view after aspiration of fluid. (An: annular ring; Mh: handle of malleus; Um: umbo)

5. *Grommet insertion*: Shah ventilation tube is placed on the tympanic membrane close to the incision with tip of the shoe facing anterosuperiorly using an alligator forceps. The projecting flange/shoe is gently pushed within the tympanum using the forceps and a smooth curved or angled pick is used to negotiate the tube entirely inside by gently pushing from its posterior aspect.

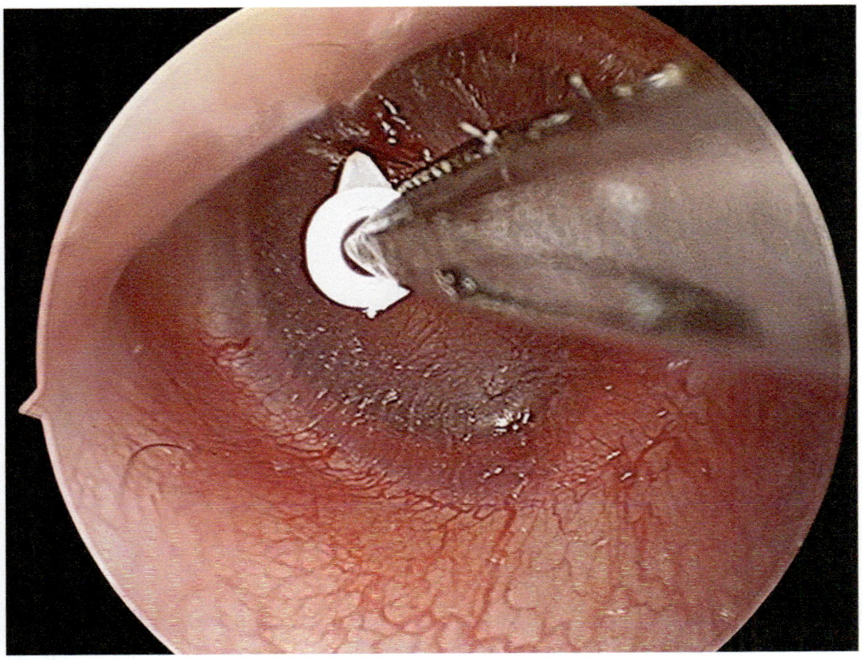

Fig. 6A: Grommet being introduced with alligator forceps.

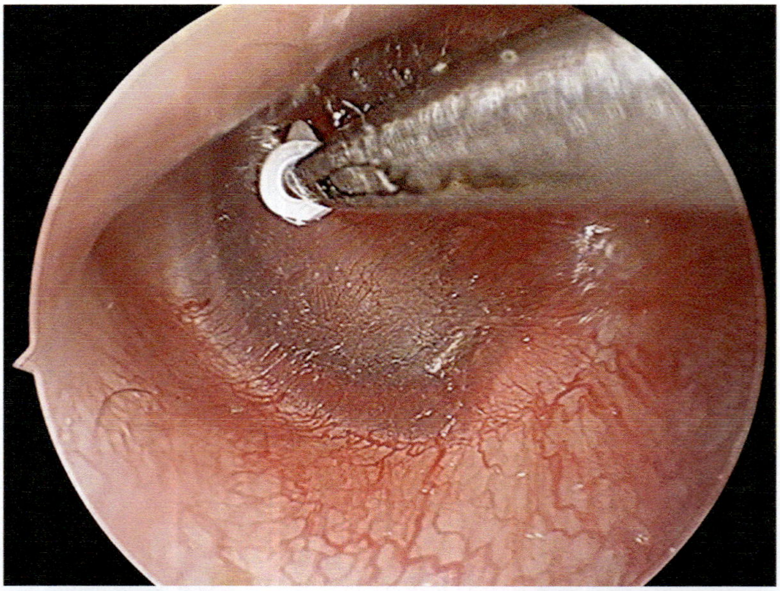

Fig. 6B: Shoe of the grommet being glided into tympanum.

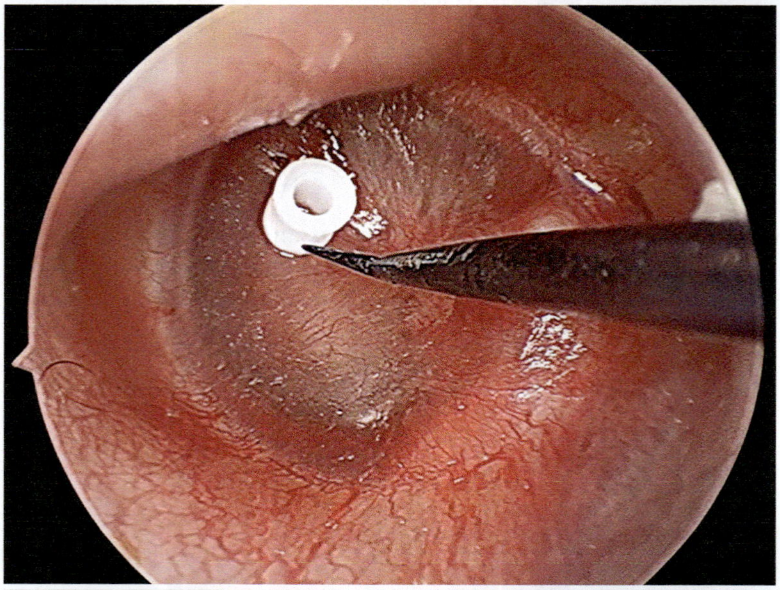

Fig. 6C: Grommet being negotiated using angled pick.

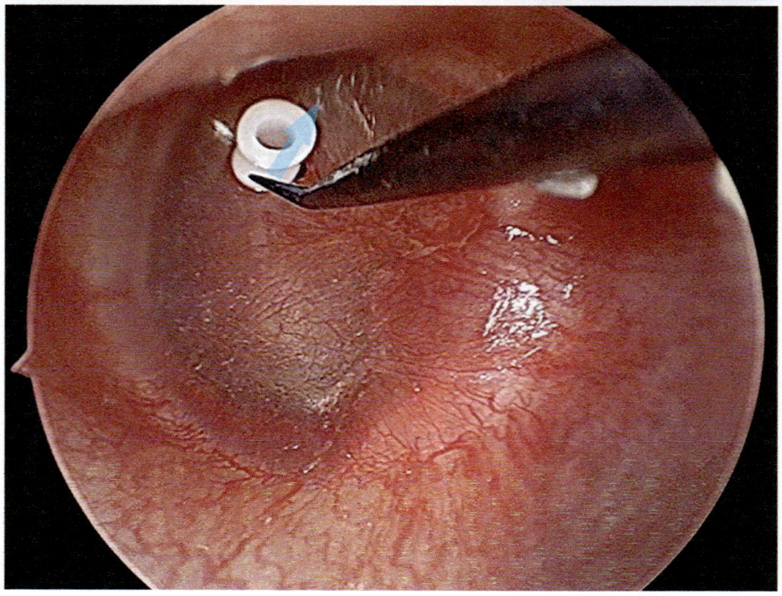

Fig. 6D: Grommet being gently pushed on its posterior aspect.

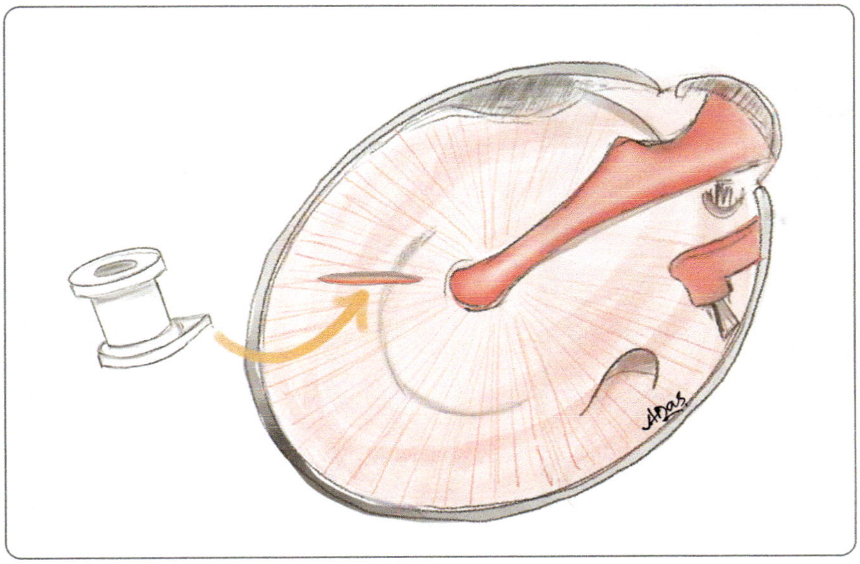

Fig. 7A: Site of placement of grommet.

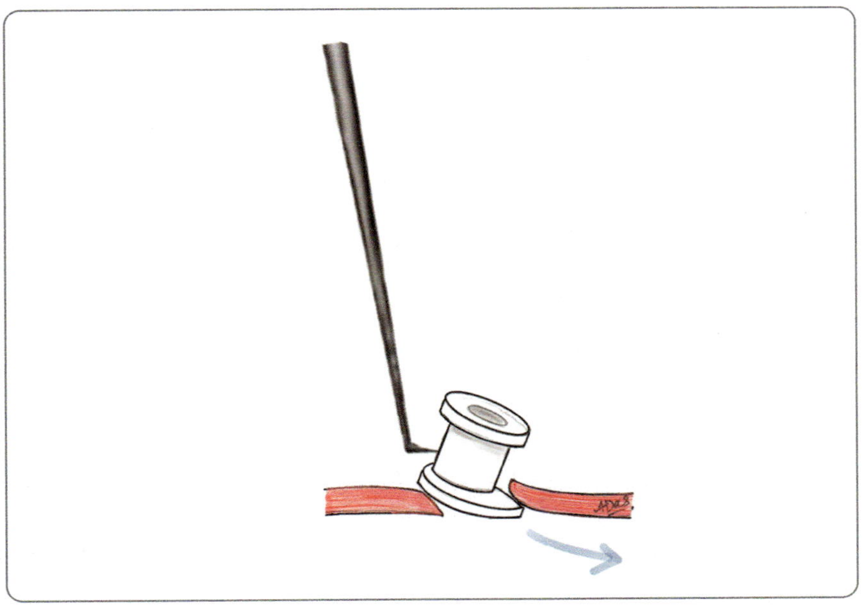

Fig. 7B: Use of angled pick to gently push on posterior aspect of grommet.

A tube placed anteriorly is also associated with a reduced but nonsignificant reduction in persistent perforation compared to a tube placed posteriorly in the tympanic membrane (1.8% vs. 3.7%).[5]

Placement of the grommet anteroinferiorly compared with placement posteroinferiorly lengthens the time a Shepard ventilation tube remains in situ (80% vs. 45% at 6 months and 30% vs. 15% at 12 months)[4] but the longer a tube stays *in situ*, the higher the chance of complications, including plugging of the lumen, infection, thinning, and collapse of the tympanic membrane with possible retraction and permanent perforation.[6]

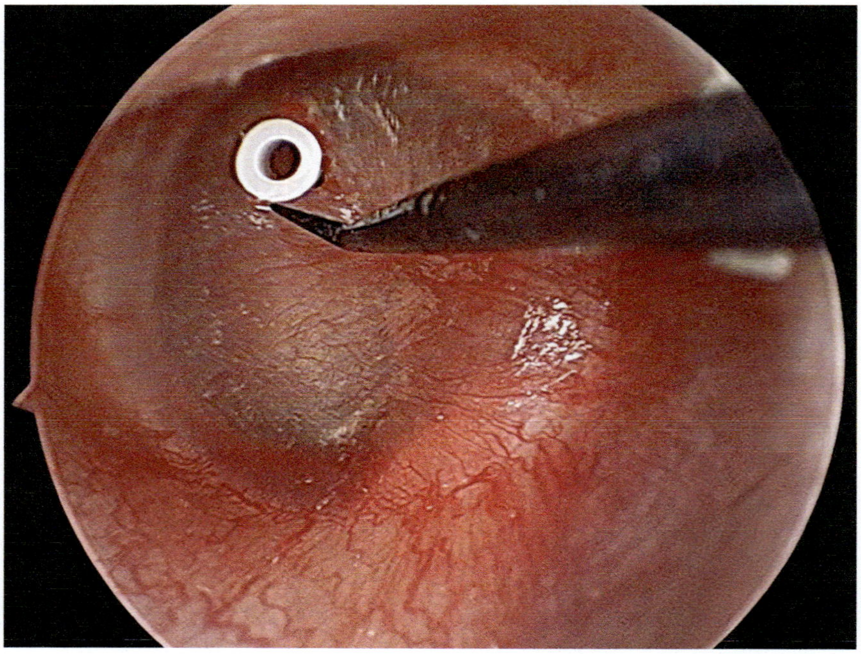

Fig. 8A: Palpation (from sides) using fine pick to ensure snuggly fitting the tube onto the tympanic membrane.

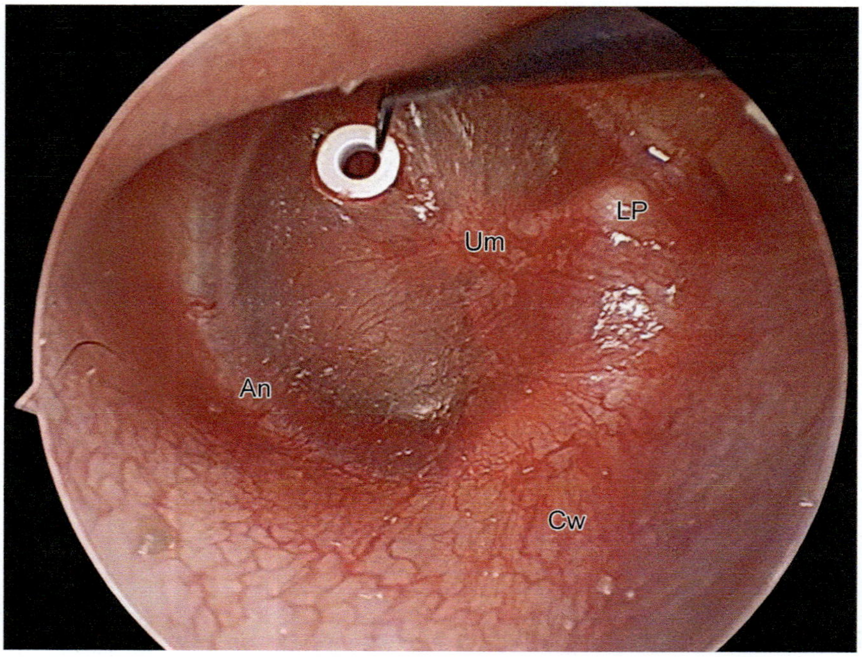

Fig. 8B: Palpation (from top) using fine pick to ensure snuggly fitting the tube onto the tympanic membrane.
(An: annular ring; LP: lateral process of malleus; Um: umbo; Cw: canal wall)

It is advisable not to place any gel foam or cotton pledget at the opening of the grommet as it incites further inflammation and plugging of the tube.

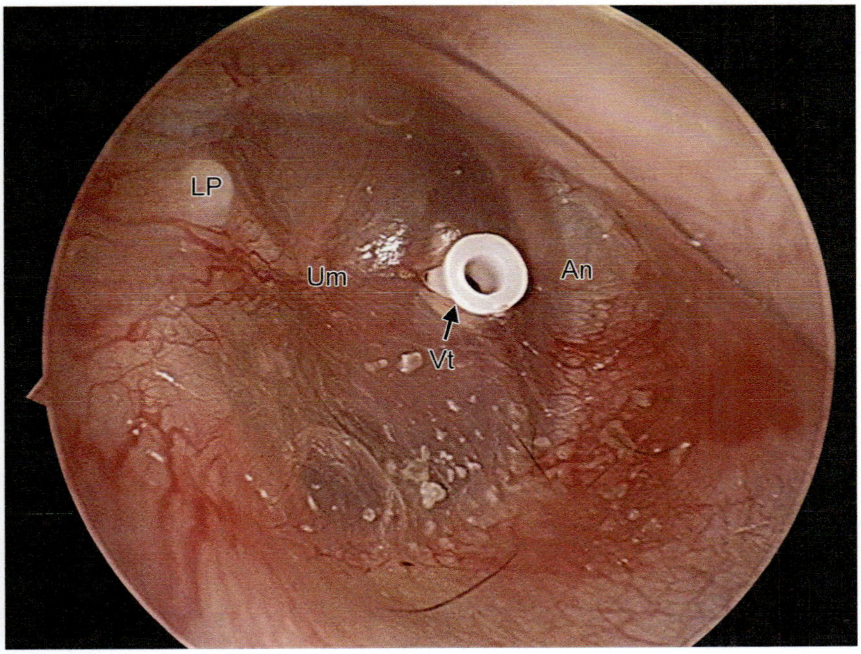

Fig. 9A: Final view after placement of ventilation tube (grommet) on right ear with reference to landmarks: Intraoperative view. (An: annular ring; LP: lateral process of malleus; Um: umbo; Vt: ventilation tube)

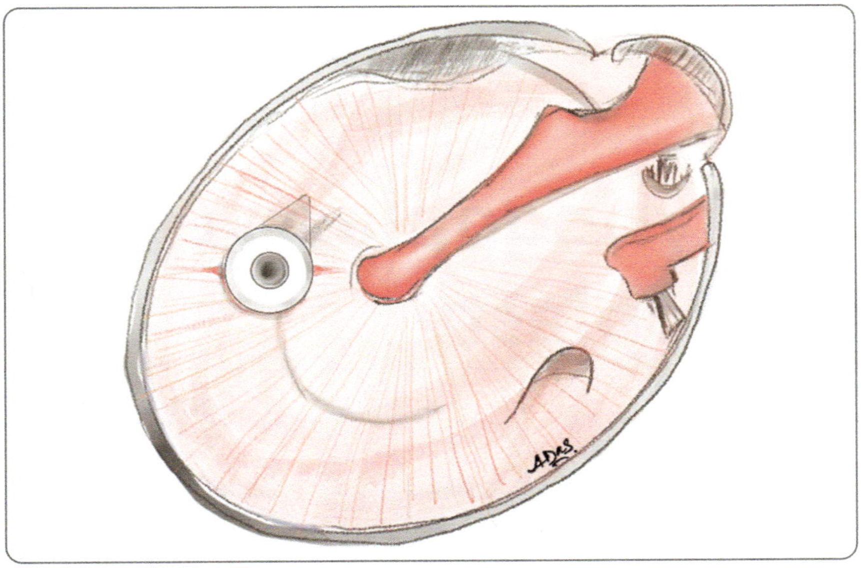

Fig. 9B: Final view after placement of ventilation tube (grommet) on left ear with reference to landmarks: Pictorial depiction.

REFERENCES

1. Orchik DJ, Dunn JW, McNutt L. Tympanometry as a predictor of middle ear effusion. Arch Otolaryngol. 1978;104:4-6.
2. Guttenplan MD, Tom WC, DeVito MA, Handler SD, Wetmore RF, Potsic WP. Radial versus circumferential incision in myringotomy and tube placement. Int J Pediatr Otorhinolaryngol. 1991;21:211-5.
3. Amer HS, El-anwar MW, Elfeky AE. The efficacy of adjuvant intratympanic steroid treatment for otitis media with effusion in children. Int Arch Otorhinolaryngol. 2016; 20(3):244-7.
4. Laina V, Pothier DD. Should we aspirate middle-ear effusions prior to insertion of ventilation tubes? J Laryngol Otol. 2006;120: 818-21.
5. Heaton JM, Bingham BJG, Osbourne J. A comparison of performance of Shepard and Sheehy collar button ventilation tubes. J Laryngol Otol. 1991;105:896-8.
6. Weigel MT, Parker MY, Goldsmith MM, Postma DS, Pillsbury HC. A prospective randomized study of four commonly used tympanostomy tubes. Laryngoscope. 1989; 99:252-6.

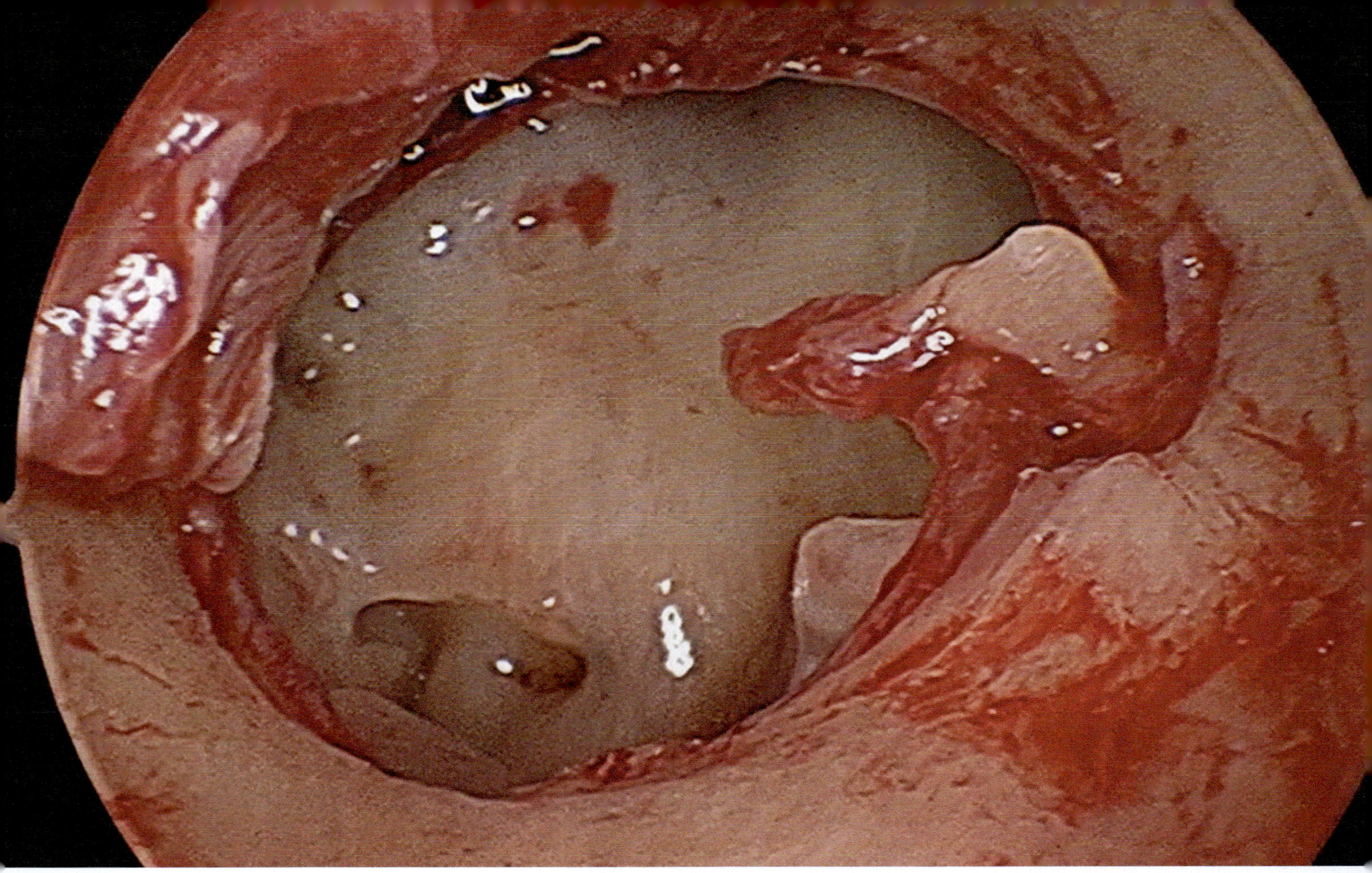

CHAPTER 7

Endoscopic Myringoplasty/ Tympanoplasty

Arindam Das, Sandipta Mitra

Chapter Outline

IMPORTANT DEFINITIONS

Myringoplasty is defined as the reconstruction of perforated tympanic membrane.

Tympanoplasty is defined as the surgical procedure performed to reconstruct hearing mechanism of middle ear.

INTRODUCTION

Otologic surgeries encompass a vast spectrum of surgeries ranging from myringoplasty, ossicular chain reconstruction, stapes surgery to epitympanic exploration, atticotomy, and mastoidectomy, which may be performed either endoscopically or microscopically.

In this chapter, we shall discuss one of the most important surgeries that should be mastered by all otologic surgeons, which forms the foundation of all otologic surgeries.

Reconstruction of tympanic membrane is one of the oldest otologic procedures, dating back to the 17th century, done by Banzer using pig's bladder.[1] Since its inception, tympanoplasty has undergone immense modifications in terms of surgical techniques as well as grafting materials.[2] Mucosal variety of chronic otitis media is the most common variety of chronic otitis media that is encountered by otologists in their day-to-day practice. Tympanoplasty being the mainstay of treatment for mucosal variety of chronic otitis media, all otologic surgeons must be proficient in this particular type of surgery.

Postaural, endaural, and transcanal are well-established approaches of tympanoplasty. Among these, endaural and transcanal approaches were devised to avoid the surgical scar and hence make it more cosmetically acceptable, in spite of having a number of surgical disadvantages such as compromised visibility and accessibility. Clear visualization of anterior annulus and protympanum is necessary for successful grafting.

Herein comes the role of endoscopic approach, which has been established as the most functional technique, having definite advantages over the conventional microscopic approach. Over several decades, thousands of articles and reviews have been published every year showing its clear edge over conventional microscopic technique.

INDICATIONS OF ENDOSCOPIC TYMPANOPLASTY

- Clinically diagnosed cases of chronic otitis media of mucosal variety
- Traumatic perforation not healing spontaneously
- Part of other otologic surgeries

SURGICAL RATIONALE AND ITS PHYSIOLOGICAL BASIS

- *Scarless*: Grafting materials are harvested either from:
  - Temporalis fascia via a small incision masked above the hairline
  - Tragal cartilage/perichondrium harvested via incision behind the tragus which is well hidden.
- *Excellent visibility*:
  - Panoramic view, visualization of the intricate details, and ability to look around corners
  - Entire tympanic membrane with all its quadrants and annulus can be visualized as a whole.
- *Visualization of protympanum and Eustachian tube area*:
  - Protympanum and Eustachian tube orifice can be clearly visualized using endoscope.
  - This is of importance during graft placement since it is often the cause of graft failure in the postoperative period.
- *Middle ear inspection*:
  - Ossicular chain, middle ear mucosa, and ventilation pathways can be clearly visualized in details using 0° and angled scopes.
  - No bone removal is required for visualization of hidden corners and incudostapedial complex.
- *More functional*
- *Less time consuming*
- *Minimizes complications*
- *Less chances to miss subtle ossicular chain erosion*
- *On detection of additional pathology such as ventilation fold blockage, it can be easily converted to endoscopic epitympanic exploration (EEE), without the need for additional instrumentation* (See Chapter 9 "Endoscopic Epitympanic Exploration")

Steps of Surgery

Patient Preparation

- *Anesthesia*:
  - Local anesthesia is preferred.
  - General anesthesia may be used in special circumstances such as apprehensive patients and pediatric patients.
    - *Local infiltration: 2% Xylocaine with 1:100,000 adrenaline is used.*
  - *Sites of infiltration*:

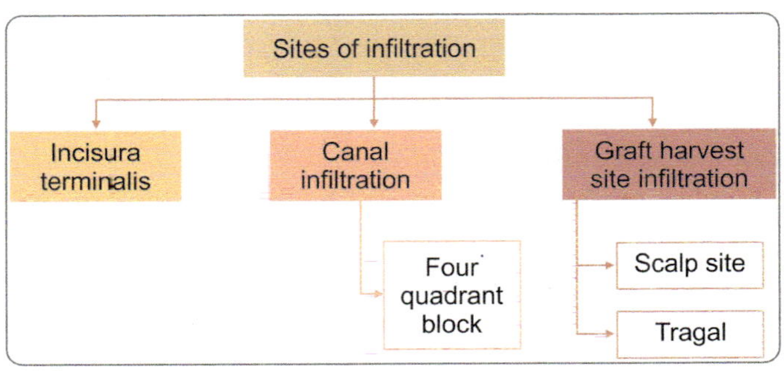

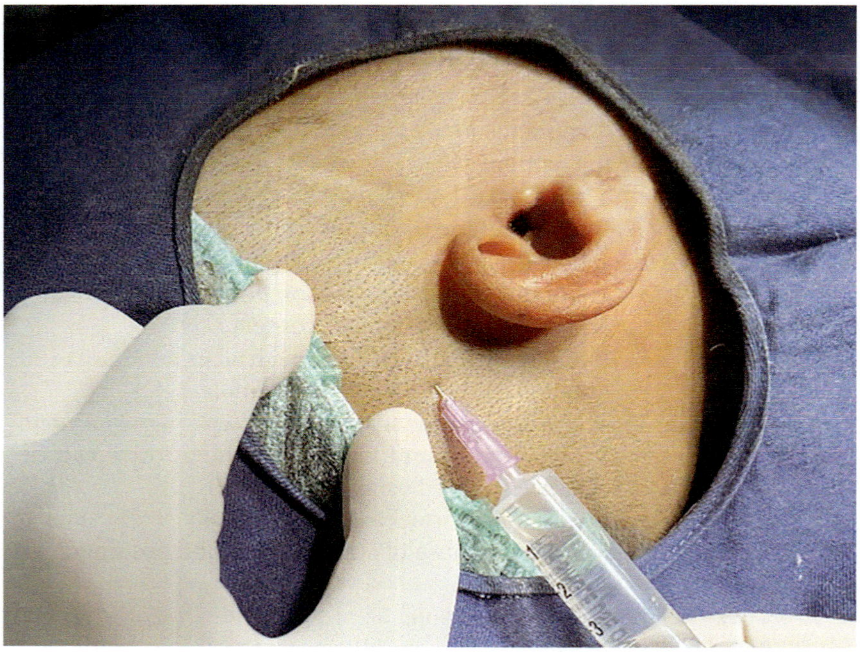

Fig. 1A: Local infiltration at the site of temporalis fascia harvest over the scalp just above the hairline (right ear): Aspirate before infiltration to avoid intravenous injection.

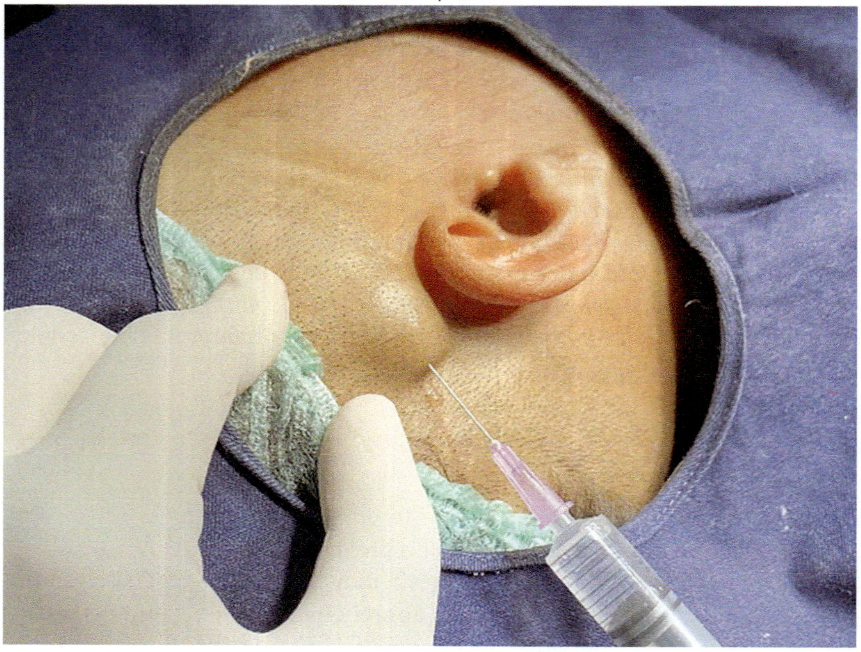

Fig. 1B: Local infiltration at the site of temporalis fascia harvest over the scalp just above the hairline (right ear).

PEARL

The piston of the syringe should always be withdrawn to avoid inadvertent intravascular infiltration of local anesthetic solution, which may have devastating consequences.

Four Quadrant Block

- 0.5 mL of local anesthetic solution is injected in each quadrant.
- The beveled face of the needle should be introduced facing the bone at or above the bony cartilaginous junction to inject the solution in the subperiosteal layer.

TIP

- Posterior quadrant infiltration should be done via the postaural groove.
- One should note the tenting of the canal skin by tip of the needle prior to injecting the solution.
  - This is essential for proper local anesthesia and to avoid bleb formation.

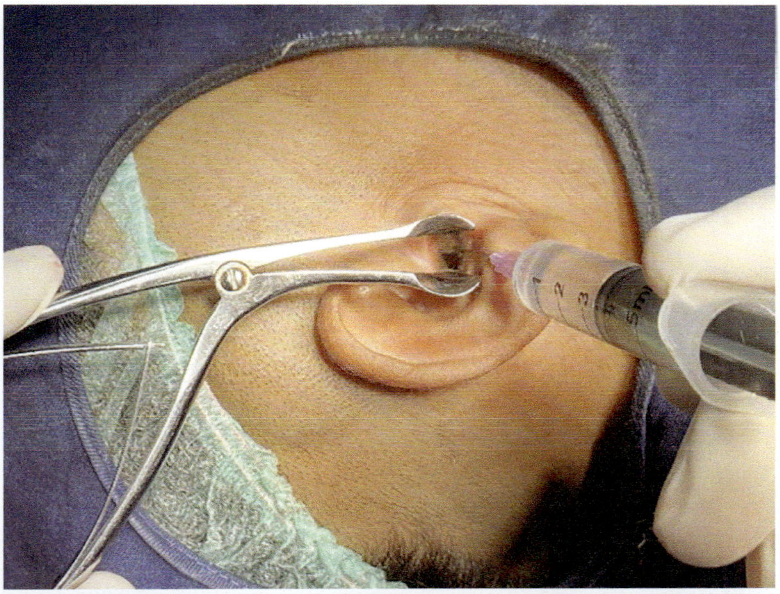

Fig. 2A: Sites of local anesthetic infiltration at anterior canal wall.

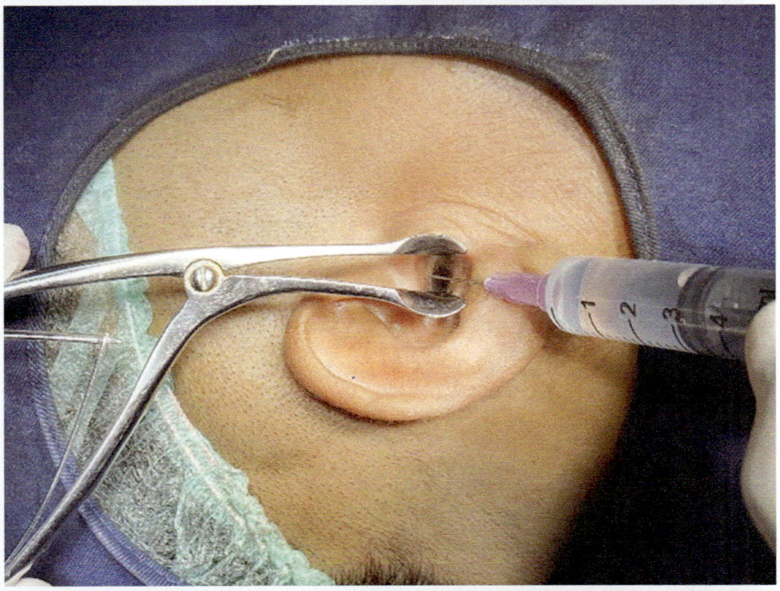

Fig. 2B: Sites of local anesthetic infiltration at superior canal wall.

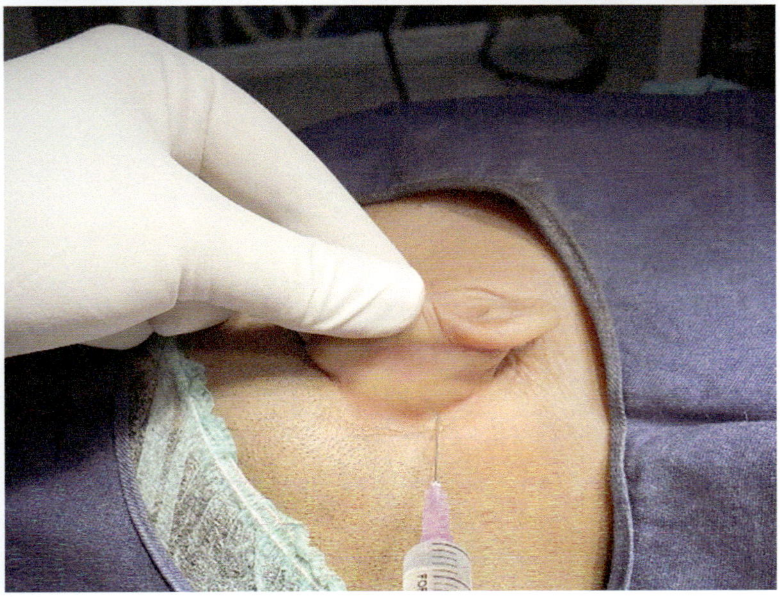

Fig. 2C: Sites of local anesthetic infiltration at postauricular region (For posterior canal wall).

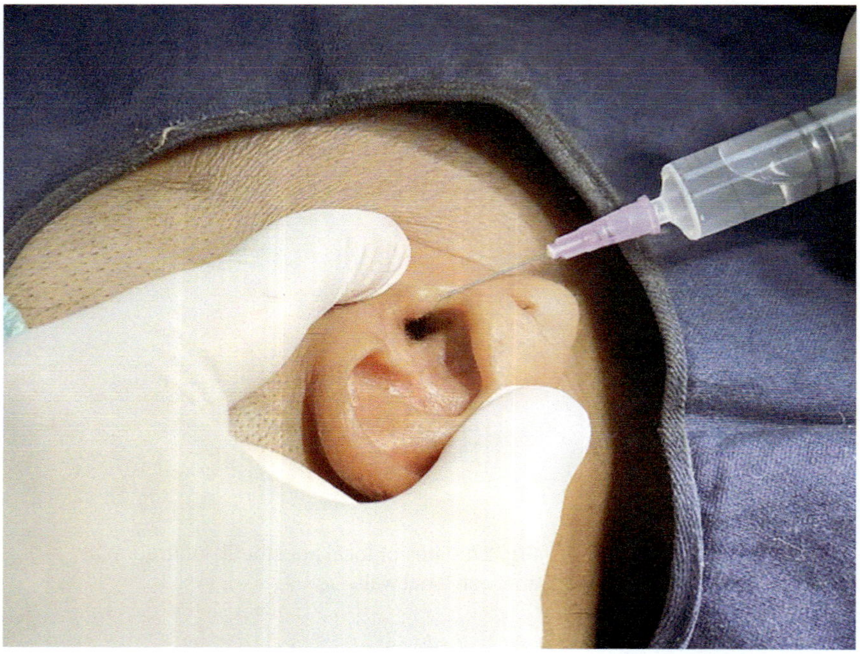

Fig. 2D: Sites of local anesthetic infiltration at tragal cartilage harvest site.

Ear Packing and Surface Anesthesia

- Middle ear mucosa is highly pain-sensitive, having multiple innervations (tympanic plexus and Jacobson's nerve)
- Surface anesthesia gives extra advantage in terms of analgesia and intraoperative patient comfort
- 4% Xylocaine with 1:1,000 adrenaline is used.
- *Advantages*:
  - Surface anesthesia
  - Excellent vasoconstriction
  - Mucosal decongestion
- Ear is packed with a cotton pledget soaked in anesthetic solution.

PEARL

- Following infiltration, the anesthetic solution accumulates in the subperiosteal space causing bleb formation and narrowing of canal dimensions leading to a fish-mouth appearance.
- Ear packing helps in dissipation of the local anesthetic in proper space and opens up the canal dimensions due to tamponade effect

- This packing is done 5–10 minutes prior to making the incision.

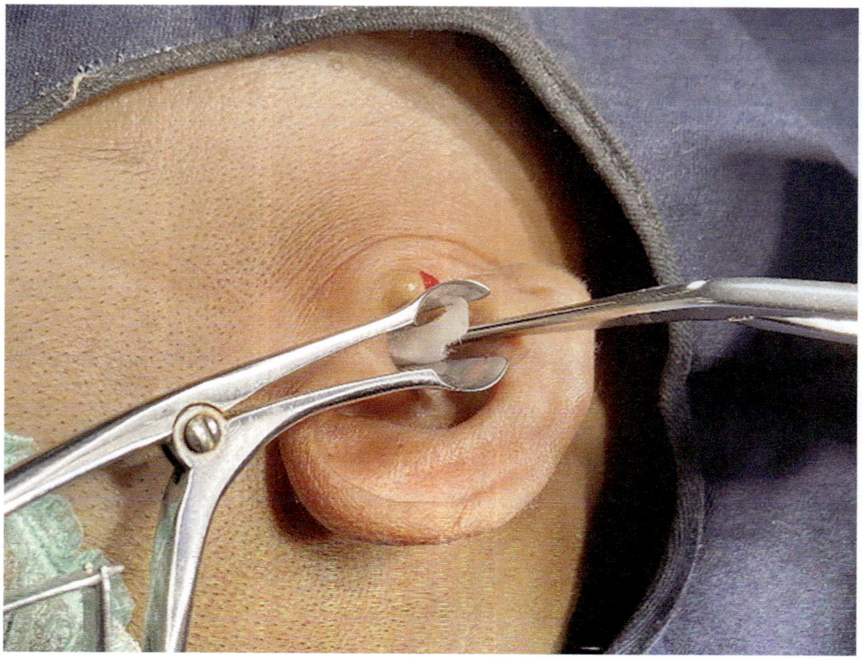

Fig. 3A: Packing of external auditory canal following four-quadrant local anesthetic infiltration.

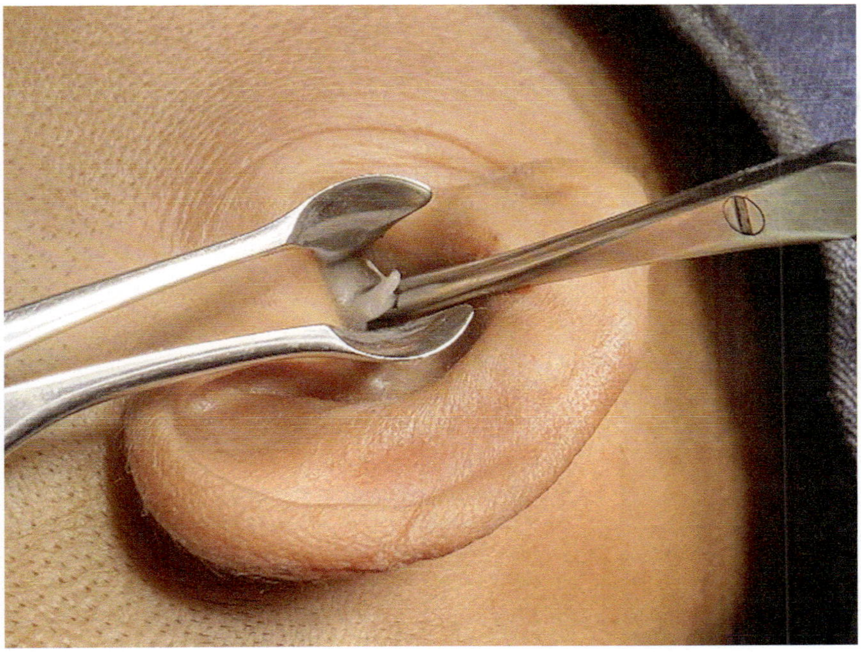

Fig. 3B: Packing of external auditory canal following four-quadrant local anesthetic infiltration: Close-up view.

Tranexamic Acid Protocol

Tranexamic acid protocol is followed to minimize intraoperative bleeding. Slow intravenous tranexamic acid bolus (10 mg/kg) half an hour before the start of surgery followed by infusion (5 mg/kg/hour). The infusion is prepared in normal saline. (See Chapter 2 "Principles of Endoscopic Ear Surgery" for further details).

Canal Hair Removal

- External canal hairs (especially in male patients with dense hair growth) may obscure the visualization and cause repeated soiling of endoscope tip during surgery.
- The medial part of external auditory canal is packed with a cotton pledget.
- A curved iris scissor is used to trim the hairs.
- The convex surface of the scissors is placed along the curvature of the canal and the hairs are trimmed.
- After thorough saline irrigation and suction, the cotton pledget is removed carefully.

Stay Suture

- *Aim*: To straighten the curvature of the external auditory for better visibility and easy instrumentation
- 1-0 nonabsorbable suture material (nylon) is passed through bony-cartilaginous junction and retracted posteriorly and clamped with drape sheet
- Prior to its application, the surgeon should assess the visibility by retracting the pinna posteriorly and laterally and check the exposure.
- If a significant improvement is noted by this maneuver, the suture is applied.

FRESHENING OF MARGINS OF PERFORATION

- Pathophysiologically, permanent perforation is defined as epithelial migration along the margins of perforation.
- Margins undergo endarteritis, become thickened, avascular, and covered by squamous epithelium
- Adequate margins need to be removed with a sharp instrument such as sickle knife and microscissors.

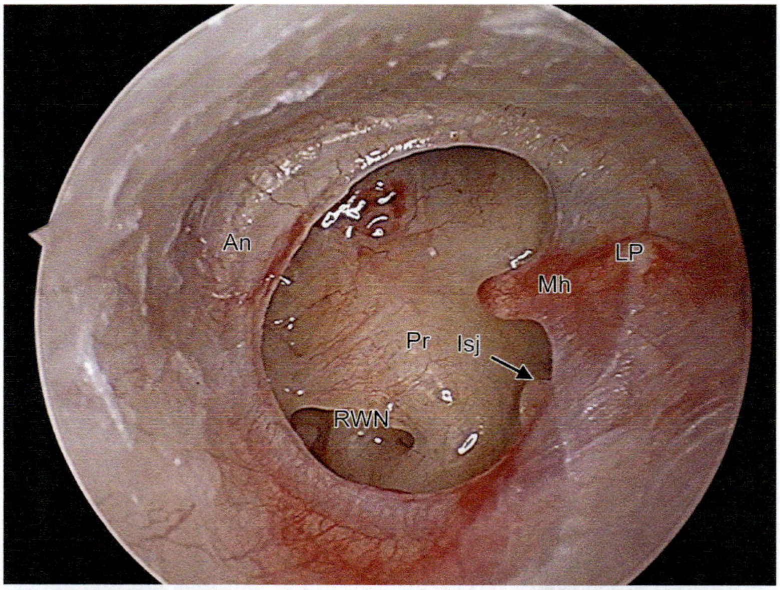

Fig. 4A: Otoendoscopy and visualization of the margins of perforation (left ear).
(An: annulus; Isj: incudostapedial joint; LP: lateral process; Mh: malleus handle; Pr: promontory; RWN: round window niche)

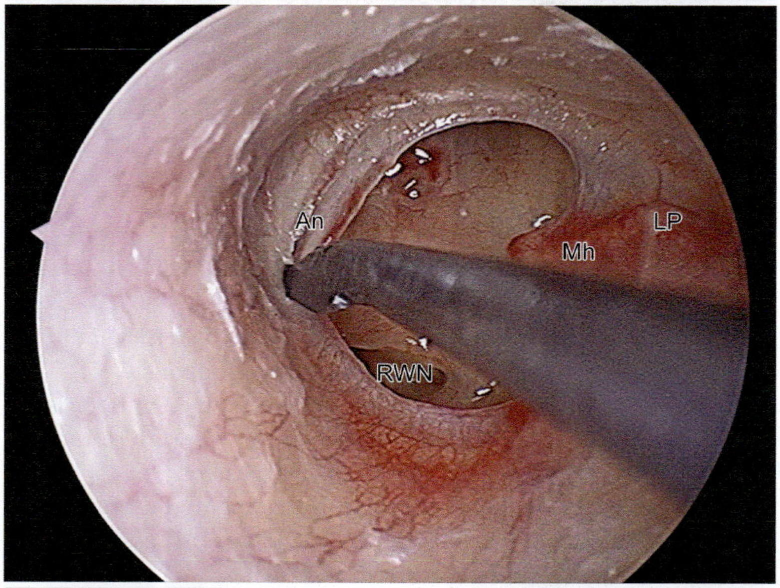

Fig. 4B: Freshening of margins of perforation using sickle knife.
(An: annulus; LP: lateral process; Mh: malleus handle; RWN: round window niche)

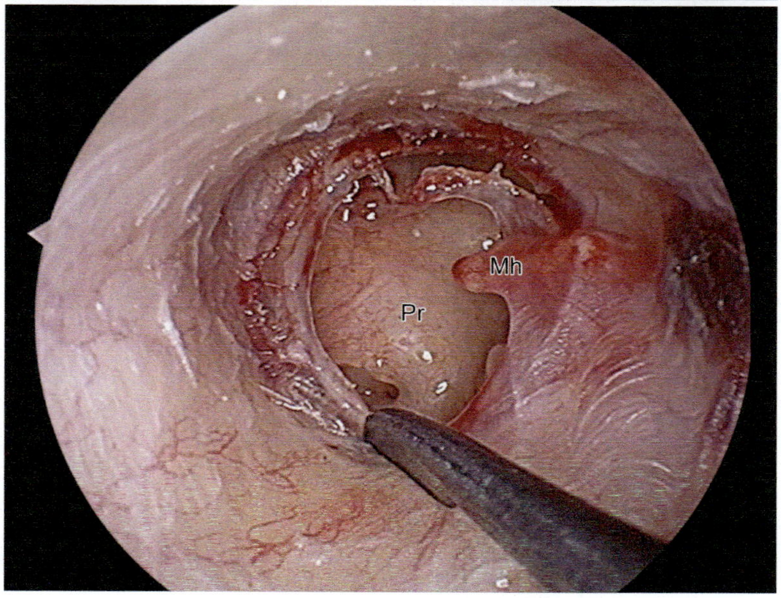

Fig. 4C: Rim of epithelium being incised along the margin of perforation.
(Mh: malleus handle; Pr: promontory)

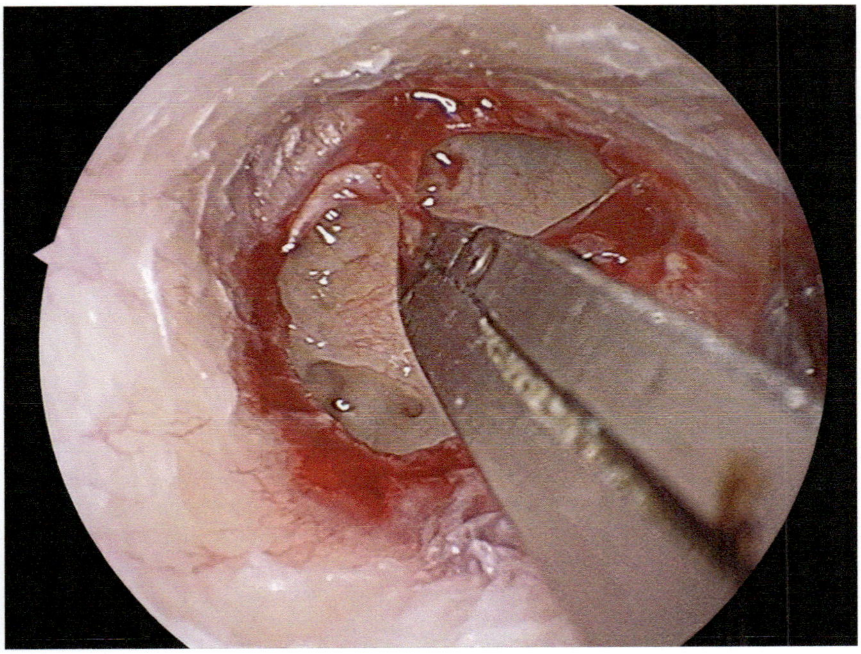

Fig. 4D: Final separated rim of epithelium being taken out using alligator forceps.

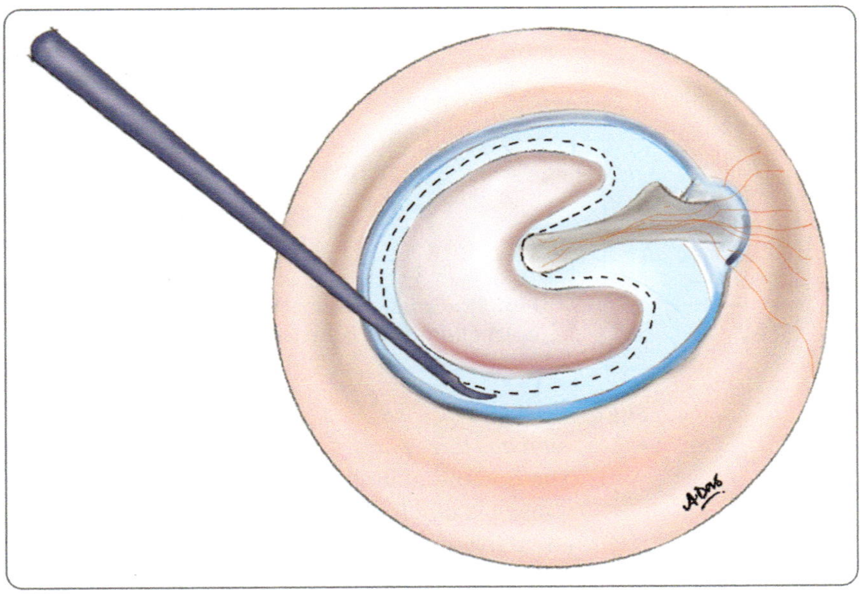

Fig. 4E: Pictorial depiction of freshening of margin of tympanic membrane perforation.

TIP

- In subtotal perforation, often there may be a very narrow strip of anterior margin.
- However, the surgeon should not hesitate to de-epithelize this narrow strip, in the fear of damaging the annulus.
- One should be very cautious about the tip of the sharp instrument while freshening the margin, which is often not directly visualized and may inadvertently injure the middle ear mucosa.

PEARL

- Margin freshening is one of the most vital steps influencing the graft take-up as it helps in proper epithelialization over the scaffold
- After freshening, bleeding from the cut margins is a good sign of viability and guides the amount of tissue to be removed.

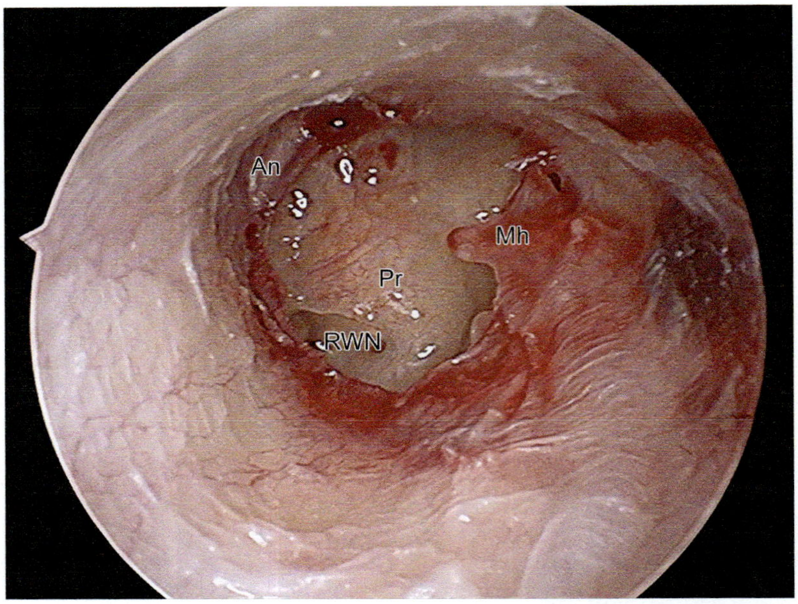

Fig. 5A: Remnant of tympanic membrane following freshening of margins. Note the fresh bleeding at the edges after permanent epithelium has been incised. (An: annulus; Mh: handle of malleus; Pr: promontory; RWN: round window niche)

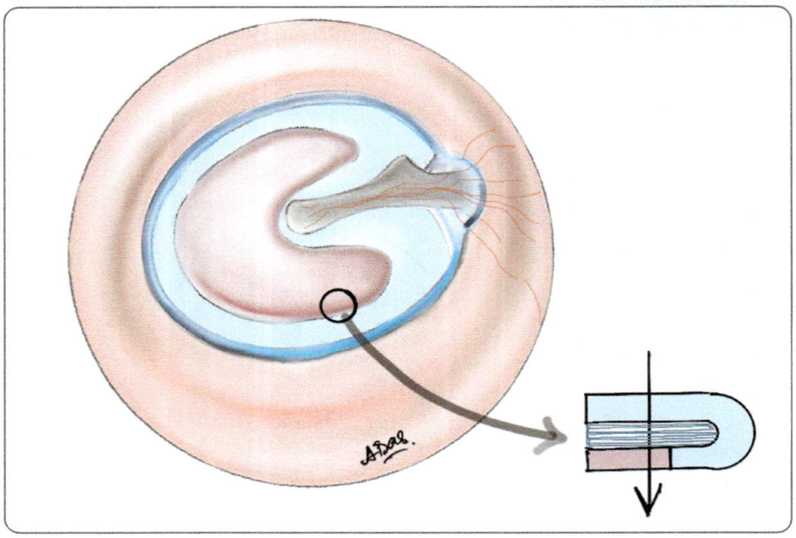

Fig. 5B: Cross-sectional depiction of permanent epithelium that is incised during freshening of margins.

INCISION

- Prior to placement of incision, one should palpate the annulus for proper judgment of depth and distance at which incision is to be placed
- Adequate length is vital as:

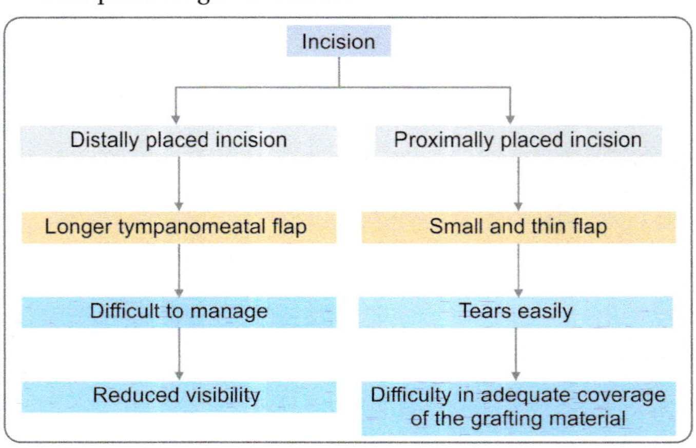

- *Site of incision*:
  - *Incision has three parts*:
    1. The horizontal limb is fashioned at a distance of about 4–6 mm from the annulus with the help of a circular knife.
    2. The superior incision is placed in continuity with the horizontal limb and is extended further anterior to lateral process of malleus.
    3. The inferior limb is positioned at 6 o'clock position, 1 mm away from the inferior annulus and joins the lower border of the horizontal limb.

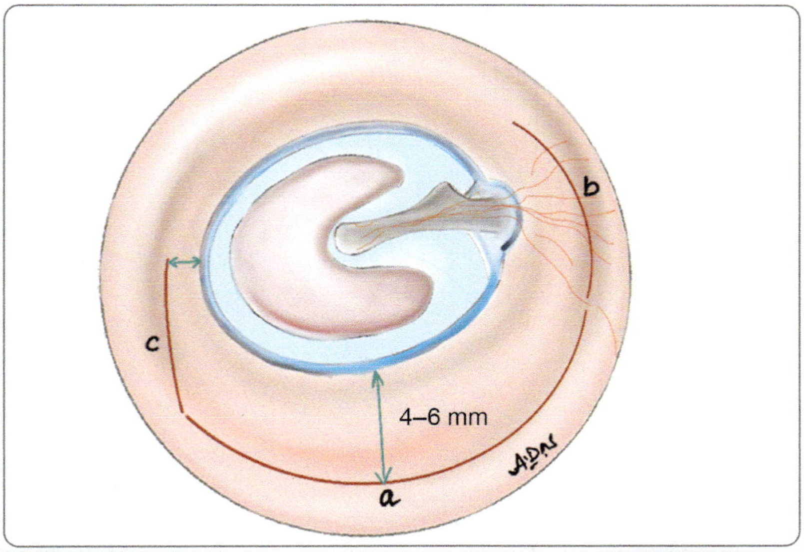

Fig. 6A: Pictorial depiction showing the surface markings of the limbs of incision (left ear).

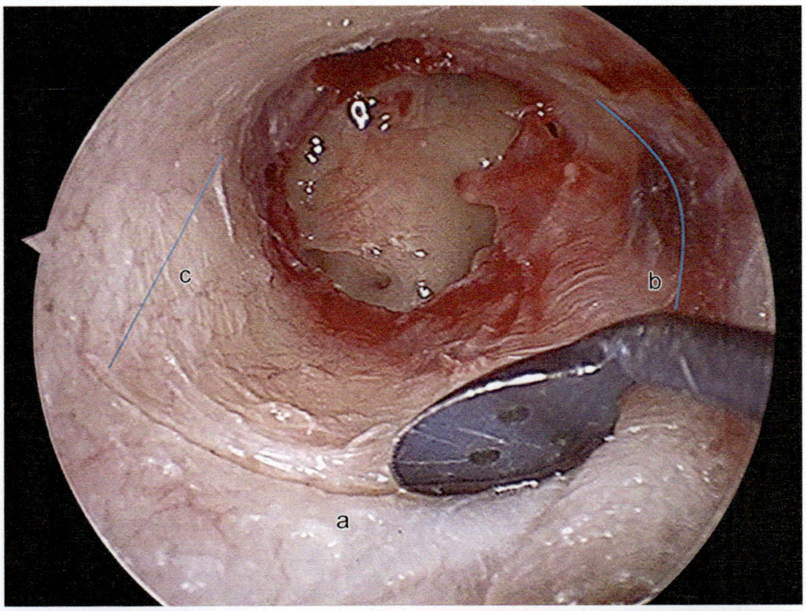

Fig. 6B: Intraoperative marking of the three limbs of incision (a, b, c).

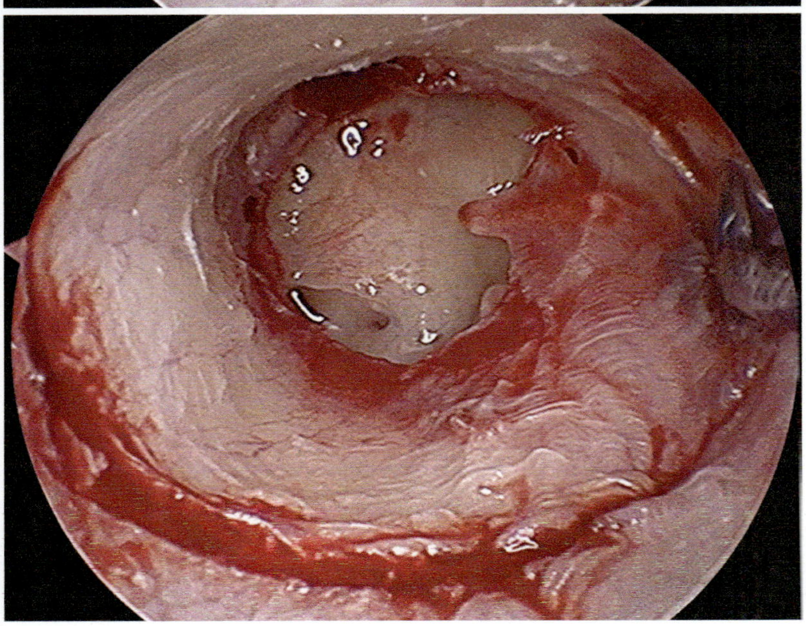

Fig. 6C: Superior limb of incision being marked with a side knife.

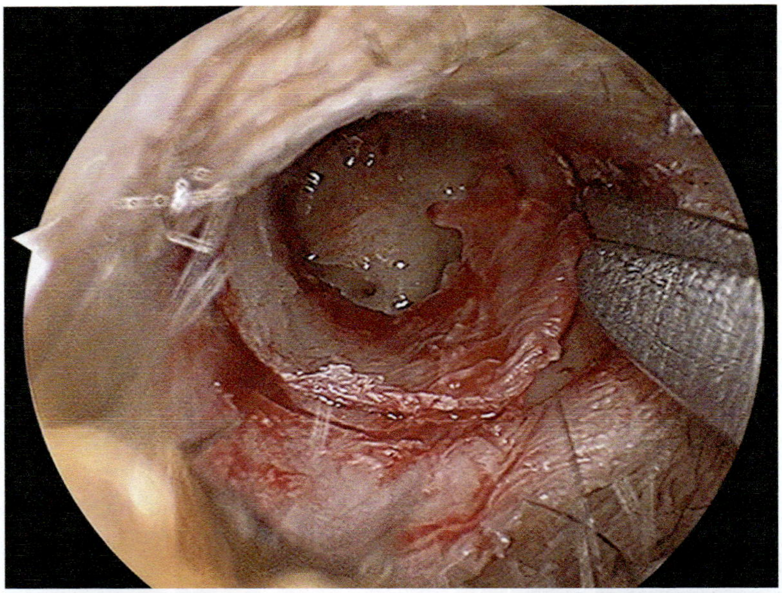

Fig. 6D: Thicker posterosuperior part of the flap being sharply cut.

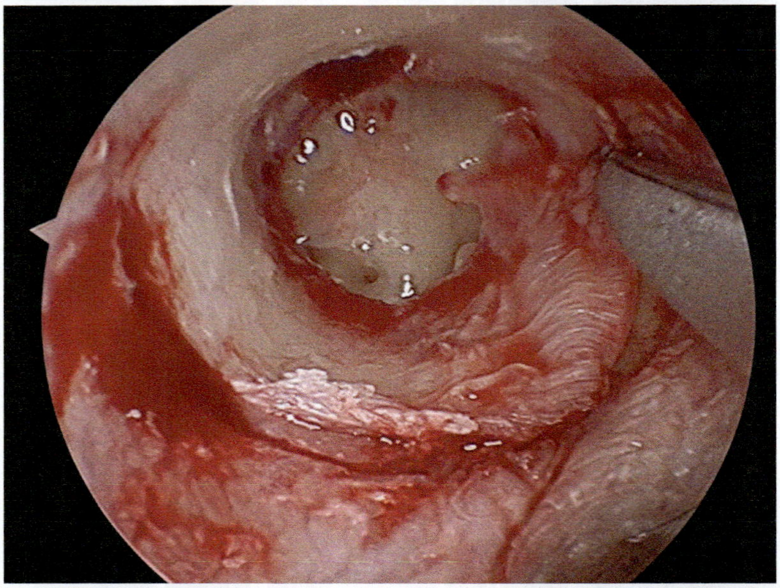

Fig. 6E: Thicker posterosuperior part of the flap being sharply cut (Use of iris scissor).

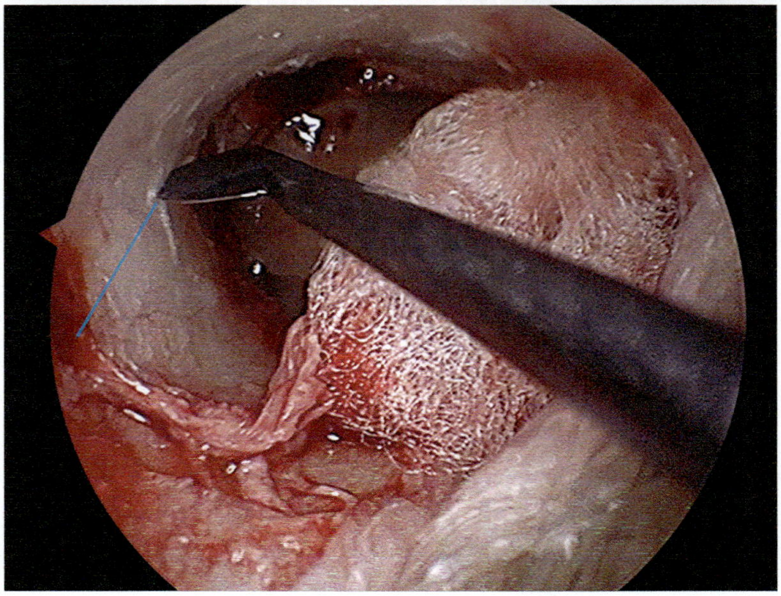

Fig. 6F: Inferior limb of the incision being marked.

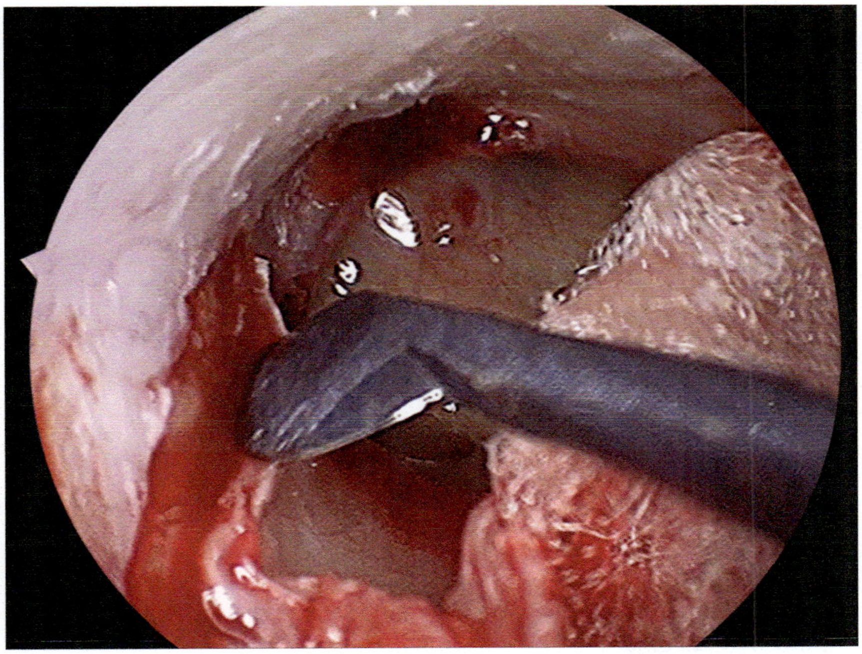

Fig. 6G: Elevation of the inferior limb of incision.

> **TIP**
>
> A sharp instrument should be used to make the incisions in order to avoid laceration of the canal skin margin.
> - Incisions should be made bone-deep
> - Posterosuperior part of the flap is thicker than the rest of the flap and needs to be sharply cut using a curved iris scissors.
> - Inferior vertical limb usually bleeds. Such bleeding should be controlled with adrenaline-soaked cotton pledgets before elevating the flap.
> - Many authors advocate the use of diathermy knife for flap incision to avoid bleeding
> - However, we usually avoid the use of diathermy for incision as it causes more tissue loss and delays healing

FLAP ELEVATION

- Tympanomeatal flap must be elevated slowly and meticulously.
- Adrenaline-soaked cotton pledgets are used during elevation of the flap, to control the bleeding.
- Suction instruments (circular and side-knife) may be used depending on the situation.
- Such instruments must be kept ready in hand.
- Flap is often tightly adherent to the underlying suture line.
- At such sites, the flap should be sharply cut in order to elevate it from the underlying bone.

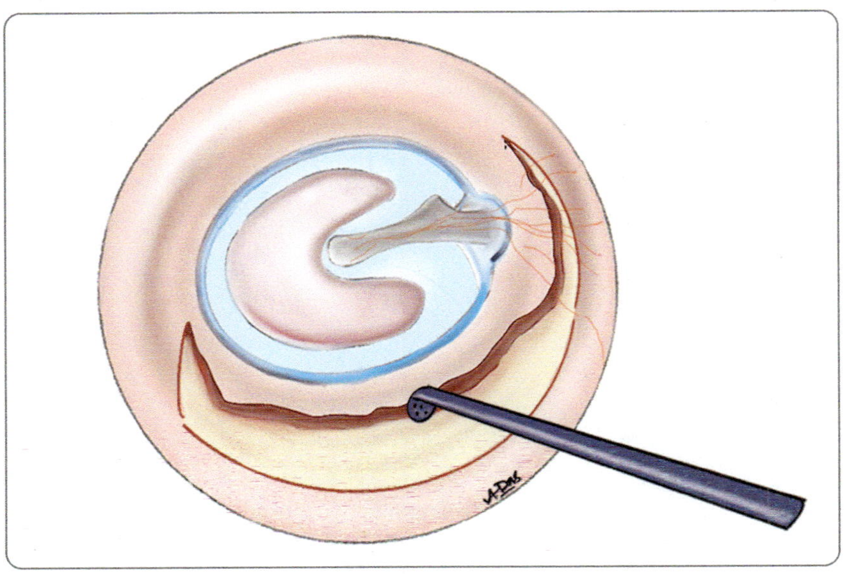

Fig. 7A: Pictorial depiction of tympanomeatal flap elevation.

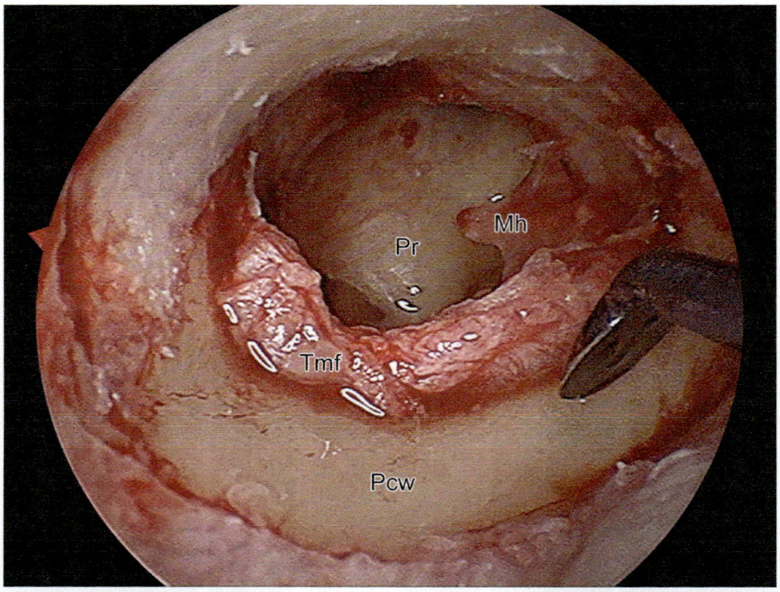

Fig. 7B: Tympanomeatal flap being elevated using a round knife.
(Mh: malleus handle; Pcw: posterior canal wall; Pr: promontory; Tmf: tympanomeatal flap)

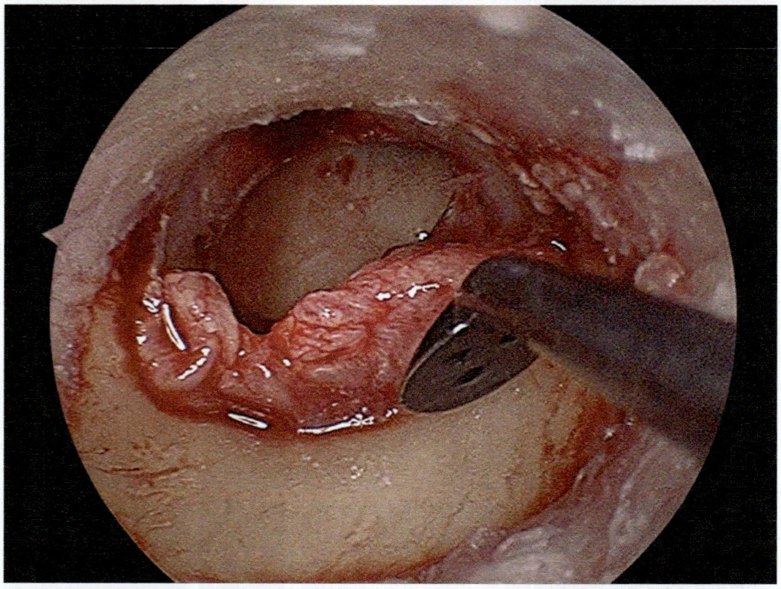

Fig. 7C: Tympanomeatal flap being elevated towards annulus using a round knife.

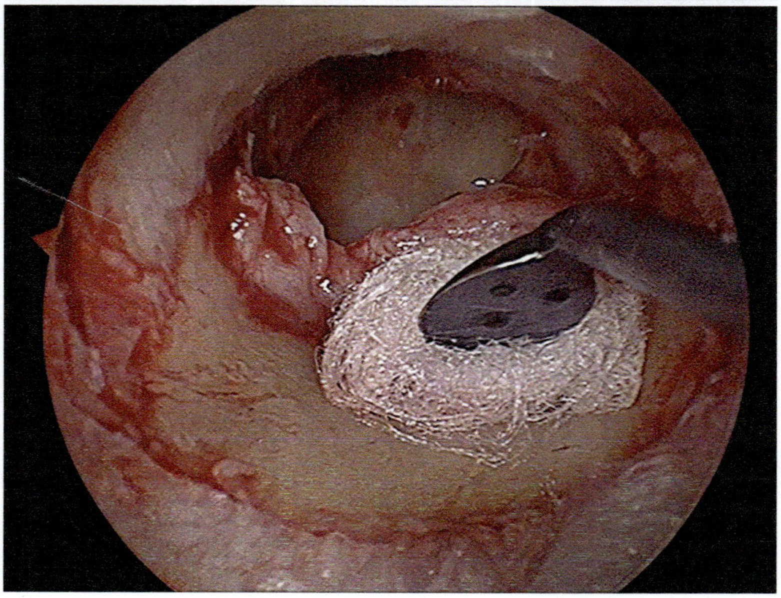

Fig. 7D: Intermittent use of adrenaline-soaked cotton balls to keep the field clear as well as protect the flap from undue pressure.

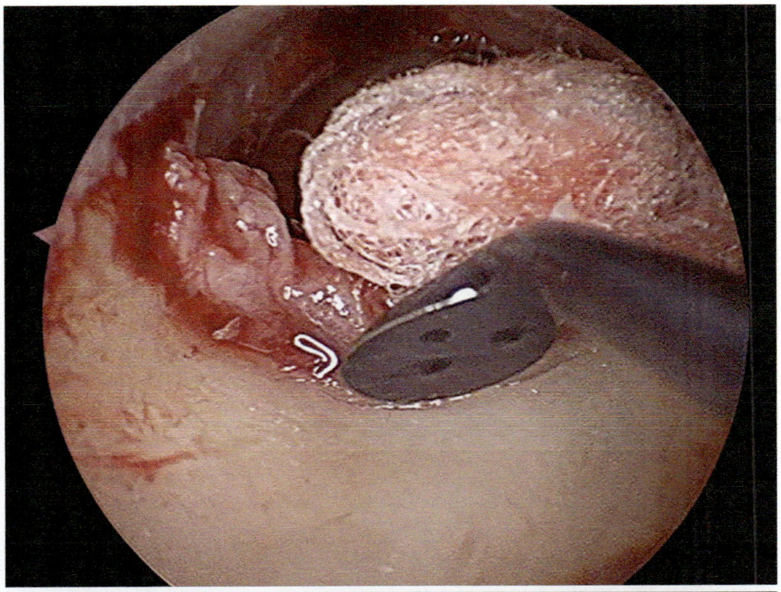

Fig. 7E: Cotton kept aside to check for the extent of elevation.

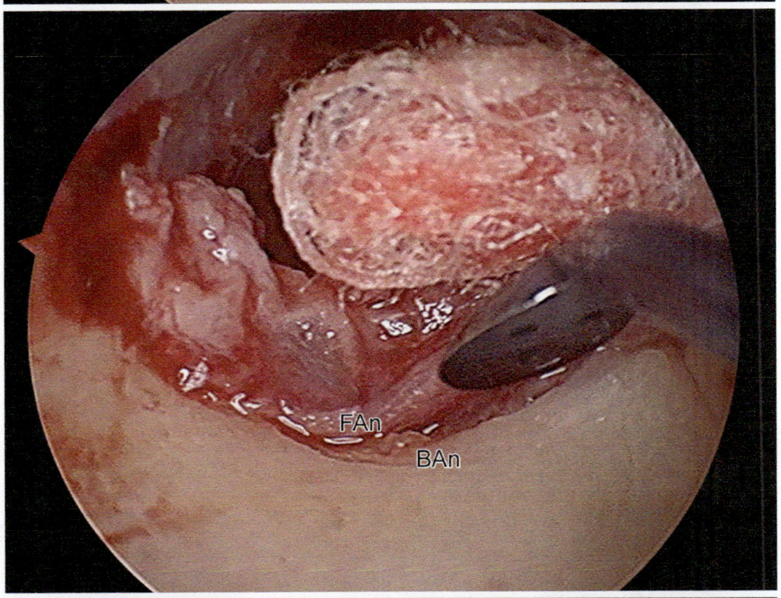

Fig. 7F: Dissection continued until the junction of fibrous and bony annulus is reached.
(BAn: bony annulus; FAn: fibrous annulus)

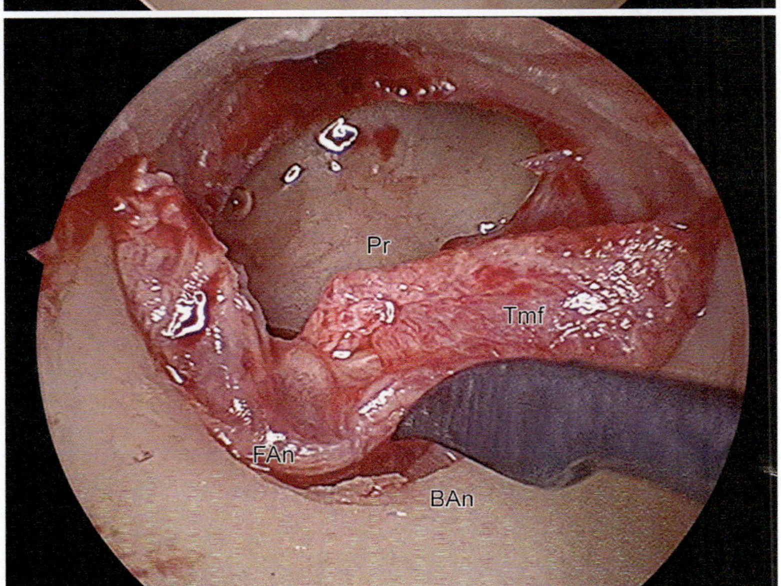

Fig. 7G: A sharp sickle knife is insinuated in-between the fibrous and bony annulus to separate them.
(BAn: bony annulus; FAn: fibrous annulus; Pr: promontory; Tmf: tympanomeatal flap)

- On reaching the bony annulus, one should pack the canal and wait for a minute.
- This increases the visibility of the annulus which must be clearly visualized before proceeding further.
- Annulus elevator and sickle knife are used to dissect in the plane between the fibrous and bony annulus till the chorda tympani nerve is identified.

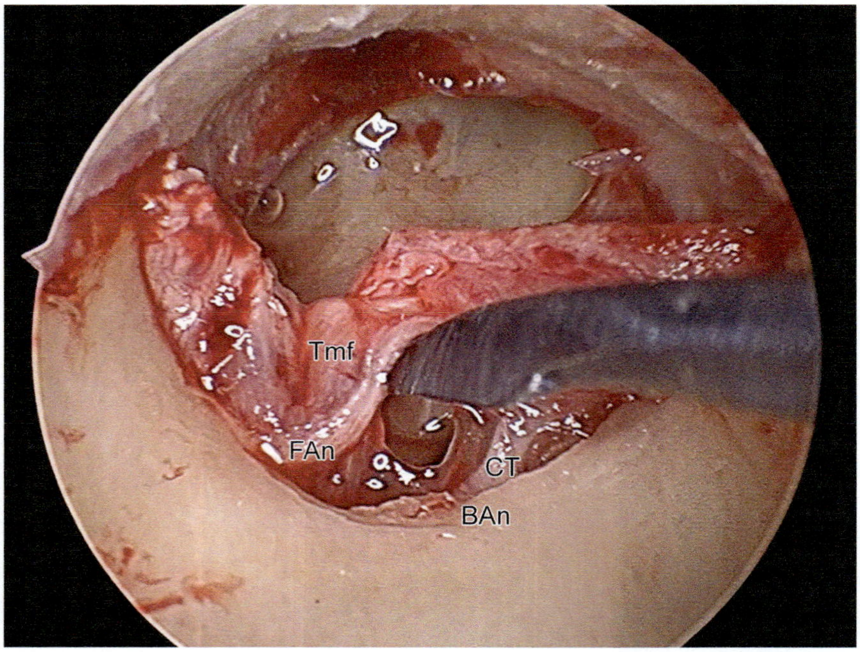

Fig. 8A: A sharp sickle knife being used to incise the middle ear mucosa and elevate the fibrous annulus.
(BAn: bony annulus; CT: chorda tympani nerve; FAn: fibrous annulus; Tmf: tympanomeatal flap)

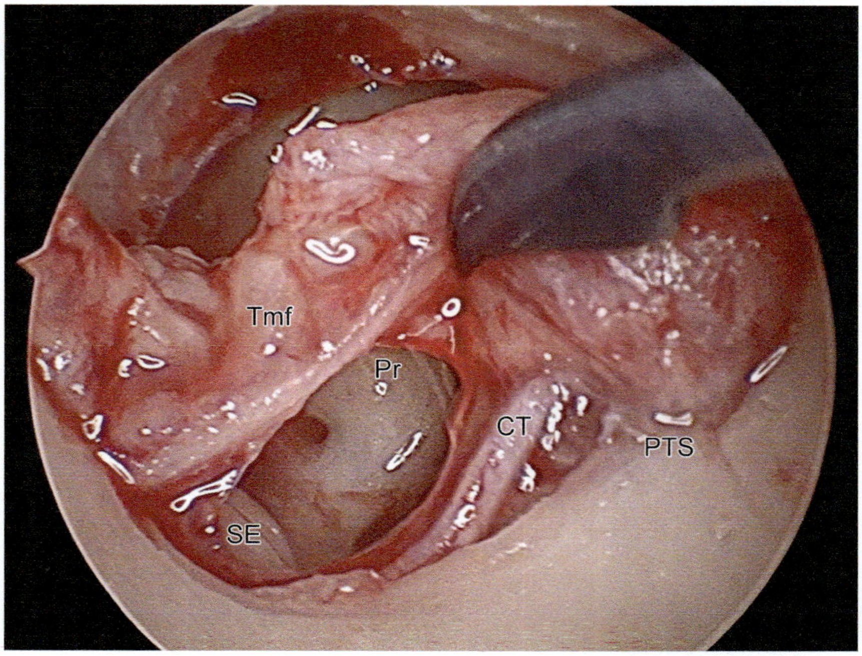

Fig. 8B: A sharp sickle knife being used to elevate the fibrous annulus further and dissect it free from chorda tympani nerve. Note the exposure of middle ear structures beneath.
(CT: chorda tympani nerve; PTS: posterior tympanic spine; Pr: promontory; Tmf: tympanomeatal flap; SE: styloid eminence)

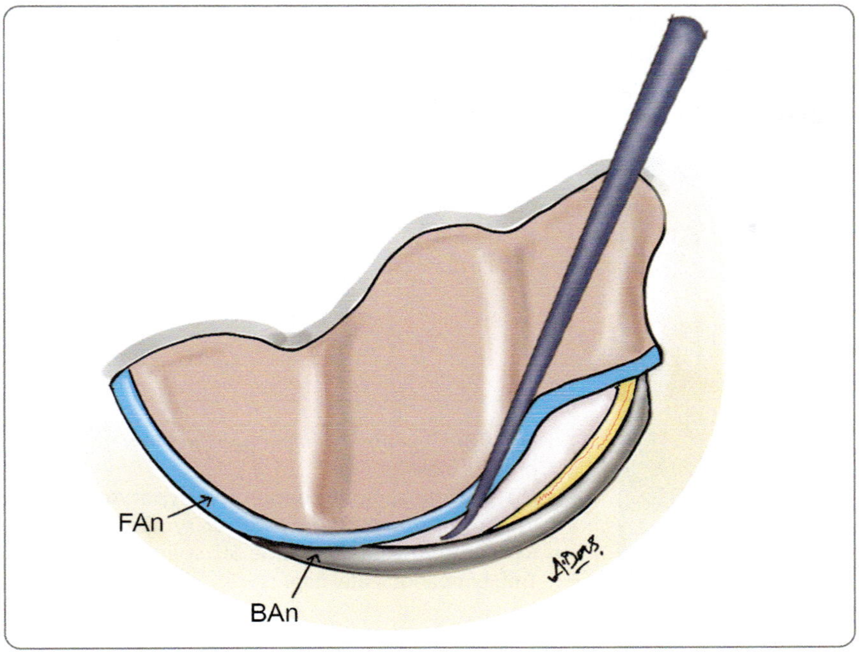

Fig. 8C: Pictorial depiction of separation of fibrous from bone annulus, dissecting the chorda tympani free.
(BAn: bony annulus; FAn: fibrous annulus)

TIP

- Sickle knife is then inserted in the plane between the annulus and the chorda tympani nerve such that the chorda is dissected free.
- The annulus, free from its bony and chordal attachments is then dissected inferiorly up to 6 o'clock.
- Superior flap elevation is one of the most challenging steps in single-handed surgery.
- Sharp side-knife is used to elevate the superior flap up to anterior tympanic spine.
- At this point of time, the lateral process of malleus is identified.
- A groove is created between the lateral process of malleus and anterior tympanic spine sharply.
- A sickle knife is inserted in the groove and incised sharply along the anterior border of handle of malleus up to umbo.

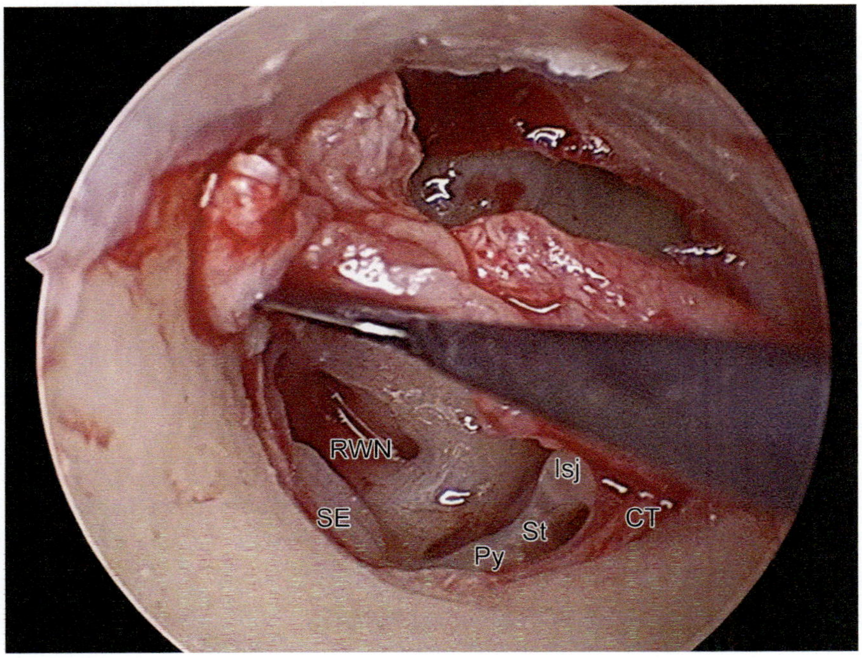

Fig. 9A: Elevation of tympanomeatal flap inferiorly.
(CT: chorda tympani nerve; Isj: incudostapedial joint; Py: processus pyramidalis; RWN: round window niche; SE: styloid eminence; St: stapedius tendon.)

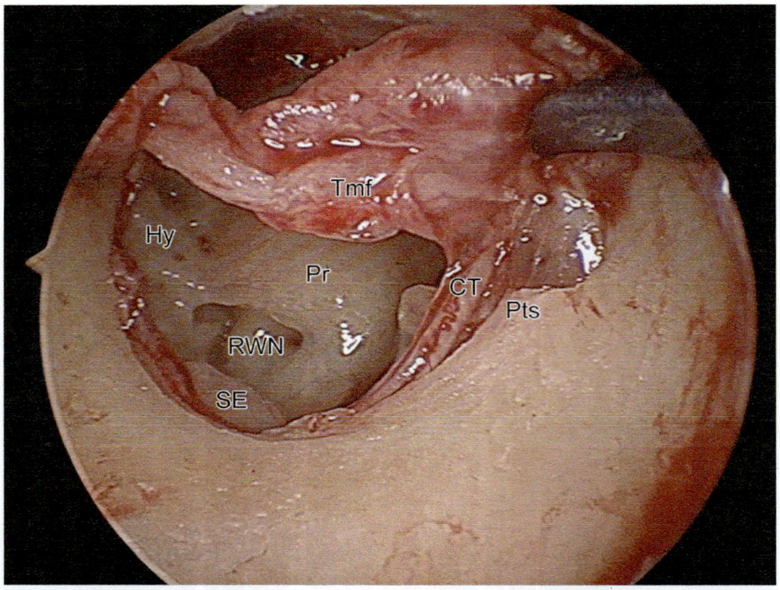

Fig. 9B: Elevation of flap superiorly toward lateral process malleus.
(CT: chorda tympani nerve; Hy: hypotympanum; Pr: promontory; Pts: posterior tympanic spine; RWN: round window niche; SE: styloid eminence; Tmf: tympanomeatal flap)

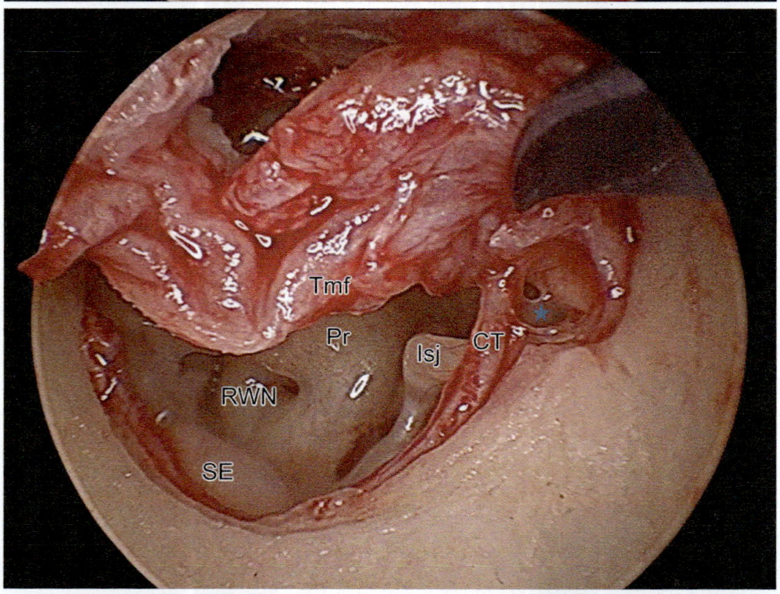

Fig. 9C: Palpation of lateral process of malleus.
(CT: chorda tympani nerve; Isj: incudostapedial joint; Pr: promontory; RWN: round window niche; SE: styloid eminence; Tmf: tympanomeatal flap)
Blue star indicates posterior pouch of von Troltsch.

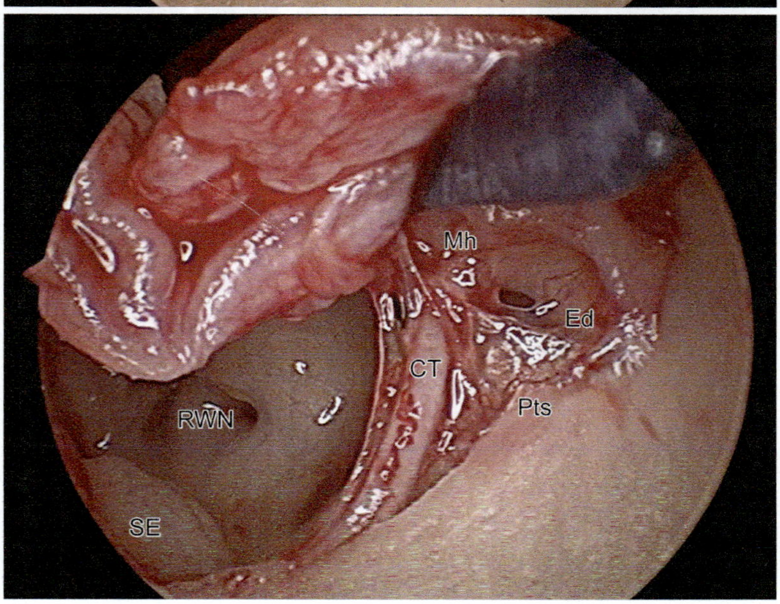

Fig. 9D: Sickle knife insinuated between anterior tympanic spine and lateral process of malleus and slid downward.
(CT: chorda tympani nerve; Ed: epitympanic diaphragm; Mh: malleus handle; Pts: posterior tympanic spine; RWN: round window niche; SE: styloid eminence)

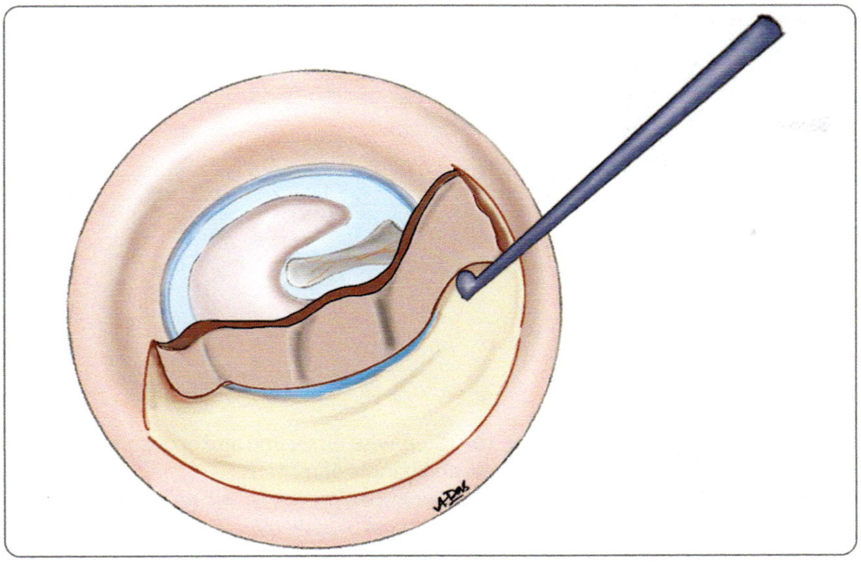

Fig. 9E: Pictorial depiction of steps of superior flap elevation.

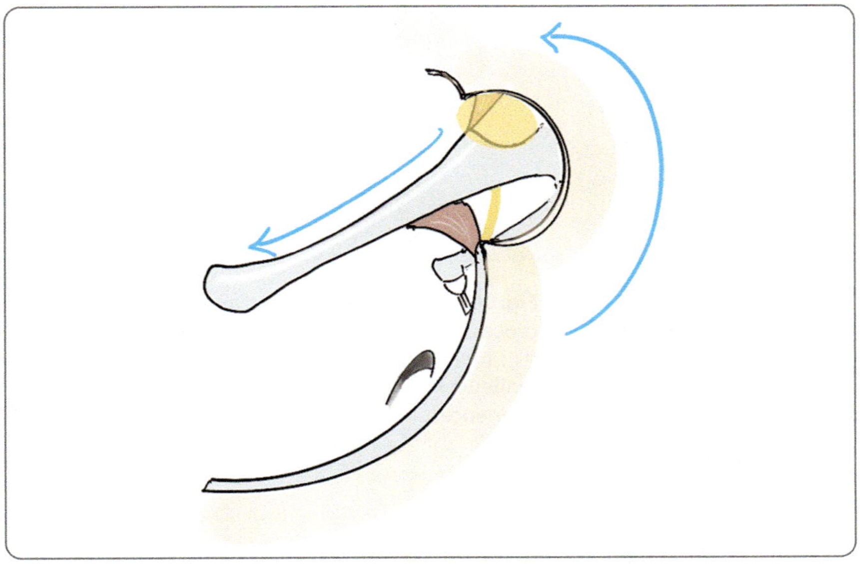

Fig. 9F: Pictorial depiction of direction of instrument movement.

PEARL

- This longitudinal axis is the strongest axis and any movement in any other direction may cause ossicular dislocation.
- Umbo contains strong fibrous attachments which need to be cut with a sharp curved iris scissors.

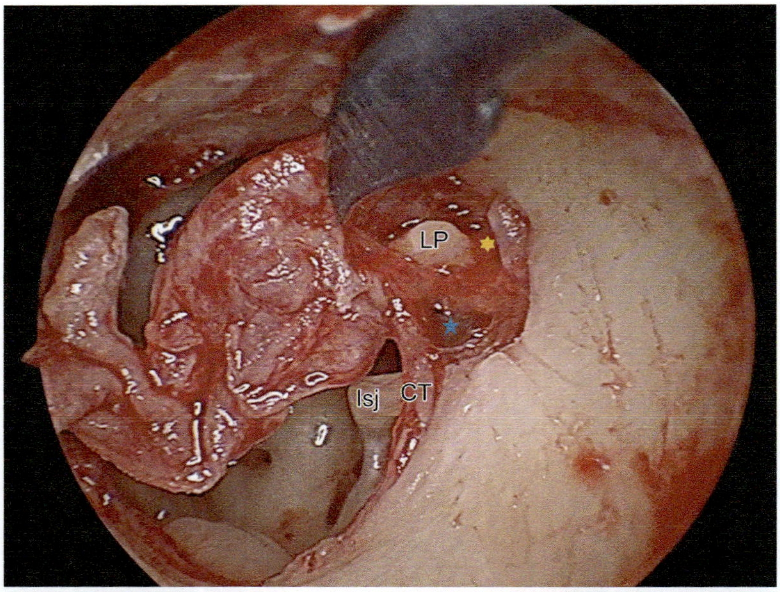

Fig. 10A: Step-wise dissection and exposure of lateral process and handle of malleus.
(CT: chorda tympani nerve; Isj: incudostapedial joint; LP: lateral process of malleus)
Yellow star—Prussak's space
Blue star—posterior pouch of von Troltsch

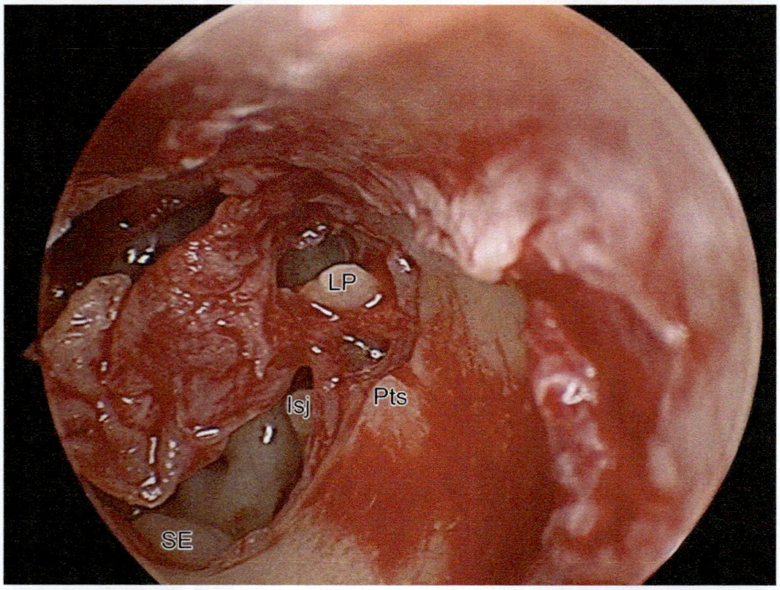

Fig. 10B: Step-wise dissection and exposure of lateral process and handle of malleus.
(Isj: incudostapedial joint; LP: lateral process of malleus; Pts: posterior tympanic spine; SE: styloid eminence)

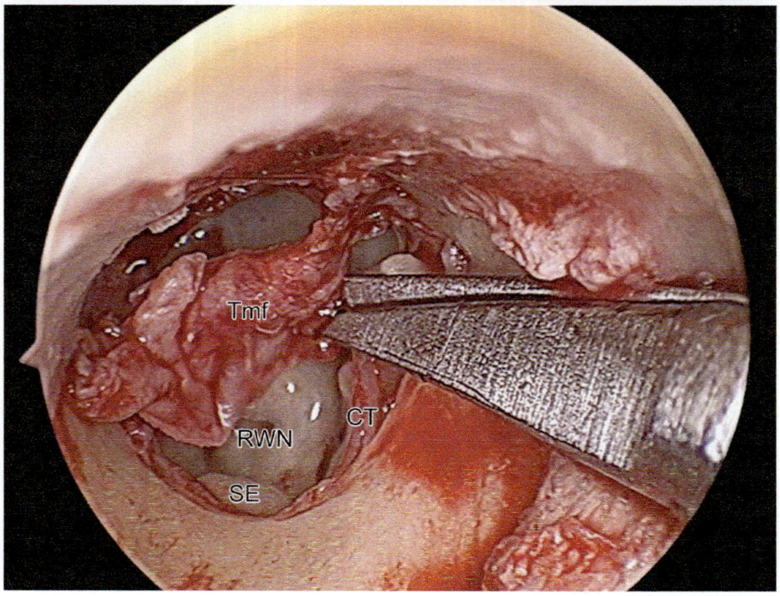

Fig. 10C: Step-wise dissection and exposure of lateral process and handle of malleus. (Sharp dissection at the level of umbo).
(CT: chorda tympani nerve; RWN: round window niche; SE: styloid eminence; Tmf: tympanomeatal flap)

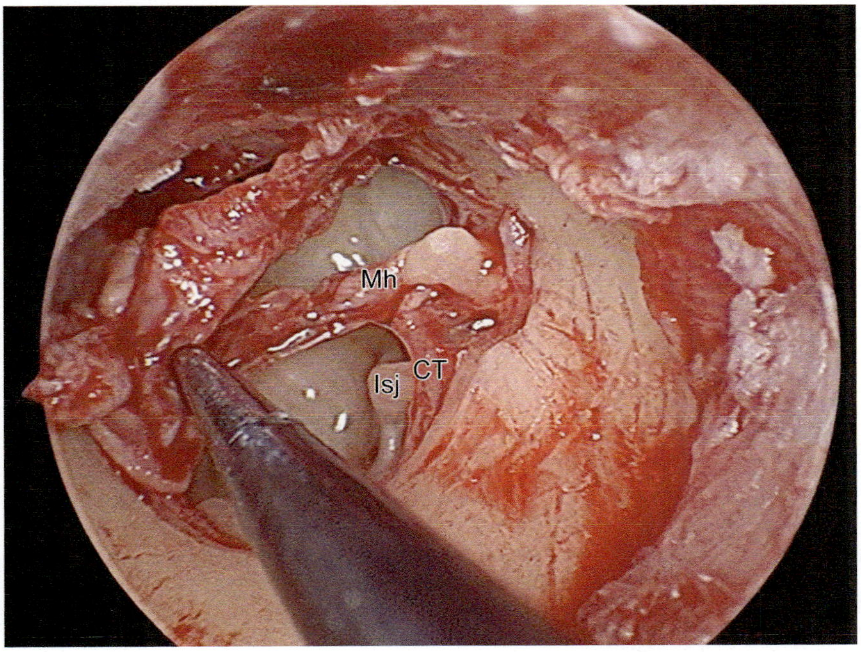

Fig. 10D: Step-wise dissection and exposure of lateral process and handle of malleus (sharp dissection at umbo using sickle knife).
(CT: chorda tympani nerve; Isj: incudostapedial joint; Mh: malleus handle)

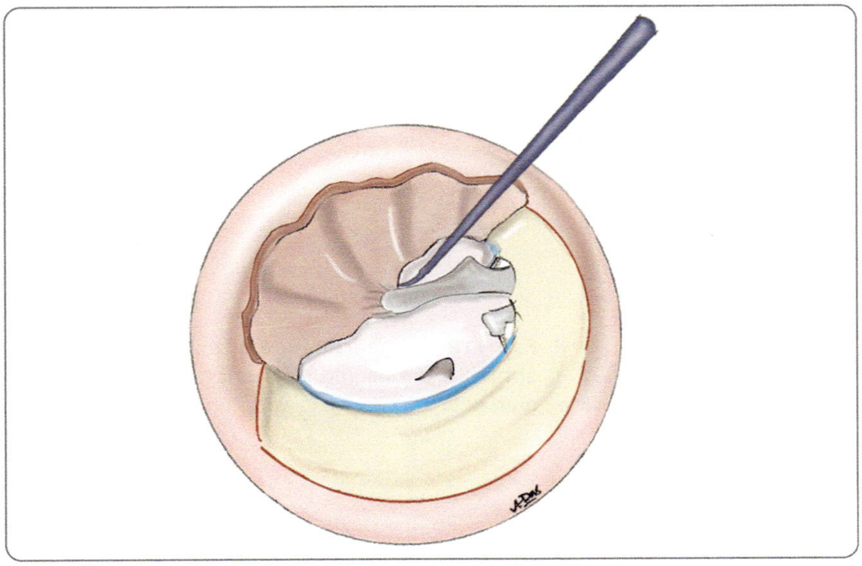

Fig. 10E: Pictorial depiction.

TIP

- Intermittent saline irrigations are necessary to wash away blood clots, epithelial debris and to decrease the middle ear temperature.

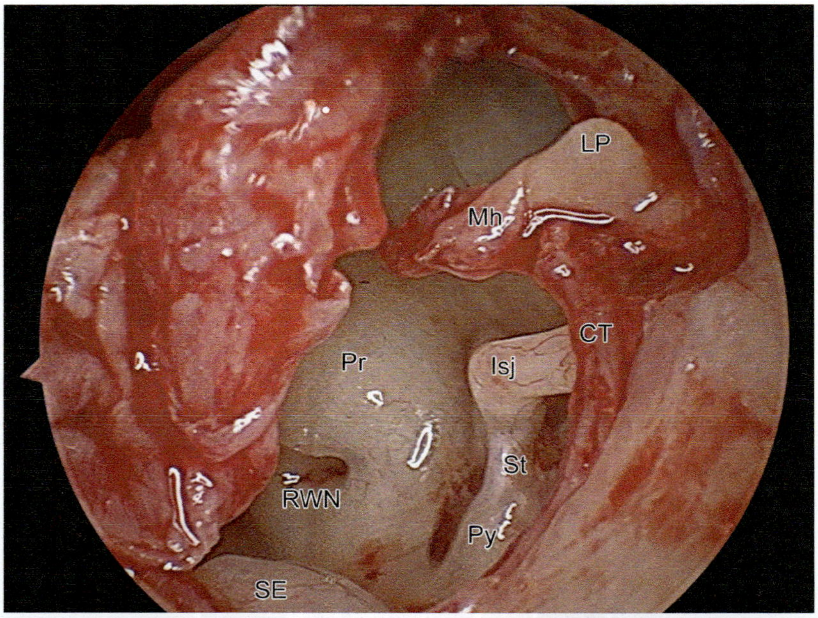

Fig. 11A: Intraoperative view of middle ear structures following exposure of handle of malleus.
(CT: chorda tympani nerve; Isj: incudostapedial joint; LP: lateral process of malleus; Mh: malleus handle; Pr: promontory; Py: processus pyramidalis; RWN: round window niche; SE: styloid eminence; St: stapedius tendon)

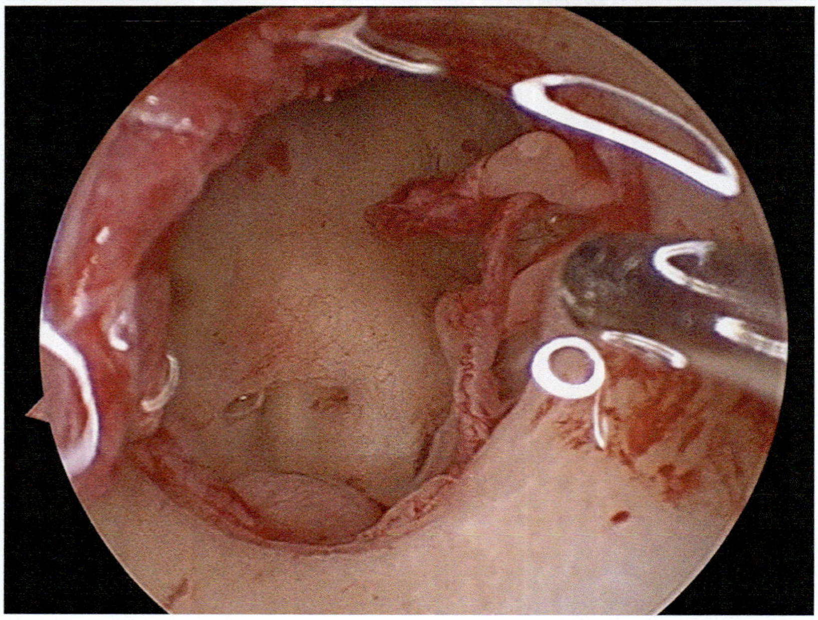

Fig. 11B: Saline irrigation of middle ear to clear epithelial debris and clots prior to preparation of graft bed.

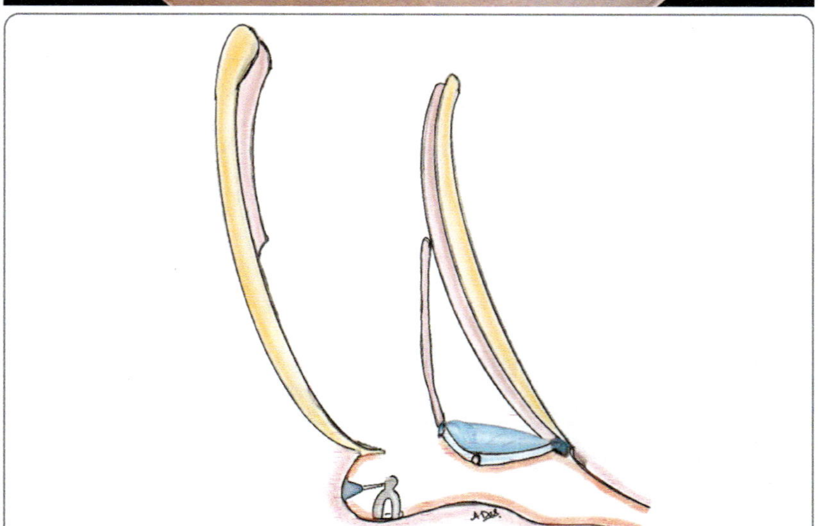

Fig. 11C: Pictorial depiction of middle ear cross section at this stage.

MIDDLE EAR INSPECTION

- *Angled scopes are used to visualize the hidden areas such as:*
  - *Protympanum and Eustachian tube orifice*
  - *Tympanic isthmus*
  - *Incudostapedial complex*
- The elevated tympanomeatal flap is placed on anterior canal wall to create adequate space between the handle of malleus and bony annulus.

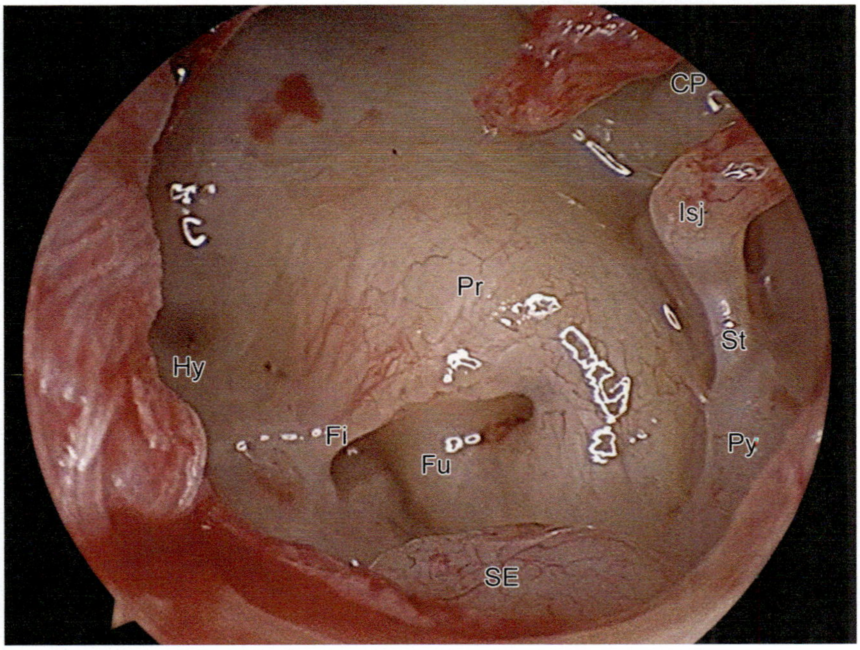

Fig. 12A: Middle ear inspection: Vital landmarks visualized with 0° endoscope.
(CP: processus cochleariformis; Fi: finiculus; Fu: fustis; Hy: hypotympanum; Isj: incudostapedial joint; Pr: promontory; Py: processus pyramidalis; SE: styloid eminence; St: stapedius tendon)

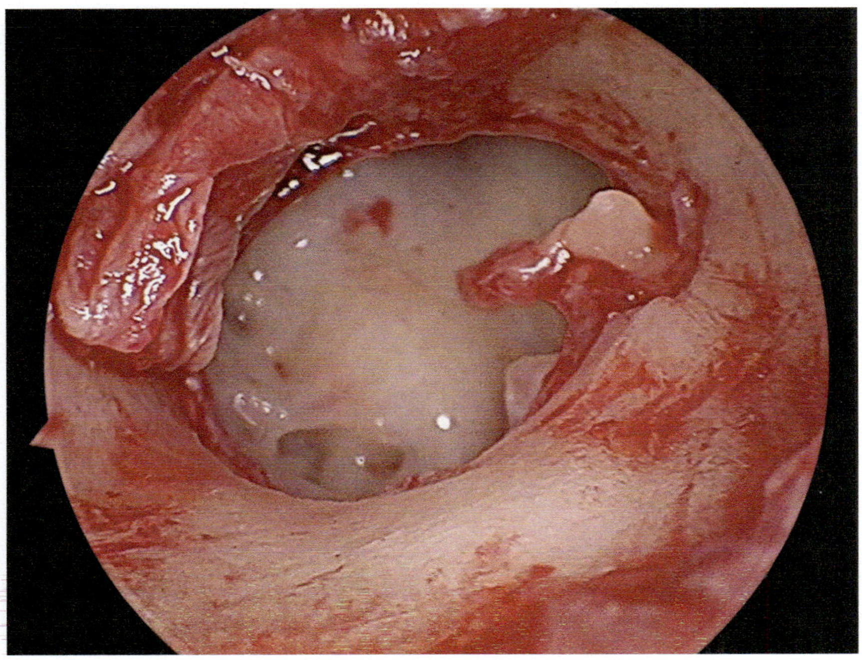

Fig. 12B: Middle ear inspection: Panoramic view of middle ear after flap elevation.

- Angled endoscope such as 30° 2.7 mm is inserted anterior to the handle of malleus.
- Hidden areas are then inspected by rotating the scope:
  - *Superiorly*: Tensor fold, supratubal recess
  - *Anteriorly*: Eustachian tube orifice
  - *Inferiorly*: Hypotympanic air cells

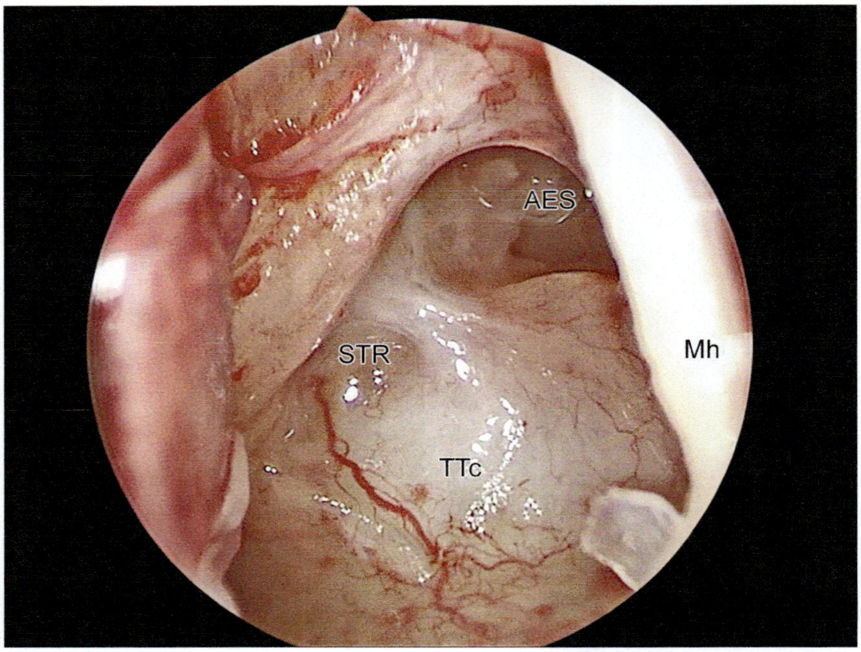

Fig. 13A: Endoscopic inspection of middle ear using angled (30°) endoscope: Scope placed anteriorly to visualize protympanum and tensor fold.
(AES: anterior epitympanic space; Mh: malleus handle; STR: supratubal recess; TTc: canal for tensor tympani)

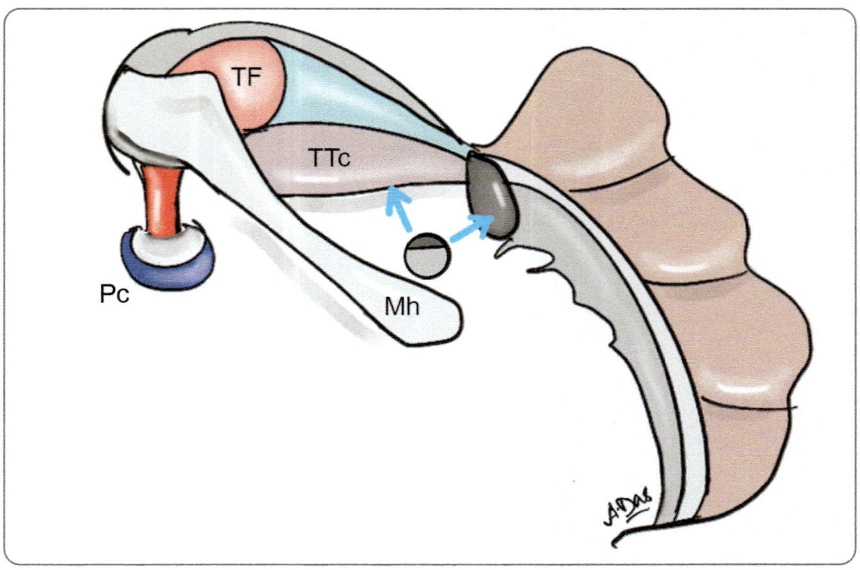

Fig. 13B: Endoscopic inspection of middle ear using angled (30°) endoscope: Scope placed anteriorly to visualize protympanum and tensor fold: Pictorial depiction.
(Mh: malleus handle; Pc: processus cochleariformis; TF: tensor fold; TTc: canal for tensor tympani)

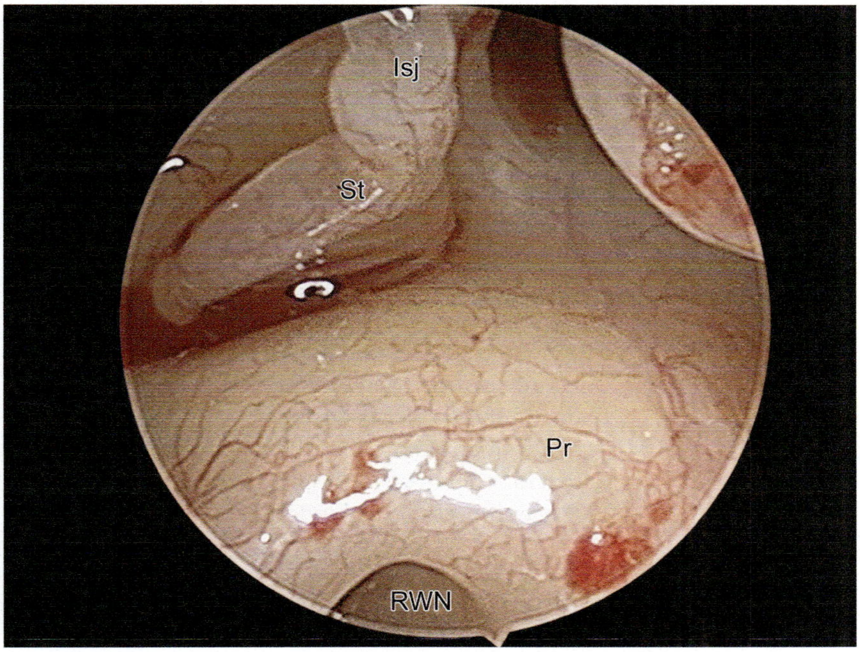

Fig. 13C: Endoscopic inspection of middle ear using angled (30°) endoscope: Scope placed posteriorly to visualize isthmus anticus, posticus and superior retrotympanum.
(Isj: incudostapedial joint; Pr: promontory; St: stapedius tendon; RWN: round window niche)

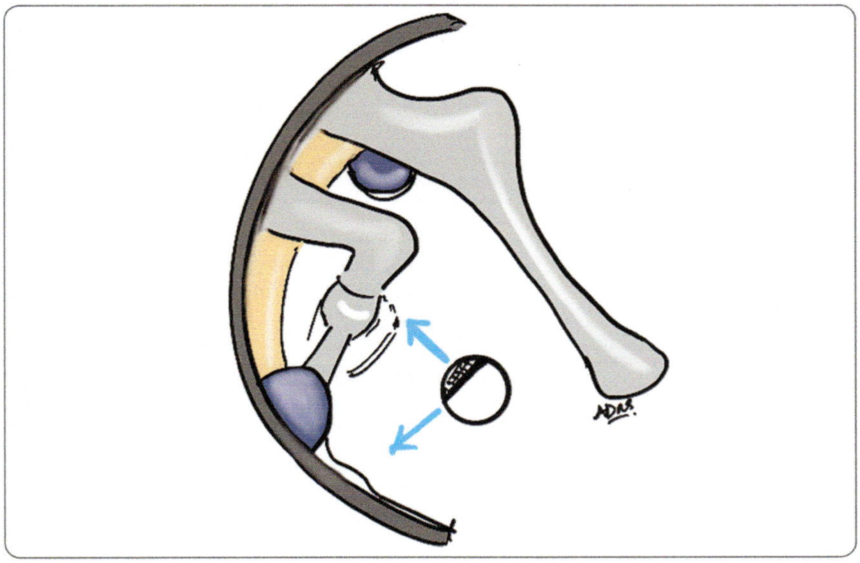

Fig. 13D: Endoscopic inspection of middle ear using angled (30°) endoscope: Scope placed posteriorly to visualize isthmus anticus, posticus and superior retrotympanum: Pictorial depiction.

- Depending on the pneumatization of supratubal recess, the position of tensor fold may be horizontal or vertical.
- A vertical tensor fold is difficult to visualize using angled endoscope.
- Angled endoscope is placed posterior to the handle of malleus and slowly rotated superiorly to visualize the anterior and posterior tympanic isthmi.
- Chorda tympani needs to be dissected inferiorly to create the space for inspection
- To inspect incudostapedial complex and retrotympanum, the scope is tilted slightly posteriorly.

PALPATION OF OSSICULAR CHAIN

- Palpation of ossicular chain is one of the most critical steps without which a tympanoplasty is incomplete.
- The ossicles are to be palpated in the proper direction exerting optimal force in order to avoid inadvertent ossicular dislocation.

- The ossicles are palpated individually using a smooth curved pick.
- Malleus mobility is checked by palpating it in a medial-to-lateral direction.
- Incus palpated in an anteroposterior direction
- Stapes is palpated in superior-to-inferior direction.
- Round window reflex must be checked at this point.

PEARL

- Normal ossicular chain mobility must be ensured prior to graft placement as mere anatomical closure of the perforation will not provide optimal audiological outcome.
- Closure of tympanic membrane perforation in the presence of an ossicular chain fixation, may in fact, worsen the hearing status.

PREPARATION OF GRAFT BED

- There are several methods of tympanic membrane grafting
- We advocate "underlay" technique of grafting
- The temporalis fascia graft is placed lateral to the handle of malleus
- *360° annulus elevation:*
    - Anterior fibrous annulus with a part of the anterior canal skin is elevated in a retrograde manner using a circular knife.
    - The circular knife is positioned in the bony annulus.
    - The knife is then used to dissect the fibrous annulus of the underlying bony annulus.
    - 1–2 mm of anterior canal skin is also elevated along with it in order to create a space beneath it for tucking in the temporalis fascia underneath.

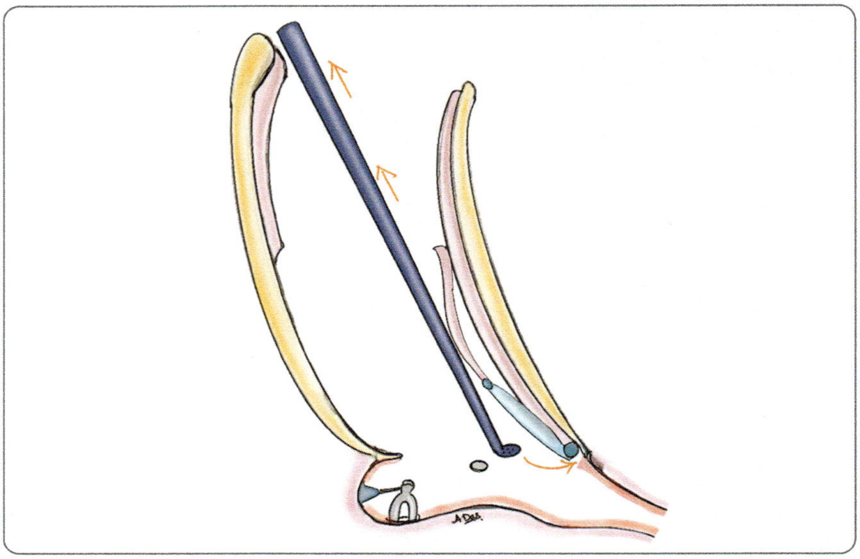

Fig. 14A: Fibrous annulus elevation to expose the anterior bony annulus: Pictorial depiction (Sagittal view).

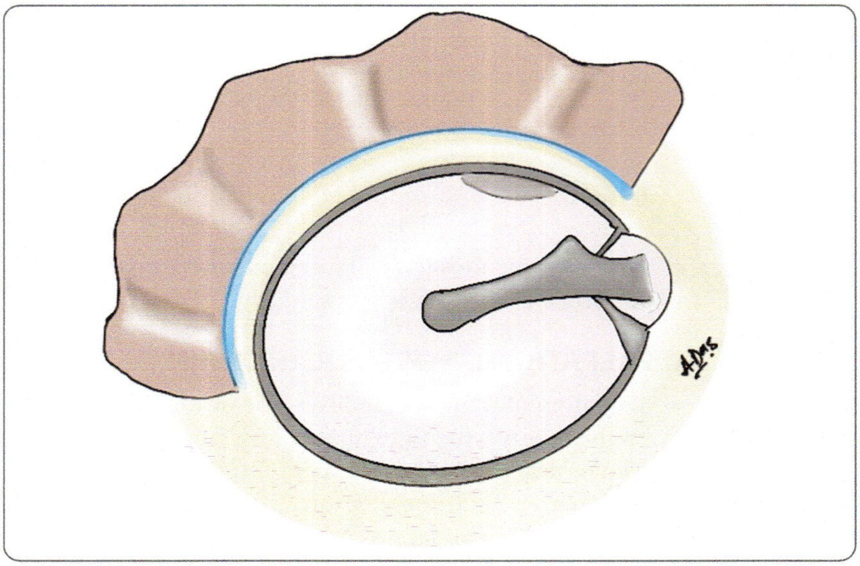

Fig. 14B: Fibrous annulus elevation to expose the anterior bony annulus: Pictorial depiction (Endoscopic view).

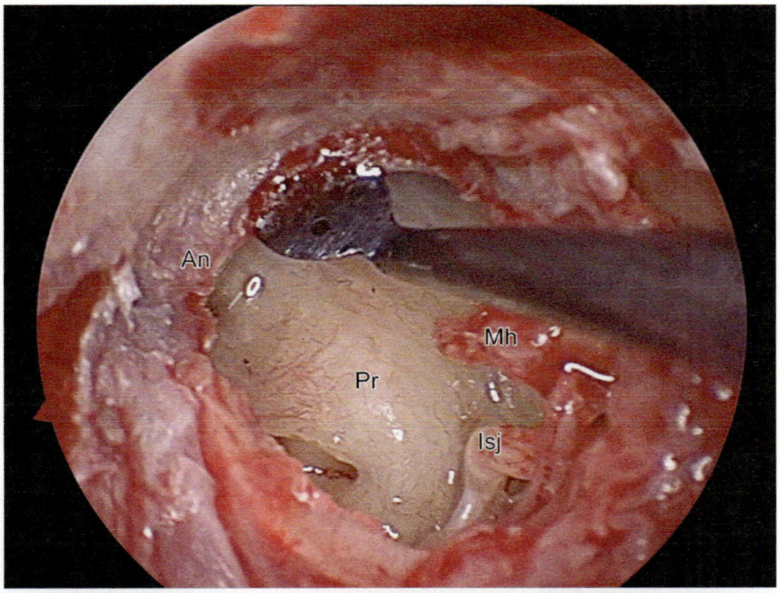

Fig. 14C: Fibrous annulus elevation to expose the anterior bony annulus: Dissection with round knife to lift the anterior fibrous annulus with anterior canal skin.
(An: annulus; Isj: incudostapedial joint; Mh: malleus handle; Pr: promontory)

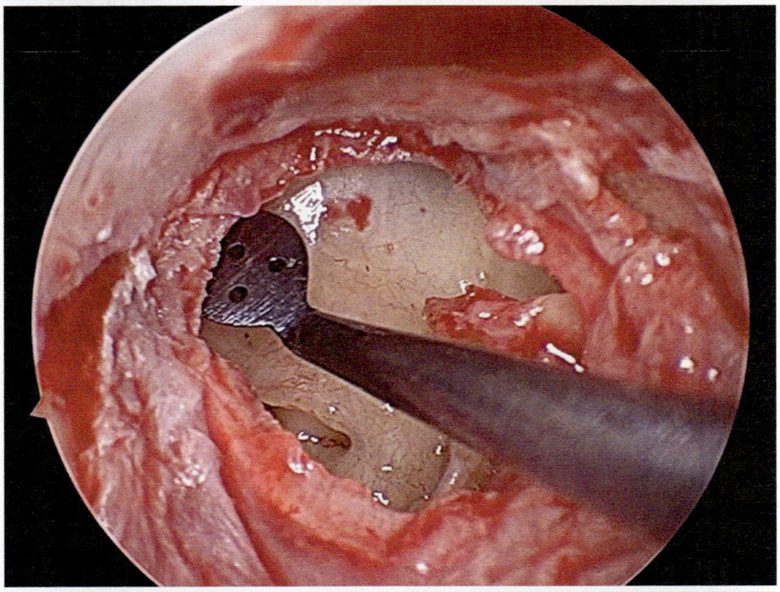

Fig. 14D: Fibrous annulus elevation to expose the anterior bony annulus: Intraoperative step-wise dissection to expose the underlying bony annulus.

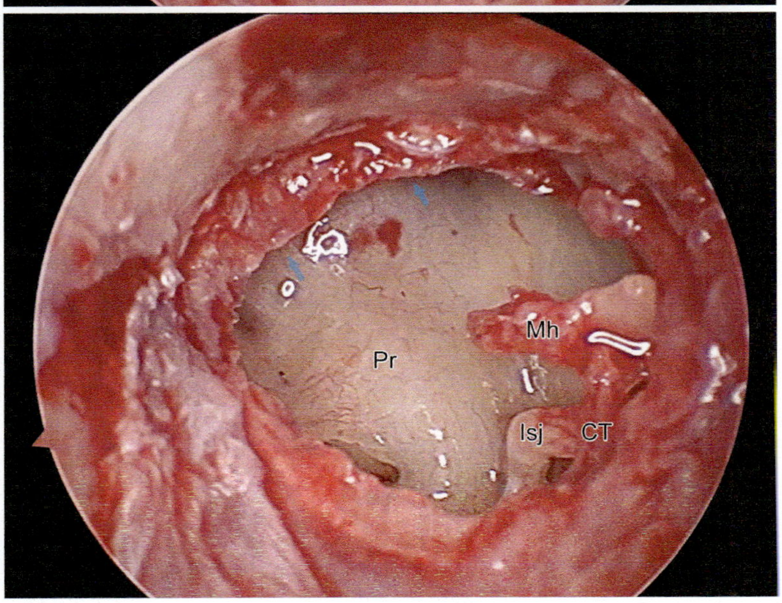

Fig. 14E: Fibrous annulus elevation to expose the anterior bony annulus: Fibrous annulus with anterior canal skin elevated.
(CT: chorda tympani; Isj: incudostapedial joint; Mh: malleus handle; Pr: promontory)

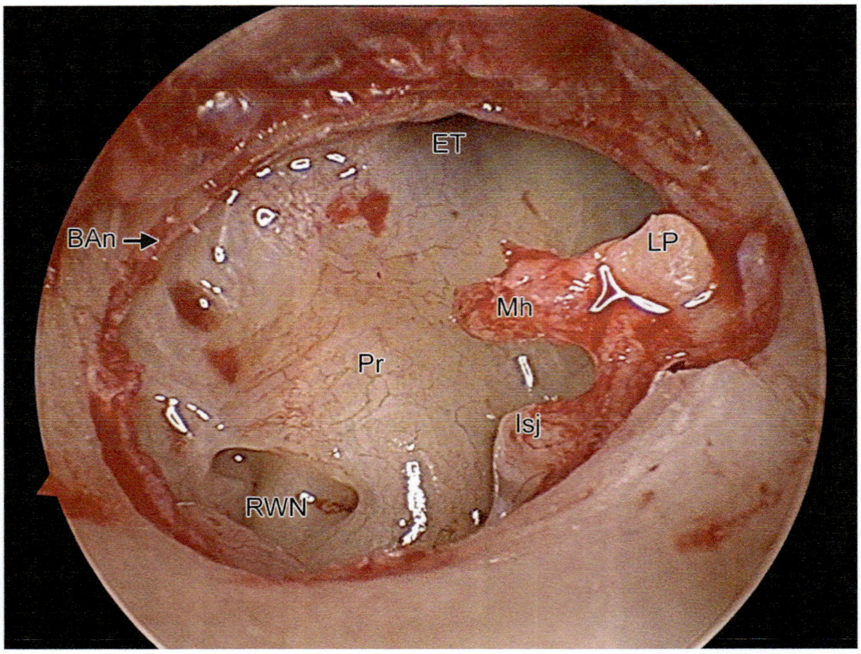

Fig. 14F: Fibrous annulus elevation to expose the anterior bony annulus: Final view after elevation of fibrous annulus all-around.
(BAn: bony annulus; ET: eustachian tube; Isj: incudostapedial joint; LP: lateral process of malleus; Mh: malleus handle; Pr: promontory; RWN: round window niche)

TIP

- Care must be taken not to damage the mucosal lining of Eustachian tube orifice and protympanum
- The annulus and flap must be preserved carefully
  - The tympanic cavity is then packed with adrenaline-soaked cotton pledget for a minute.
  - Ensuring a clear field prior to graft placement is absolutely necessary for precise placement of the graft and to avoid residual perforation.
  - Moreover, excess fluid pooled in the tympanic cavity may cause premature soakage of the graft which increases the difficulty in handling and its precise placement.

PREPARATION OF TEMPORALIS FASCIA

- *Incision*: A linear incision is made parallel to the Frankfurt plane well hidden above the hairline.
- Incision should not cross the vertical line passing through the tragus.
- This is important as anterior part of temporalis fascia is thick and densely adherent to the underlying muscle.
- Risk of injuring the superficial temporal vessels is higher if this line is crossed.

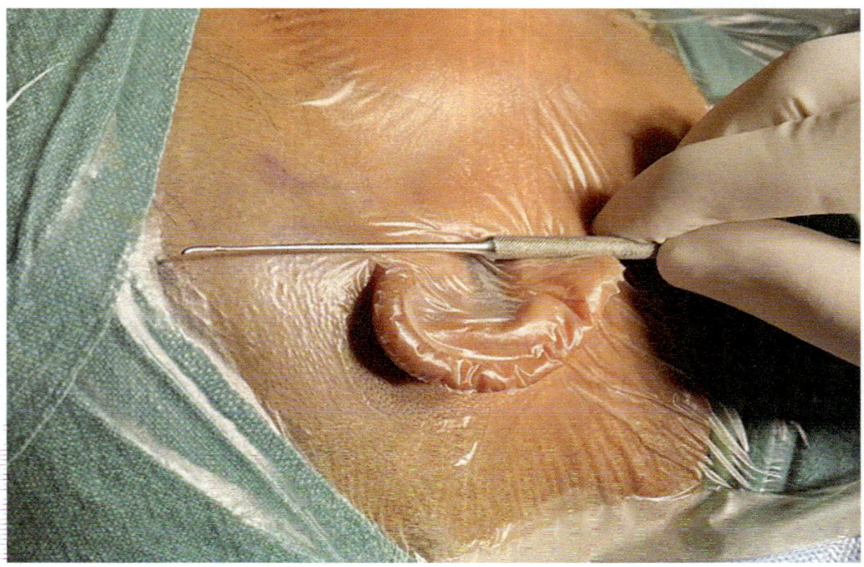

Fig. 15A: Steps of temporalis fascia harvesting: Marking of anterior-most limit beyond which lies the territory of superficial temporal artery.

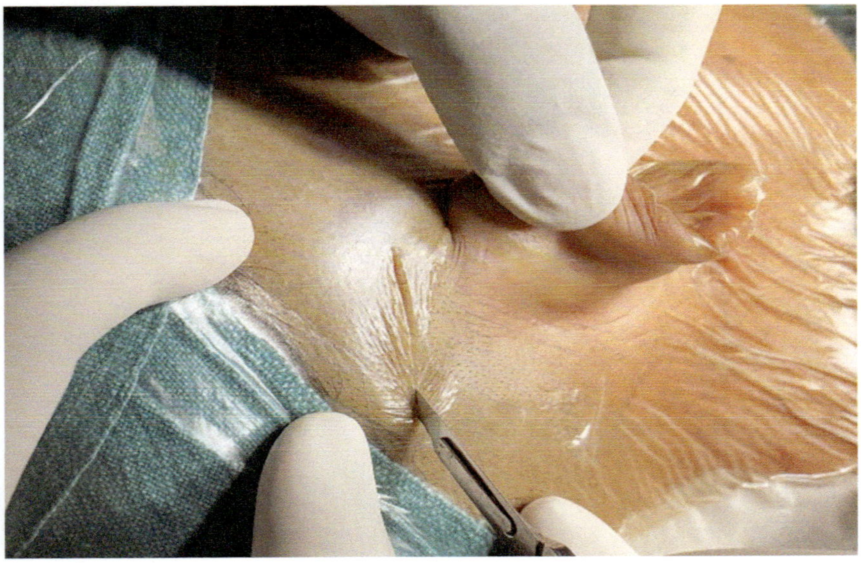

Fig. 15B: Steps of temporalis fascia harvesting: Incision of skin.

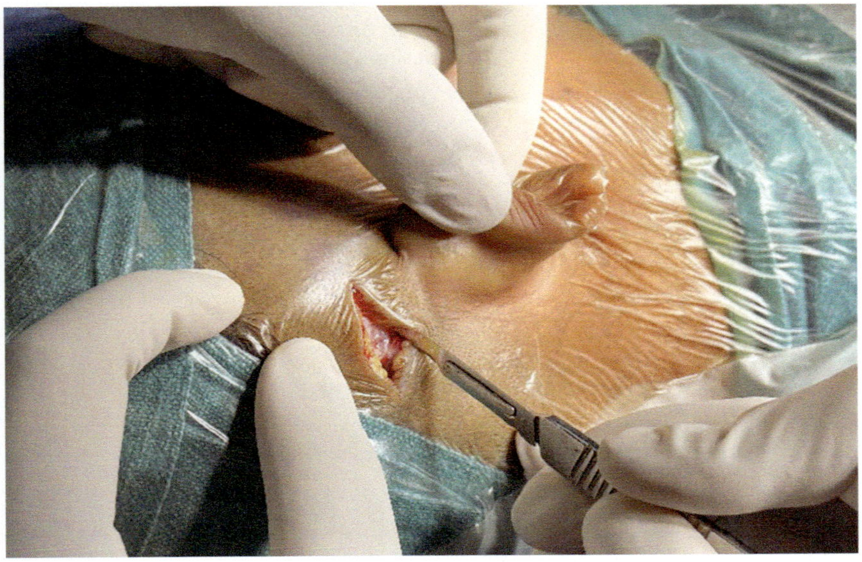

Fig. 15C: Steps of temporalis fascia harvesting: Incision of subcutaneous soft tissues.

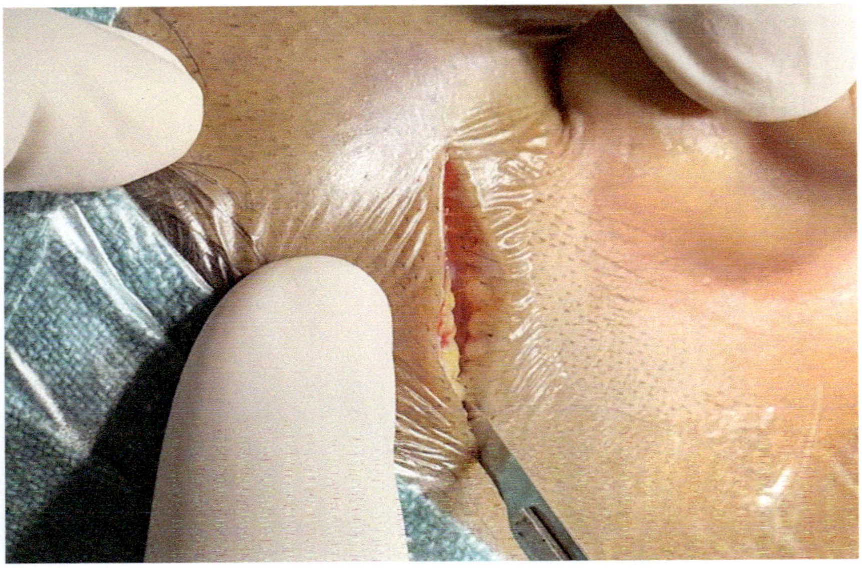

Fig. 15D: Steps of temporalis fascia harvesting: Dissection of subcutaneous soft tissues.

- Soft tissues are dissected, two-prong mastoid retractor applied.
- Normal saline injected deep to temporalis fascia for hydrodissection
- Temporalis fascia harvested
- Any muscle fiber or fat is scraped off the temporalis fascia and placed over a metallic surface to dry.

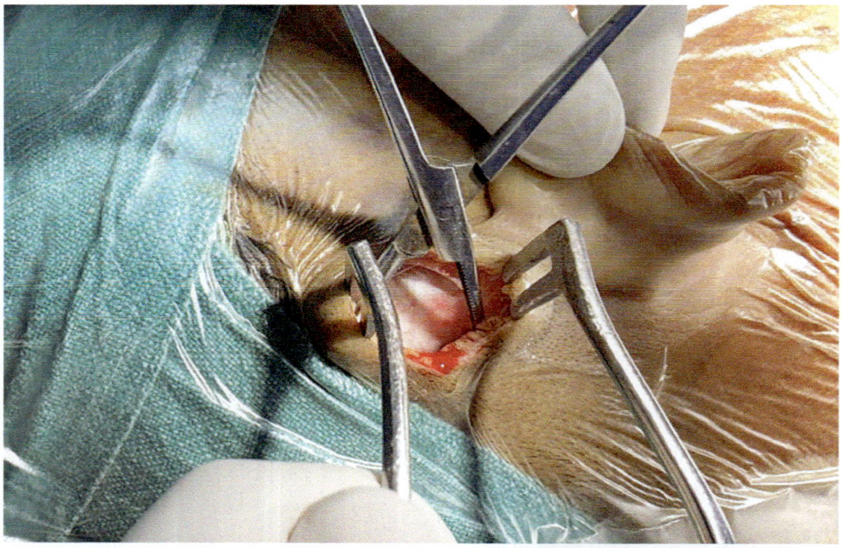

Fig. 16A: Steps of temporalis fascia harvesting: Dissection of soft tissues and exposure graft harvest site.

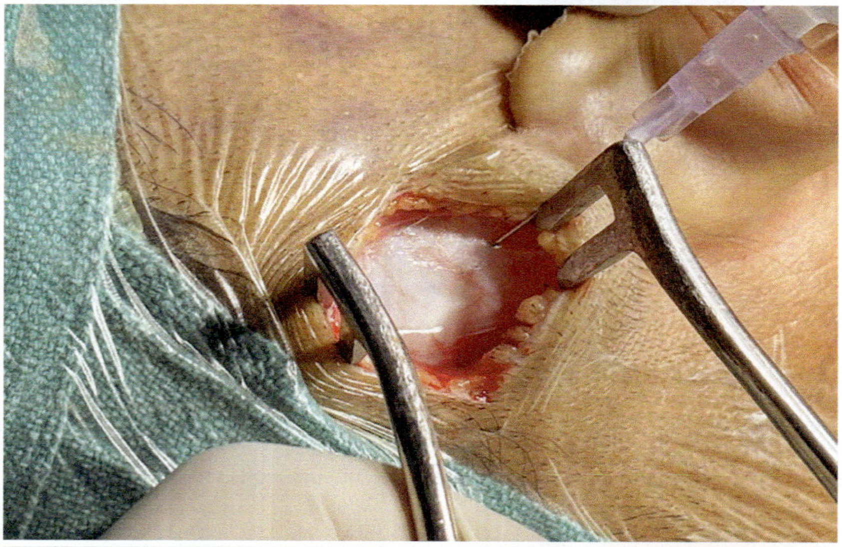

Fig. 16B: Steps of temporalis fascia harvesting: Hydrodissection using normal saline.

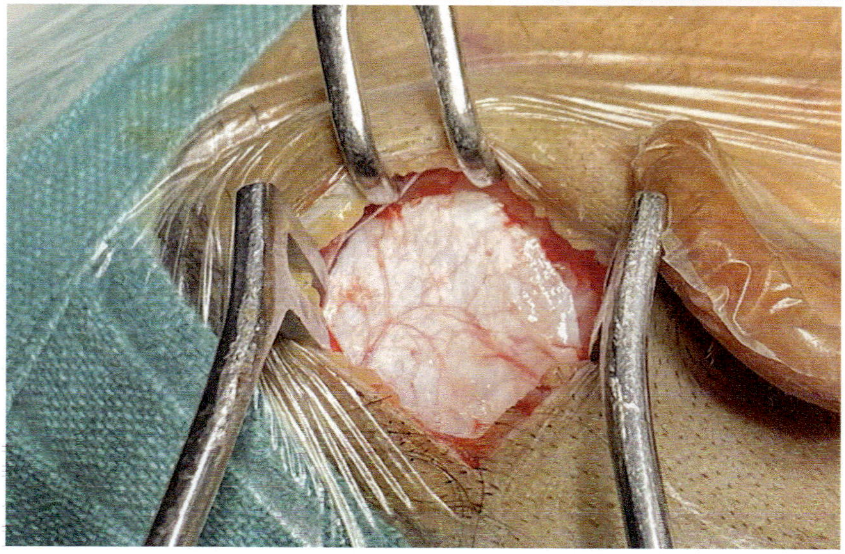

Fig. 16C: Steps of temporalis fascia harvesting: Incision all around the temporalis fascia graft.

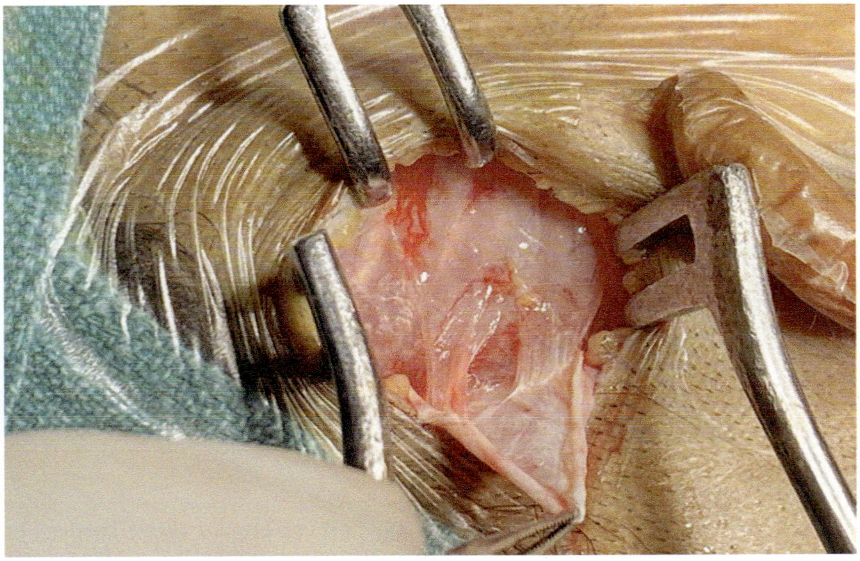

Fig. 16D: Steps of temporalis fascia harvesting: Temporalis fascia being teased off underlying muscle.

- Hot water may be used to dry the fascia faster
- Dry graft is preferred in endoscopic ear surgery as a wet graft is difficult to handle single-handedly due to surface tension.

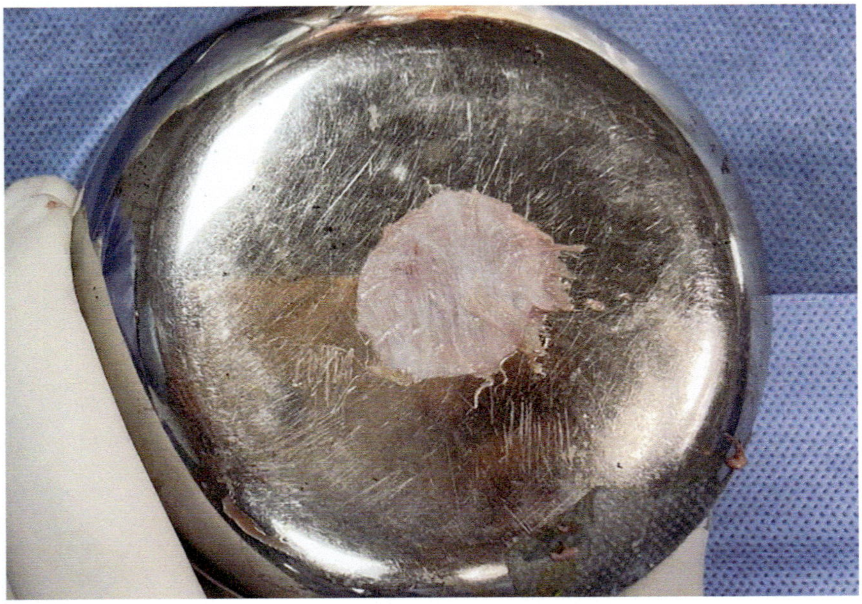

Fig. 17A: Temporalis fascia laid over a metallic surface to dry.

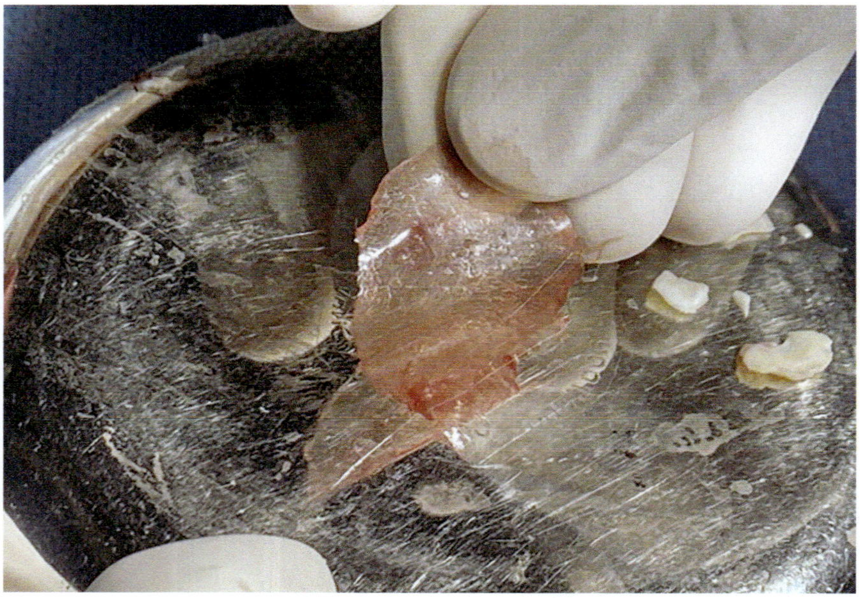

Fig. 17B: Completely dry fascia ready for grafting (Note the paper-thin nature and translucency of the dried graft).

TIP

- Adequate size is the key factor for smooth graft placement
- Larger grafts tend to get folded during placement
- Length of the fascia should be short in comparison to microscopic approach
- First attempt is the golden chance for graft placement.
- In case the fascia gets folded and needs to be removed, it should always be made dry before replacing it.

PREPARATION OF CARTILAGE-PERICHONDRIUM

- Tragal cartilage is generally used for endoscopic ear surgery.
- *Incision*: Horizontal incision is placed on the medial aspect of tragus slightly away from the edge.
- Following skin incision, the cartilage is incised in the same plane, preserving the cartilage's tip, in order to avoid any cosmetic deformity.

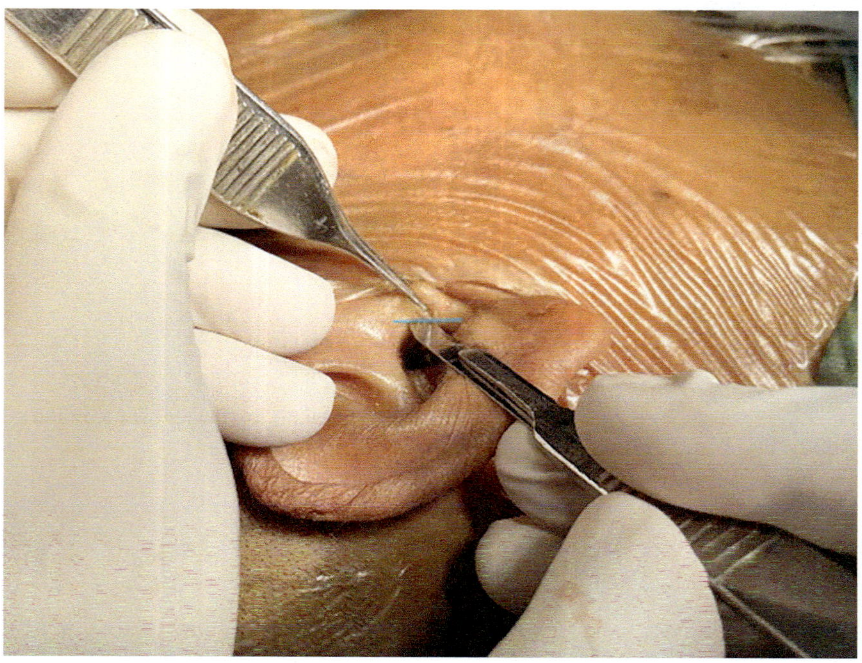

Fig. 18A: Steps of tragal cartilage harvest: Skin incision placed over medial aspect of tragus (blue line).

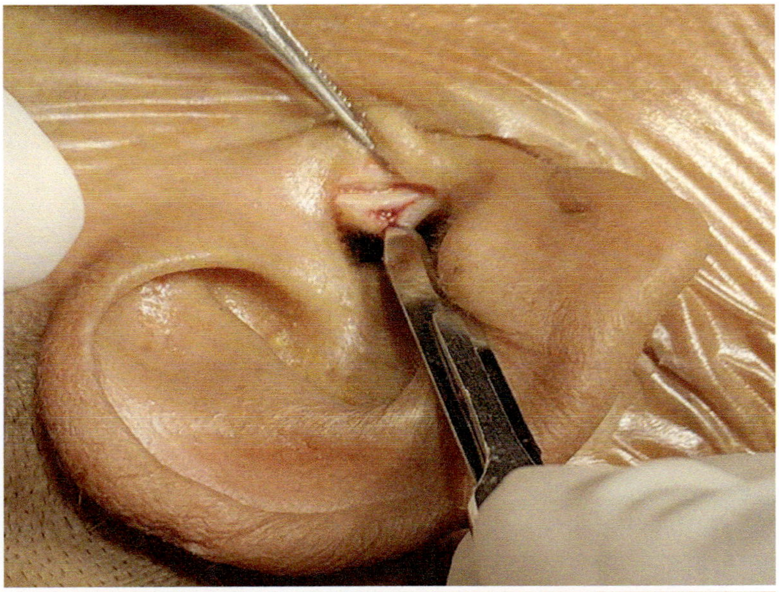

Fig. 18B: Steps of tragal cartilage harvest: Cartilage incised keeping a small strip laterally.

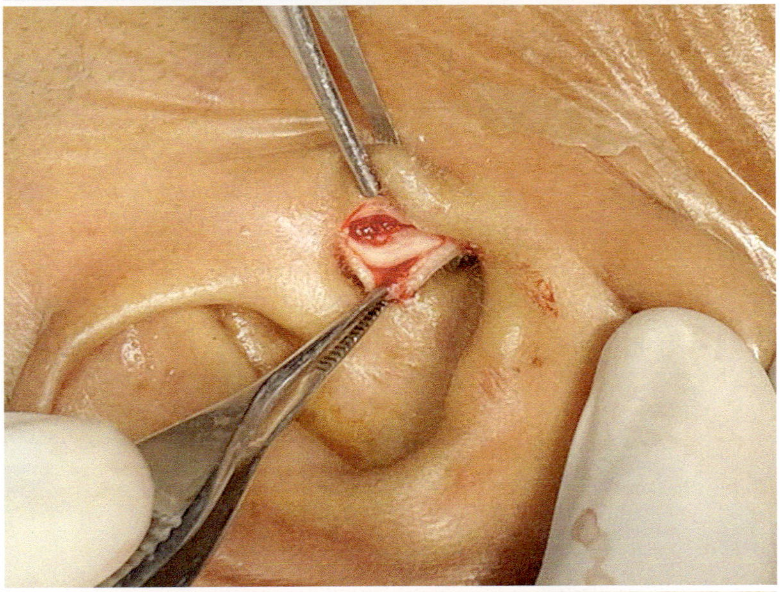

Fig. 18C: Steps of tragal cartilage harvest: Lateral strip of cartilage being retracted for proper visualization.

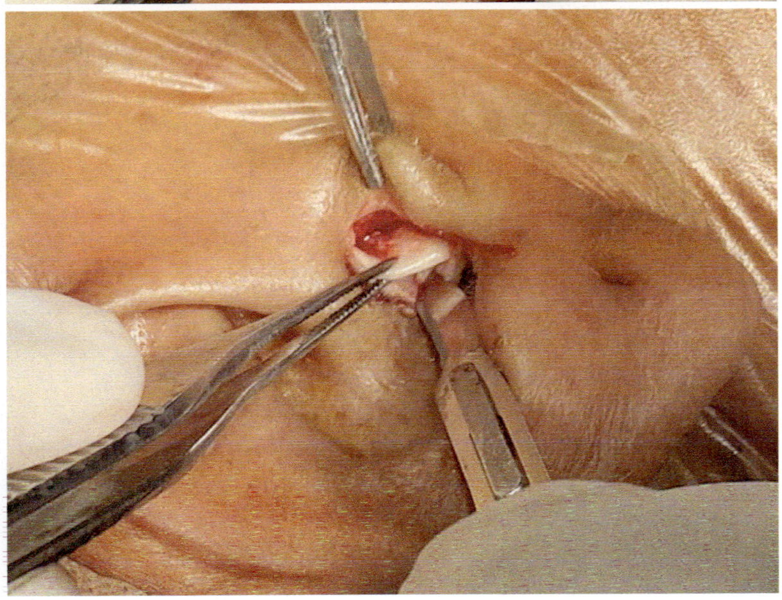

Fig. 18D: Steps of tragal cartilage harvest: Sharp dissection with knife.

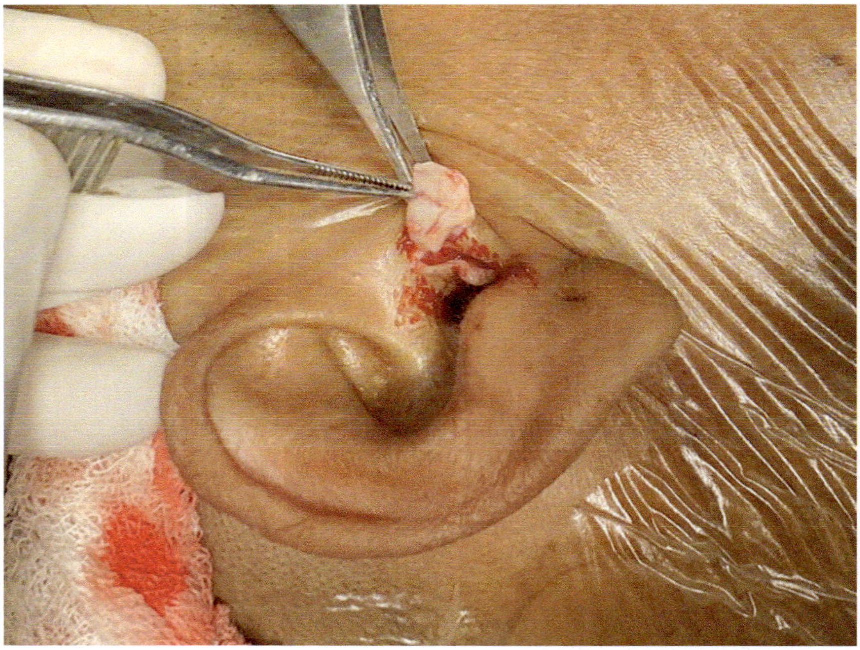

Fig. 18E: Steps of tragal cartilage harvest: Dissection and harvest.

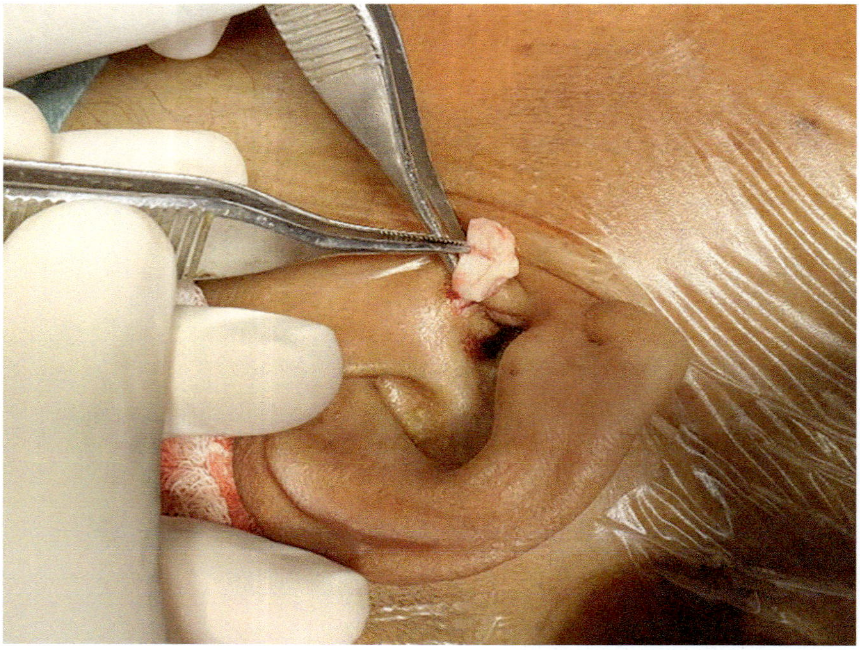

Fig. 18F: Steps of tragal cartilage harvest: Cartilage dissected out.

- Cartilage-perichondrium is harvested depending upon the size of the defect.
- Perichondrium is preserved on one side of the cartilage.
- A V-shaped slot for malleus handle is made on the superior aspect of the cartilage.

GRAFT PLACEMENT

- Single-handed graft placement (temporalis fascia) is the most difficult step of this surgery
- One should follow the proper technique of graft placement to avoid unwanted complications
- We use alligator forceps and smooth curved pick or needle for graft placement

Checklist Prior to Graft Placement

- No active bleeding
- Good field visibility
- Tympanomeatal flap properly placed on anterior canal wall
- 360° of bony annulus visible
- Dry and proper-sized graft should be ready
- Tip of the alligator should be absolutely dry

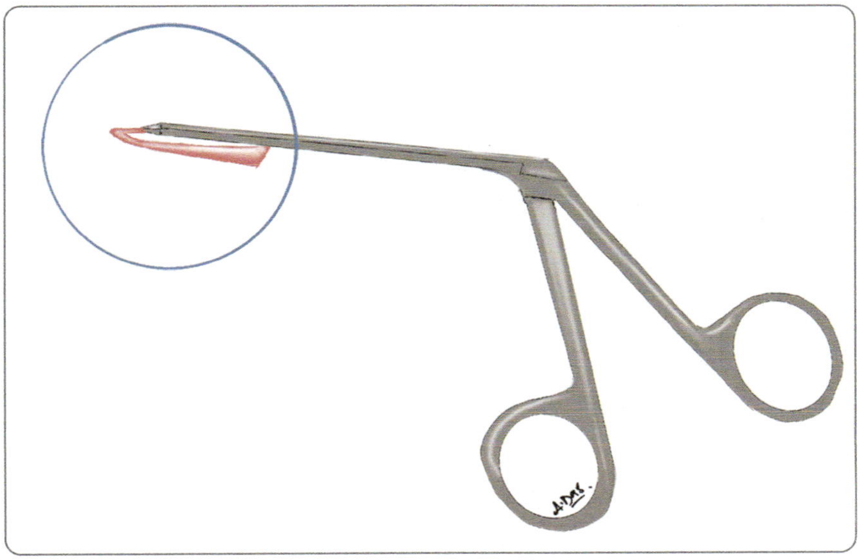

Fig. 19A: Pictorial depiction of correct method of holding the graft with the tip of an alligator forceps.

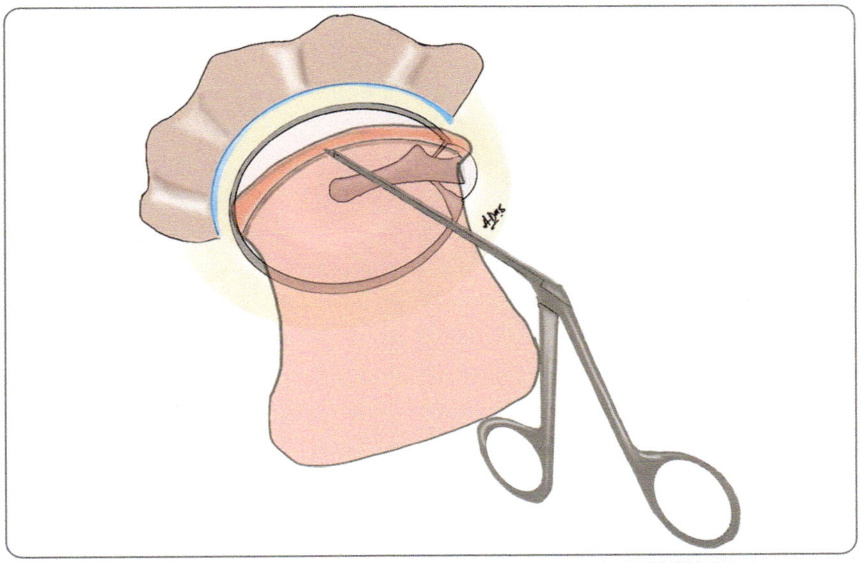

Fig. 19B: Advancement of graft.

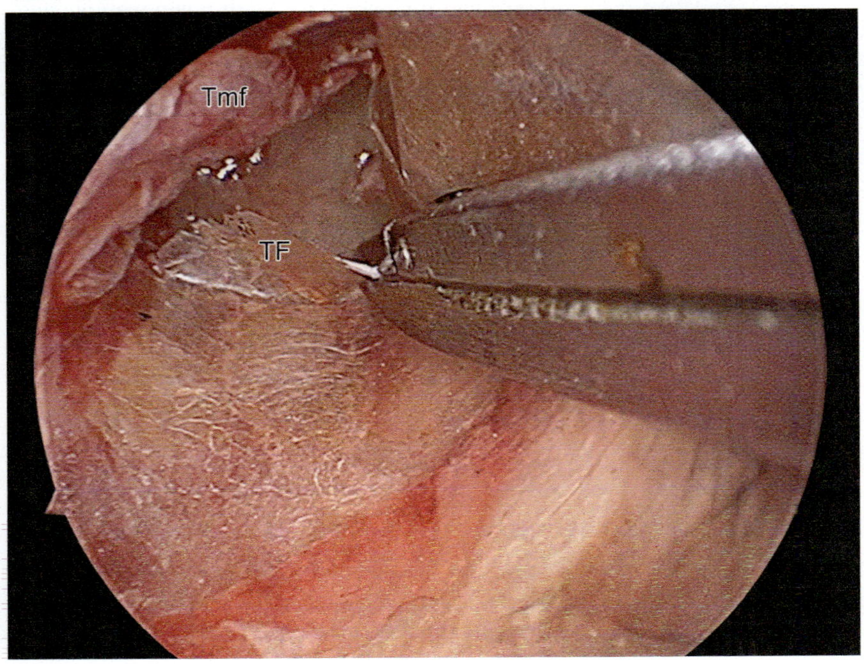

Fig. 19C: Intraoperative step-wise advancement of graft into the middle ear: Graft being advanced using alligator forceps.
(TF: temporalis fascia; Tmf: tympanomeatal flap)

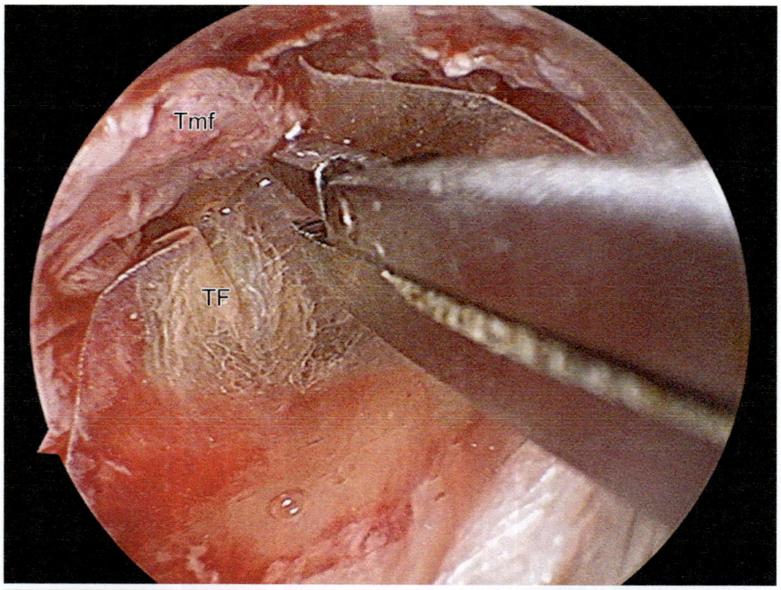

Fig. 19D: Intraoperative step-wise advancement of graft into the middle ear. Graft left off the alligator anterior to handle of malleus.
(TF: temporalis fascia; Tmf: tympanomeatal flap)

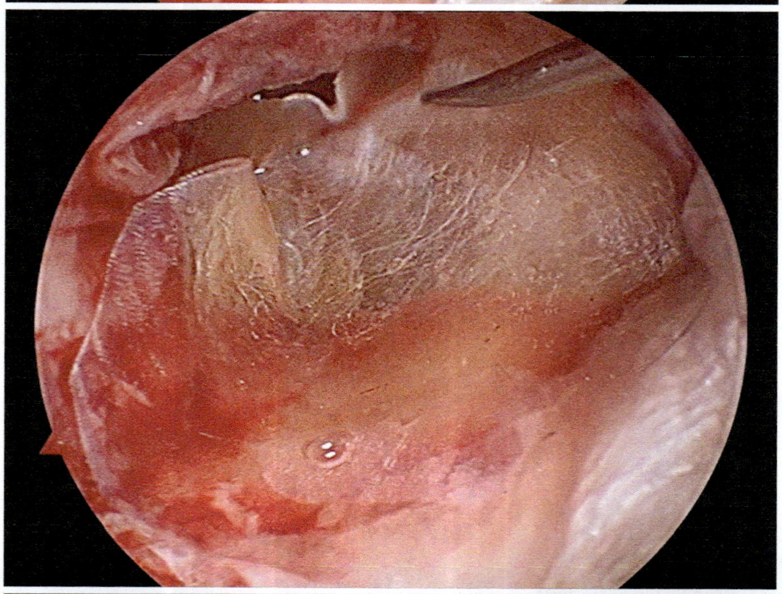

Fig. 19E: Intraoperative step-wise advancement of graft into the middle ear. Graft being manipulated using smooth curved pick.

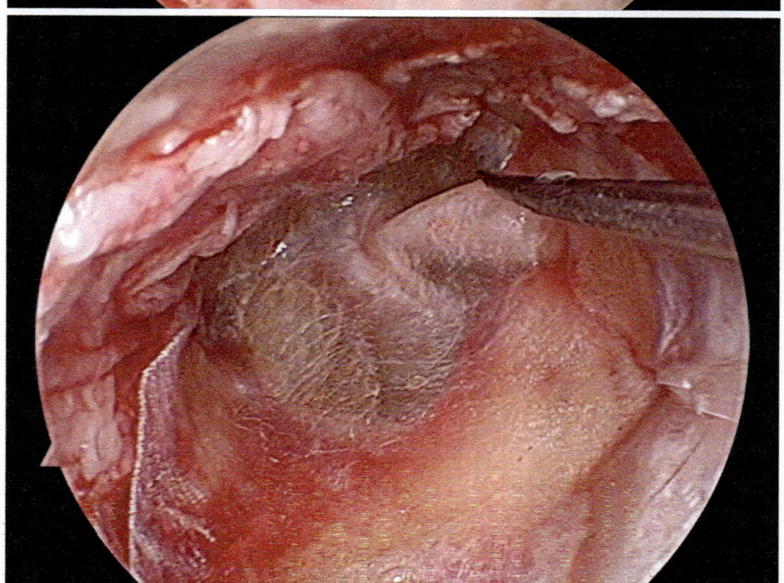

Fig. 19F: Intraoperative step-wise advancement of graft into the middle ear: Fascia being placed over lateral to handle of malleus.

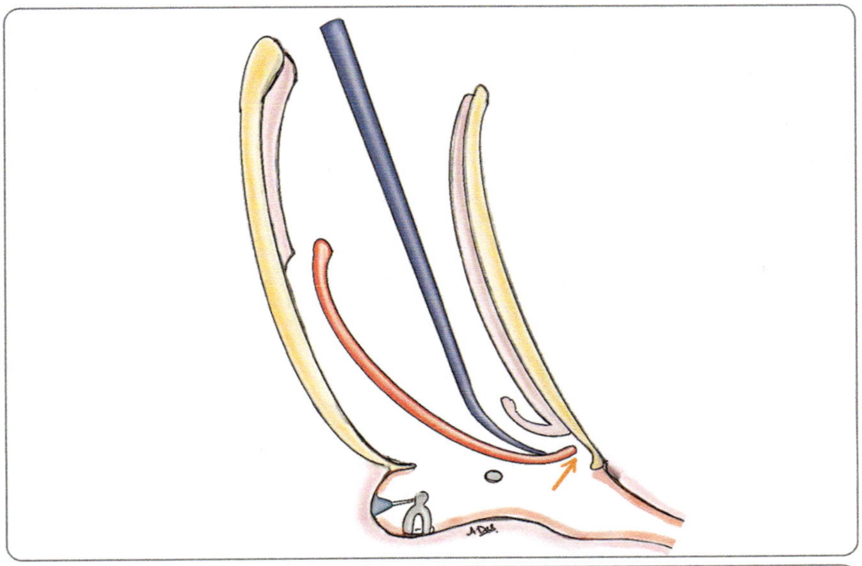

Fig. 20A: Pictorial depiction of exact position of anterior edge of graft with respect to anterior perforation margin and bony annulus.

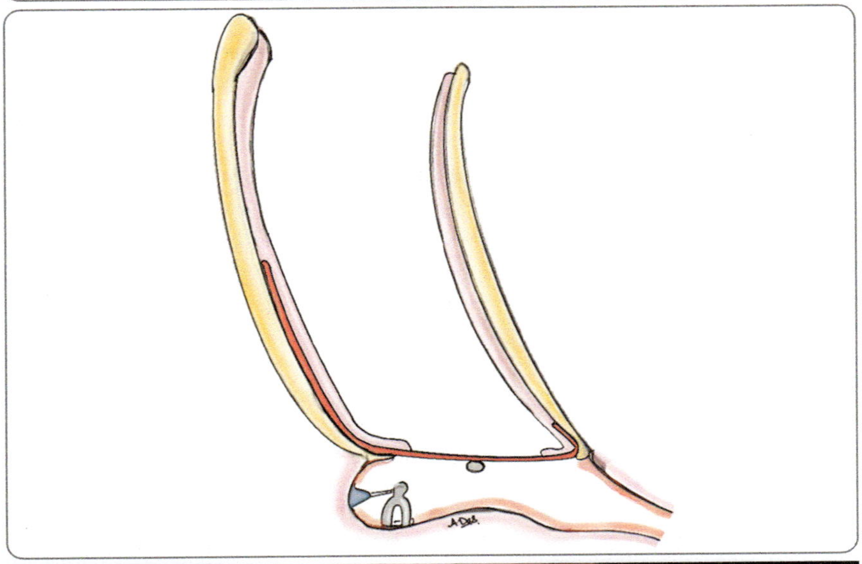

Fig. 20B: Graft position after placement of tympanomeatal flap.

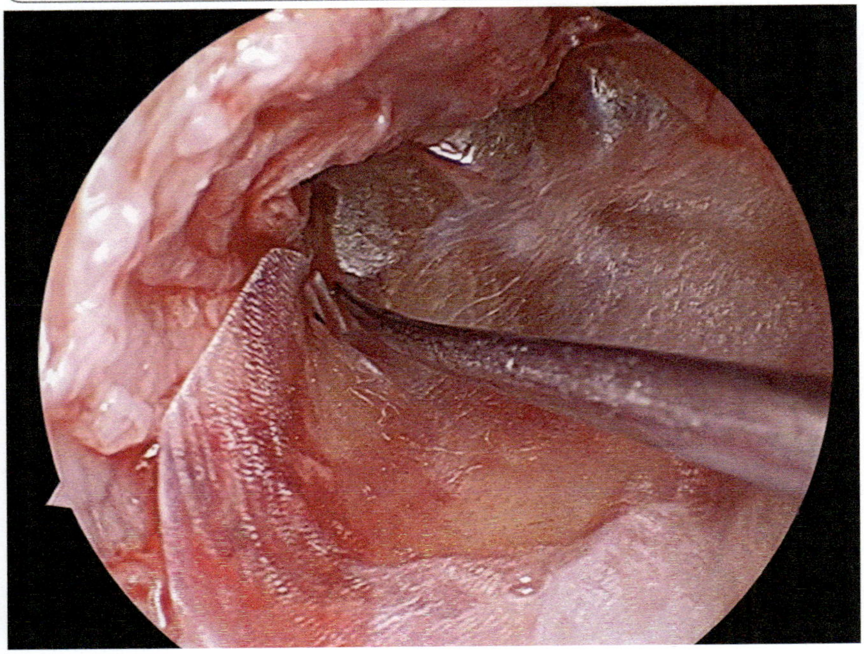

Fig. 20C: Graft being placed underneath the fibrous annulus inferiorly.

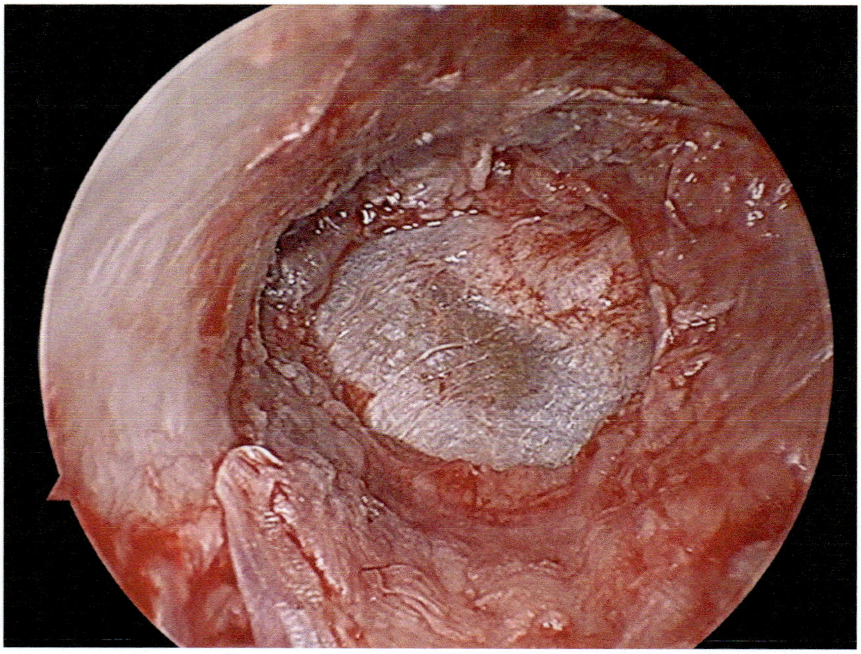

Fig. 20D: Intraoperative placement of graft and replacement of tympanomeatal flap.

PEARL

- The margin of the graft should not be held very tightly as it may not be released at proper position single-handedly
- Surface tension is extremely crucial in every otologic surgery, more so in a single-handed surgery like endoscopic ear surgery
- Surface tension is useful and makes a number of steps feasible for us. But it can be equally sinister and may cause complications in endoscopic ear surgery, especially in crucial steps such as graft placement
- The tip of the alligator is kept dry to negate this factor:
  - The tip of the dry graft is grasped lightly with alligator forceps and folded posteriorly
  - Fascia is advanced over handle of malleus.
  - The fascia is let go at the level of anterior bony annulus.
  - Smooth curved pick is used to spread the fascia over the bony annulus.
  - Tympanomeatal flap is repositioned over the temporalis fascia.
  - Cartilage-perichondrium being thicker and less malleable, it is easier to manipulate single-handedly.
  - The crux lies in appropriate size of the cartilage and proper positioning of the malleus slot
  - Middle ear is filled with antibiotic-soaked gel foam to support the cartilage graft

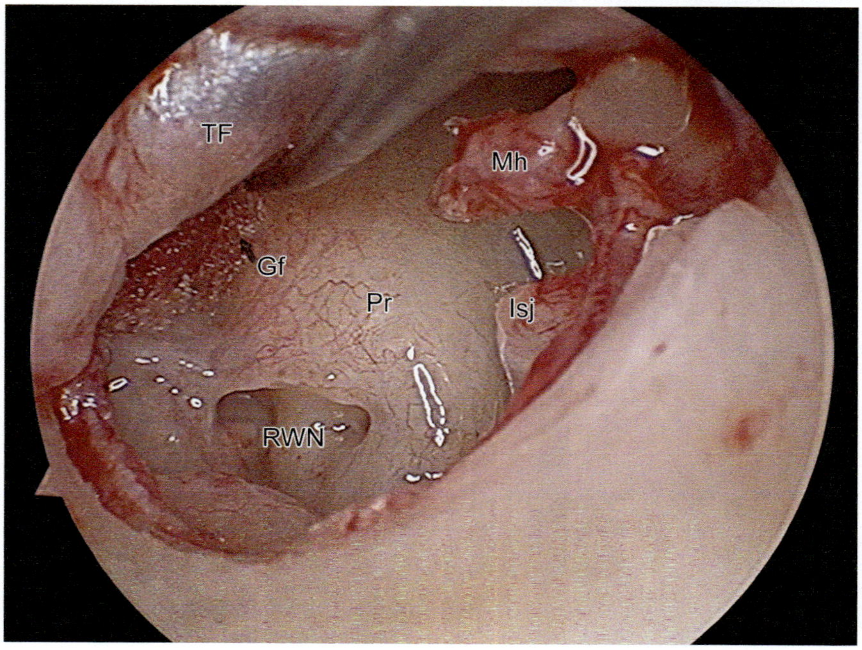

Fig. 21A: Gelfoam placement anteriorly under bony annulus to support the anterior margin. (Gf: gelfoam; Isj: incudostapedial joint; Mh: malleus handle; Pr: promontory; Rwn: round window niche; TF: temporalis fascia)

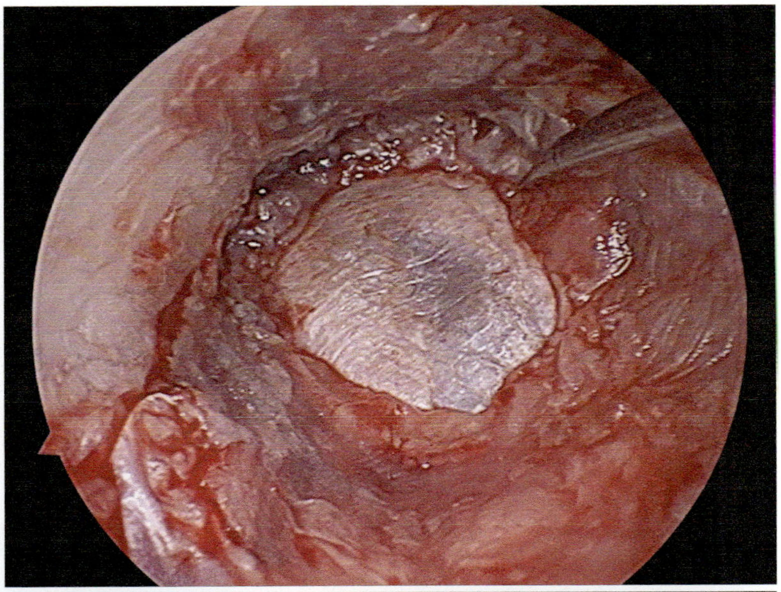

Fig. 21B: Replacement of graft-flap assembly.

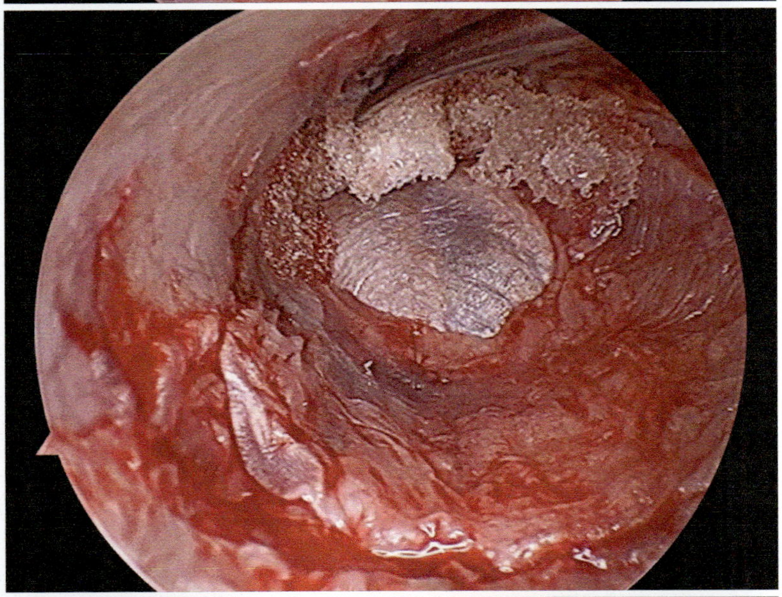

Fig. 21C: Gelfoam placement along anterior margin of the canal and along edges of canal incision.

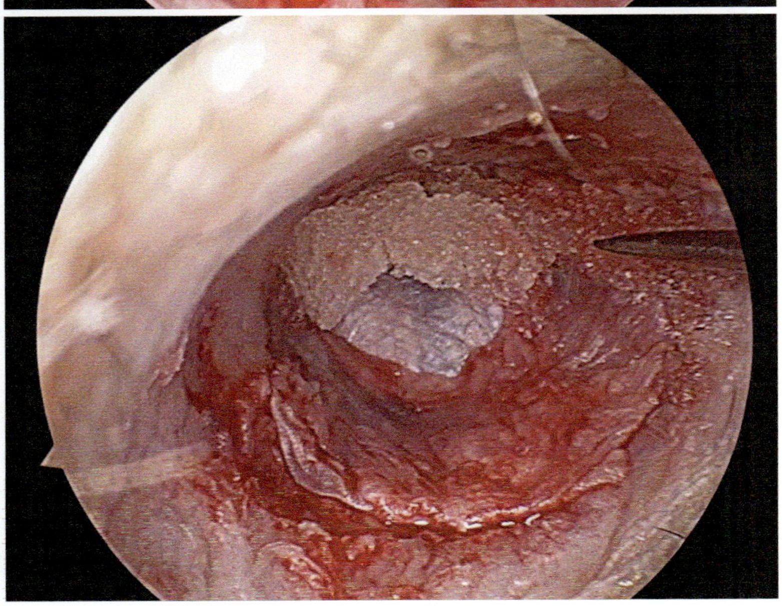

Fig. 21D: Gelfoam placement along anterior margin of the canal and along edges of canal incision.

CLOSING STEPS

- The anterior margin is closely inspected for any gap.
- In case a gap is detected, the fascia is repositioned under the anterior margin using a smooth curved pick gently.
- Antibiotic-soaked gelfoam is placed to secure the anterior margin.
- The flap-graft assembly is elevated gently to inspect the middle ear.
- Three to four small pieces of antibiotic-soaked gelfoam are placed under the bony annulus.
- The assembly is repositioned back.
- The external auditory canal is packed with similar gelfoam pieces.
- A small antibiotic ointment-soaked ribbon is used to plug the external auditory meatus.
- The graft harvest site is closed in single layer with nonabsorbable suture.

REFERENCES

1. Banzer M. Disputatio de Auditione Laesa. Wittenberge: Johannis Rohrerei; 1651.
2. Ghanad I, Polanik MD, Trakimas DR, Knoll RM, Castillo-Bustamante M, Black NL, et al. A Systematic Review of Nonautologous Graft Materials Used in Human Tympanoplasty. Laryngoscope. 2021;131(2):392-400.

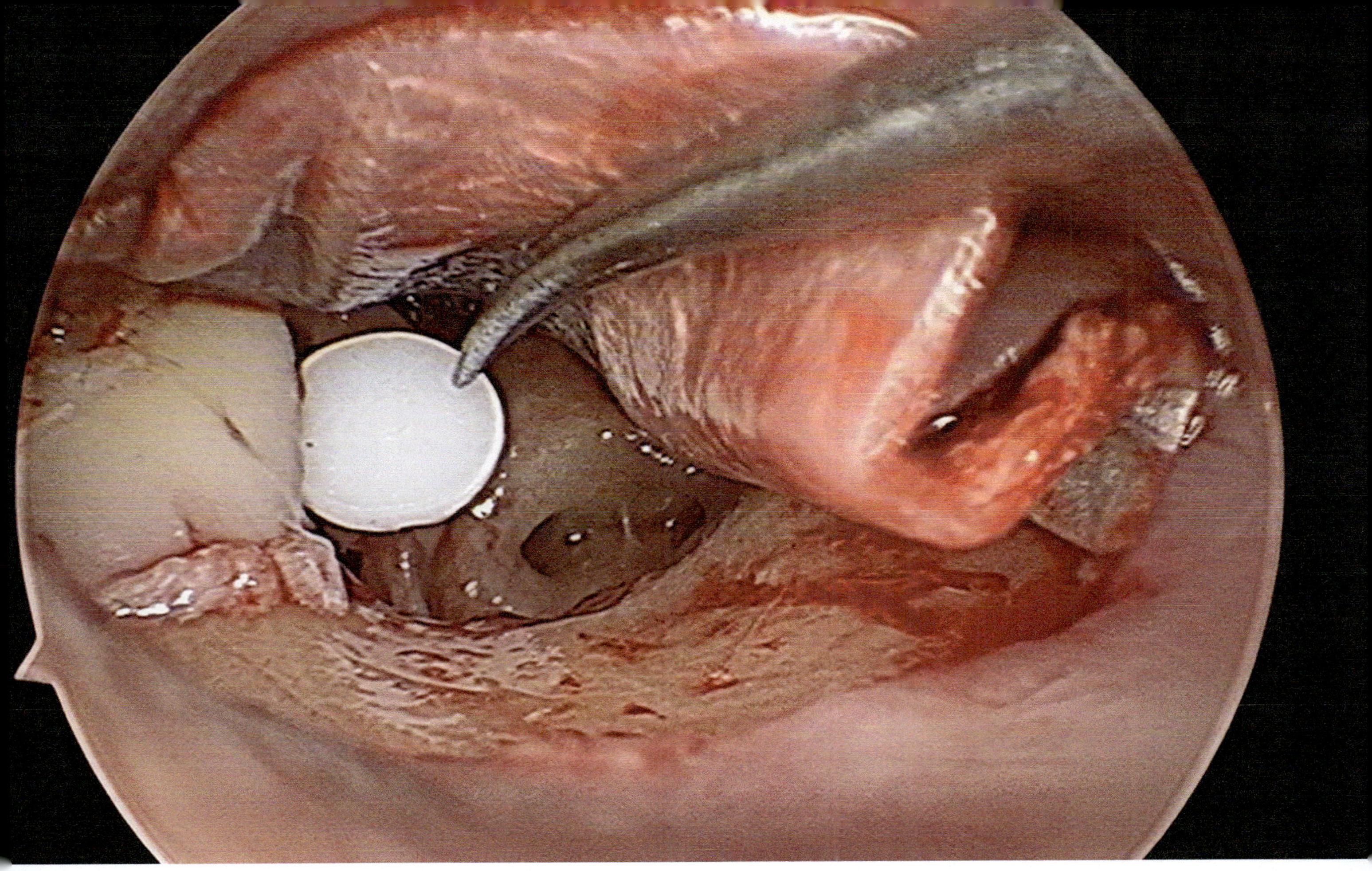

CHAPTER **8**

Endoscopic Ossiculoplasty

Arindam Das, Sandipta Mitra

Chapter Outline

INTRODUCTION

Endoscopic ossiculoplasty is ossicular chain reconstruction with the help of endoscope. There are several reasons which may give rise to ossicular chain discontinuity. These include chronic otitis media (both mucosal and squamosal varieties), trauma, etc. Apart from ossicular chain discontinuity, congenital fixation of the ossicles also warrants ossicular chain reconstruction. Incus (lenticular process > long process) happens to be the most common ossicle to get eroded by disease process followed by stapes superstructure and handle of malleus.[1]

The ossicular chain defects can be classified in a number of ways of which the *Austin-Kartush classification* is the most widely accepted. The classification was first put forward by Austin in 1971 which was later modified by Kartush in 1994.[2,3]

AUSTIN CLASSIFICATION OF OSSICULAR CHAIN DEFECTS WITH ABSENT INCUS

Group	Ossicular status	Abbreviation	Prevalence (%)
A	Malleus handle and stapes superstructure present	M+S+	60
B	Malleus handle present, stapes superstructure absent	M+S–	23
C	Malleus handle absent, stapes superstructure present	M–S+	8
D	Malleus handle and stapes superstructure absent	M–S–	8

KARTUSH MODIFICATION OF AUSTIN CLASSIFICATION OF OSSICULAR CHAIN DEFECTS

Group	Ossicular status
O	Intact ossicular chain
E	Ossicular head fixation
F	Stapes fixation

MATERIALS USED FOR OSSICULOPLASTY

Various materials have been used as grafts for ossicular chain reconstruction. Broadly, these can be biological or synthetic. Biological materials may be autografts or homografts. Commonly used biological materials are cartilage (conchal, tragal, septal spur, etc.) and ossicles. Synthetic materials may be solid plastics such as polytetrafluoroethylene (Teflon), polyethylene; solid metals like stainless steel, gold, titanium; porous sponge like plastics such as Proplast, Plastipore or ceramics like aluminum oxide, hydroxyapatite. Each has its own merits and demerits, the discussion of which is beyond the scope of this book.

GENERAL PRINCIPLES OF OSSICULOPLASTY

Merchant and Rosowski's ***TRACS*** Principles:[4]

- *Tension*:
  - Excessive laxity causes sound energy loss, displacement
  - Excessive mobility leads to scarring, adjacent ossicle erosion
  - Excessive tension-dampens sound energy, worsens hearing result
  - Implant should remain inherently stable, should not topple
  - Length of prosthesis > visible gap
- *Round-round window protection*:
  - Isolation of round window maximizes sound transmission
- *Angle*:
  - Prosthesis should contact tympanic membrane (TM)/malleus handle at 45–90° angle
  - Acute angulation leads to hearing loss
  - Avoid incus interposition if stapes head is at same height as malleus
  - Position partial ossicular replacement prosthesis (PORP)/total ossicular replacement prosthesis (TORP) as vertically as possible
- *Centered*:
  - Position prosthesis close to center of TM (catenary lever mechanism)
  - Preserve handle of malleus and incorporate it into reconstruction
  - Handle of malleus, if medialized, can be lateralized by dividing tensor tympani muscle and stretching it
- *Space*:
  - Air space around ossicular chain should be > 0.3 mL
  - Reconstruct air space to optimize hearing and prevent adhesions
  - Insert tympanostomy tube if ear tubes (ET) function compromised.

PROGNOSTICATION IN OSSICULOPLASTY

"SPITE" Method of Assessment[5]

- ***S***urgical
- ***P***rosthesis
- ***I***nfection
- ***T***issue factors
- ***E***ustachian tube factors

PRINCIPLES OF ENDOSCOPIC OSSICULOPLASTY

- *Anatomical configuration*:
  - A detailed knowledge of the three-dimensional orientation of the ossicles and their relative

configuration is imperative for a successful ossicular chain reconstruction.
- Relevant endoscopic anatomy has been described in detail in the respective chapter of this book.

- *Physiological principles*:
  - Maximal preservation of normal mucosa, mucosal folds and ligaments form the pillars of functional endoscopic ear surgery.
  - Well aerated middle-ear space without adhesions implies faster healing with minimal fibrosis that leads to early hearing improvement and hence holds the key to a successful ossicular chain reconstruction.
- *Visualization*:
  - Endoscopes by virtue of their dynamic position help in visualization of the ossicular assembly at various angles in a magnified way.
  - Thus, the configuration of each ossicle, its integrity and relative position with respect to other ossicles and surrounding critical structures such as the facial nerve, processus cochleariformis, etc., are better appreciated with the help of endoscopes (zero degree and angled scopes).
- *Confirmation of diagnosis*:
  - Diagnosis of ossicular chain erosion or discontinuity are well-diagnosed at a very early point in surgery.
  - In the presence of tympanic membrane perforation or retraction pocket, the diagnosis may be confirmed by negotiating the scope through the perforation/ retraction.
  - This avoids extra bone drilling or chorda tympani manipulation, simply for the sake of exposure
  - It is important to realize that every inch of *normal* soft tissue should be ideally preserved as they contribute to the postoperative stability of the newly constructed assembly.
- *Placement of prosthesis*:
  - The crucial step of placement of prosthesis has two parts: the transit of the prosthesis from outside to the bed where it is to be placed and placement of the prosthesis.
  - The initial step requires optimal depth perception and higher magnification for precise placement of the prosthesis.
  - In microscopic surgery, the two have to be manually adjusted by the surgeon accordingly, whereas, in endoscopic surgery it is automatically achieved by virtue of its dynamic property.
  - Moreover, clearer view of the bed, to ensure it is adequately prepared (cleared of granulations, clots, etc.) and the final fit (for example, correct fit of the stapedius tendon into the slit created on the side of a partial ossicular reconstruction prosthesis) can be easily achieved using the endoscope.
  - Every such minute detail adds to the final audiological outcome which is of paramount importance and the main goal of ossiculoplasty.

STEPS OF ENDOSCOPIC OSSICULOPLASTY

Ossiculoplasty is a part of a surgery (that may be functional endoscopic ear surgery or endoscopic mastoid surgery) designed to repair the damaged ossicles/ossicular chain aimed to restore middle ear transformer mechanism.

Depending on the surgery of which it is a part, the initial steps are done according to that primary surgery.

The sequence of steps related to ossicular chain reconstruction is as follows:

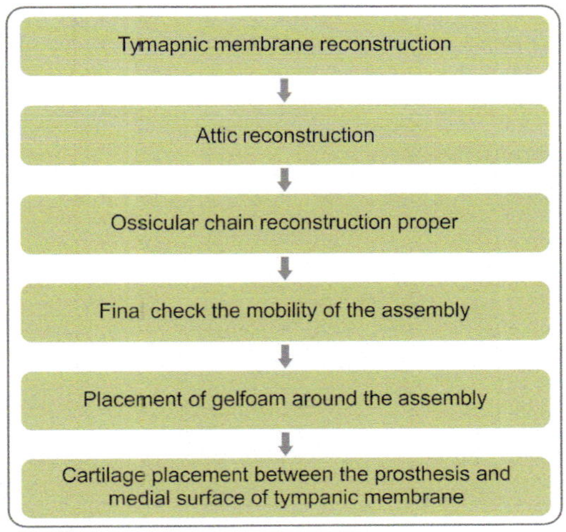

The different clinical scenarios usually encountered in day-to-day practice may be broadly classified into two basic conditions:

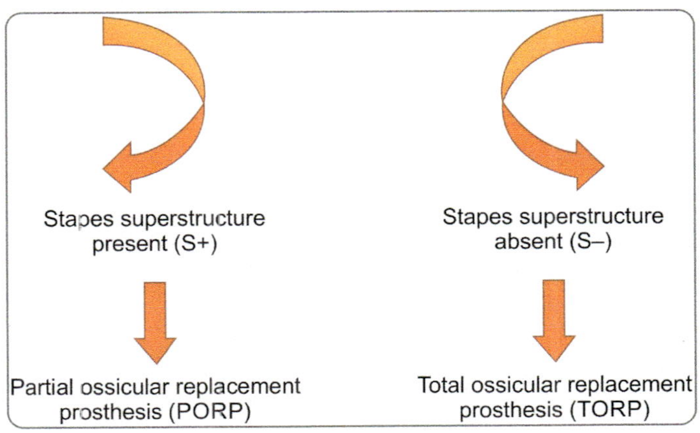

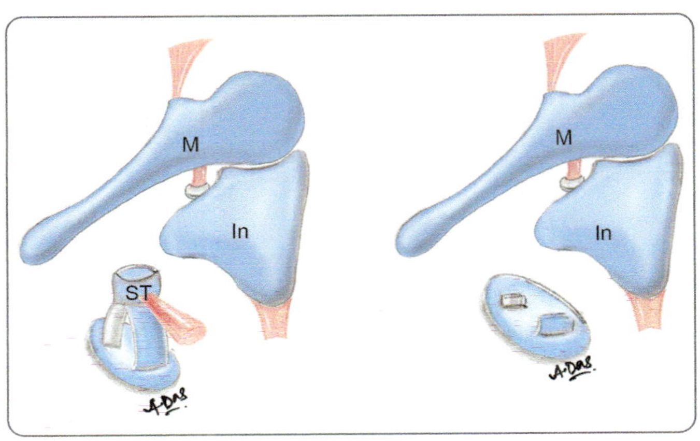

In this chapter, we have discussed two basic clinical scenarios—(1) stapes suprastructure present (left; 60%) and (2) stapes absent (right; 23%). Together, these constitute >80% of the encountered scenarios of ossicular chain status.

CLINICAL SCENARIO: STAPES SUPERSTRUCTURE PRESENT (S+); RECONSTRUCTION WITH PARTIAL OSSICULAR REPLACEMENT PROSTHESIS

- Incus remnant, if present, has to be removed in order to make space for the new assembly as well as to clear the ventilation pathways.
- A fine-tipped pick is used to disarticulate the incudomalleolar joint which is relatively resistant to inflammatory disease process and is eroded late.
- The eroded incus is then gently delivered out using alligator or cup forceps.

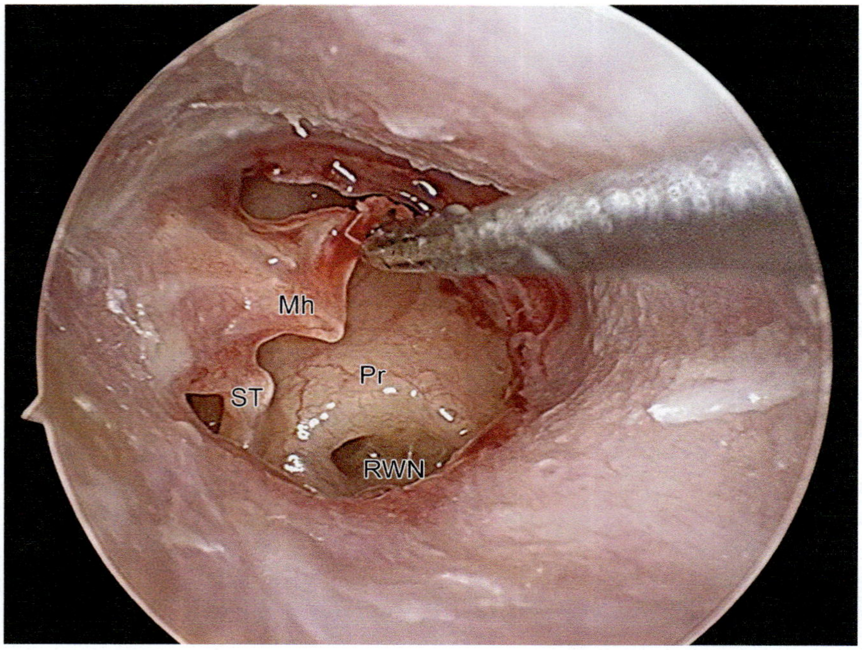

Fig. 1A: Margin of perforation being freshened. (Mh: handle of malleus; Pr: promontory; RWN: round window niche; ST: stapes)

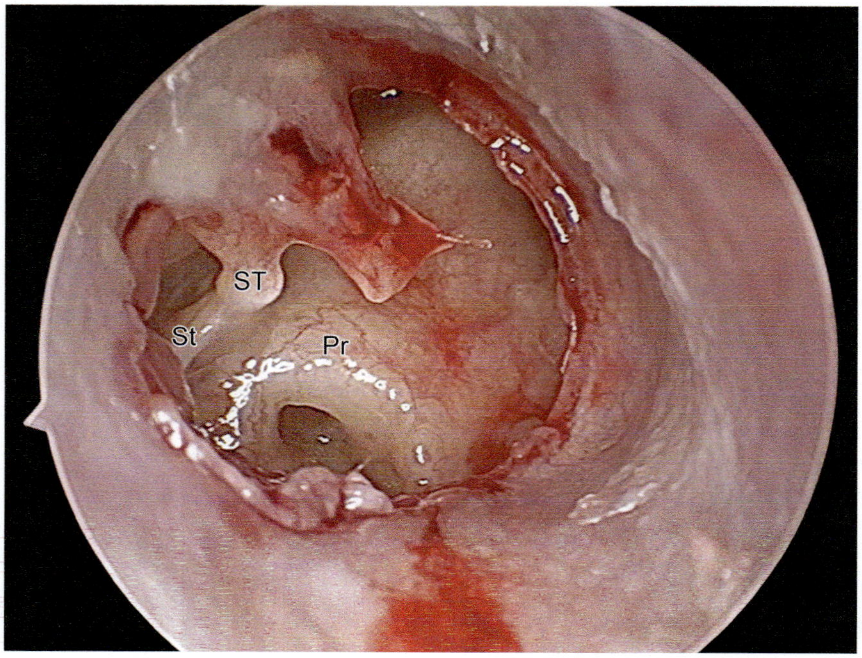

Fig. 1B: Inspection of ossicular chain status prior to tympanomeatal flap elevation. (Pr: promontory; ST: stapes; St: stapedius tendon)

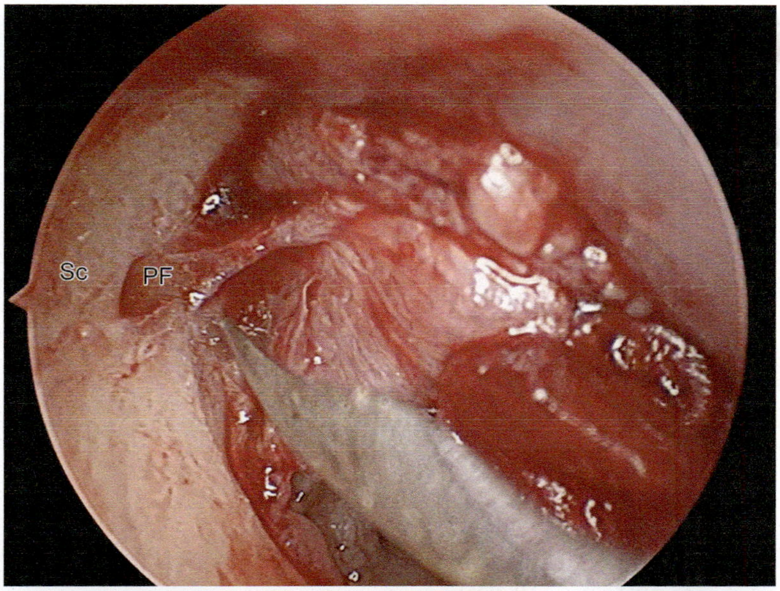

Fig. 1C: Elevation of tympanomeatal flap.
(PF: pars flaccida; Sc: scutum)

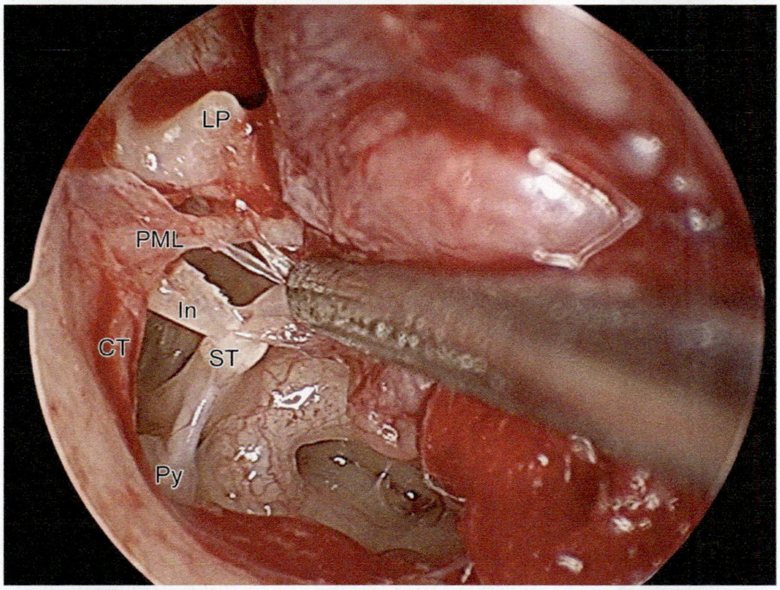

Fig. 1D: Exposure of ossicular chain after elevation of tympanomeatal flap.
(CT: chorda tympani; In: incus; LP: lateral process; PML: posterior malleolar ligament; Py: processus pyramidalis; ST: stapes)

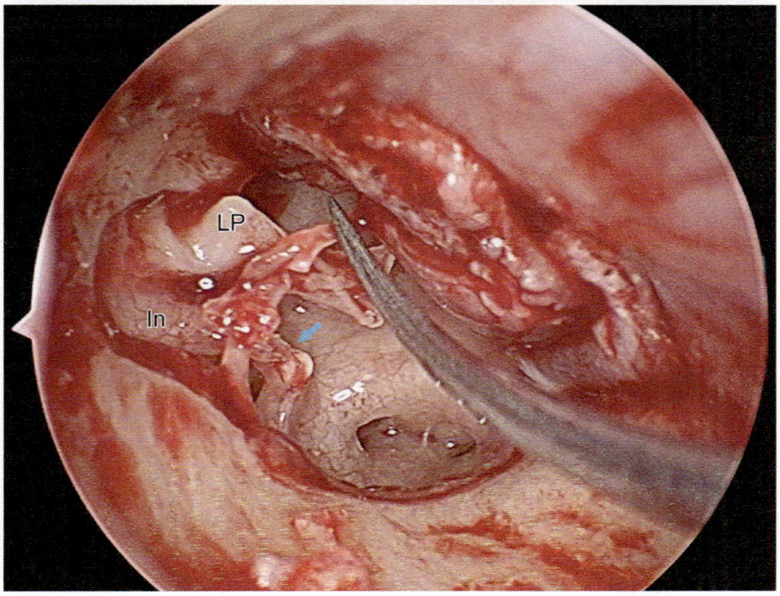

Fig. 2A: Incudostapedial joint inspected (arrow).
(In: incus; LP: lateral process)

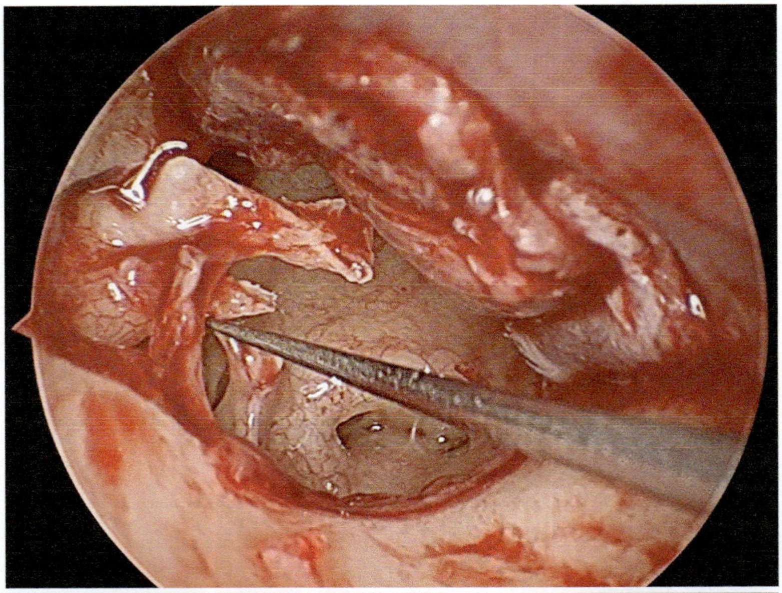

Fig. 2B: Fibrous bands dissected out using a smooth curved pick.

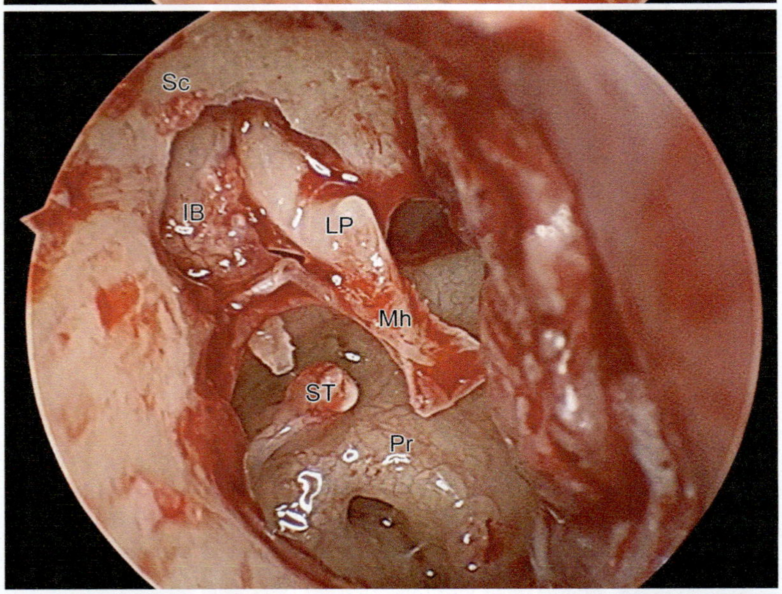

Fig. 2C: Incus body with eroded long process visualized.
(IB: body of incus; LP: lateral process; Mh: handle of malleus; Pr: promontory; Sc: scutum; ST: stapes)

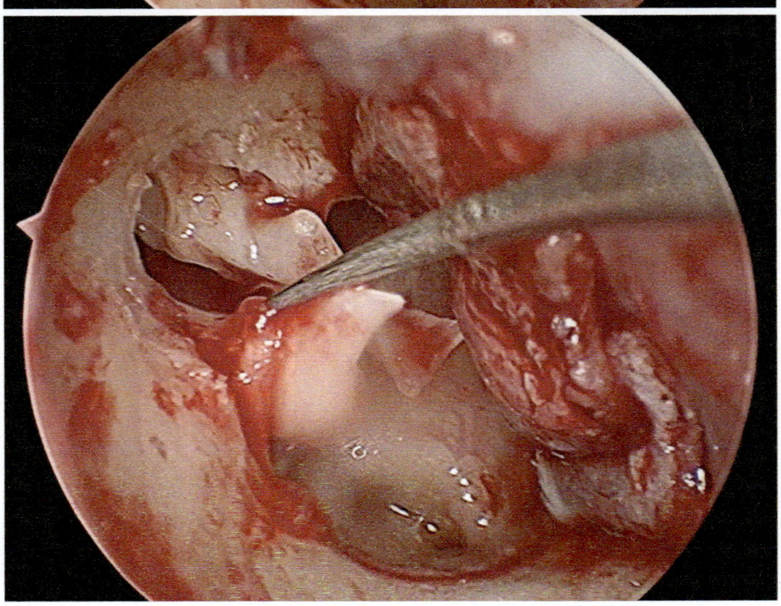

Fig. 2D: Incus being delivered out.

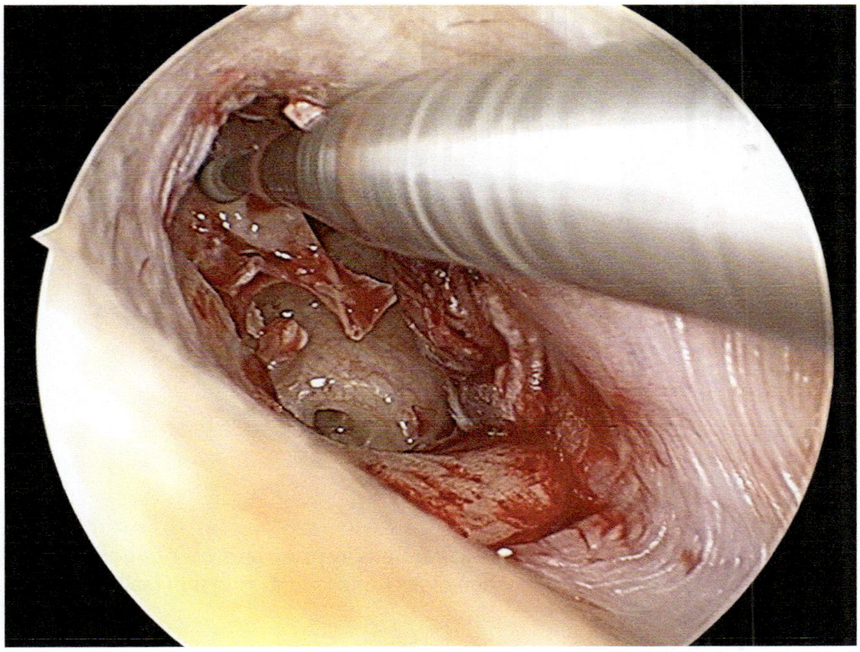

Fig. 3: Atticotomy for complete exposure of ossicular chain.

- The head of the malleus is then nipped just above the neck (where the tensor tympani attaches to it) with a malleus nipper, taking care to not damage the tensor tendon, keeping processus cochleariformis in view.

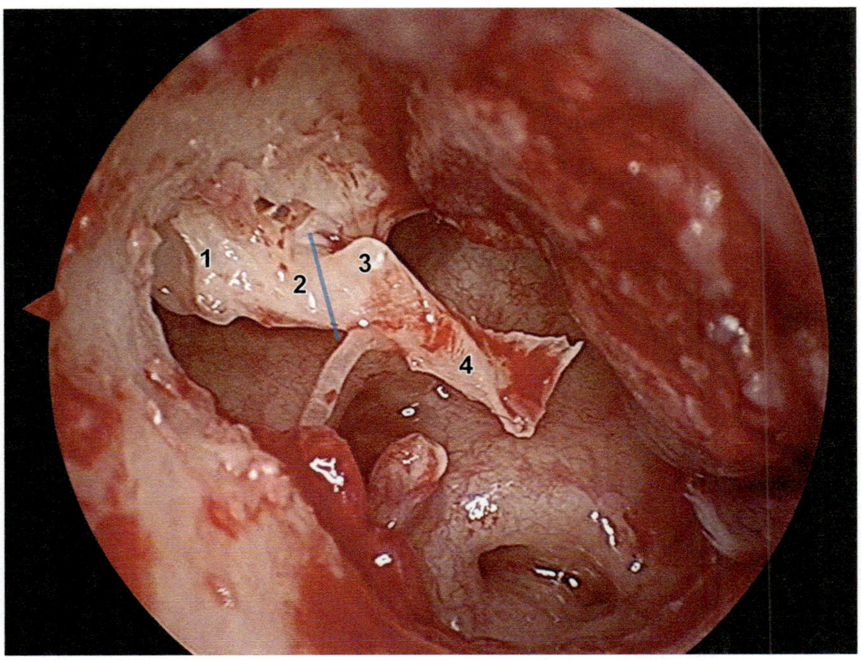

Fig. 4A: Site of nipping of malleus head (1. Head of malleus, 2. Neck, 3. Lateral process of malleus, 4. Handle of malleus).

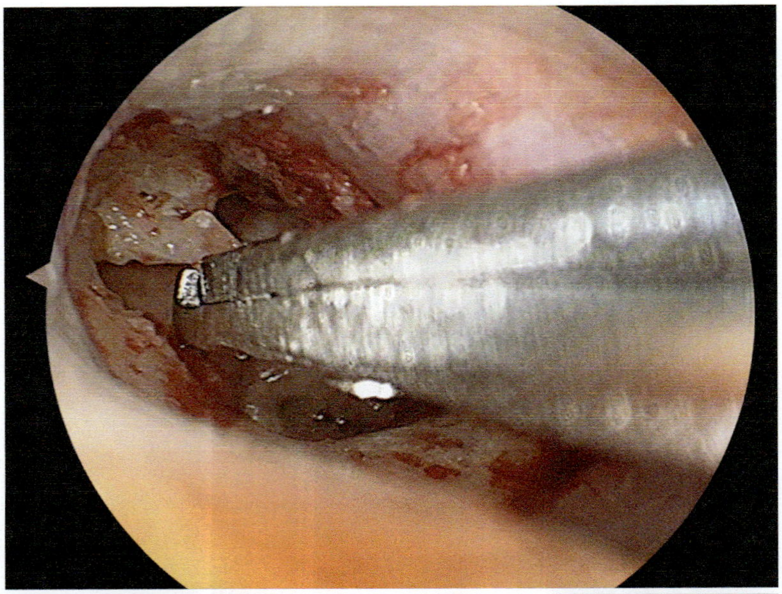

Fig. 4B: Malleus nipper being engaged at the junction of neck and lateral process of malleus.

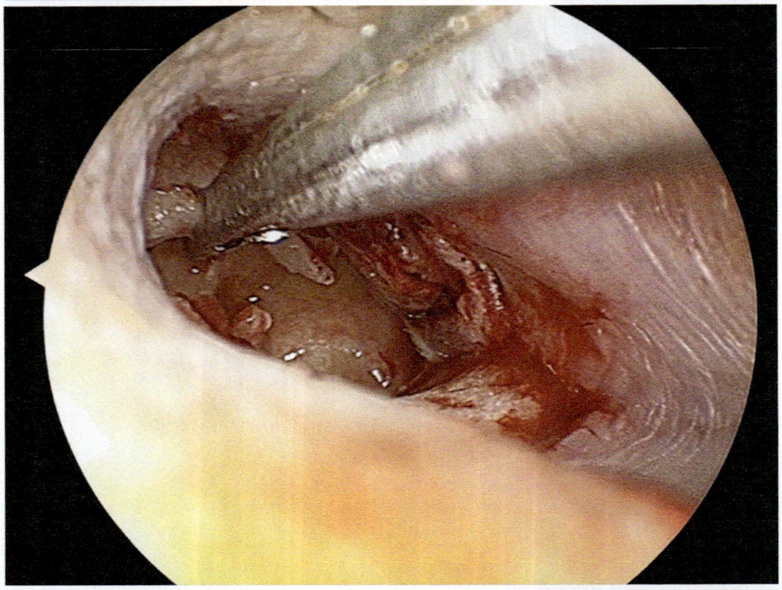

Fig. 4C: Malleus being nipped.

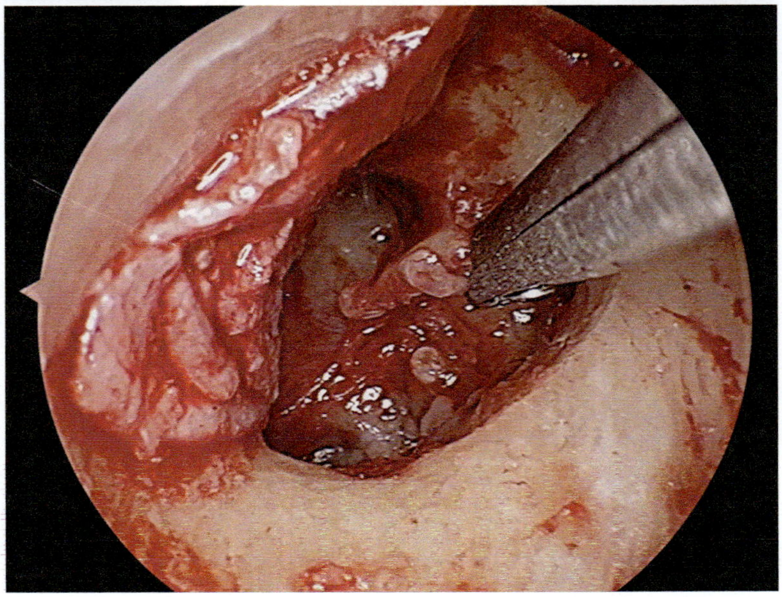

Fig. 4D: Introduction of malleus nipper in left ear.

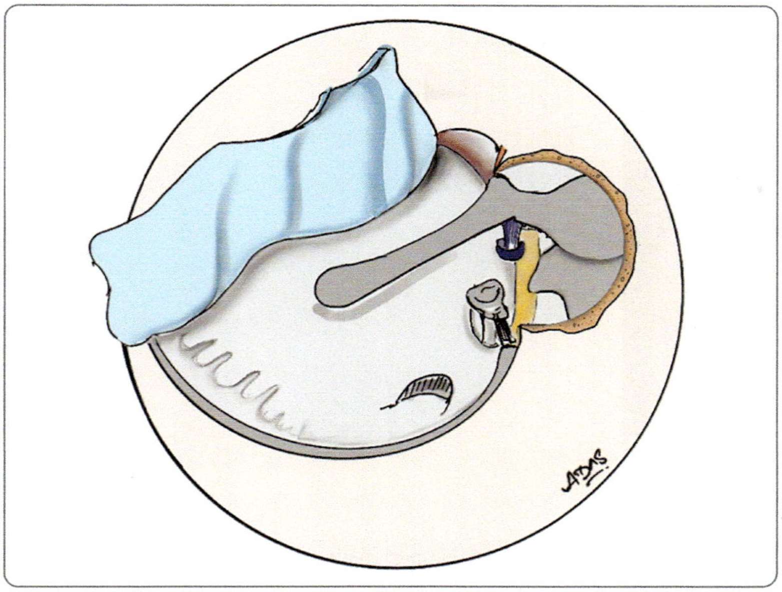

Fig. 4E: Pictorial depiction of exposed working area.

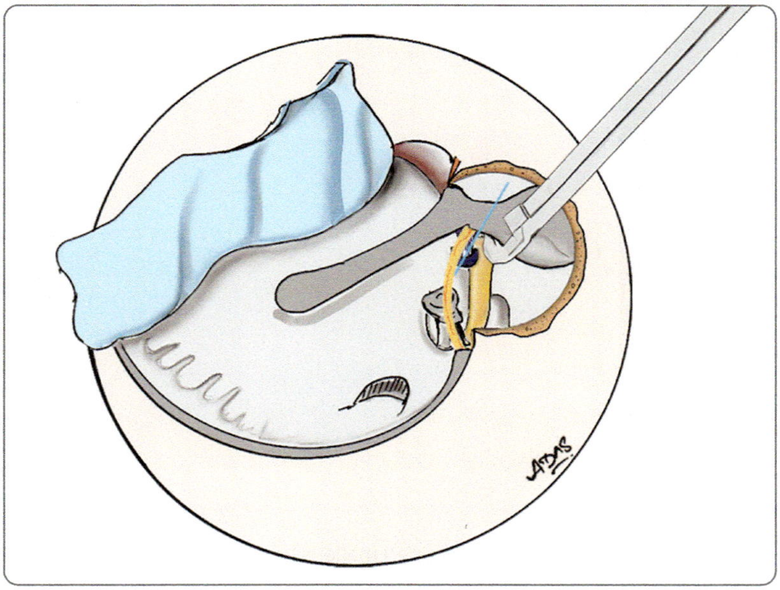

Fig. 4F: Engaging the malleus nipper at the correct site.

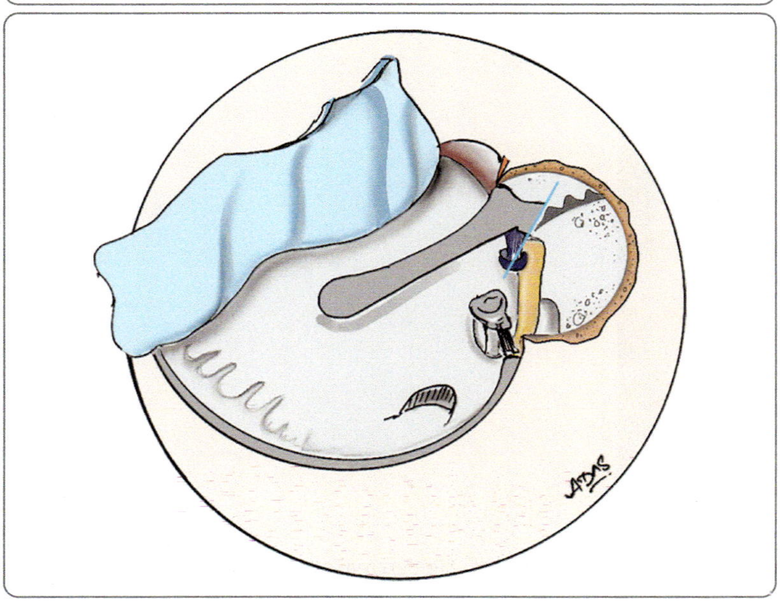

Fig. 4G: Exposure after removal of malleus head.

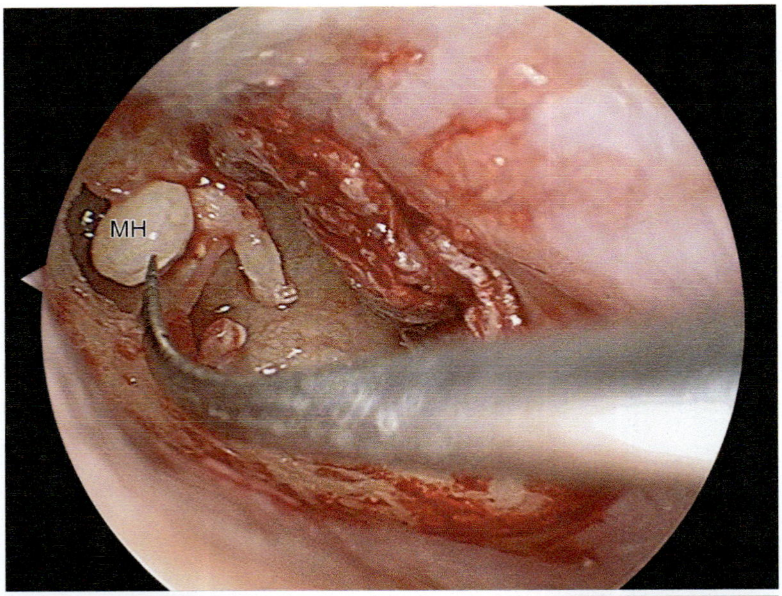

Fig. 5A: Nipped malleus head (MH) being manipulated using smooth curved pick (right ear).

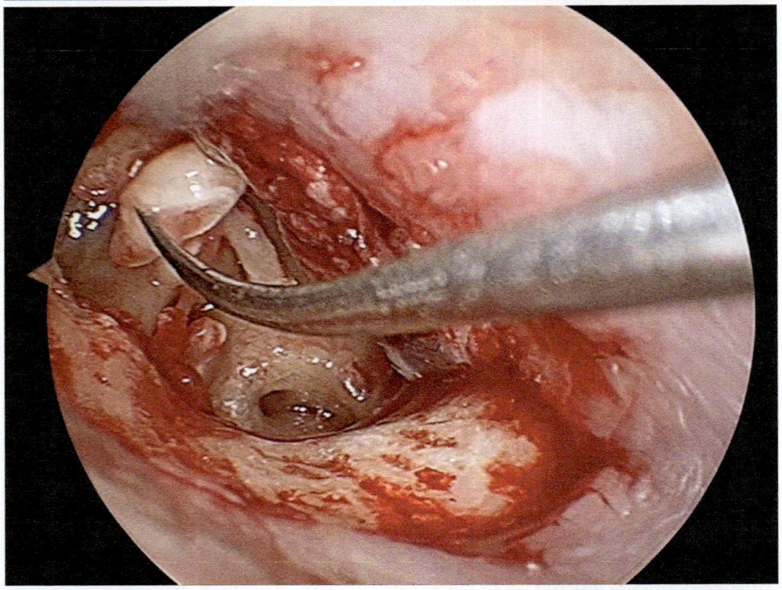

Fig. 5B: Nipped malleus head (MH) being delivered out (right ear).

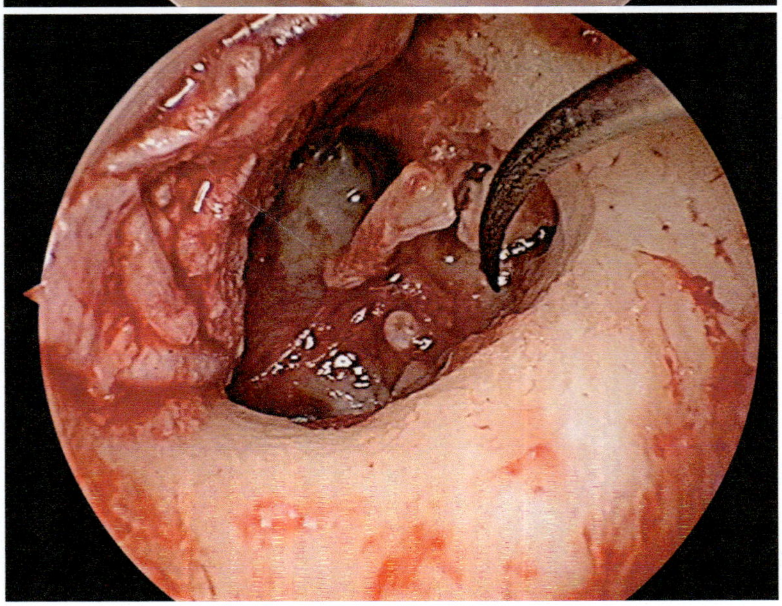

Fig. 5C: Nipped malleus head being manipulated using smooth curved pick (left ear).

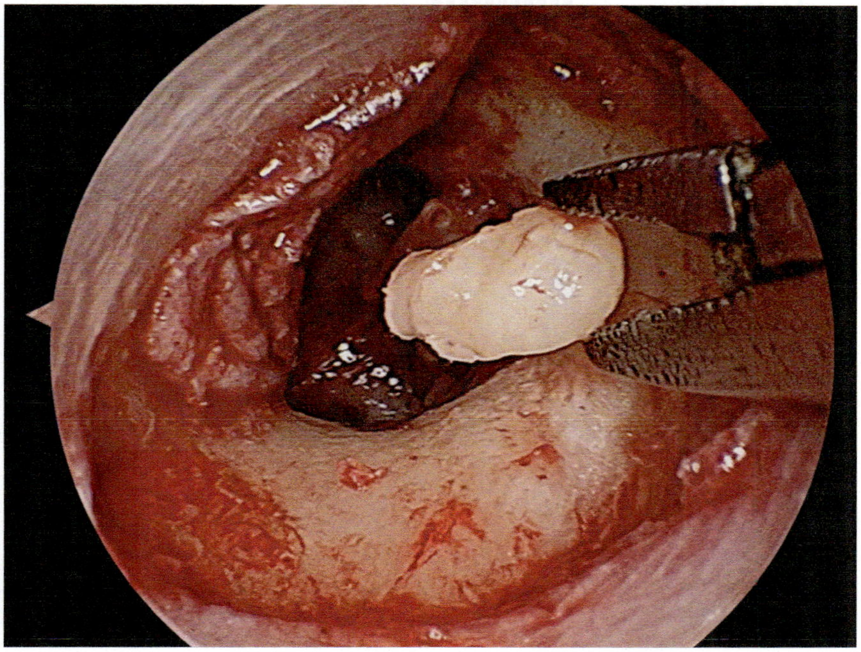

Fig. 5D: Nipped malleus head being delivered out using alligator forceps (left ear).

PEARL **NIPPING THE HEAD OF MALLEUS**

The advantages of this step are:

- Better visualization of the *anterior epitympanic space* and *protympanum*
- Clearance of any disease (cholesteatoma or granulations blocking the additional anterior pathway/tensor fold)
- Next, the bed for the ossicular chain reconstruction has to be prepared meticulously

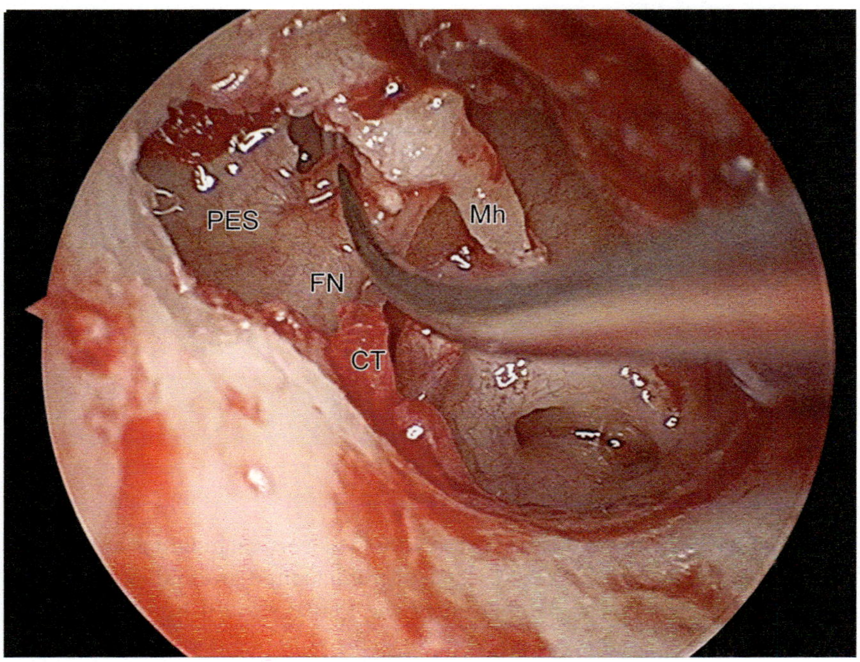

Fig. 6A: Dissection of anterior epitympanic space through the atticotomy window.
(CT: chorda tympani; FN: facial nerve; Mh: malleus handle; PES: posterior epitympanic space)

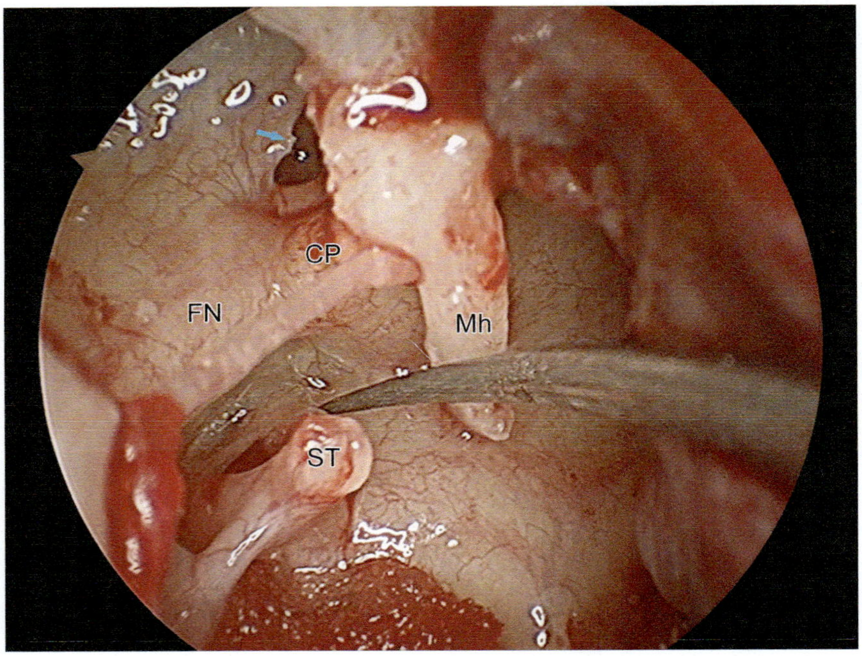

Fig. 6B: Inspection of epitympanic space. (CP: cochleariform process; FN: facial nerve; small arrow: Cog; Mh: malleus handle)

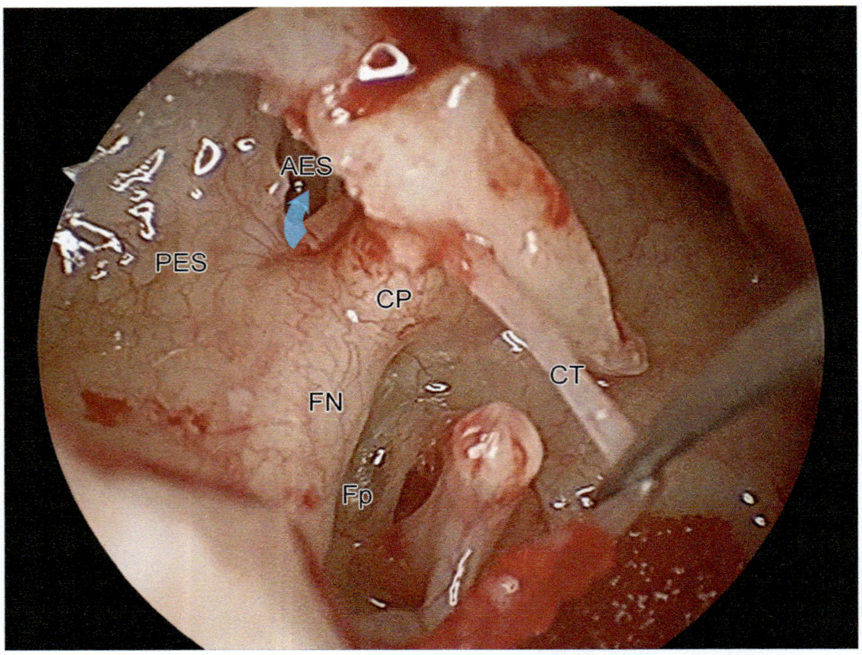

Fig. 6C: Inspection of anterior epitympanic space (Curved arrow) and tensor fold through the atticotomy window. (AES: anterior epitympanic space; CP: cochleariform process; CT: chorda tympani; FN: facial nerve; Fp: footplate; PES: posterior epitympanic space)

PEARL **PREPARATION OF THE BED OF THE ASSEMBLY**

- Often florid granulations are found to cover the stapes footplate and its adjacent area
- These granulations need to be cleared for proper stability of the newly reconstructed assembly
- A piece of dry gelfoam is used to gently wipe the area around the stapes superstructure and then gently passed in between the crura to clear the granulations

TIP

- All movements of and around the ossicles must be in the proper direction to avoid iatrogenic ossicular dislocation.

- *Preparation of prosthesis:* The vertical height is measured with the help of a custom designed graduated dissector. The vertical limb of the PORP should be of the same length. A number 11 scalpel blade is used to sharply create a "V"-shaped *slit in the posterior aspect of the vertical limb*. This slit is made to ensure a snug fit of the *stapedius tendon* inside it, thus making the assembly more stable.

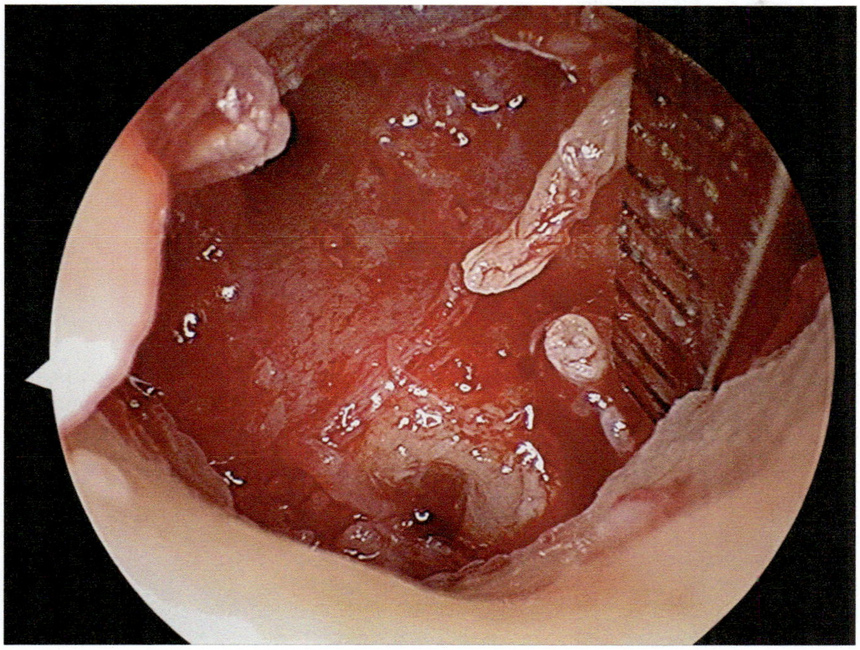

Fig. 7A: Measurement of the length of prosthesis in situ using graduated dissector (From footplate).

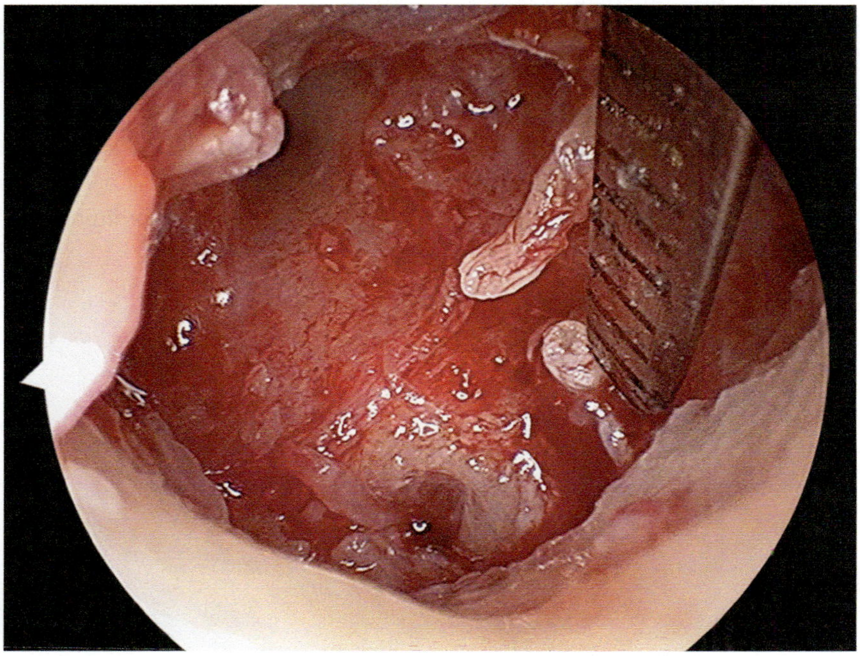

Fig. 7B: Measurement of the length of prosthesis in situ using graduated dissector (From stapes head).

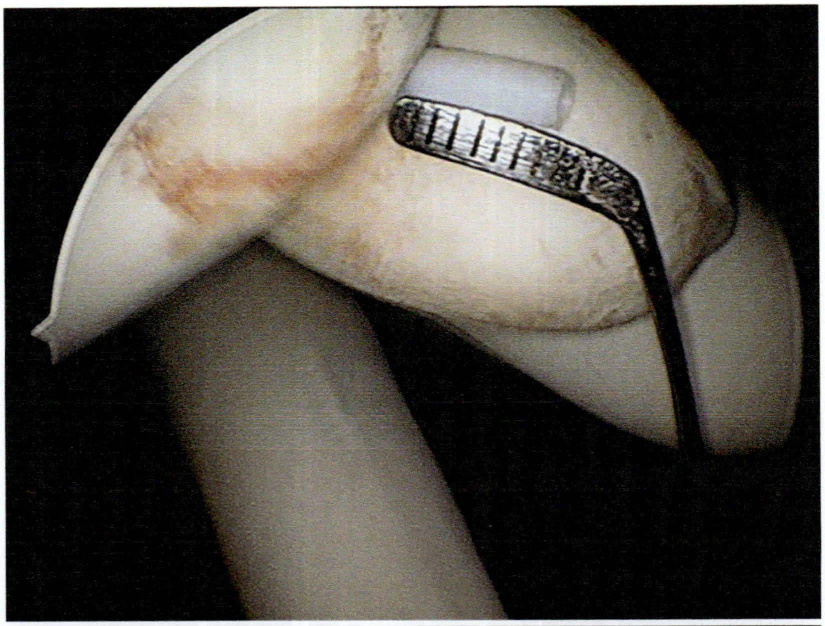

Fig. 7C: Measurement of length of prosthesis prior to trimming according to the appropriate length.

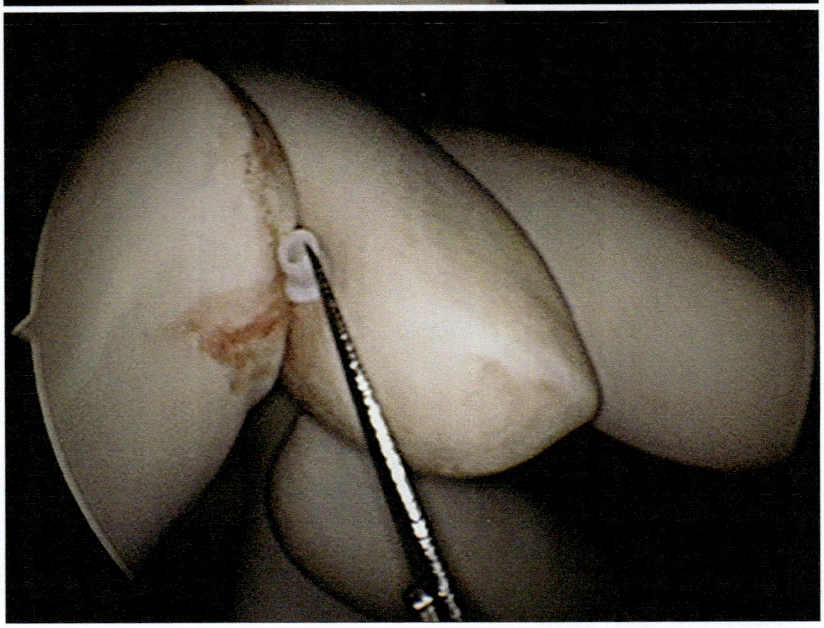

Fig. 7D: Creating a V-shaped slit for fitting the tendon of stapedius.

PEARL **RELEVANT ANATOMICAL MEASUREMENTS FOR OSSICULOPLASTY**

Capitulum is usually 1–2 mm, vertical height from footplate is 4–5 mm. Distance between stapes and malleus is usually 3–4 mm.

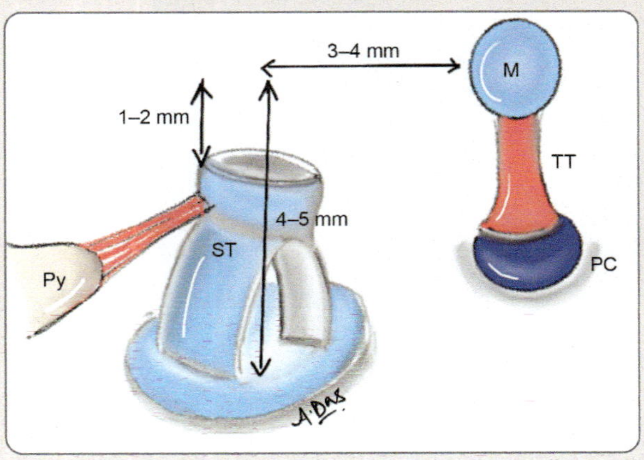

- *Placement of prosthesis:* The prosthesis is carried anterior to the stapes suprastructure with the help of a suction tip or an alligator forceps and then pulled backward over it, using a smooth curved pick. The inner groove of the vertical limb is placed atop the stapes superstructure, with the slit for stapedius placed posteriorly to fit in the stapedial tendon. It is then adjusted with the help of a fine pick for optimal fit. Gelfoam pieces are placed around the assembly to stabilize it.

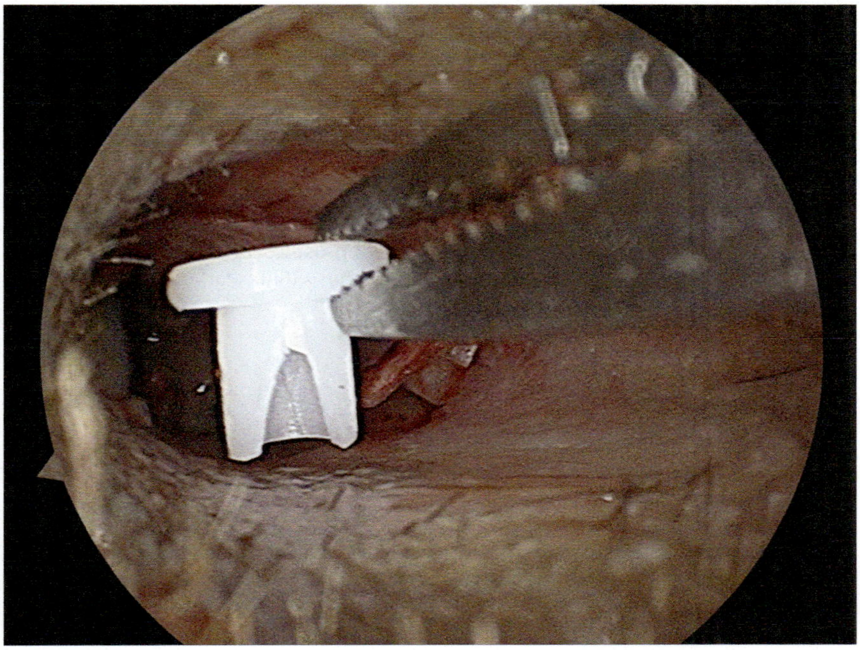

Fig. 8A: Method of prosthesis placement: Holding the prosthesis using alligator forcep.

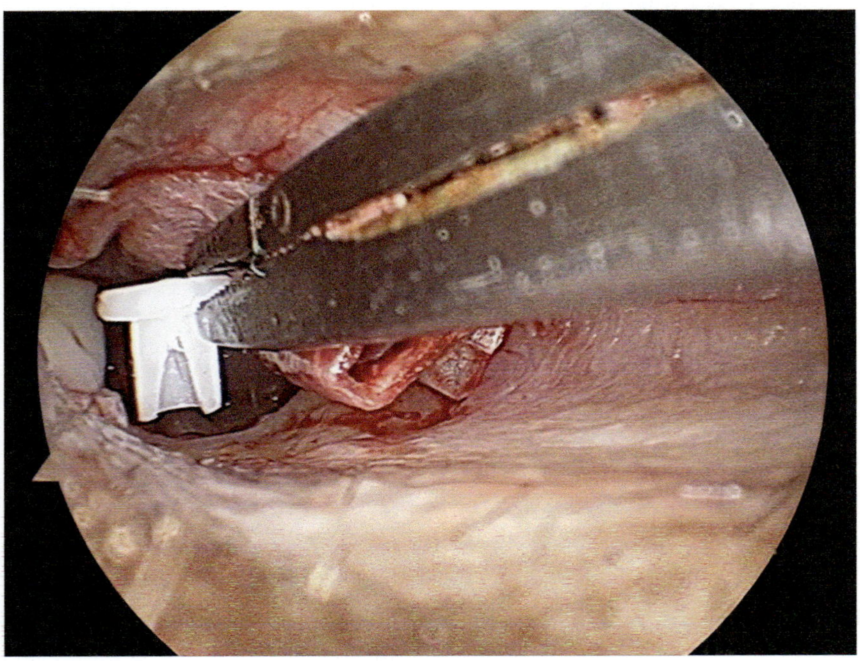

Fig. 8B: Method of prosthesis placement: Advancement of prosthesis into middle ear.

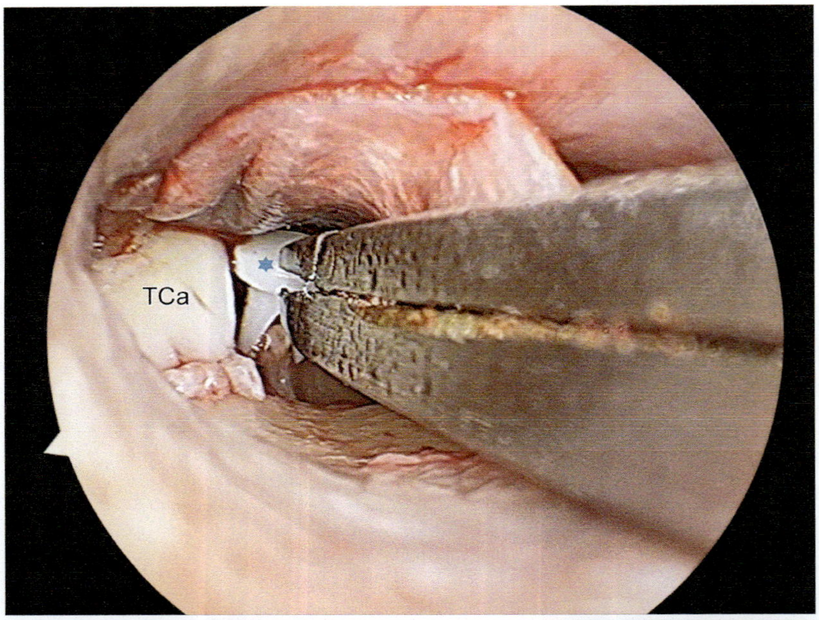

Fig. 8C: Method of prosthesis placement: Placement of prosthesis (Blue star) over stapes head. (TCa: tragal cartilage)

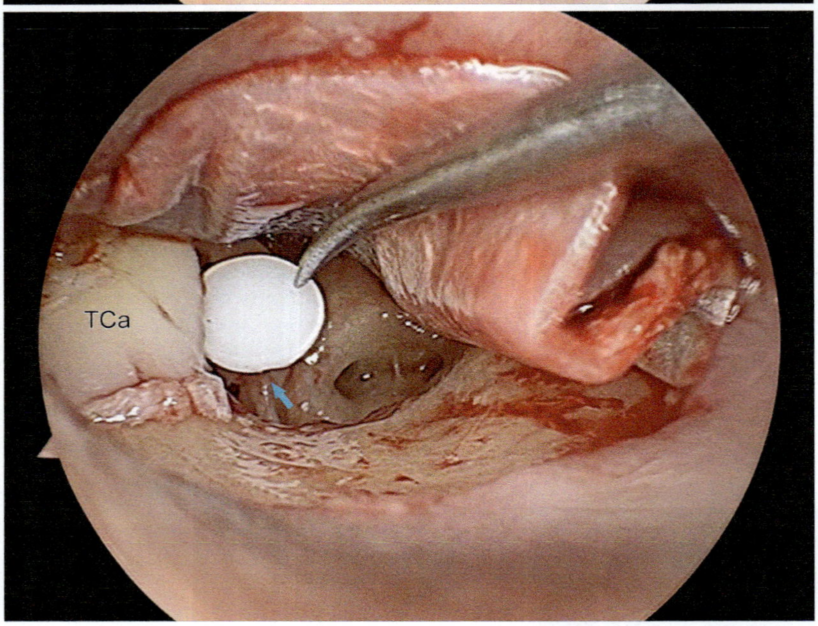

Fig. 8D: Method of prosthesis placement: Final positioning with the help of a smooth, curved pick. Arrow: Slit of prosthesis fitting over stapedius tendon. (TCa: tragal cartilage)

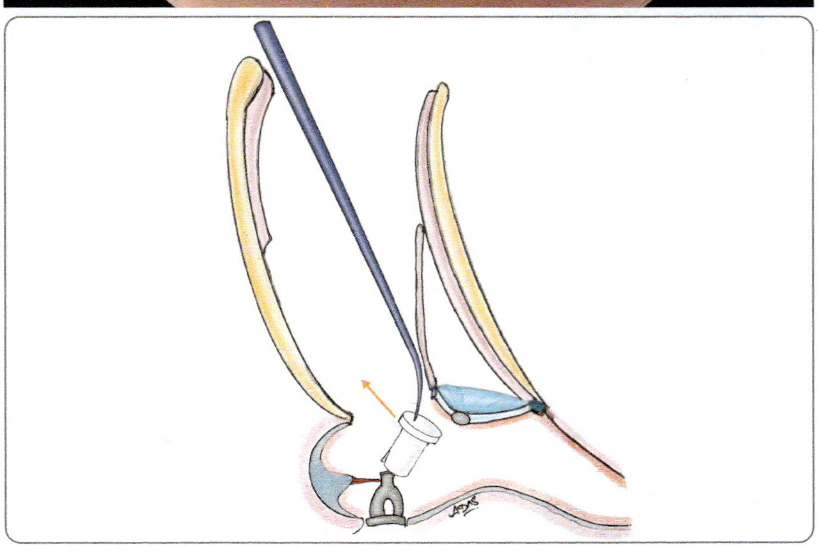

Fig. 8E: Pictorial depiction of method of placement of prosthesis in-situ (Sagittal view).

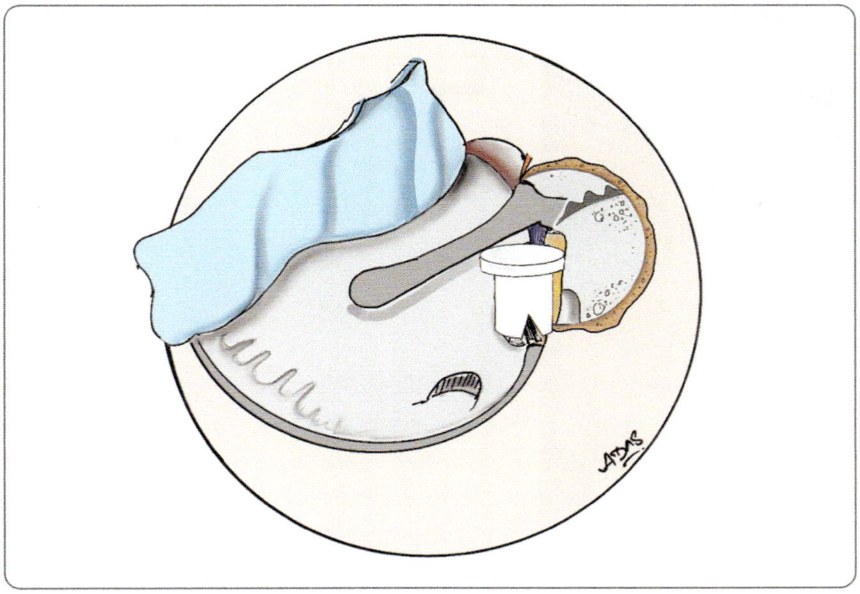

Fig. 8F: Pictorial depiction of method of placement of prosthesis in-situ (Endoscopic view).

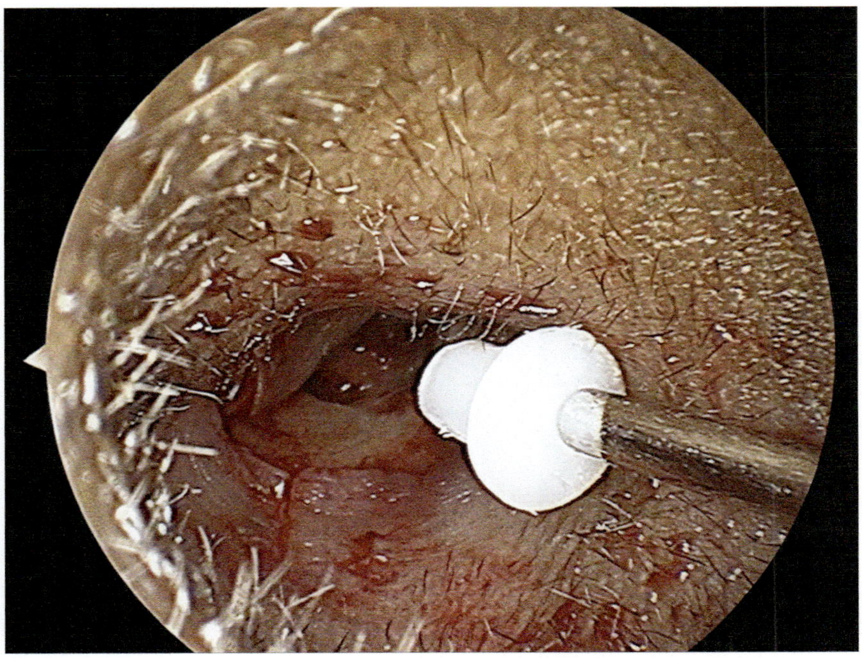

Fig. 9: Alternative method of carrying the prosthesis using a suction tip.

- *Round window reflex:* After the prosthesis has been placed, gentle pressure is exerted over the PORP with a micro-instrument and the corresponding reflection near the round window is visualized. This ensures that a proper conduction is taking place and that the prosthesis is in the correct position.

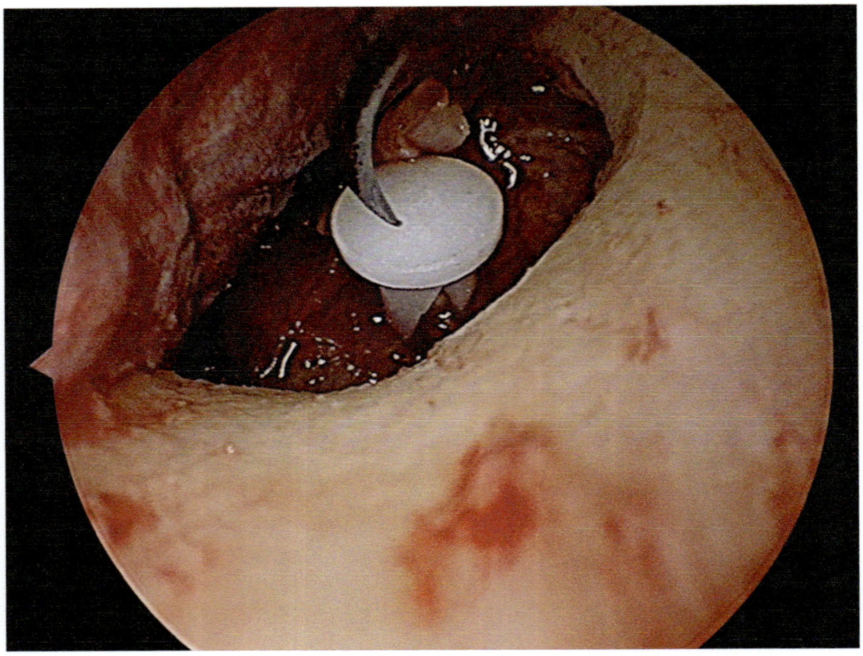

Fig. 10: Method of checking the round window reflex with a fine-tipped microinstrument (*Note* the shiny reflection below which moves with exertion of pressure over the prosthesis).

- *Cartilage cap over PORP:* A small piece of cartilage cap (usually tragal) is placed over the PORP, between the PORP and the tympanic membrane graft in order to prevent a foreign body reaction and subsequent extrusion of the prosthesis, due to direct contact with the tympanic membrane

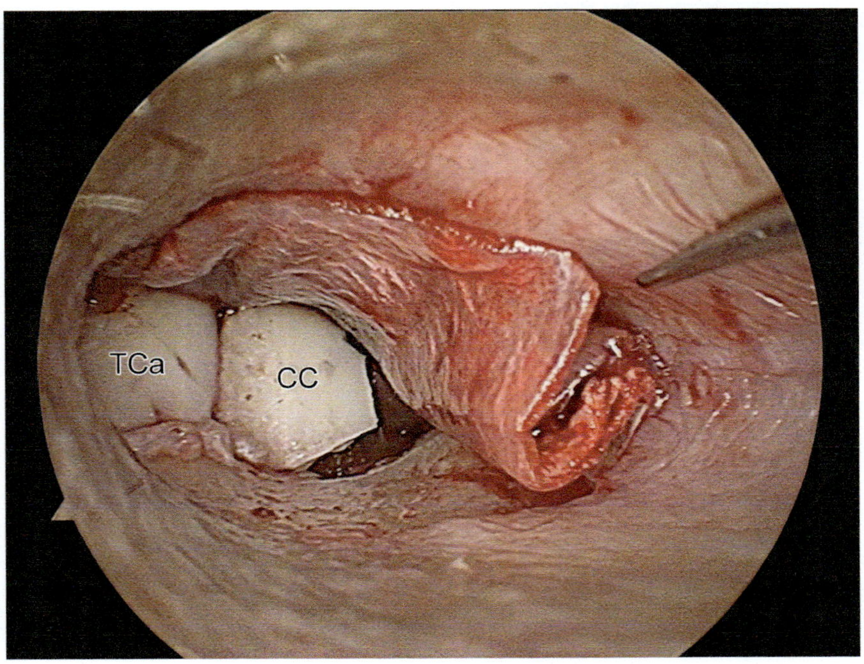

Fig. 11A: Placement of cartilage cap (CC) over prosthesis (*Note* that attic has been reconstructed with tragal cartilage (TCa).

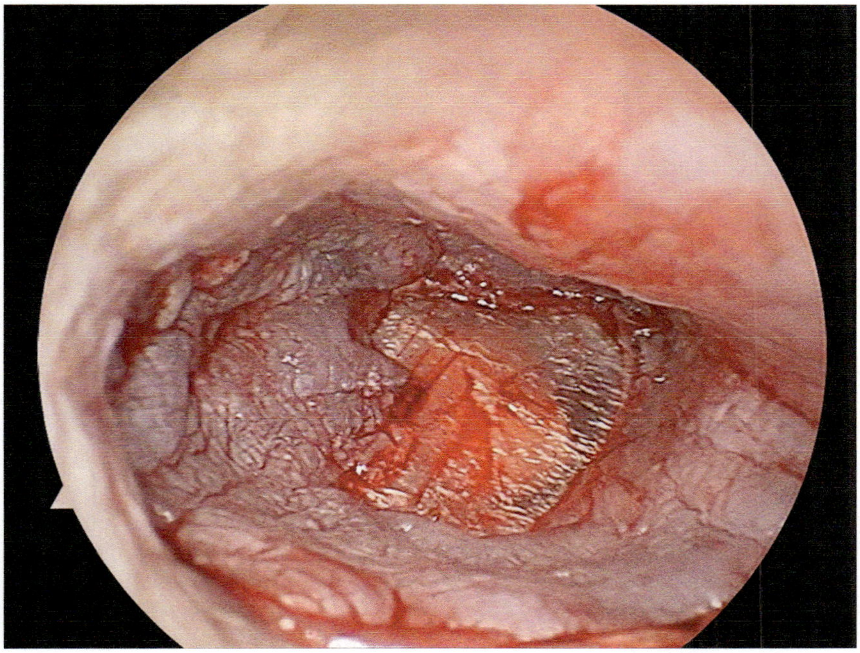

Fig. 11B: Final view after graft and tympanomeatal flap in position.

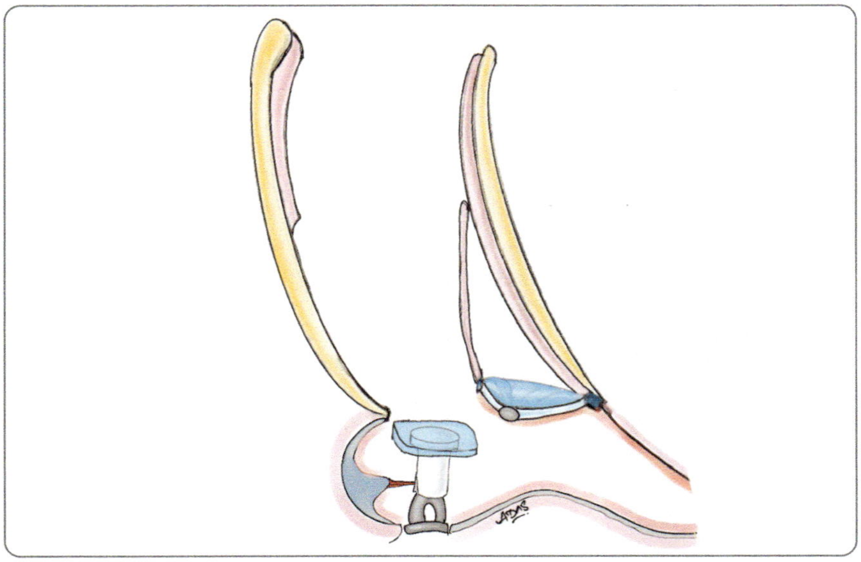

Fig. 11C: Pictorial depiction of cartilage cap over prosthesis.

CLINICAL SCENARIO: STAPES SUPERSTRUCTURE ABSENT (S−); RECONSTRUCTION WITH TOTAL OSSICULAR RECONSTRUCTION PROSTHESIS

The initial steps are same as in case of the previous clinical scenario.

- *Preparation of prosthesis:* The length of the TORP is gauged in a similar way as in PORP.
- *Preparation of cartilage shoe:* A ring of cartilage is fashioned from a tragal cartilage, used to stabilize the TORP over the footplate. This is known as cartilage shoe. The harvested piece of tragal cartilage, free of its perichondrium, is perforated at its center with a 0.9 mm microtrephine. The outer margin is then fashioned according to the configuration of the footplate.

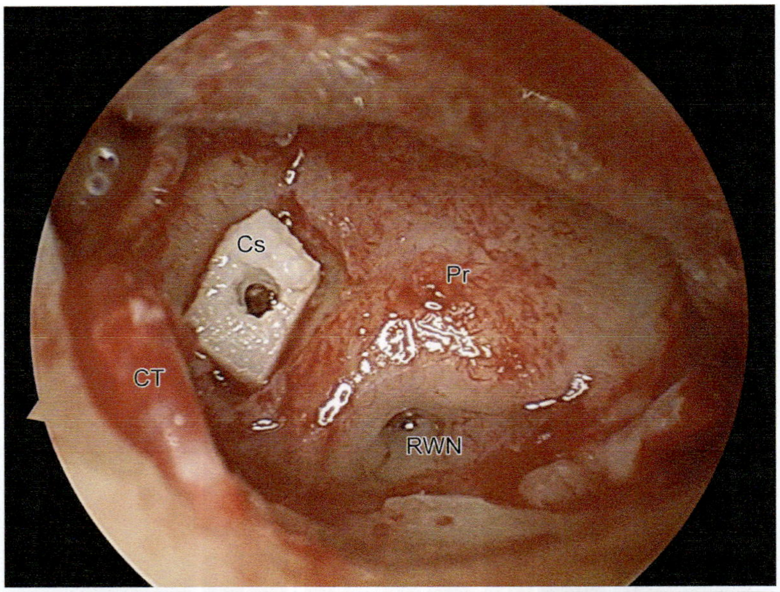

Fig. 12A: Placement of cartilage shoe over footplate. (Pr: promontory; RWN: round window niche; CT: chorda tympani nerve Cs: cartilage shoe)

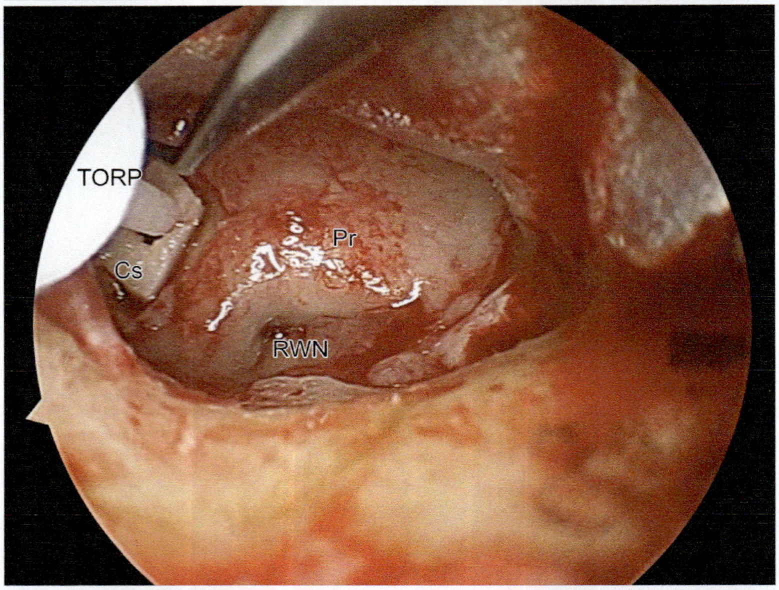

Fig. 12B: Prosthesis placement over cartilage shoe: lower end of TORP being manipulated using angled pick.
(Cs: cartilage shoe; Pr: promontory; RWN: round window niche; TORP: total ossicular replacement prosthesis)

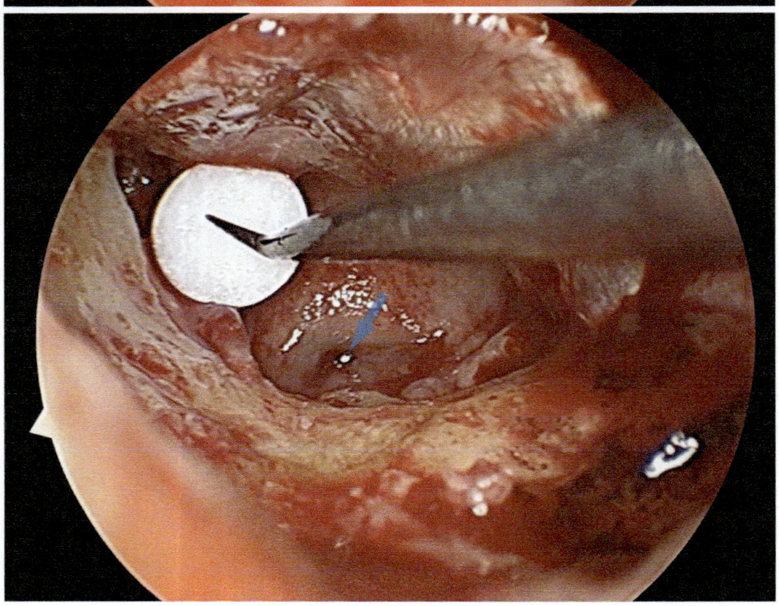

Fig. 12C: After proper placement of the prosthesis, round window reflex (Blue arrow) being checked.

- *Prosthesis placement:* The cartilage shoe is placed over the footplate (bed prepared already, described previously). The TORP is then carried to the site of reconstruction and placed over the cartilage shoe, already in place. Gelfoam pieces are placed around the assembly to further stabilize it.
- *Round window reflex*
- *Cartilage cap over TORP*

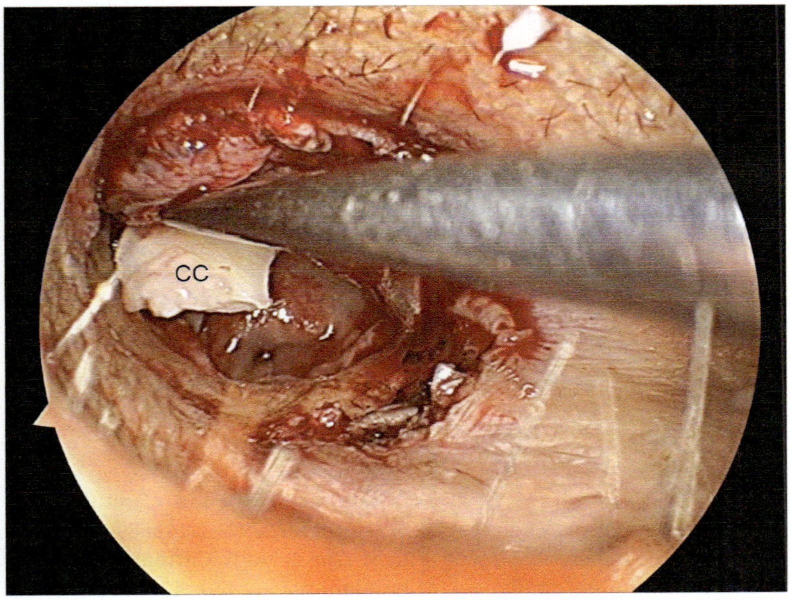

Fig.12D: Cartilage cap being placed between TORP and temporalis fascia graft.
(CC: Catrilage cap)

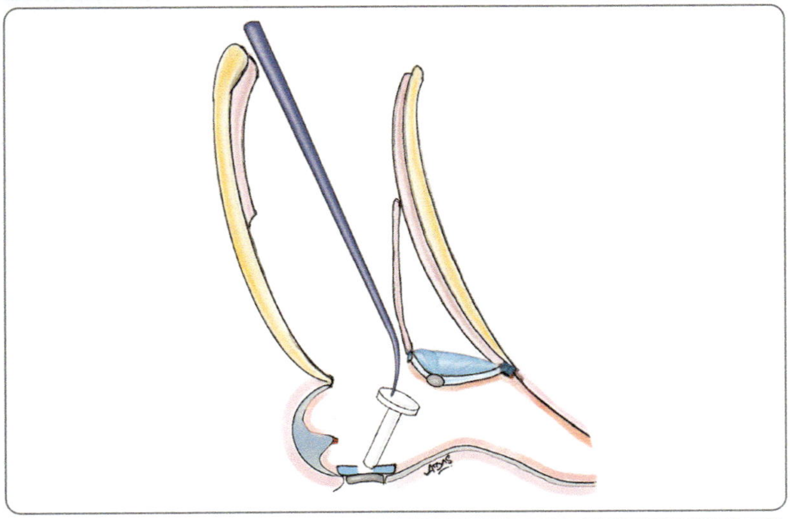

Fig. 13A: Pictorial depiction of placement of TORP over cartilage shoe (CS).

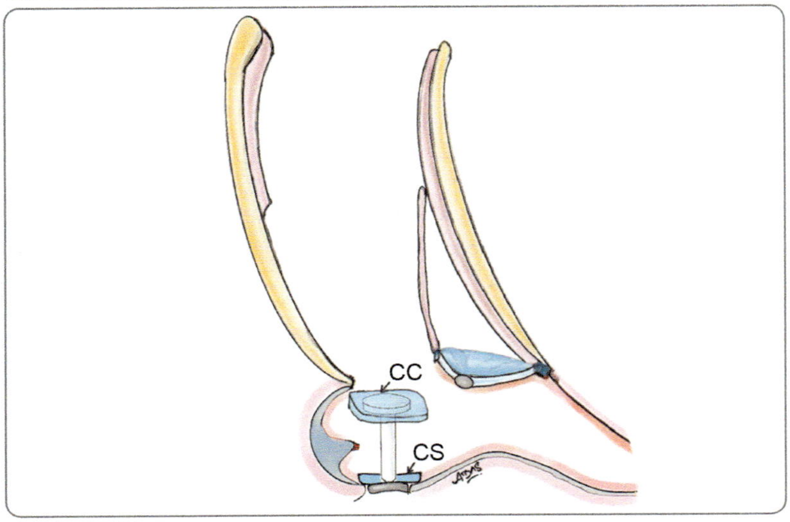

Fig. 13B: Pictorial depiction of placement of cartilage cap (CC) over TORP.

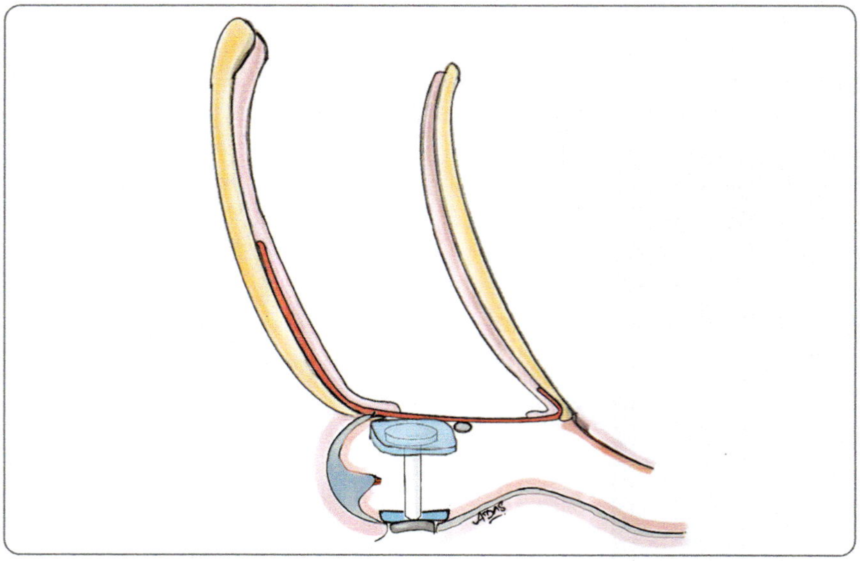

Fig. 13C: Final position of graft and tympanomeatal flap over prosthesis.

REFERENCES

1. Varshney S, Nangia A, Bist SS, Singh RK, Gupta N, Bhagat S. Ossicular chain status in chronic suppurative otitis media in adults. Indian J Otolaryngol Head Neck Surg. 2010;62(4):421-6.
2. Austin DF. Ossicular reconstruction. Otolaryngol Clin North Am. 1972;5(1):145-60.
3. Kartush JM. Ossicular chain reconstruction. Capitulum to malleus. Otolaryngol Clin North Am. 1994;27(4):689-715.
4. Merchant SN, McKenna MJ, Rosowski JJ. Current status and future challenges of tympanoplasty. Eur Arch Otorhinolaryngol. 1998;255(5):221-8.
5. Black B. Ossiculoplasty prognosis: the spite method of assessment. Am J Otol. 1992;13(6):544-51.

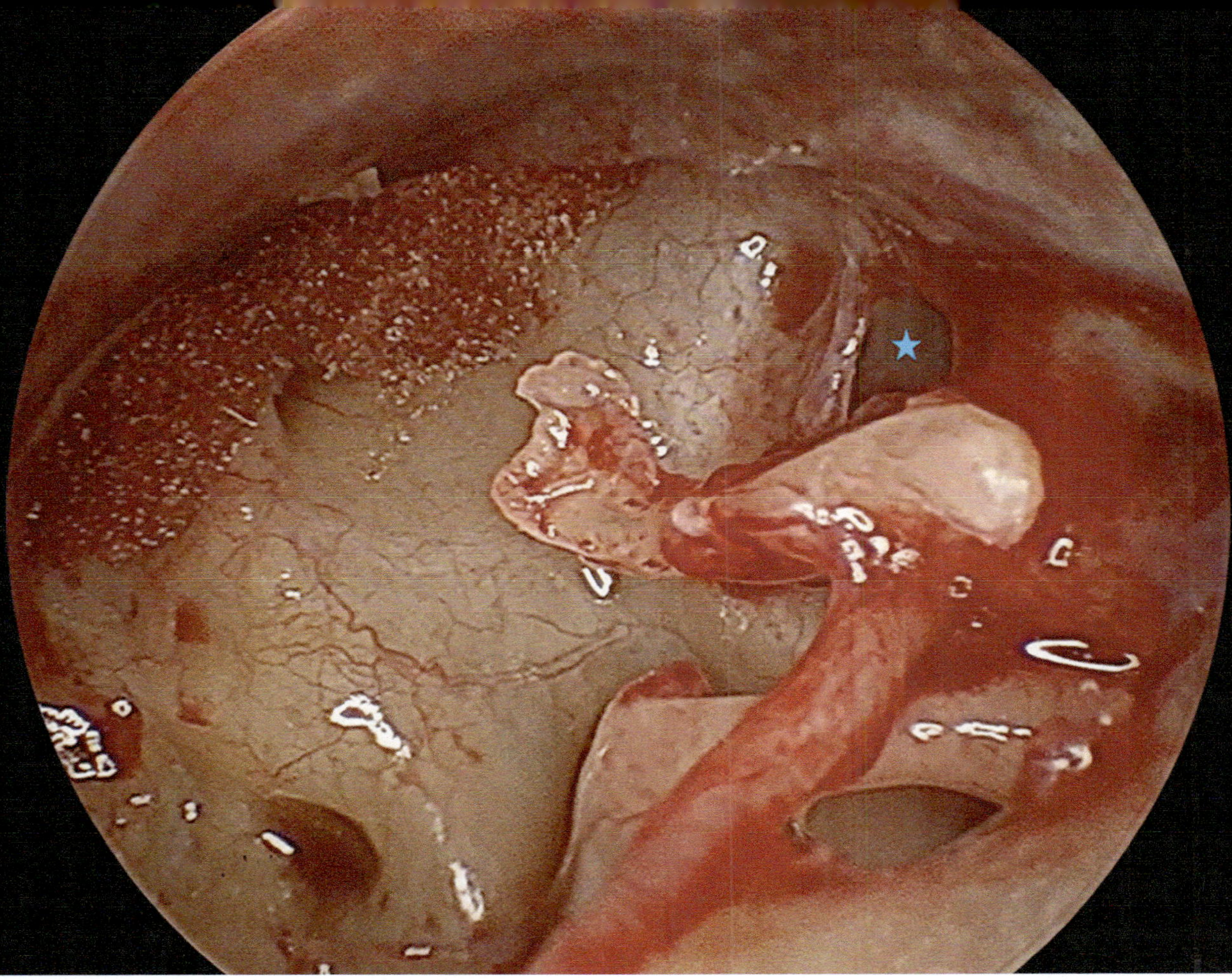

CHAPTER **9**

Endoscopic Epitympanic Exploration

Arindam Das, Sandipta Mitra

Chapter Outline

INTRODUCTION

The epitympanum is ventilated by two major (isthmus anticus and posticus) and one additional anterior route (incomplete tensor fold).[1] The anterior isthmus lies between the processus cochleariformis and the incudostapedial joint. The posterior isthmus lies between the incudostapedial joint and processus pyramidalis. The additional anterior pathway exists when the tensor fold is incomplete. A complete tensor fold with blockage of the tympanic isthmi may present with selective epitympanic dysventilation syndrome.[2] The understanding and visualization of the ventilation pathways is of paramount importance in the treatment of mucosal chronic otitis media where failure to address the pathology in these critical areas may result in reperforation or re-retraction.

INDICATIONS OF ENDOSCOPIC EPITYMPANIC EXPLORATION

- Clinically diagnosed cases of chronic otitis media of active mucosal variety
- Intraoperative diagnosis of ventilation pathway blockage during middle ear inspection in tympanoplasty

SURGICAL RATIONALE AND ITS PHYSIOLOGICAL BASIS

- Mucosal chronic otitis media is associated with inflammation and subsequent hypertrophy of the middle ear mucosal folds
- The hypertrophied mucosal folds block the normal ventilation pathways and impede the natural aeration of the epitympanic spaces
- Mere reconstruction of the tympanic membrane perforation or cortical mastoidectomy without addressing the ventilation pathway blocks lead to surgical failure and disease recurrence
- Endoscopic epitympanic exploration is mucosa-preserving, minimally invasive approach involving minimal bone curettage for exposure of the isthmi and use of soft atraumatic dissection technique with gelfoam for disease clearance.[3]

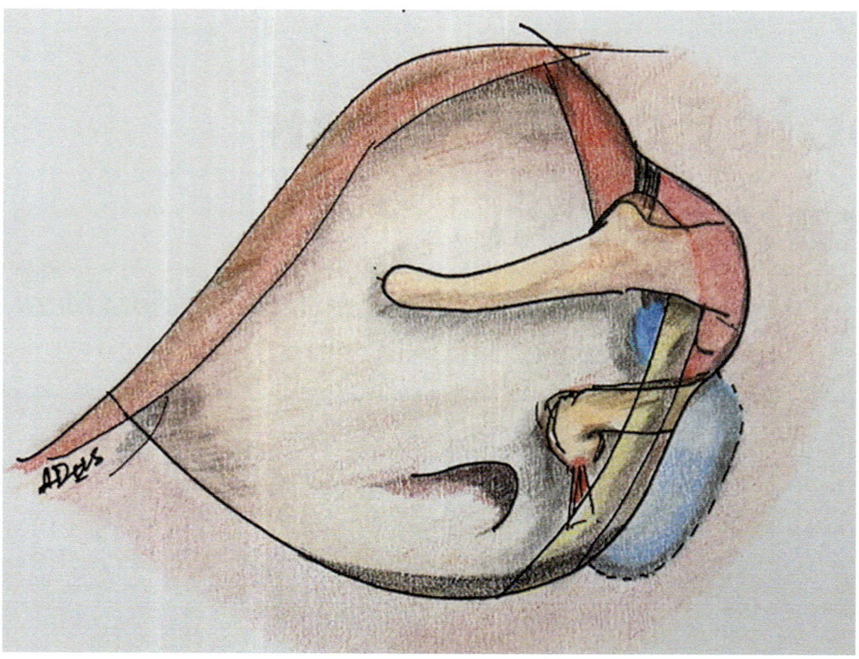

Fig. 1A: Endoscopic epitympanic exploration surgical technique: Schematic depiction of bone to be drilled for exposure.

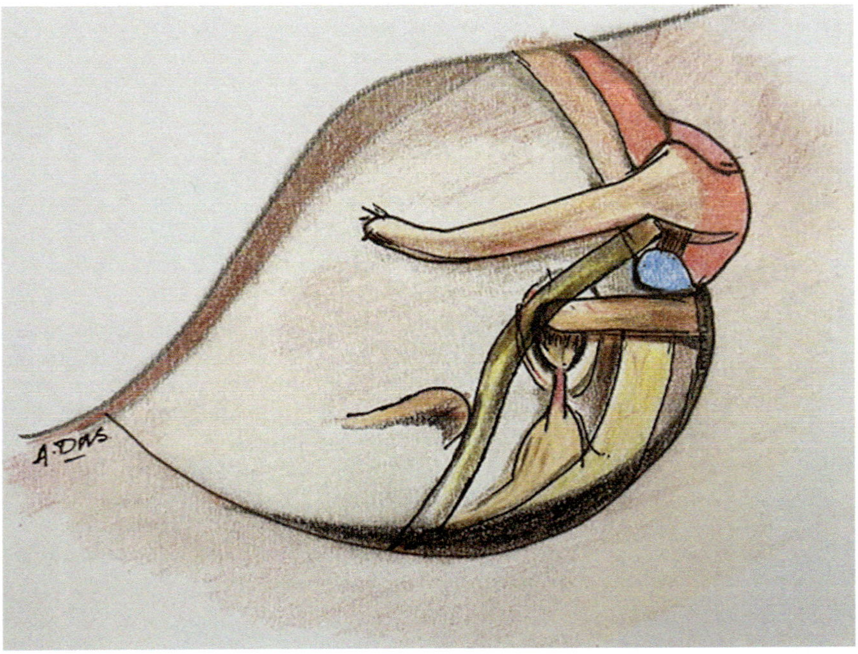

Fig. 1B: Endoscopic epitympanic exploration surgical technique: View after exposure.

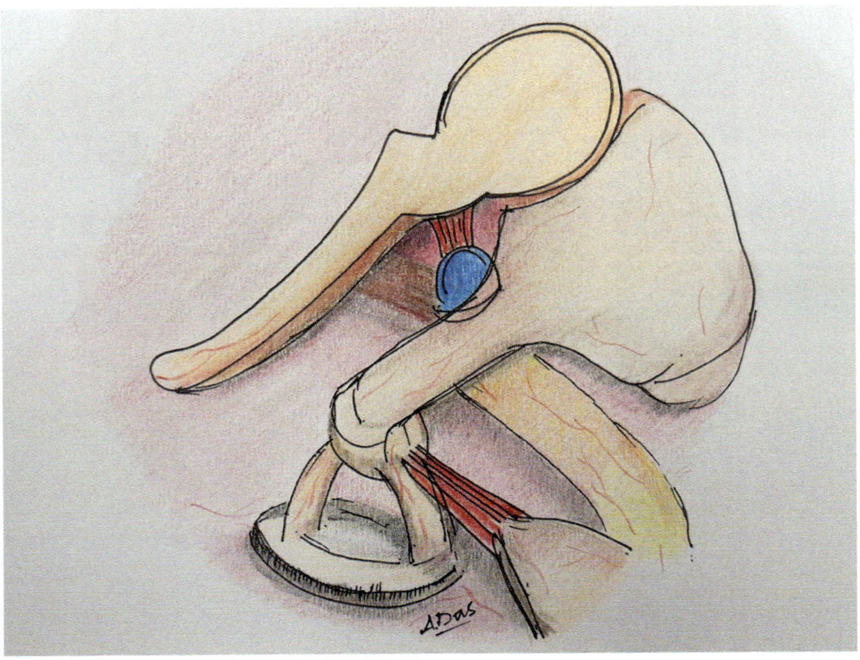

Fig. 1C: Endoscopic epitympanic exploration surgical technique: Angled (30 degree) view of ossicular chain upon adequate exposure.

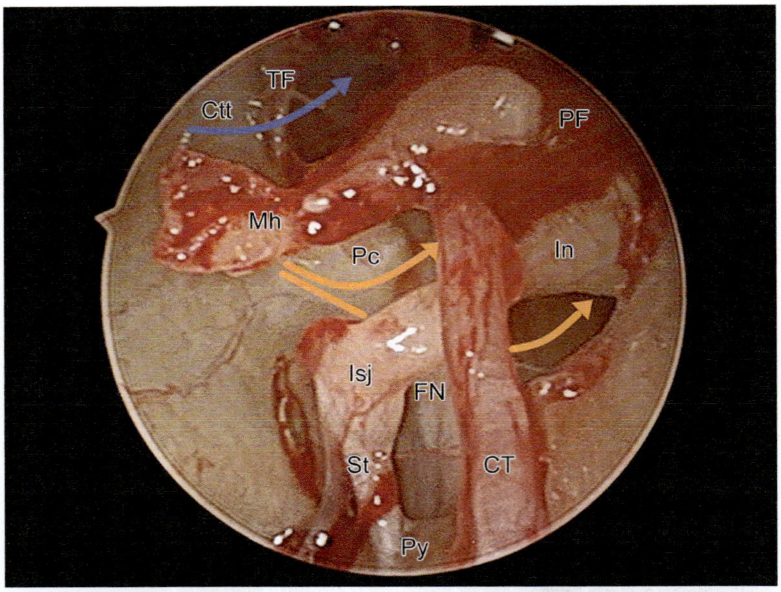

Fig. 2A: Left ear endoscopic epitympanic exploration with 2.7 mm 30-degree endoscope. Blue arrow depicts the anterior-most ventilation pathway through the tensor fold; orange arrows depict the isthmi anticus and posticus.
(CT: chorda tympani; TTc: canal for tensor tympani; FN: facial nerve; In: incus; Isj: incudostapedial joint; Mh: malleus handle; Pc: processus cochleariformis; PF: pars flaccida; Py: processus pyramidalis; St: stapedial tendon; TF: tensor fold)

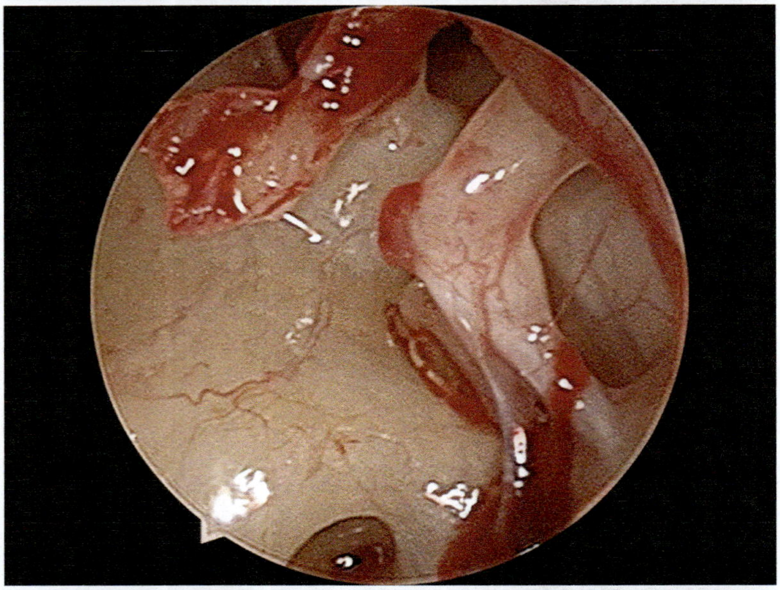

Fig. 2B: 30-degree angled endoscope being manipulated to get close-up view of the isthmi.

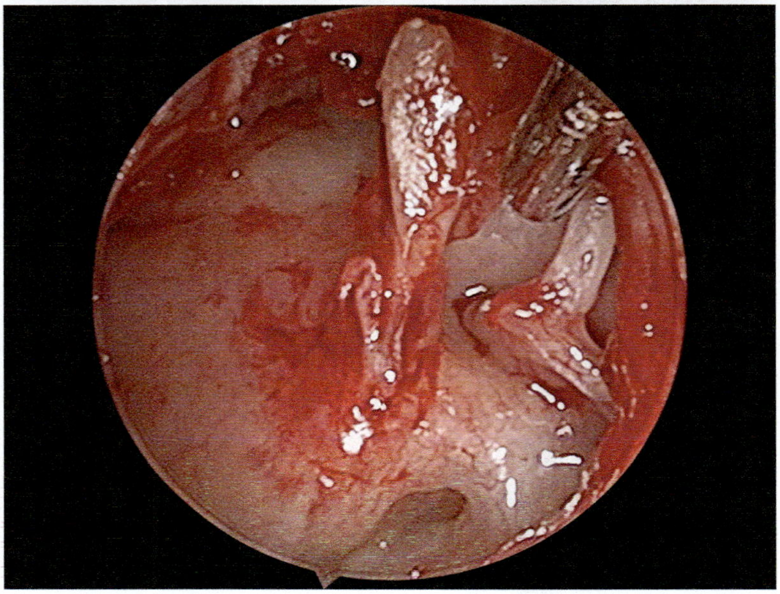

Fig. 2C: Placement and manipulation of the angled endoscope to view both anterior and posterior ventilation pathways.

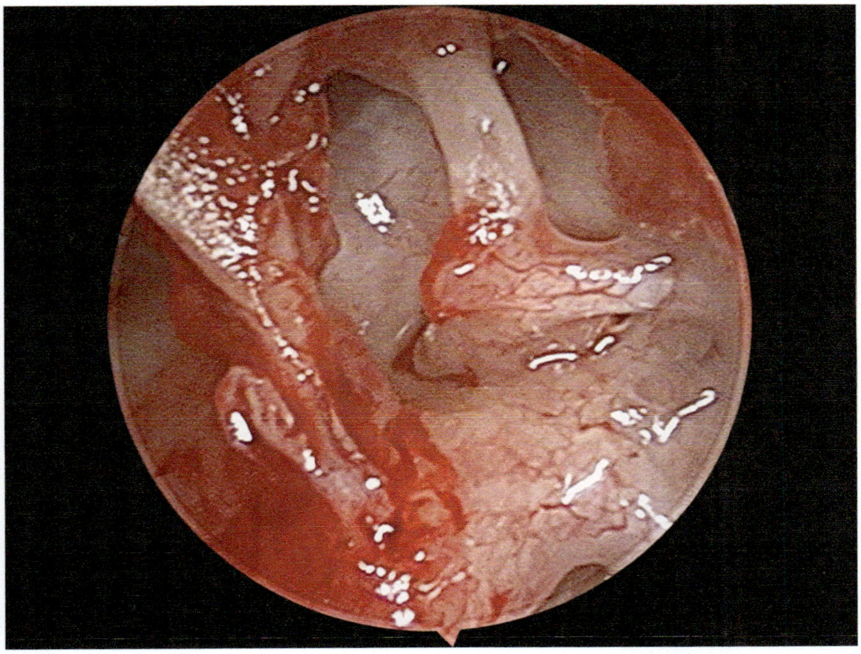

Fig. 2D: 30-degree close view of incudo-stapedial joint.

Steps of Surgery

1. Margin of tympanic membrane perforation is freshened

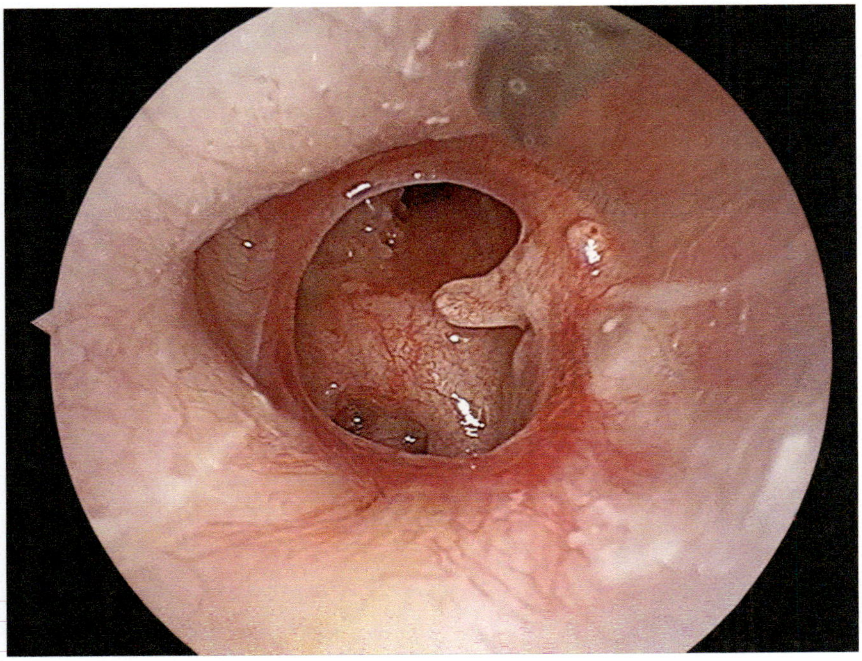

Fig. 3A: Inspection of tympanic membrane perforation.

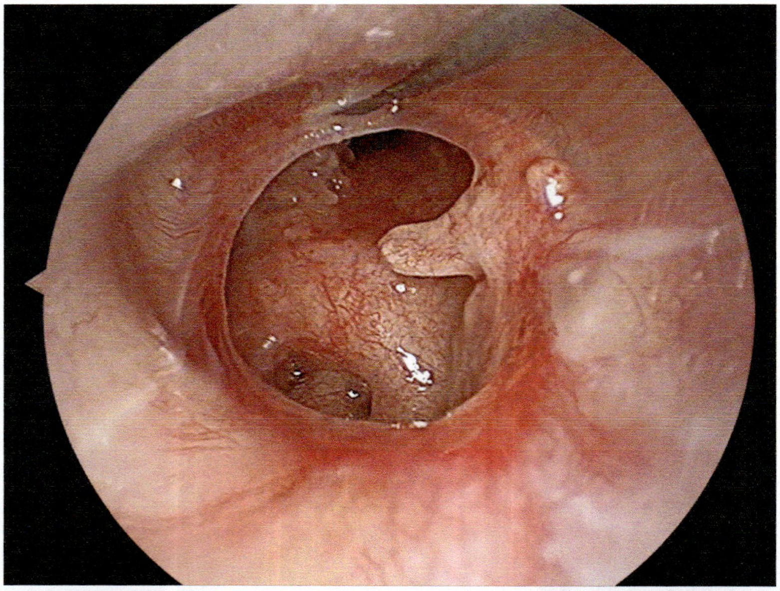

Fig. 3B: Freshening of margins of perforation. Anterior part of the margin.

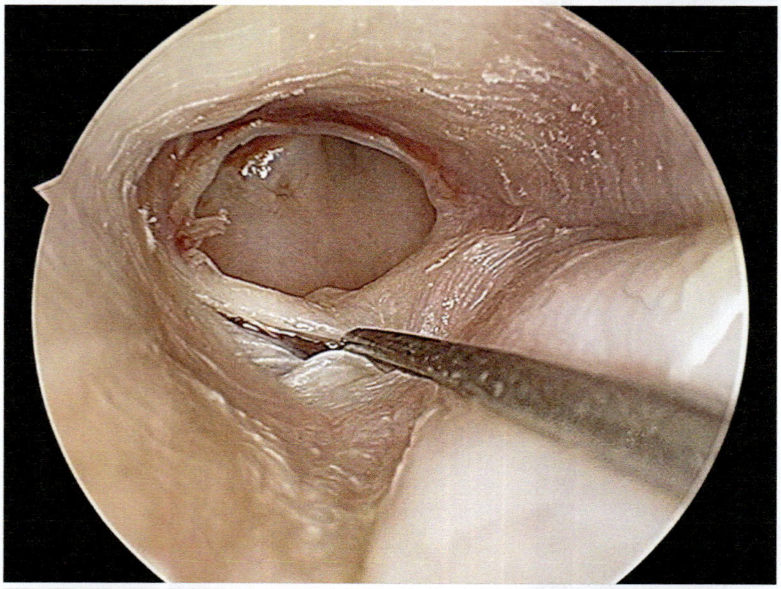

Fig. 3C: Freshening of margins of perforation. Posterior part of the margin.

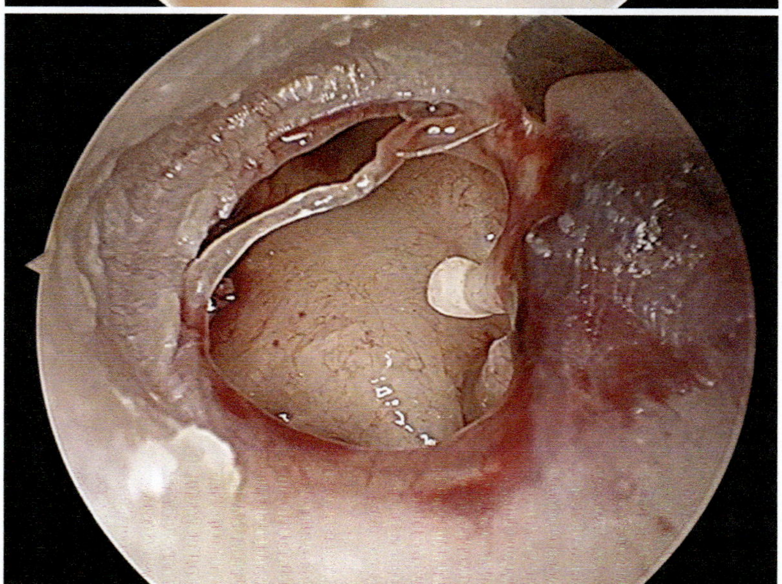

Fig. 3D: Freshening of margins of perforation. Anterosuperior area.

2. Superior incision in the external auditory canal wall is made anterior to the lateral process of malleus
   - Inferior incision is made at 6 "O" clock position

PEARL

Such an anterior placement of the superior incision ensures proper exposure of the anterior epitympanic space and the area around the tensor fold.

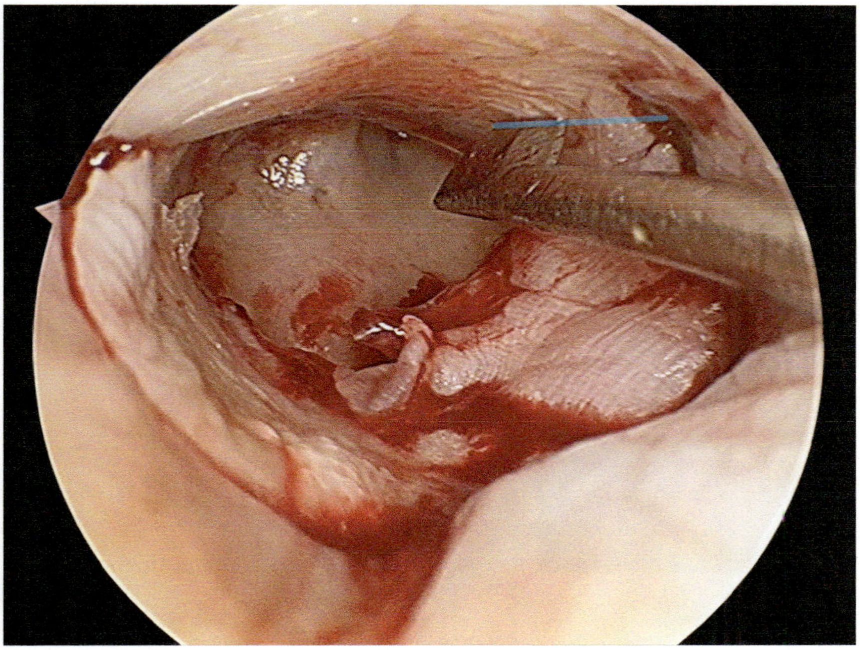

Fig. 4A: Anterior most limit of superior incision.

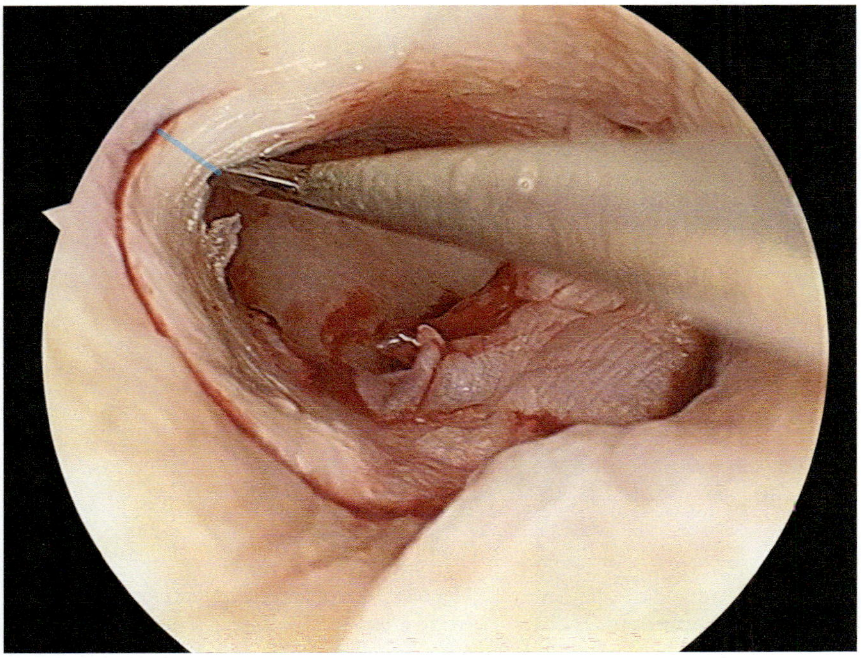

Fig. 4B: Anterior most limit of inferior incision (left ear).

3. Tympanomeatal flap is elevated.

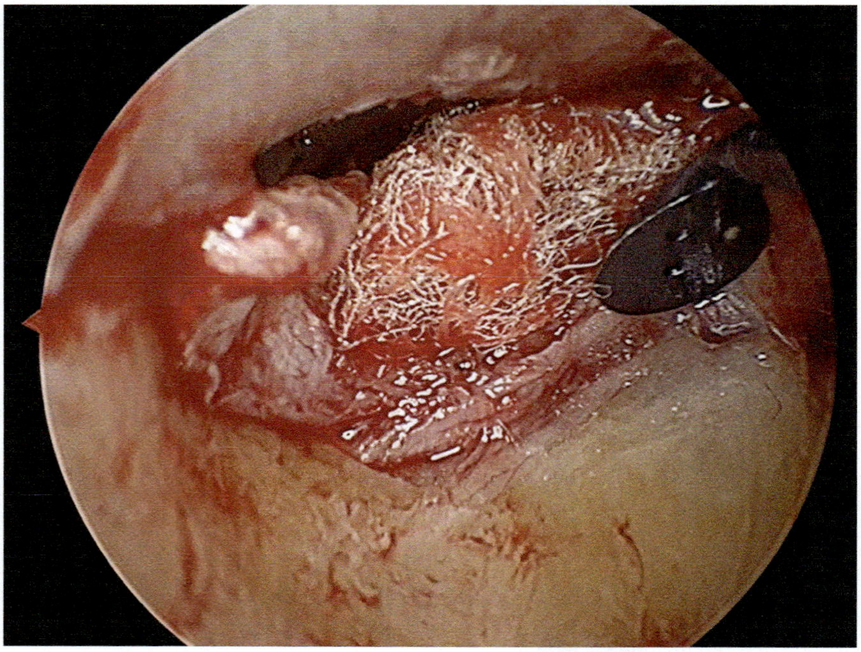

Fig. 5A: Steps of flap elevation. Up to annulus.

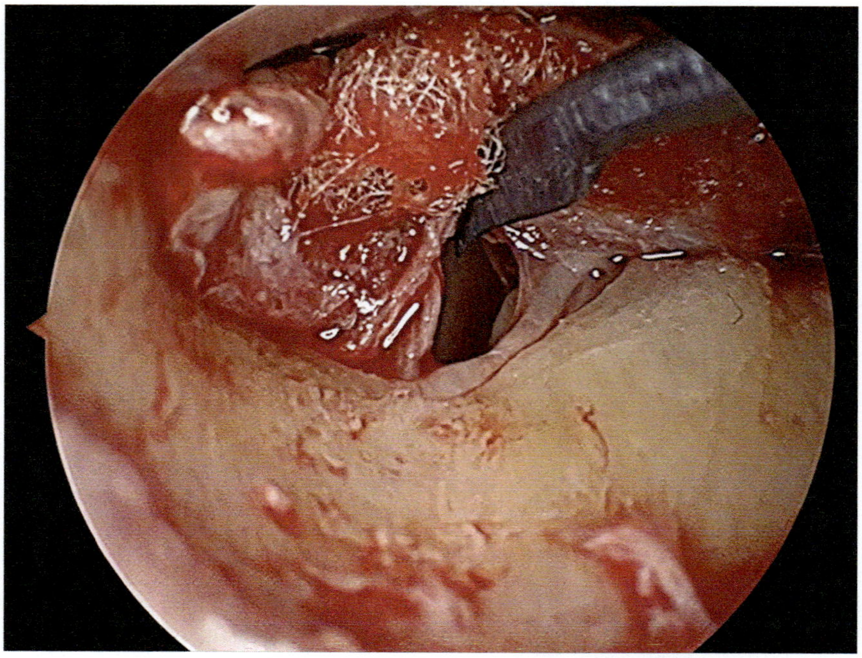

Fig. 5B: Steps of flap elevation. Fibrous annulus being lifted

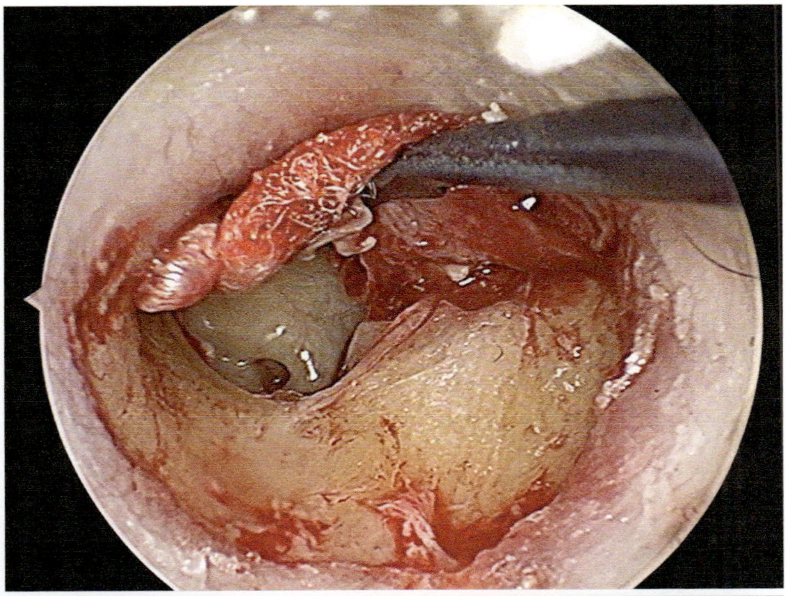

Fig. 5C: Steps of flap elevation. Flap elevated up to lateral process of malleus.

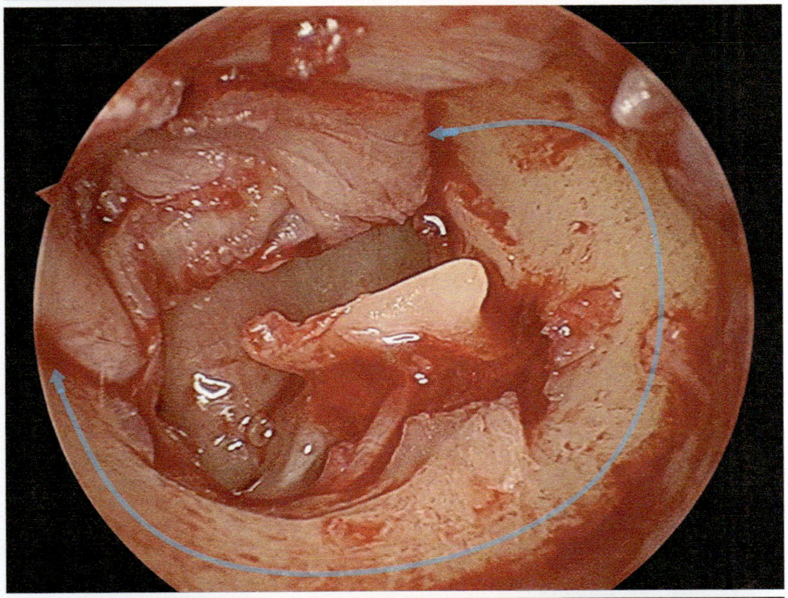

Fig. 5D: Arc of exposure.

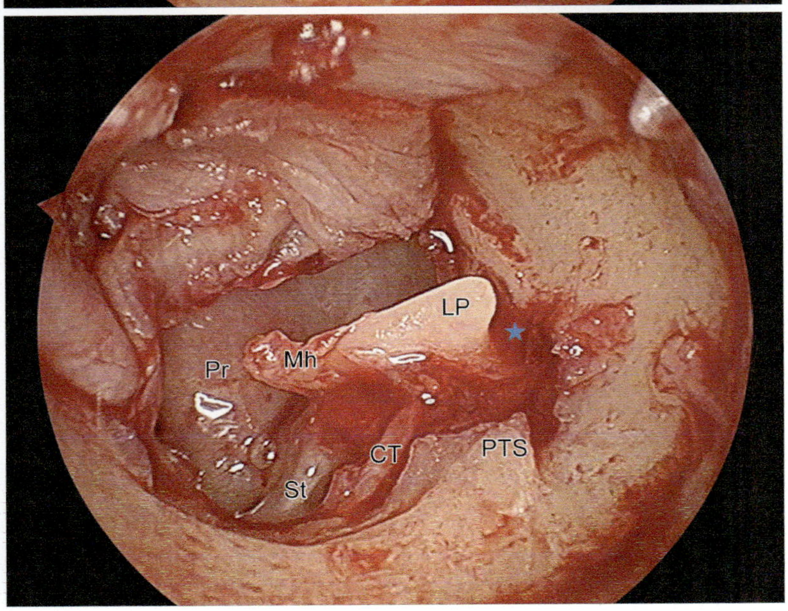

Fig. 5E: Visualization of important landmarks.
(CT: chorda tympani; Mh: malleus handle; LP: lateral process of malleus; Pr: promontory; PTS: posterior tympanic spine; St: stapedial tendon)
Blue star: Prussak's space

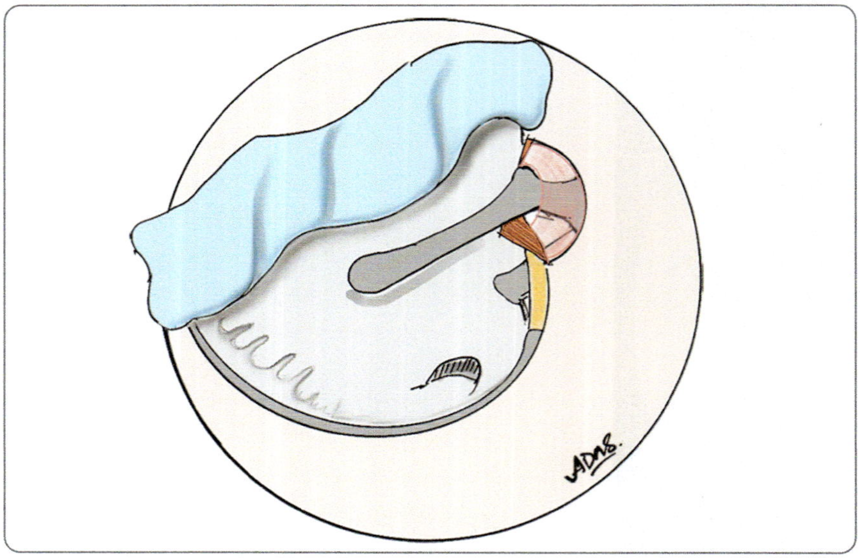

Fig. 5F: Pictorial depiction of view after flap elevation.

4. The chorda tympani nerve is dissected free from the posterior malleolar ligament and posterior tympanic spine. The posterior malleolar ligament is divided with a sharp pick or sickle.

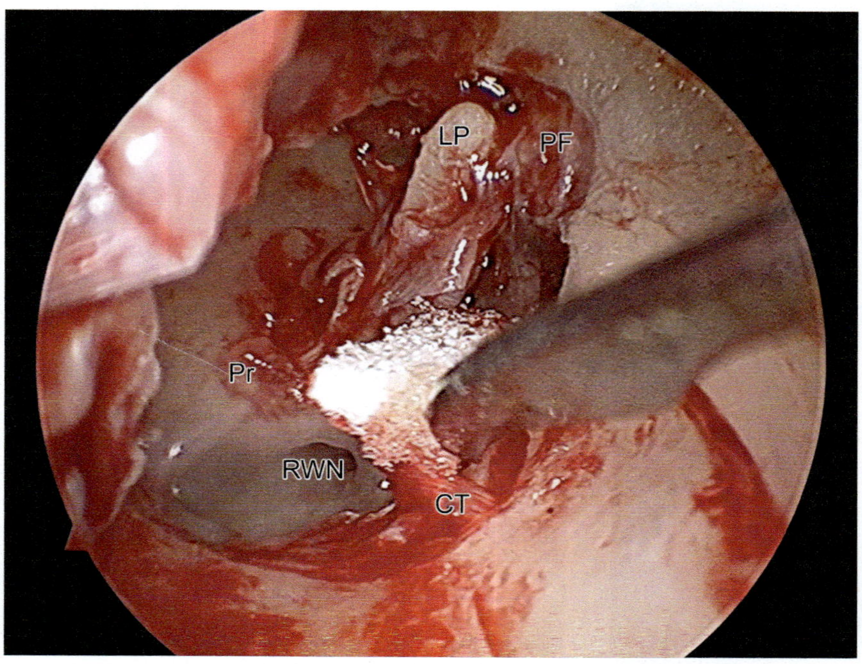

Fig. 6A: Steps of dissection of chorda tympani. (CT: chorda tympani; LP: lateral process of malleus; Pr: promontory; PF: pars flaccida; RWN: round window niche)

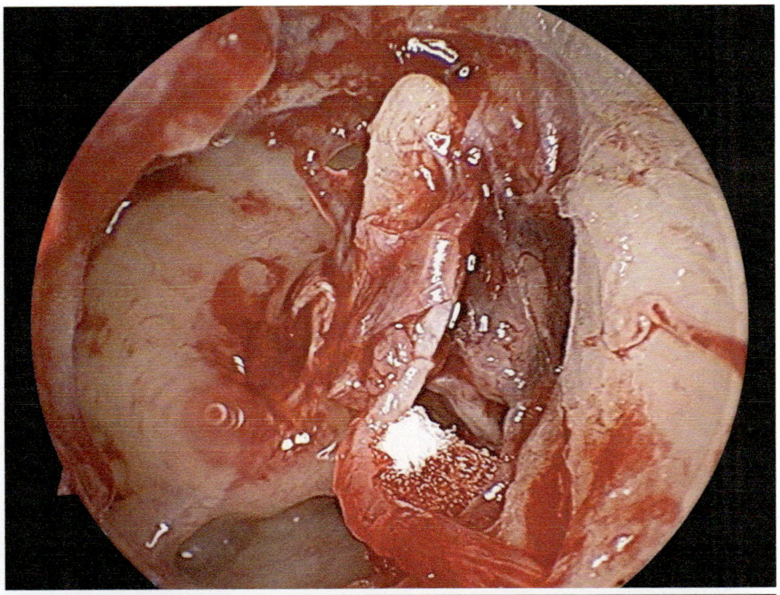

Fig. 6B: Steps of dissection of chorda tympani. Dissection of chorda tympani from epitympanic diaphragm using gelfoam.

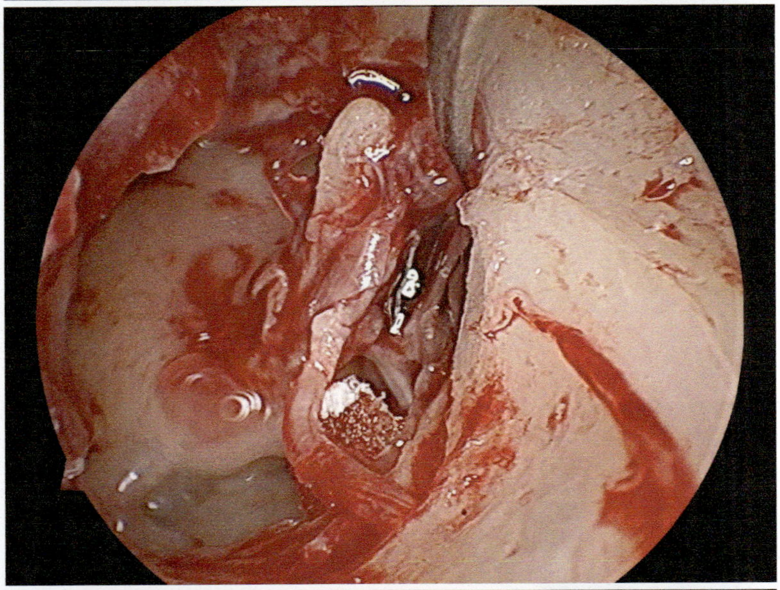

Fig. 6C: Epitympanic diaphragm being dissected using curved pick.

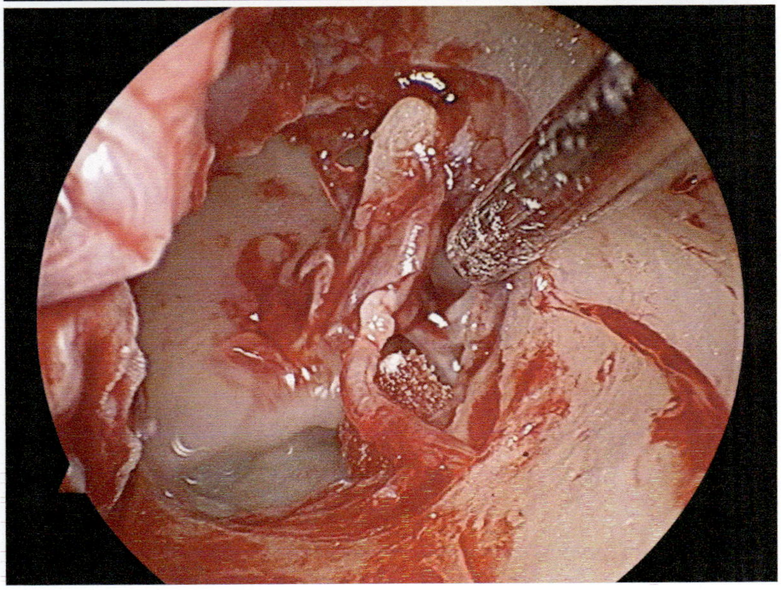

Fig. 6D: Gentle suction being used to clear the area.

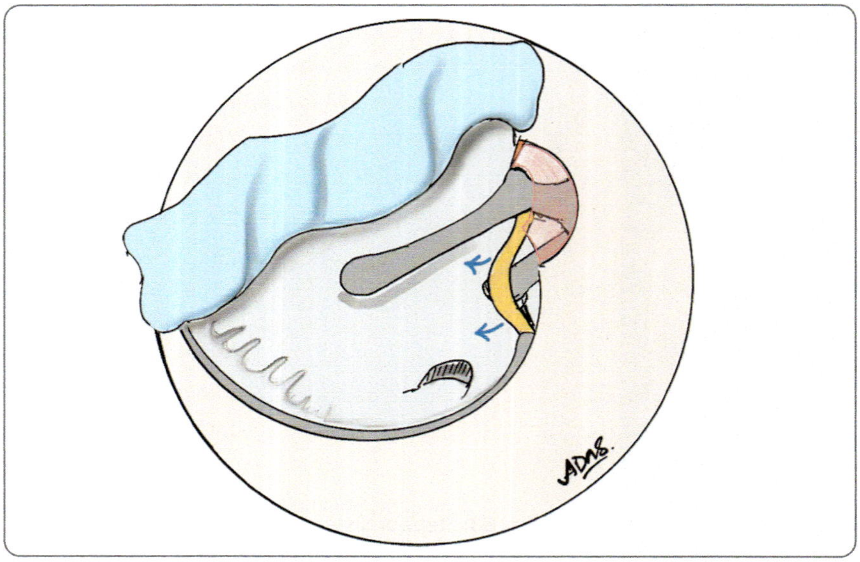

Fig. 6E: Pictorial depiction of direction of chorda tympani reflection.

5. At the same time, the chorda tympani is gently dissected from the surrounding hypertrophied mucosa with the help of dry gelfoam and pushed inferiorly.

After the chorda has been dissected, the ossicular chain status is confirmed.

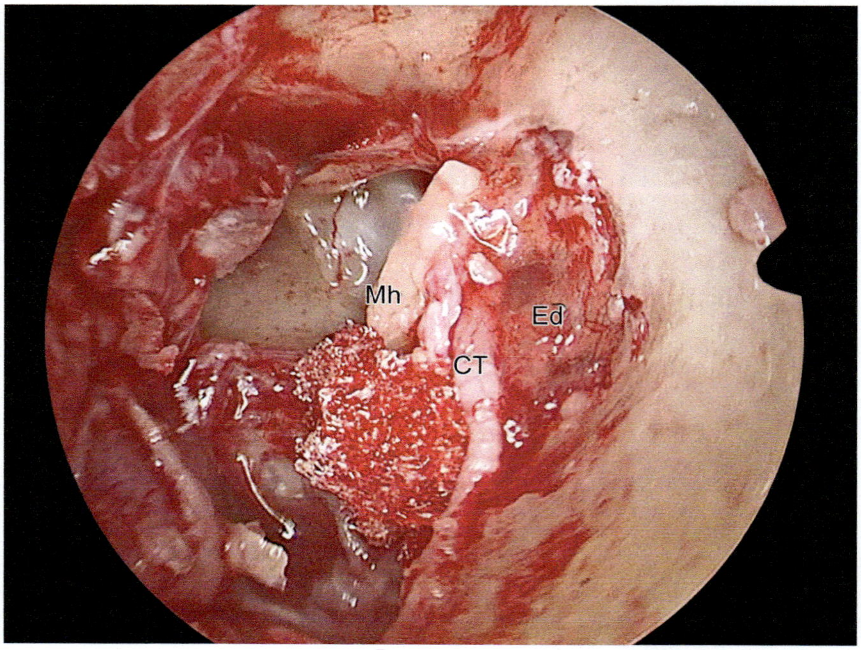

Fig. 7A: Separation of chorda tympani from surrounding mucosal folds.
(Mh: malleus handle; CT: chorda tympani; Ed: epitympanic diaphragm)

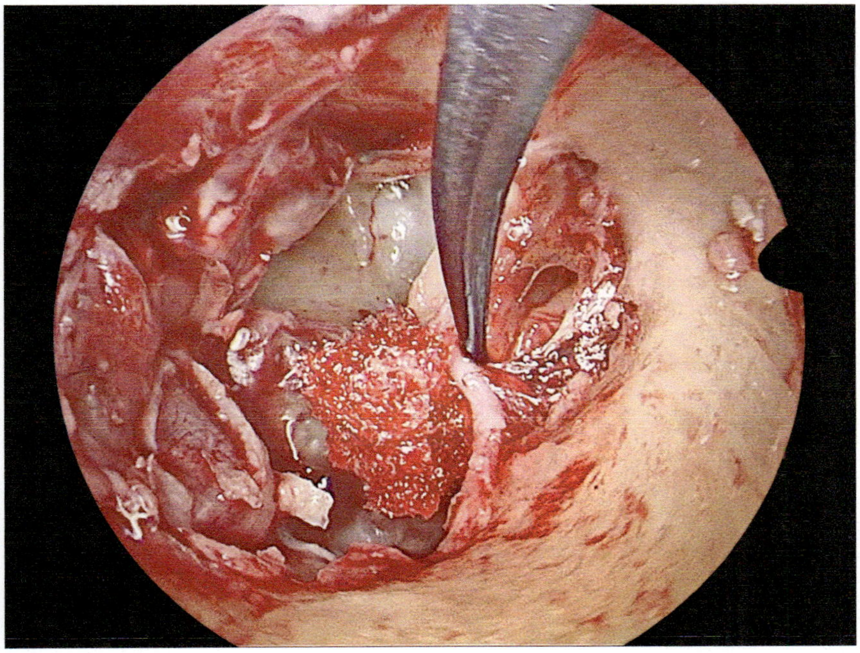

Fig. 7B: Separation of chorda tympani from surrounding mucosal folds.

6. Based on the extent of disease assessed, the bone of the posterosuperior canal wall and lateral attic wall are curetted out.

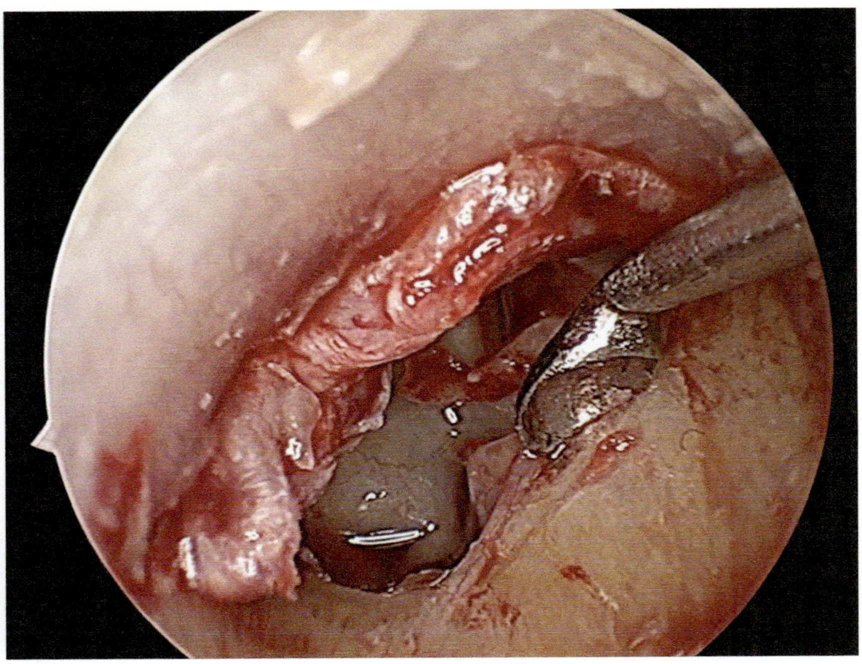

Fig. 8A: Curettage of posterosuperior canal wall (Note the direction of the instrument).

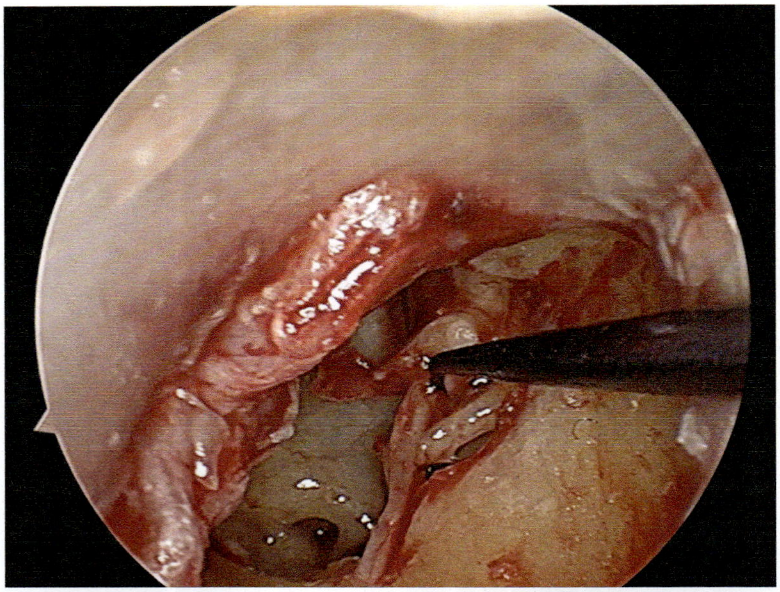

Fig. 8B: Chorda tympani reflected away from the working area.

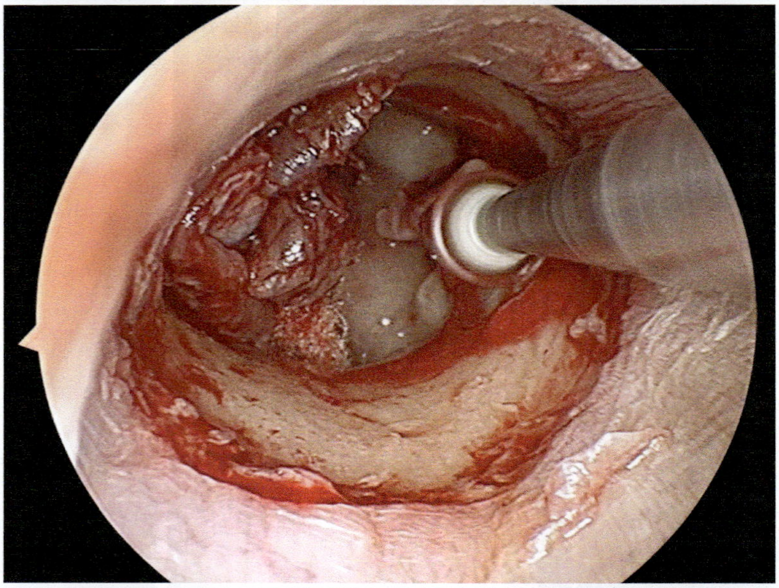

Fig. 8C: 2 mm diamond burr used to drill the thick posterosuperior canal bone.

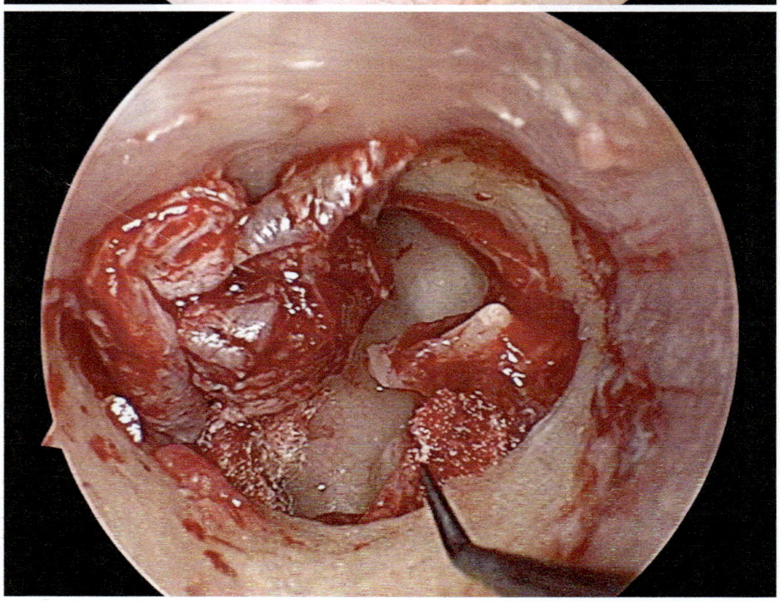

Fig. 8D: Further clearance of the posterosuperior region mucosal folds with gelfoam soaked in adrenaline.

PEARL

The bone is often found to be dense, hard and cannot be curetted out easily. In such cases, initial few layers of the bone are drilled slowly and carefully using a 2 mm diamond burr to a point that the shadow of the underlying ossicular heads are seen. Thereafter, the egg-shell bone is curetted out with a House curette.

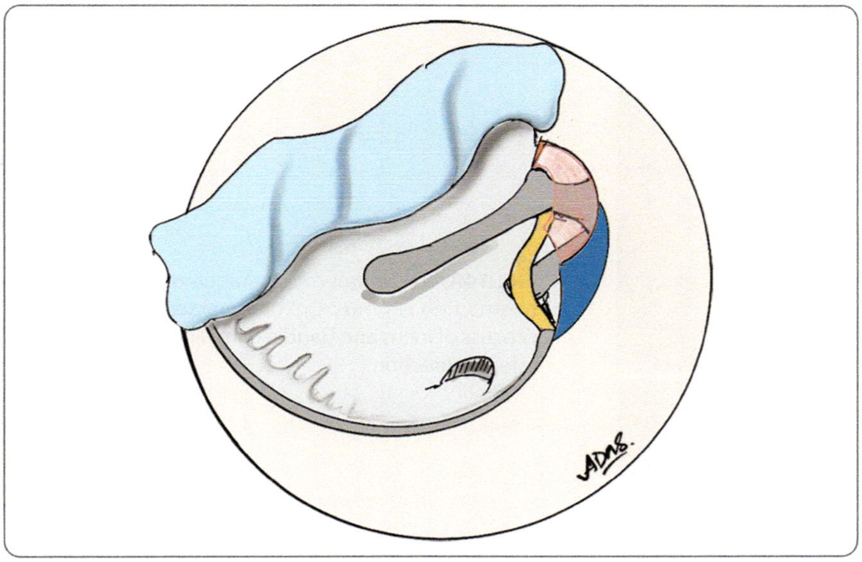

Fig. 9A: Pictorial depiction of extent of posterosuperior canal bone needed to be removed.

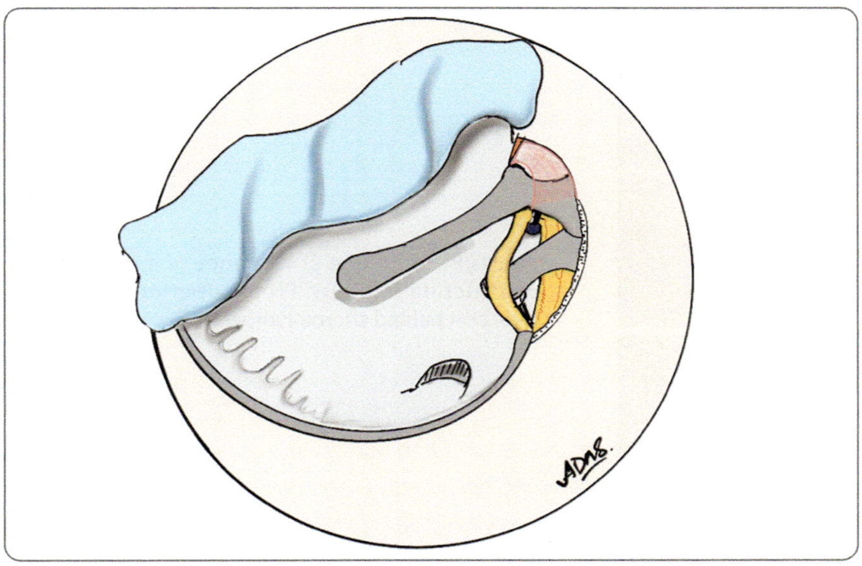

Fig. 9B: Resultant exposure.

7. The edematous, hypertrophied mucosa engulfing the ossicular chain is then dissected gently using gelfoam.

PEARL

Use of dry gelfoam aids in dissection of the diseased mucosa by virtue of its hygroscopic action with minimal pressure on the ossicles.

PEARL

The mucosa directly over the surface of the ossicles should not be stripped off as it carries a part of the blood supply to the ossicles in it.

- The subsequent dissection of the isthmi is done with 30-degree angled endoscope
- The endoscope is lodged inferiorly and curved superiorly to obtain an inferior-to-superior view of the pathways
- Dry gelfoam is then gradually passed around the ossicles to clear the blocked ventilation routes.

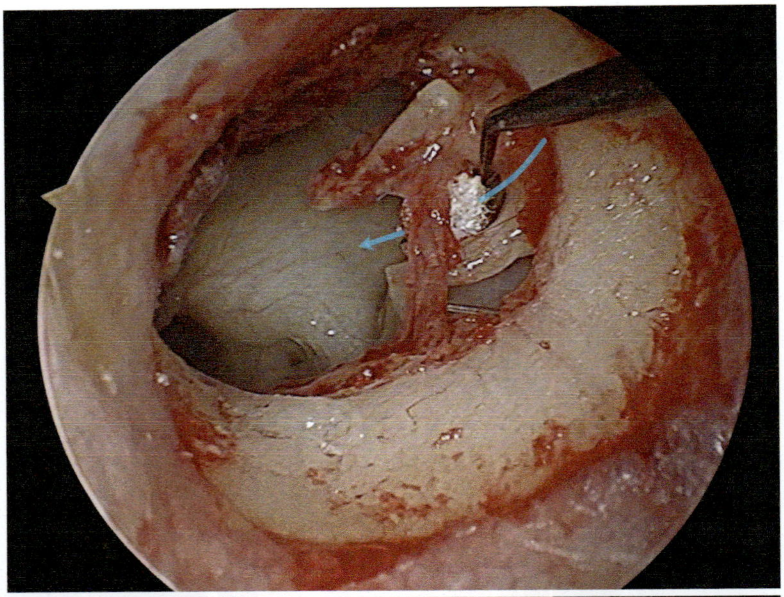

Fig. 10A: Technique of clearance of mucosal folds obstructing isthmus: Gelfoam passed between long process of incus and handle of malleus,in superior-to-inferior direction.

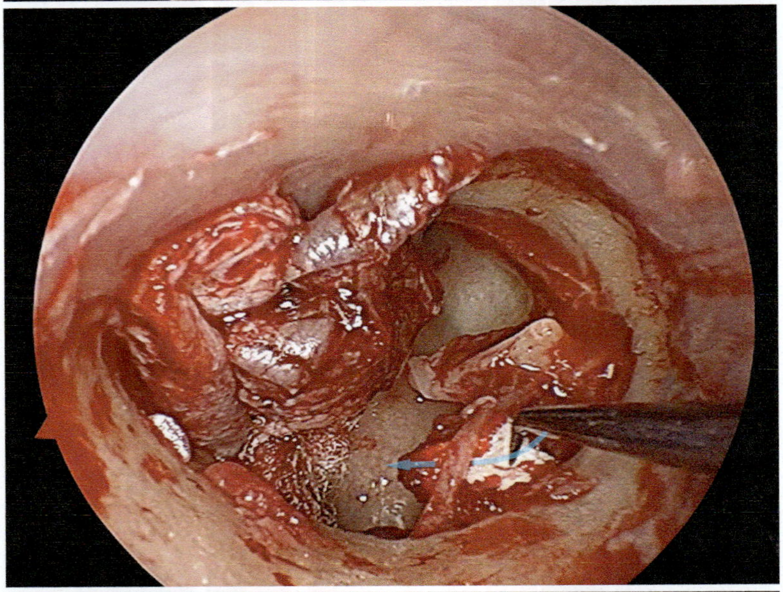

Fig. 10B: Technique of clearance of mucosal folds obstructing isthmus: From superior to inferior direction behind chorda tympani.

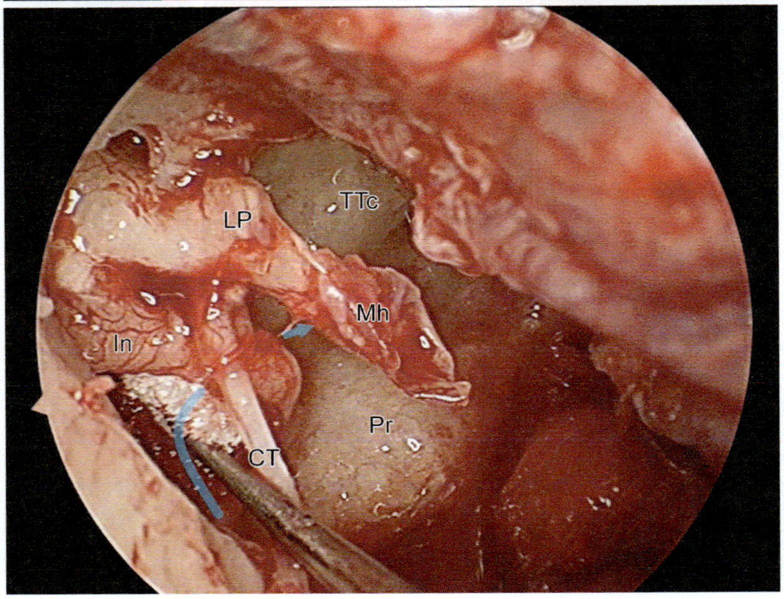

Fig. 10C: Technique of clearance of mucosal folds obstructing isthmus: Gelfoam passed underneath incus long process from posterior to anterior direction.

(TTc: canal for tensor tympani; LP: lateral process of malleus; Mh: malleus handle; In: incus; Pr: promontory; CT: chorda tympani)

PEARL THREE-PASS TECHNIQUE OF ISTHMUS CLEARANCE

In this technique, dry gelfoam is used to dissect tissues by passing:

- Between long process of incus and handle of malleus, medial to chorda tympani, in superior-to-inferior direction
- Posterior to incus long process, medial to chorda tympani, in superior-to-inferior direction
- Medial to incus, between incus and horizontal segment of facial nerve, in posterior-to-anterior direction.

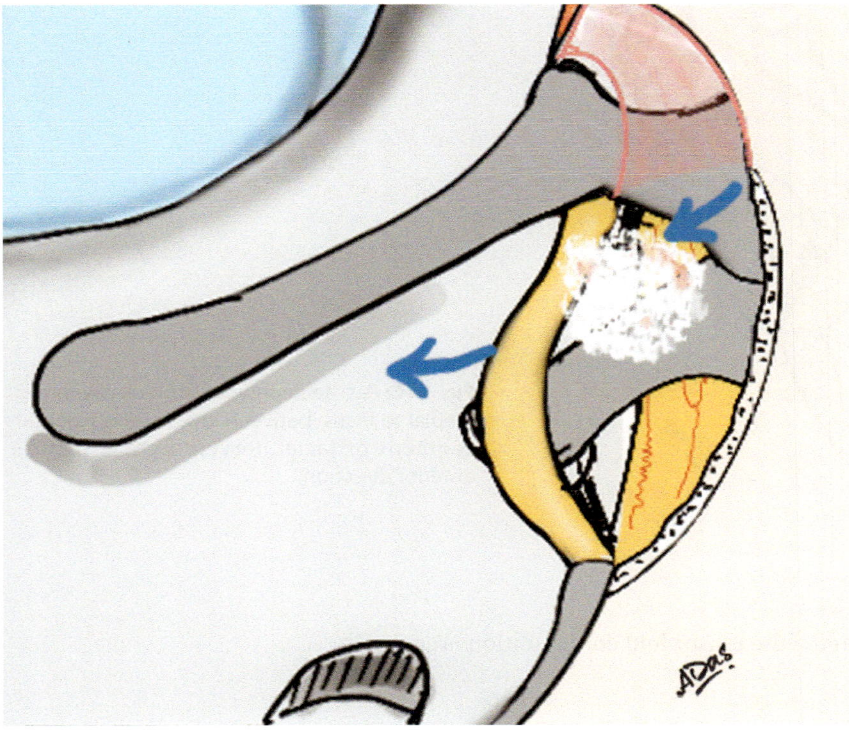

Fig. 11A: Pass technique of isthmus clearance: Between long process of incus and handle of malleus, medial to chorda tympani, in superior-to-inferior direction.

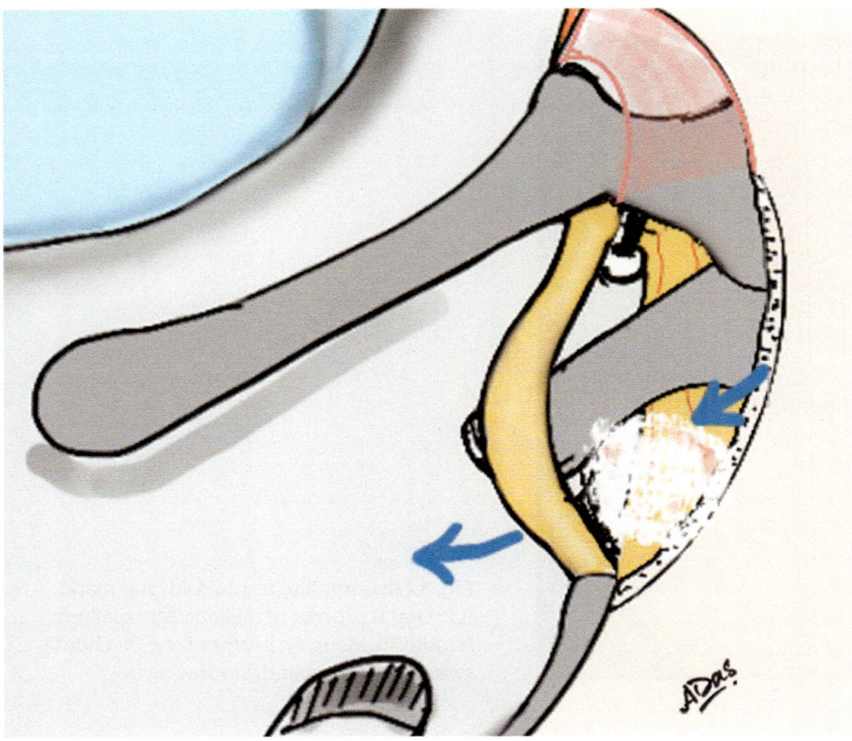

Fig. 11B: Pass technique of isthmus clearance: Posterior to incus long process, medial to chorda tympani, in superior-to-inferior direction.

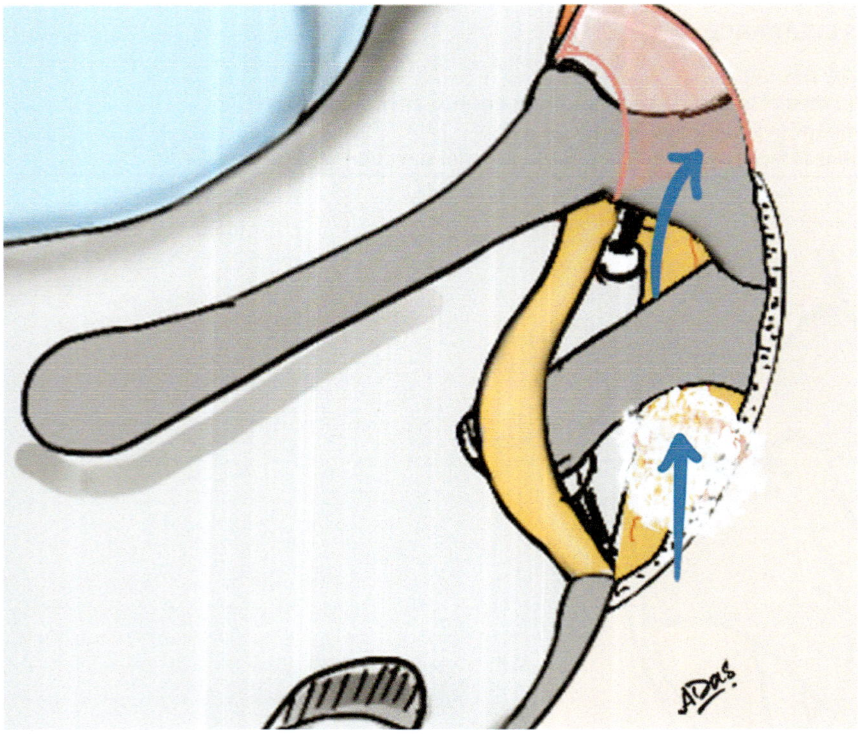

Fig. 11C: Pass technique of isthmus clearance: Medial to incus, between incus and horizontal segment of facial nerve, in posterior-to-anterior direction.

8. The additional anterior pathway is then restored if the tensor fold configuration is complete.

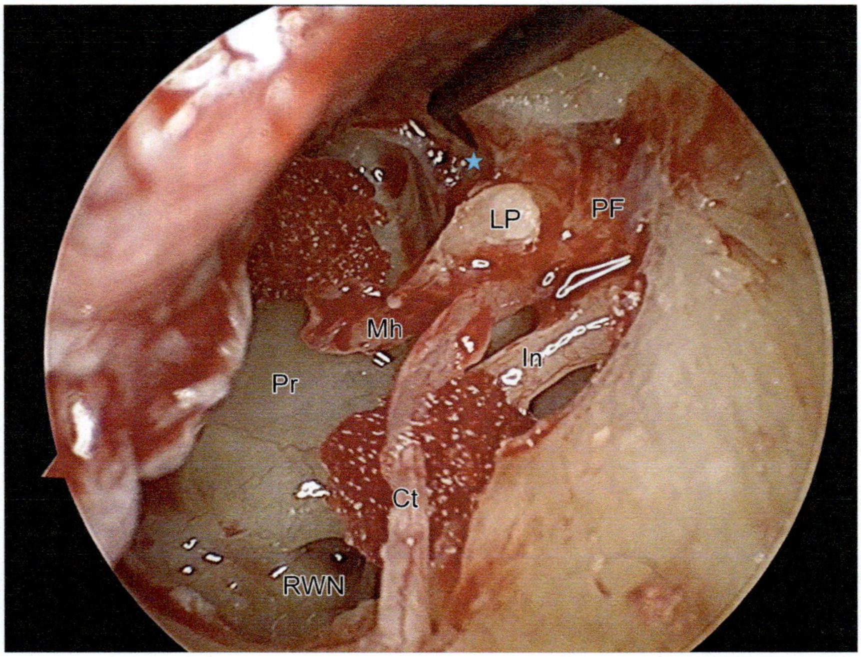

Fig. 12A: Complete tensor fold (star mark). (LP: lateral process of malleus; Mh: malleus handle; In: incus; Pr: promontory; Ct: chorda tympani; RWN: round window niche)

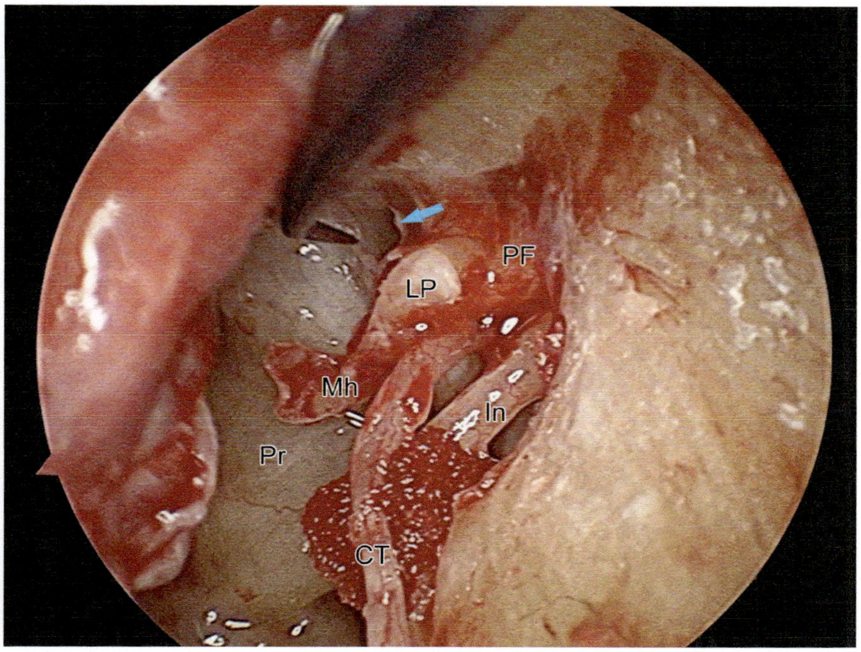

Fig. 12B: Additional anterior pathway cleared (arrow).
(LP: lateral process of malleus; Mh: malleus handle; In: incus; Pr: promontory; CT: chorda tympani; PF: pars flaccida)

- In this case, the angled scope is placed anteriorly in the inferior quadrant of protympanum and angulated superiorly to view the tensor fold
- Thereafter, similar gelfoam-dissection techniques are applied to clear the route
- Curved dissectors are also used in this step.

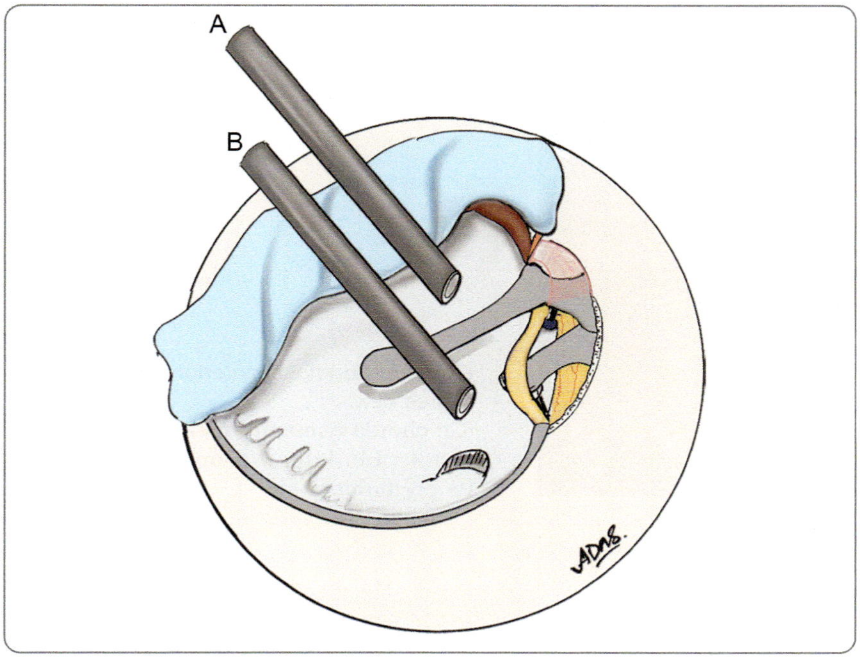

Fig. 13: Placement of angled endoscope (30-degree, 2.7 mm) anterior (A) and posterior (B) to handle of malleus.

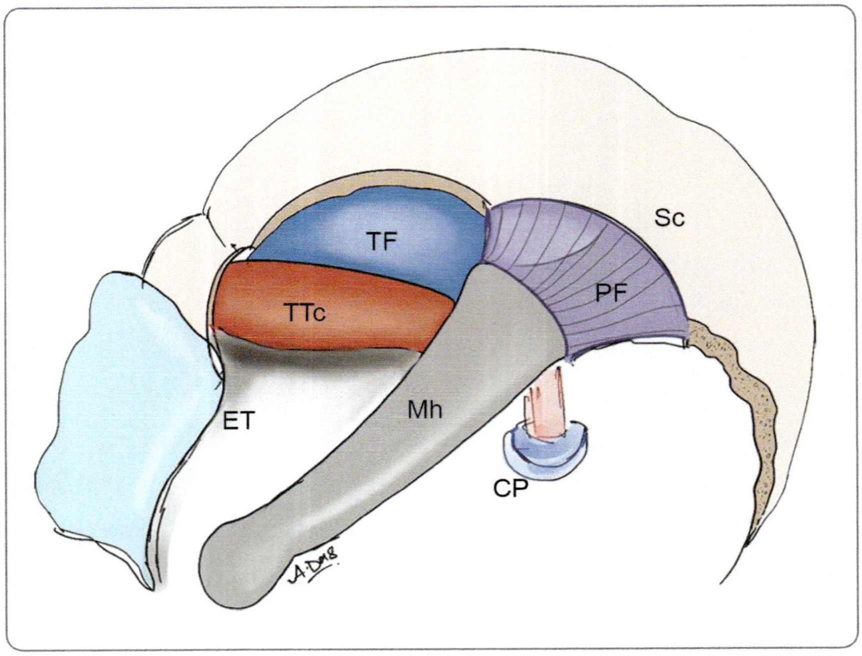

Fig. 14: Disposition of mucosal folds.
(CP: processus cochleariformis; ET: Eustachian tube; Mh: malleus handle; PF: pars flaccida; Sc: scutum; TF: tensor fold; TTc: canal for tensor tympani)

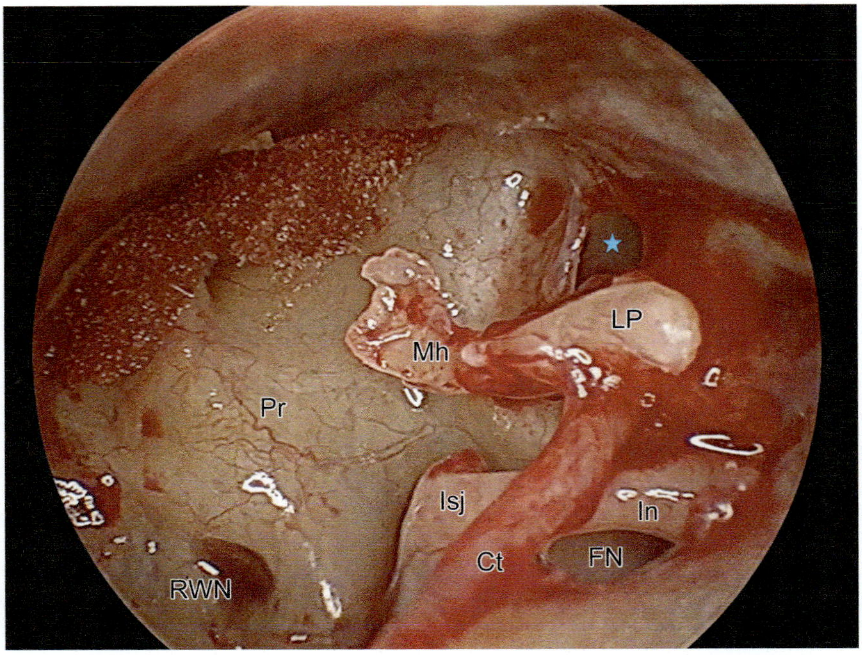

Fig. 15A: Additional anterior pathway: zero-degree view.
(Ct: chorda tympani In: incus; Mh: malleus handle; LP: lateral process of malleus; Pr: promontory)

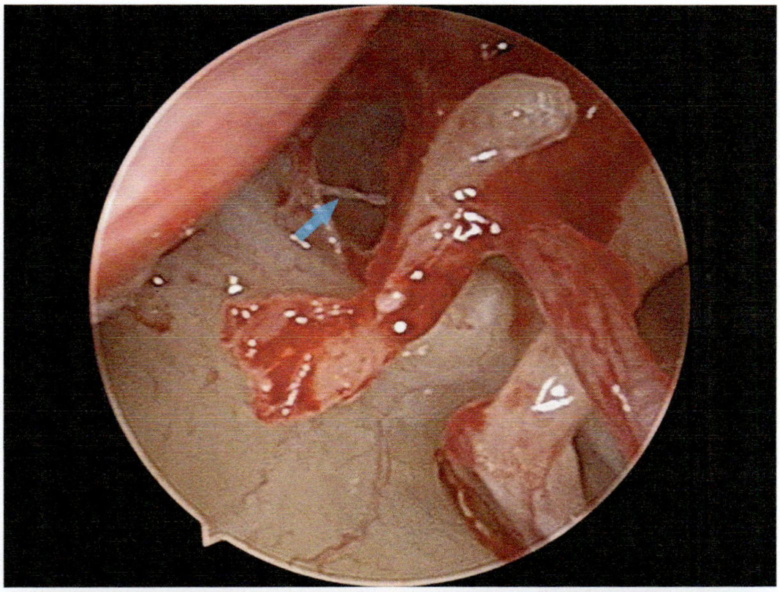

Fig. 15B: 30-degree endoscopic view.

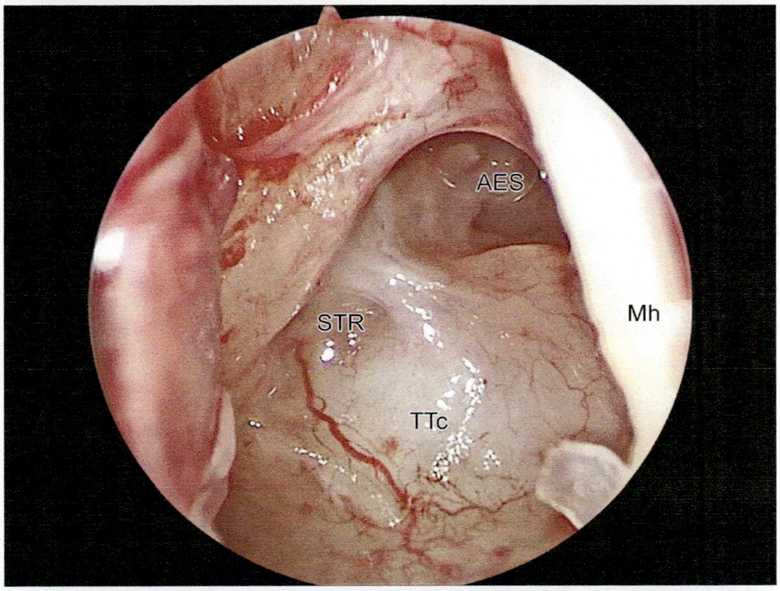

Fig. 15C: View of anterior epitympanic space with 45-degree endoscope.
(AES: anterior epitympanic space; STR: supratubal recess; TTc: canal for tensor tympani; Mh: malleus handle)

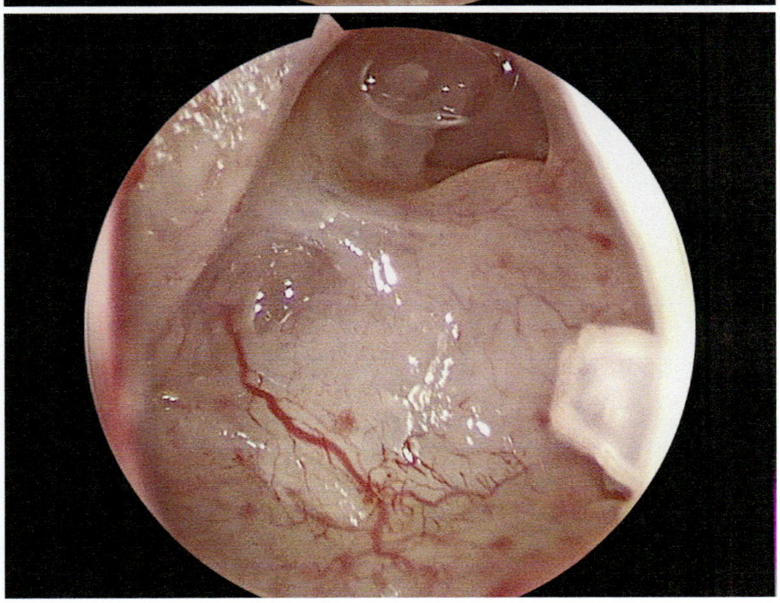

Fig. 15D: View of anterior epitympanic space with 70-degree endoscope.

PEARL

Throughout dissection, controlled and gentle movements need to be maintained to prevent iatrogenic ossicular chain mobilization and high-frequency SNHL, as the ossicular chain remains articulated (if intact).

9. The area of bone drilling/curettage is reconstructed with a piece of tragal cartilage-perichondrium harvested locally.
10. Tympanic membrane reconstruction is done.

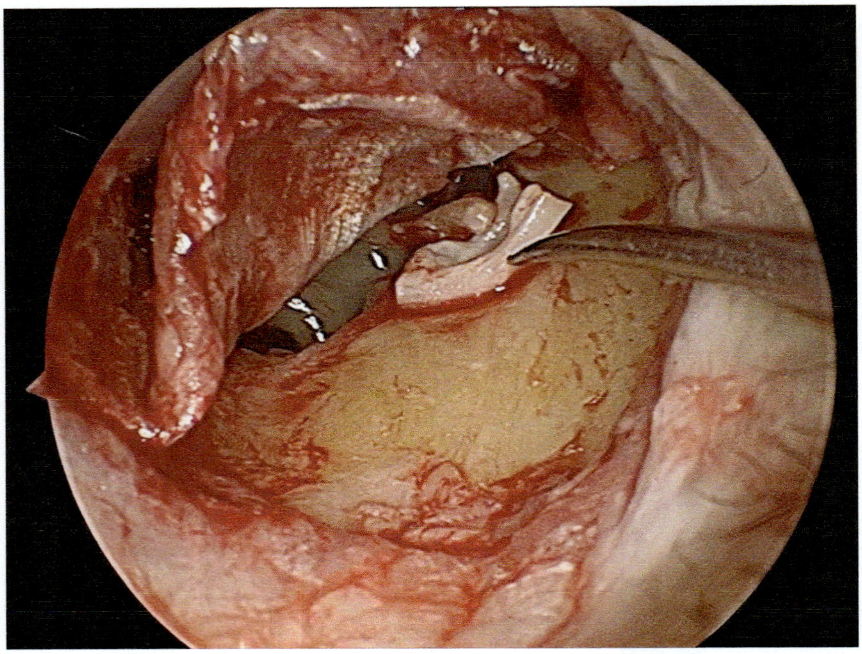

Fig. 16: Reconstruction of posterosuperior canal wall defect with tragal cartilage.

REFERENCES

1. Marchioni D, Molteni G, Presutti L. Endoscopic anatomy of the middle ear. Indian J Otolaryngol Head Neck Surg. 2011;63:101-13.
2. Marchioni D, Alicandri-Ciufelli M, Molteni G, Artioli FL, Genovese E, Presutti L. Selective epitympanic dysventilation syndrome. Laryngoscope. 2010;120:1028-33.
3. Das A, Mitra S, Hazra S, Sengupta A. Endoscopic epitympanic exploration in mucosal chronic otitis media: is canal wall up mastoidectomy really needed? J Laryngol Otol. 2021; 135(1):39-44.

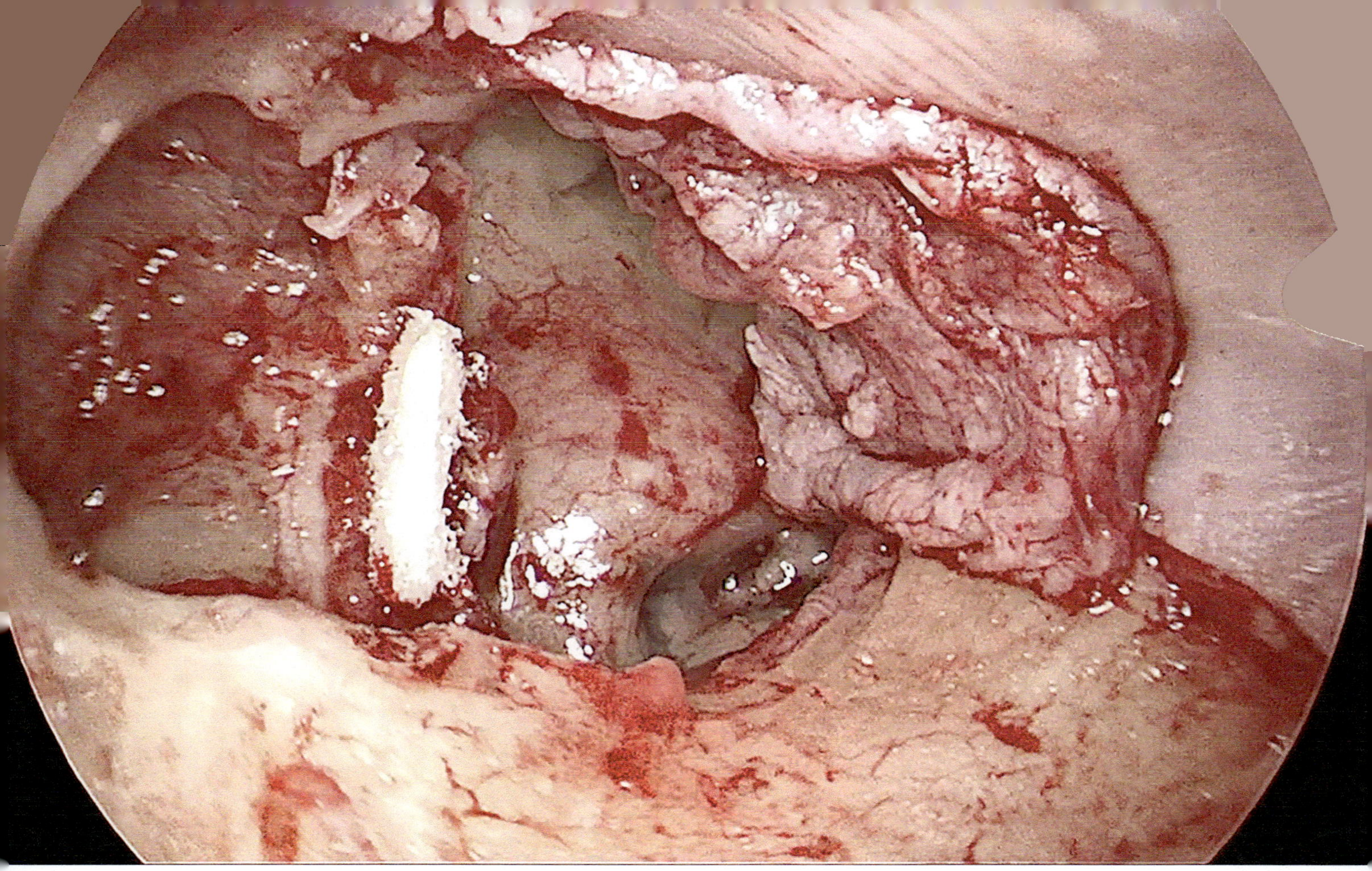

CHAPTER **10**

Endoscopic Transcanal Atticotomy

Arindam Das, Sandipta Mitra

Chapter Outline

INTRODUCTION

Atticotomy is the surgical procedure in which the epitympanum is exposed by removal of the lateral attic wall.

Classically, atticotomy is done with the help of microscope by drilling the bone of the zygomatic arch layer by layer, exposing the lateral bony attic wall also called the scutum, which is finally removed to expose the attic or the epitympanum.

PRINCIPLE OF ENDOSCOPIC TRANSCANAL ATTICOTOMY AND ITS DIFFERENCE WITH MICROSCOPIC ATTICOTOMY

Points of Difference	***Microscopic Atticotomy***	***Endoscopic Transcanal Atticotomy***
Anatomical site of bone drilling	Bone of zygomatic arch drilled from lateral to medial	Endoscope being able to bypass the lateral most bone, only the medial part, that is, the scutum is drilled
Amount of bone drilling	More	Less
Exposure	Less, in spite of more bone drill	More, in spite of less bone removal owing to magnified view and use of angled scopes
Complications	More chances of: • Tegmen damage • Chorda tympani damage	Less chances of: • Tegmen damage • Chorda tympani damage

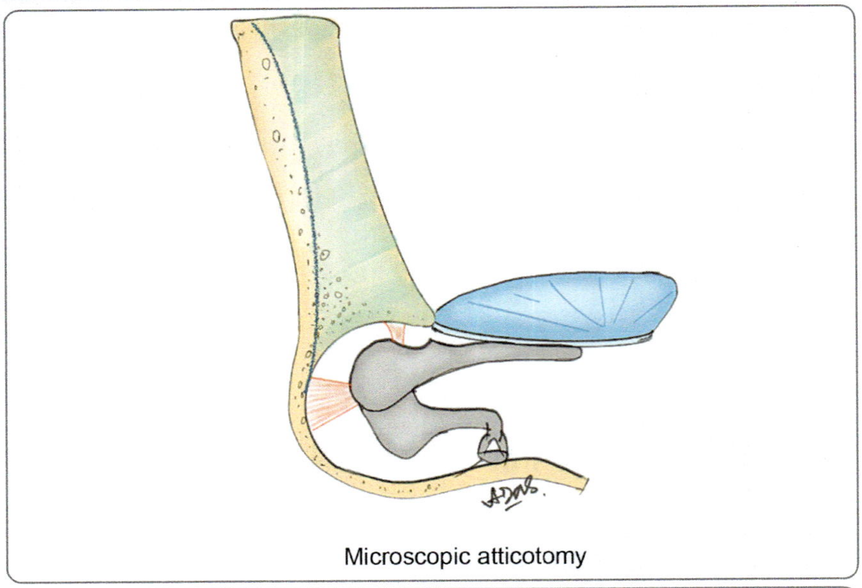

Fig. 1A: Extent of bone removal for adequate exposure: Microscopic atticotomy-entails complete drilling of bone from lateral to medial.

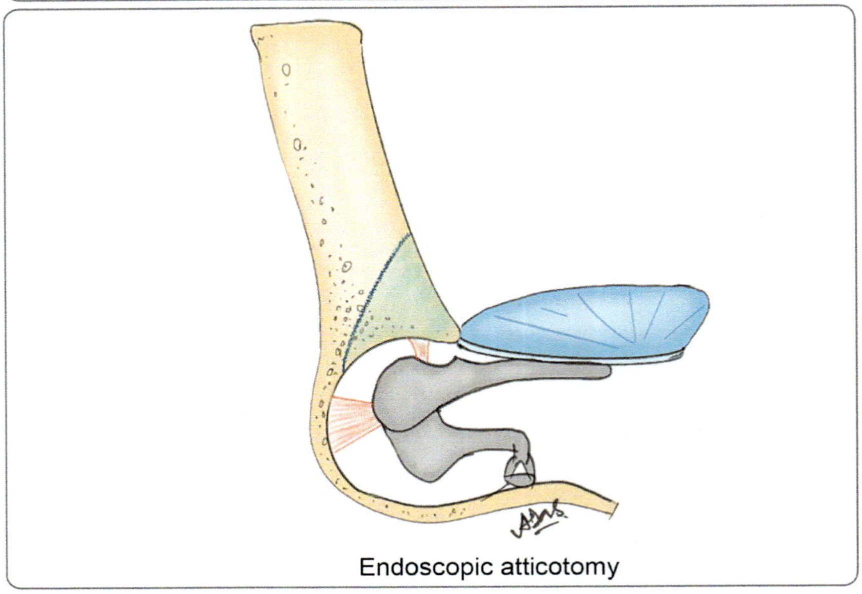

Fig. 1B: Extent of bone removal for adequate exposure: Endoscopic atticotomy-only medial aspect of the bone is to be removed for exposure.

Difference between endoscopic epitympanic exploration, endoscopic atticotomy and endoscopic mastoidectomy:

Points of difference	***Endoscopic epitympanic exploration***	***Endoscopic atticotomy***	***Endoscopic mastoidectomy***
Nature of surgery	Minimally invasive	More conservative	Comparatively less conservative
Extent of bone drilling	None or minimal, followed by use of angled scope to visualize the landmarks	Full exposure of incudomalleolar joint	Full exposure of the entire epitympanic space (AES + PES) with enlargement of aditus
Anatomical limits	Handle of malleus and long process of incus	Anterior and posterior epitympanic space	Aditus and ampullary end of lateral semicircular canal

Indications of endoscopic transcanal atticotomy:

- Limited attic and mesotympanic cholesteatoma
- Retraction pocket extending into attic
- Ossicular chain reconstruction
- Tympanosclerosis involving the ossicles, anterior and posterior epitympanic spaces
- Endoscopic facial nerve decompression surgery.

Contraindications of endoscopic transcanal atticotomy: Disease extending beyond the ampullary end of lateral semicircular canal.

- Rationale behind surgery:
  - The disease process itself does the majority of the job
  - The posterosuperior canal wall and the scutum is often found already eroded by the disease itself
  - Hence, excess bony work is often not required and endoscopes render direct access to the working area easily
  - Preservation of ossicular chain (when found intact) is possible with endoscopic approach.[1]

STEPS OF SURGERY

1. Incision

Incision has three parts. A superior limb, an inferior limb and a horizontal limb connecting the two. The horizontal limb is fashioned at a distance of about 5–6 mm from the annulus with the help of a circular knife. The inferior limb is positioned at 6 O' clock position, 1 mm away from the inferior annulus and joins the lower border of the horizontal limb. The superior incision is placed keeping a width of 1 mm and is extended further anteriorly upto the Eustachian tube.

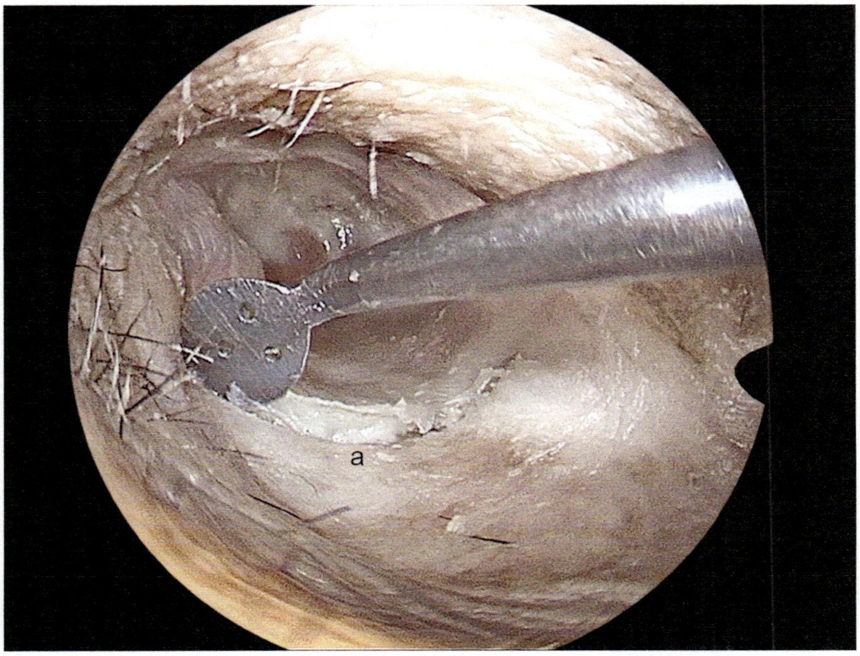

Fig. 2A: Step of canal incision: a—horizontal limb.

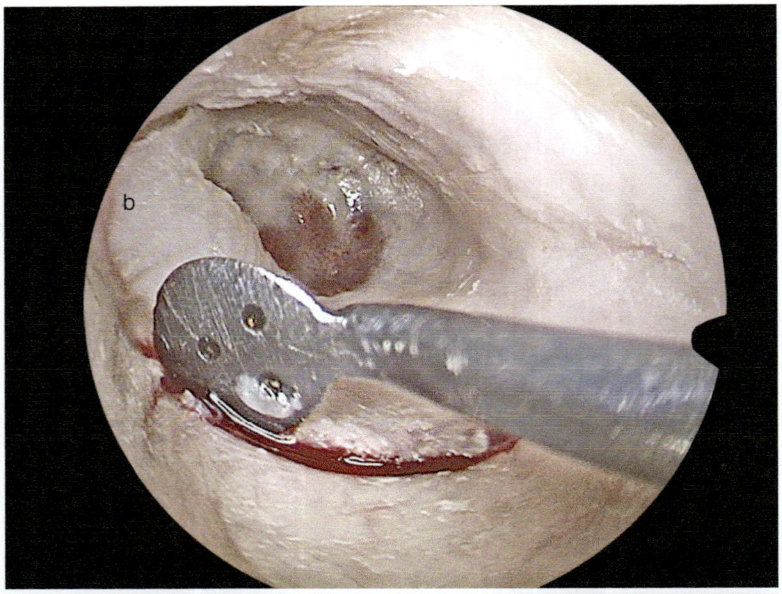

Fig. 2B: Step of canal incision: b—superior limb.

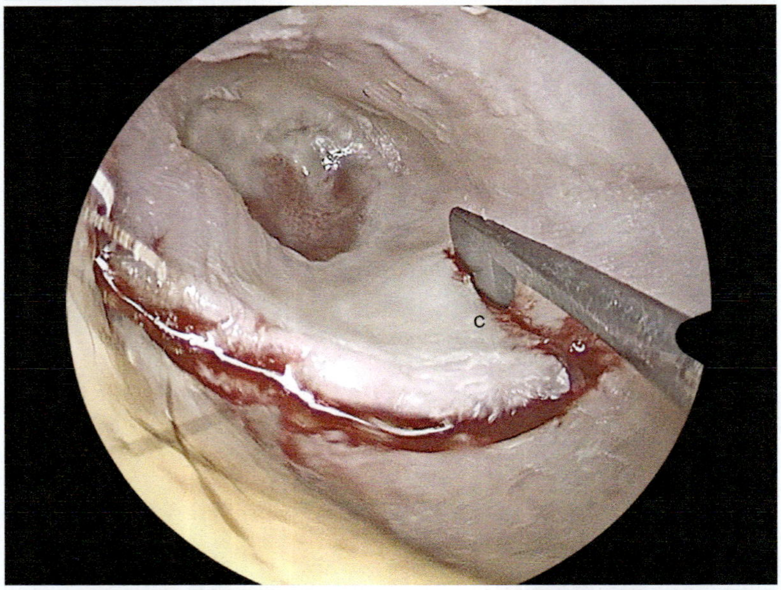

Fig. 2C: Step of canal incision: c—inferior limb.

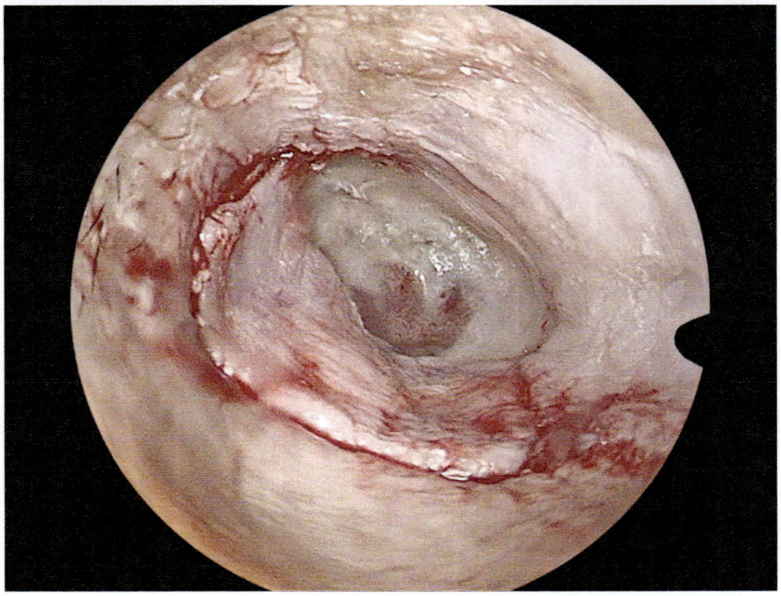

Fig. 2D: Steps of canal incision: All parts of canal incision placed.

TIP **SUPERIOR LIMB OF THE INCISION**

- It is important to fashion the superior limb of the incision carefully
- Firstly, the vascular strip has to be preserved and hence it is placed keeping a width of 1 mm
- Secondly, it is extended far anteriorly beyond the lateral process of malleus upto Eustachian tube
- This is to ensure the entire lateral attic wall upto anterior epitympanum is adequately exposed, which is the main working area for this surgery

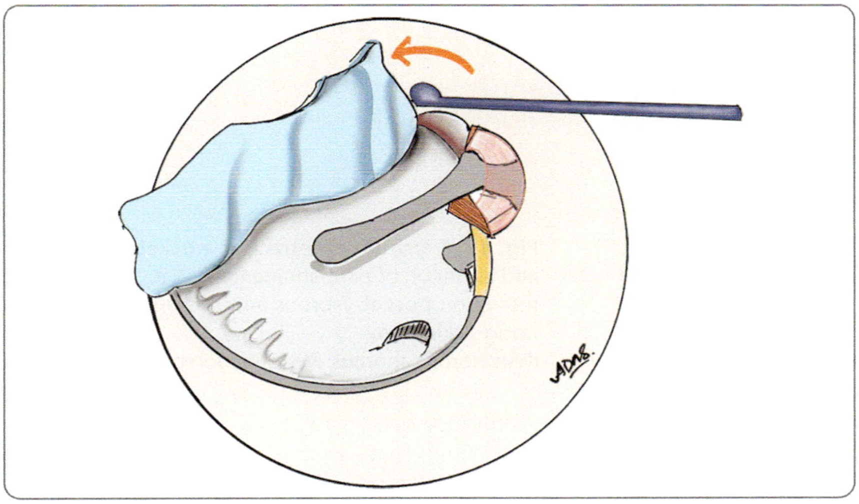

Fig. 3: Extension of superior limb of incision anterior to lateral process of malleus up to Eustachian tube.

2. Flap Elevation

- The initial steps of flap elevation remain the same as other endoscopic procedures.
- On the reaching the annulus, the technique changes.
- In case of retraction pocket, the flap has to be sharply cut at the junction of the diseased pocket and normal tympanic membrane. The normal segment is then tucked inferiorly as described previously.
- After careful elevation of the flap, it is tucked inferiorly in the hypotympanum to protect it from the rotating burr tip.

PEARL

- The retraction pocket may be adhered to the underlying ossicles or other important structures. Hence, the retraction pocket should not be pulled blindly
- Close inspection of the sac is necessary to ascertain its extensions and attachments as well as condition of the underlying ossicular chain

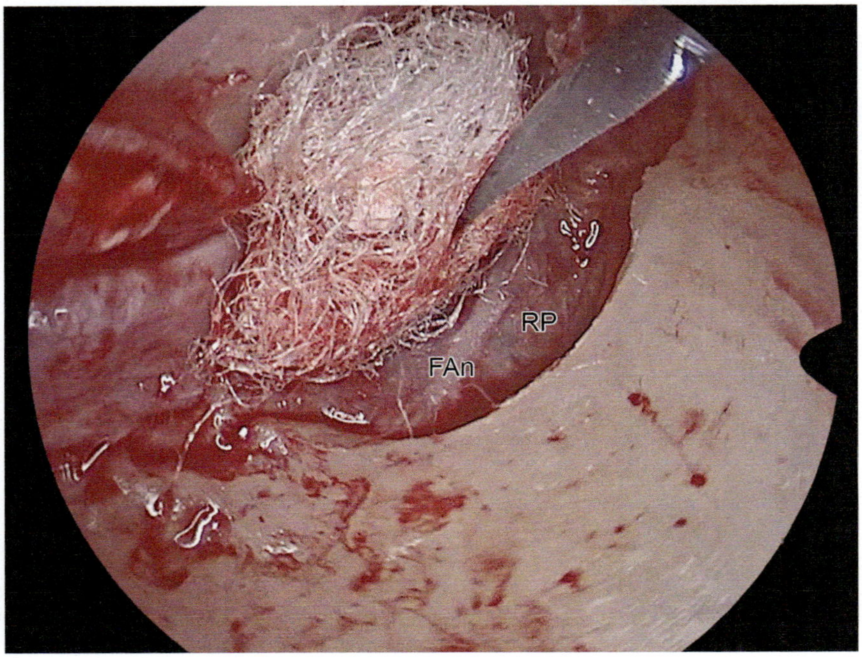

Fig. 4A: Exposure of retraction pocket: Dissection and elevation of tympanomeatal flap for exposure of retraction pocket.
(FAn: fibrous annulus; RP: retraction pocket)

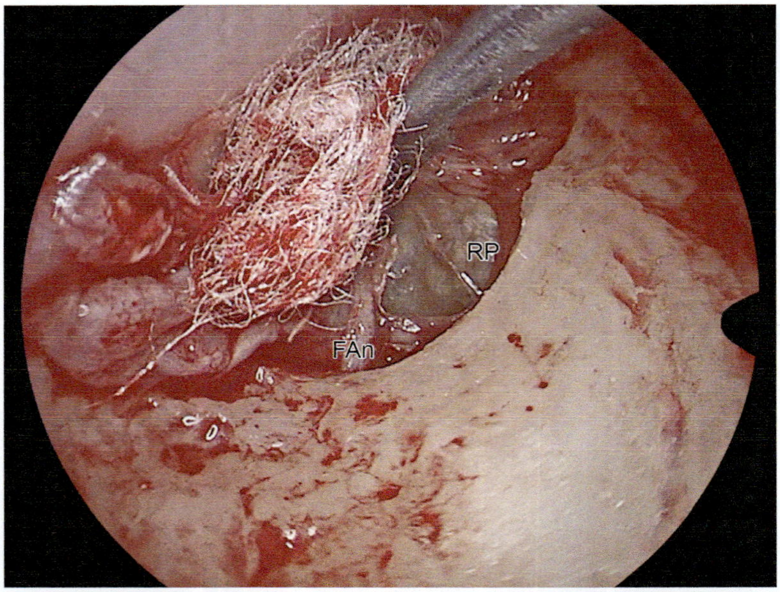

Fig. 4B: Exposure of retraction pocket: Dissection and elevation of tympanomeatal flap for exposure of retraction pocket. Fibrous annulus being dissected using sickle knife.
(FAn: fibrous annulus; RP: retraction pocket)

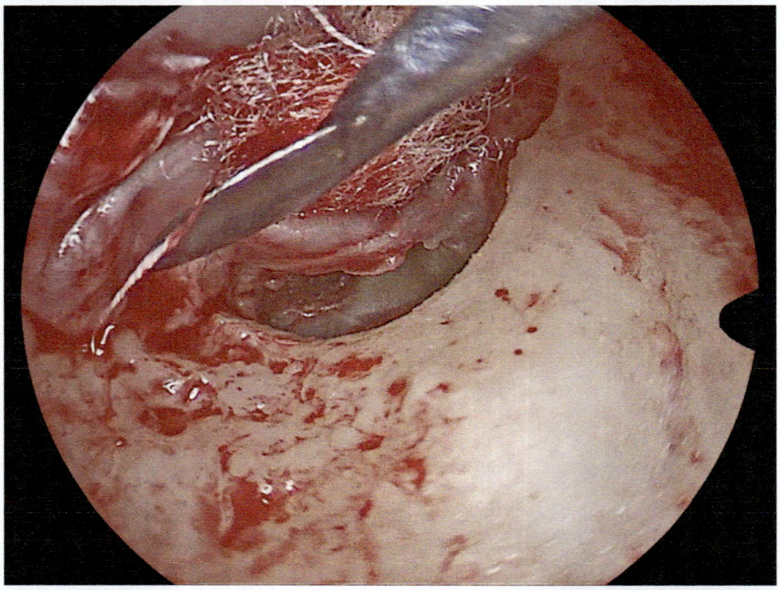

Fig. 4C: Exposure of retraction pocket: Dissection and elevation of tympanomeatal flap for exposure of retraction pocket (Note the elevation of fibrous annulus inferiorly).

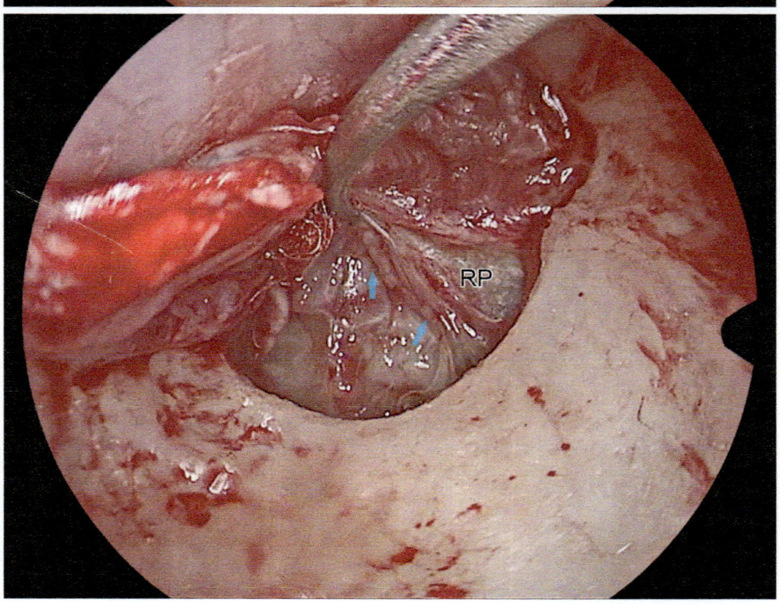

Figs. 4D: Exposure of retraction pocket: Retraction pocket being dissected off middle ear mucosa.
(RP: retraction pocket)

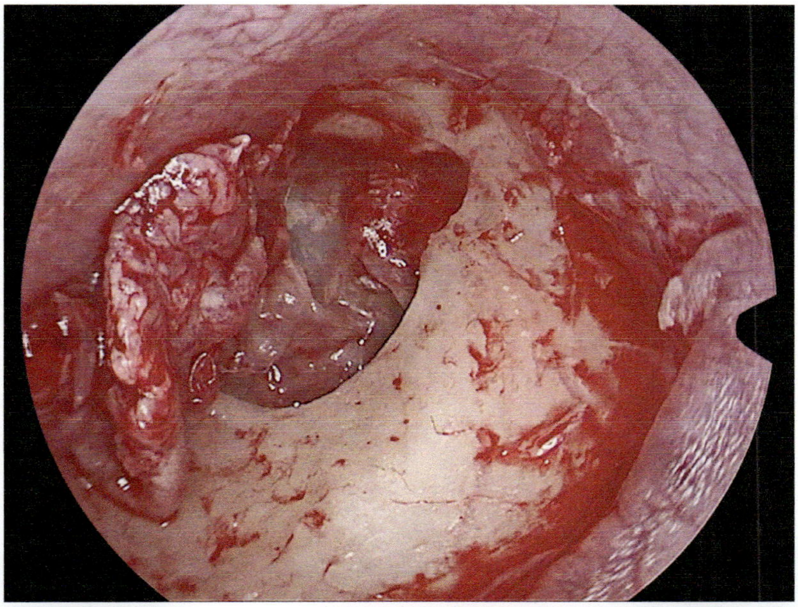

Fig. 4E: Exposure of retraction pocket: Flap separated from retraction pocket.

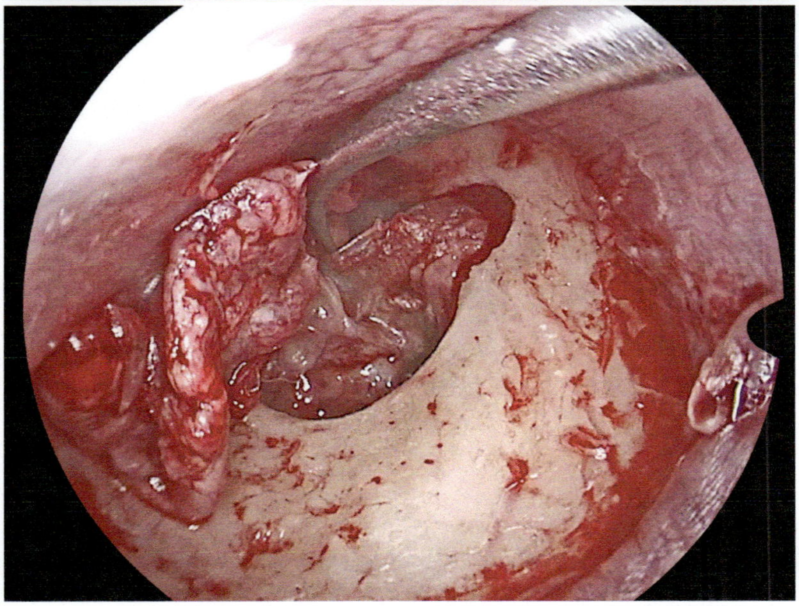

Fig. 4F: Exposure of retraction pocket: Dissection of retraction pocket from the remnant tympanic membrane with a sharp tipped microinstrument.

3. Dissection of Retraction Pocket

Prior to dissection of retraction pocket, ossicular chain status has to be confirmed.

The following possibilities are:

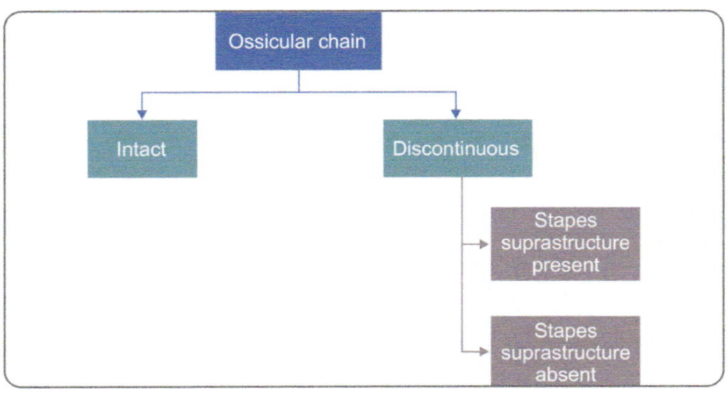

- Most commonly, the incus long process is found to be eroded
- In that case, the incus is taken out
- Before further dissection, the retraction pocket has to be exposed entirely and this requires bone drilling.

TIP

Retraction pocket has to be dissected using suction instruments (suction pick or dissector). In case such instruments are not available, careful dissection should be done using 45-degree or smooth curved pick with adrenaline-soaked cotton balls.

Dissection starts from supra-labyrinthine area, continuing over facial nerve, oval window or stapes suprastructure (depending on ossicular status) upto promontory.

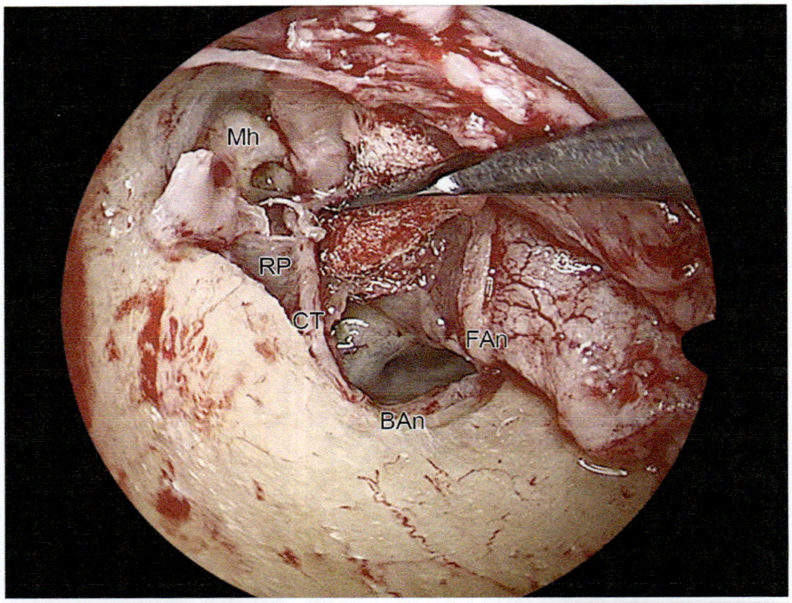

Fig. 5A: Retraction pocket dissection and exposure of middle ear structures (Note the use of cotton-ball to dissect the flap away toward hypotympanum).
(BAn: bony annulus; CT: chorda tympani; FAn: fibrous annulus; Mh: handle of malleus; RP: retraction pocket)

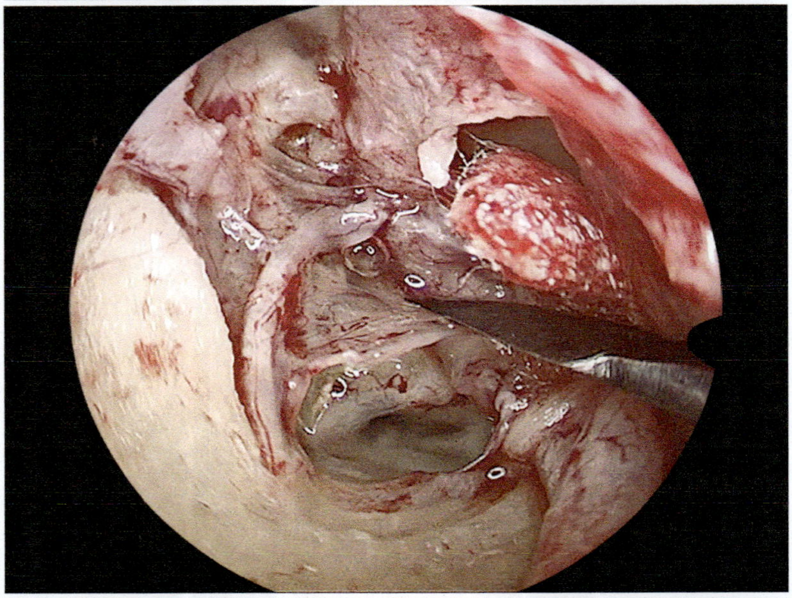

Fig. 5B: Retraction pocket dissection and exposure of middle ear structures using sickle knife.

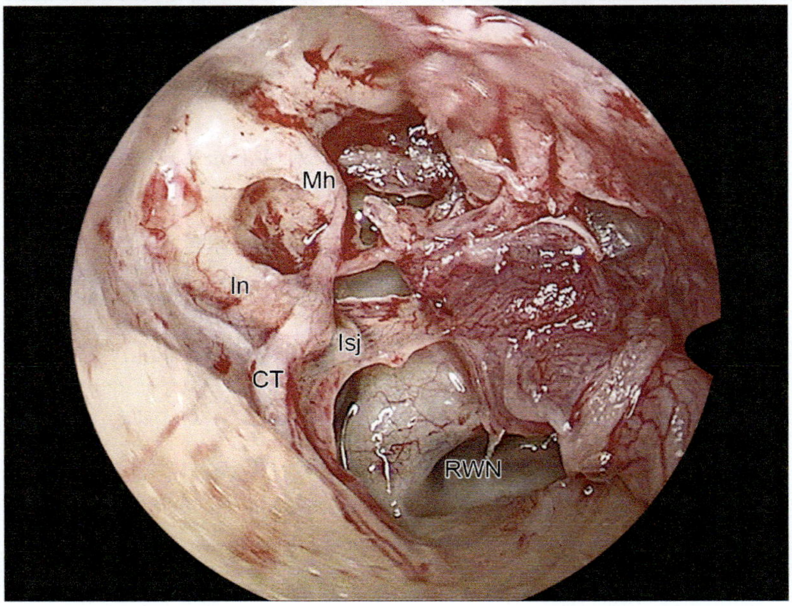

Fig. 5C: Retraction pocket dissection and exposure of middle ear structures: Retraction pocket being dissected out from incudostapedial complex.
(CT: chorda tympani; In: incus; Isj: incudostapedial joint; Mh: handle of malleus; RWN: round window niche)

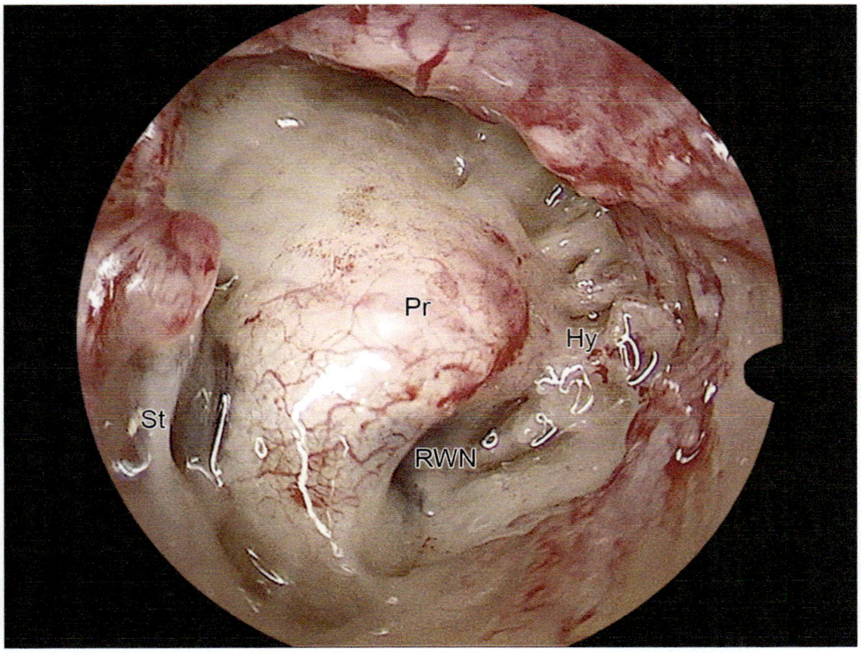

Fig. 5D: Retraction pocket dissection and exposure of middle ear structures: Final view. (Hy: hypotympanum; Pr: promontory; RWN: round window niche; St: stapedius tendon)

PEARL

- One should always try to remove the retraction pocket in continuity, avoiding remnant epithelium in the middle ear cleft
- Endoscopes provide the best possible view of sinus tympani and facial recess. Hence, complete dissection of the retraction pocket out of these hidden areas can be done easily

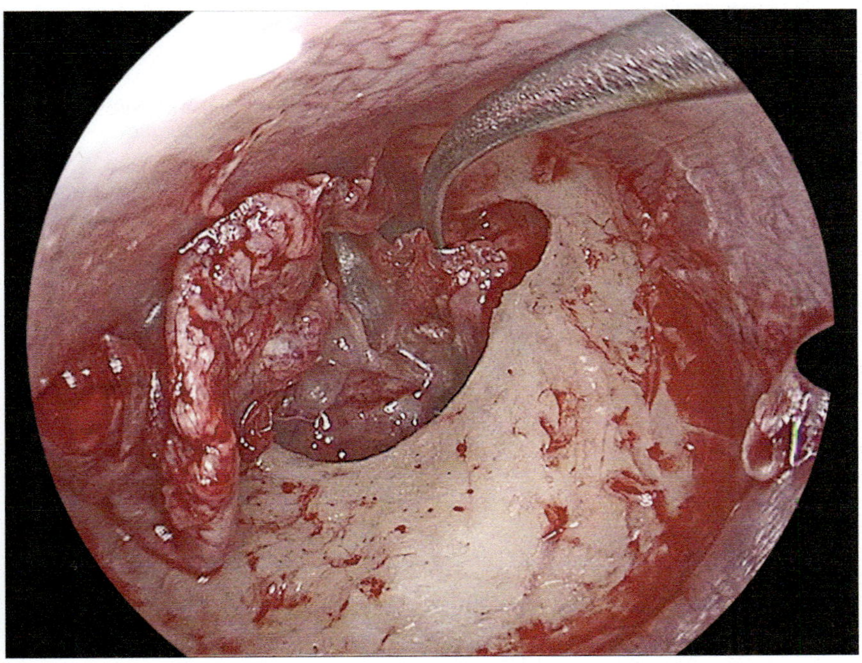

Fig. 6A: Separation of retraction pocket from surrounding ossicles and remnant tympanic membrane.

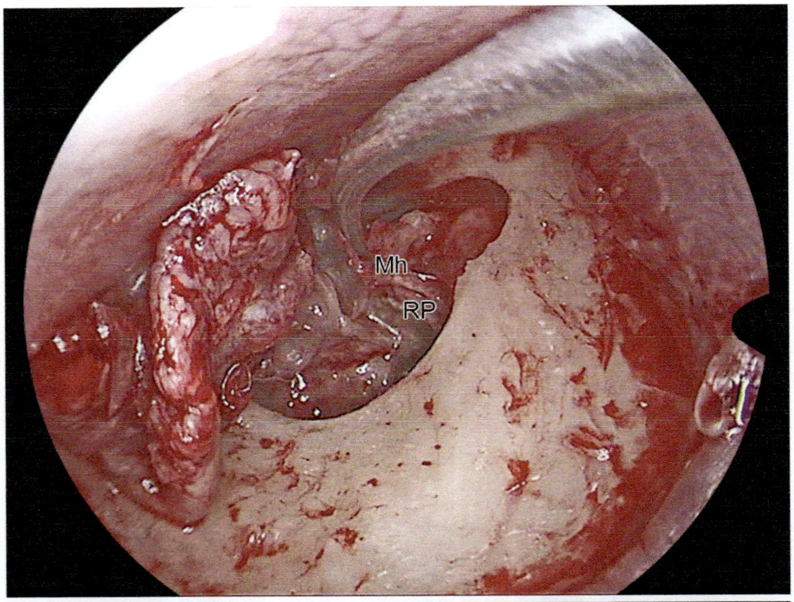

Fig. 6B: Separation of retraction pocket from surrounding ossicles and remnant tympanic membrane : Separation from handle of malleus.
(Mh: malleus handle, RP: retraction pocket)

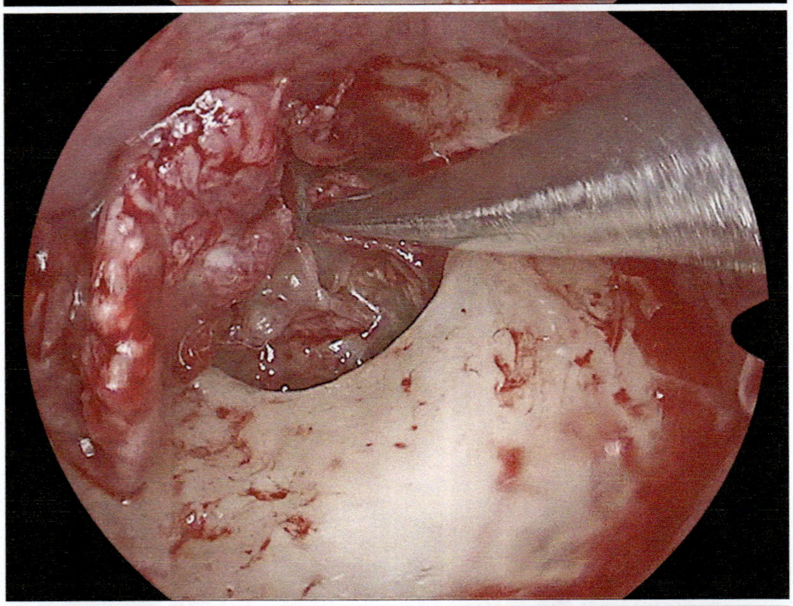

Fig. 6C: Separation of retraction pocket from surrounding ossicles and remnant tympanic membrane. Using iris scissor for sharp dissection.

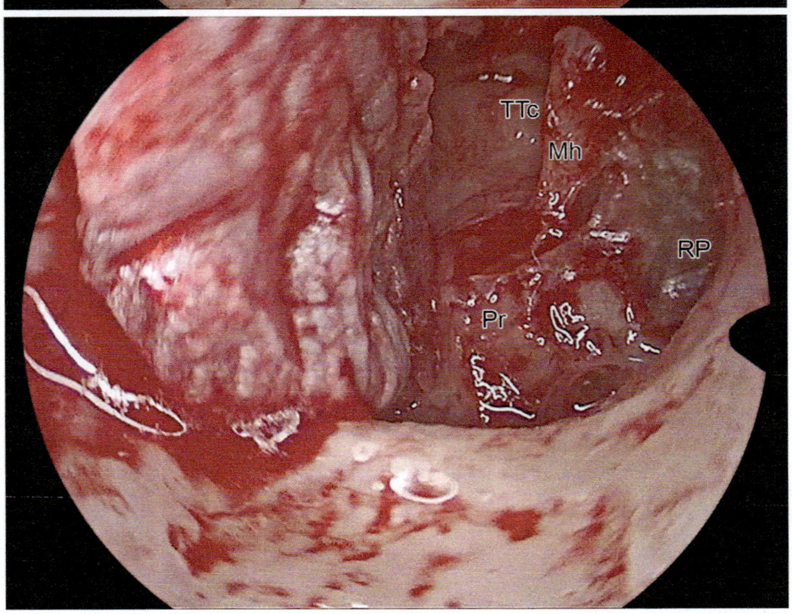

Fig. 6D: Separation of retraction pocket from surrounding ossicles and remnant tympanic membrane (Final view).
(Mh: malleus handle, RP: retraction pocket; Pr: promontory; TTc: canal for tensor tympani)

4. Bone Drilling

The exposed bone of the lateral attic wall is then drilled with a 2–2.3 mm diamond burr, layer by layer.

- The entire bone need not be drilled. It is only thinned such that the final egg-shell of bone can be removed using a House curette.

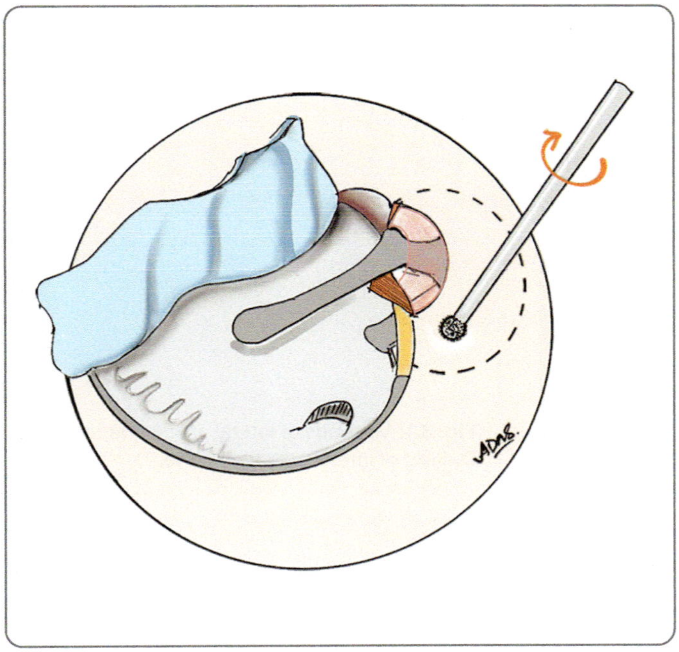

Fig. 7A: Drilling of lateral attic wall till an egg-shell of bone remains (Endoscopic view).

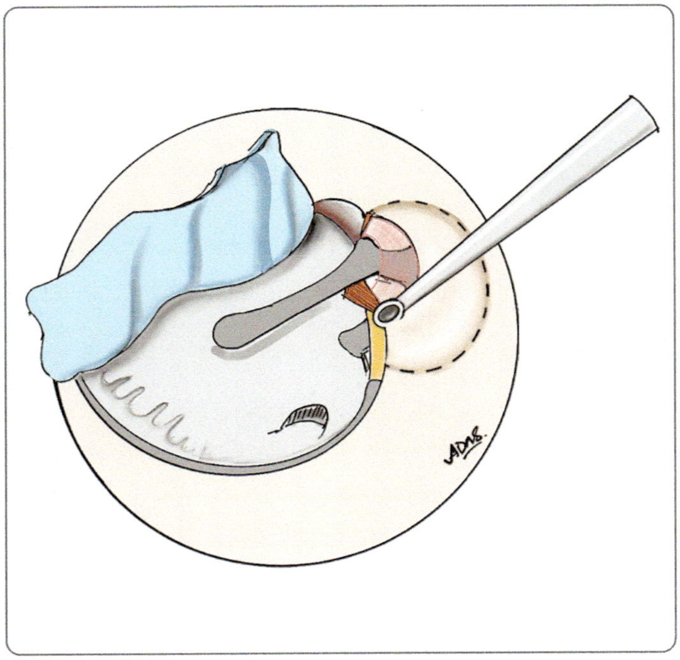

Fig. 7B: House curette used to remove the egg-shell bone to expose the attic (Endoscopic view).

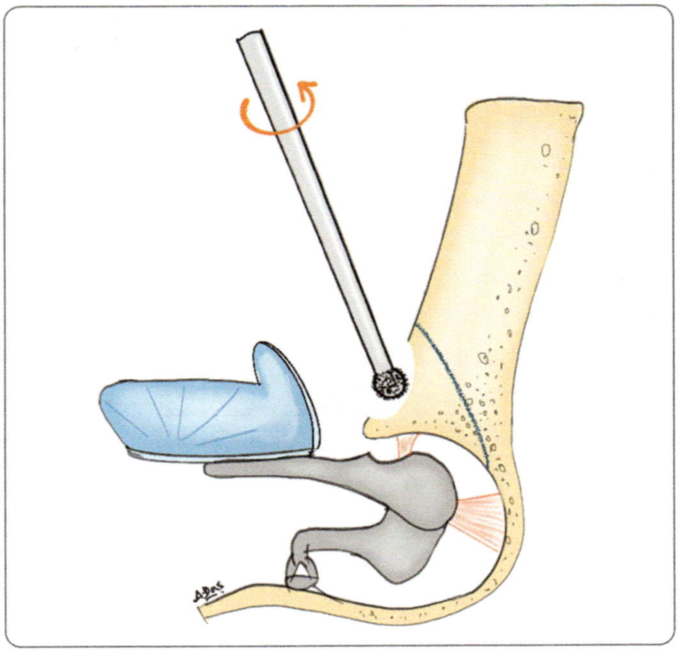

Fig. 7C: Drilling of lateral attic wall till an egg-shell of bone remains (Sagittal view).

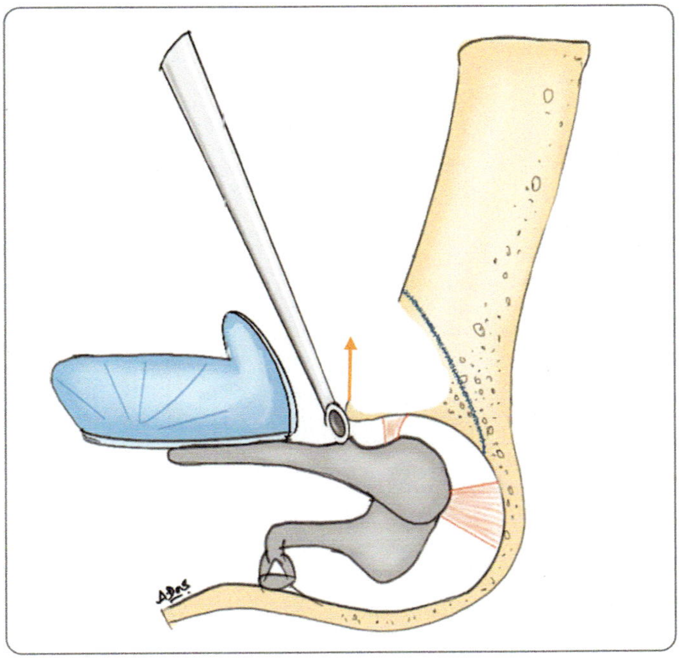

Fig. 7D: House curette used to remove the egg-shell bone to expose the attic (Sagittal view).

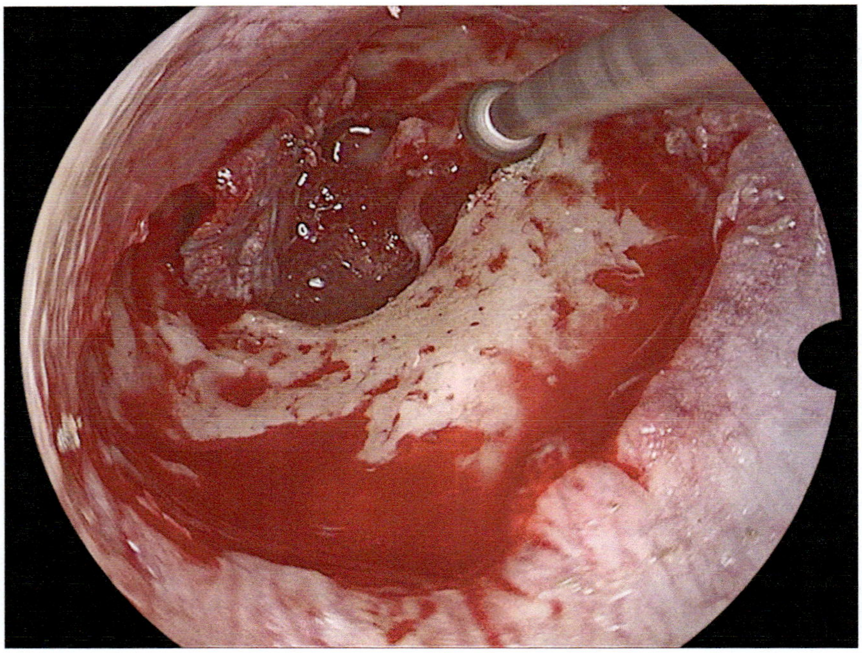

Fig. 8A: Methods of lateral attic bone removal: Drilling of lateral attic wall bone.

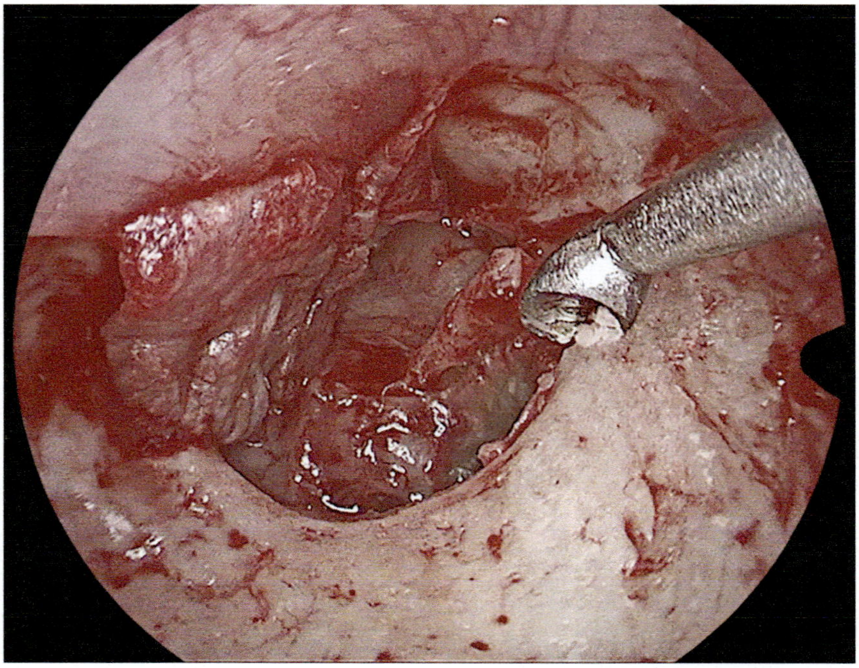

Fig. 8B: Methods of lateral attic bone removal: Method of curettage of lateral attic wall bone.

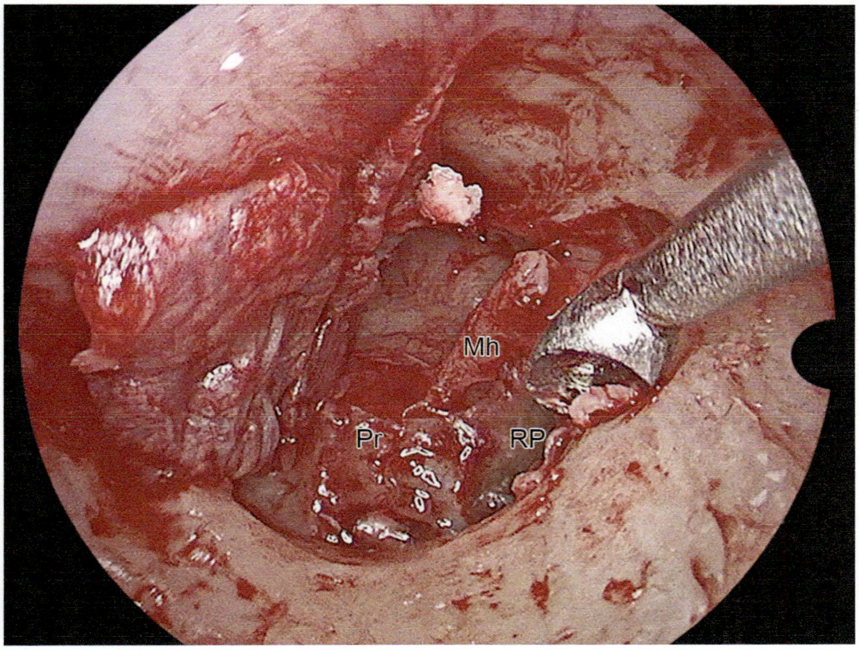

Fig. 8C: Methods of lateral attic bone removal: Method of curettage of lateral attic wall bone. (Mh: malleus handle; Pr: promontory; RP: retraction pocket)

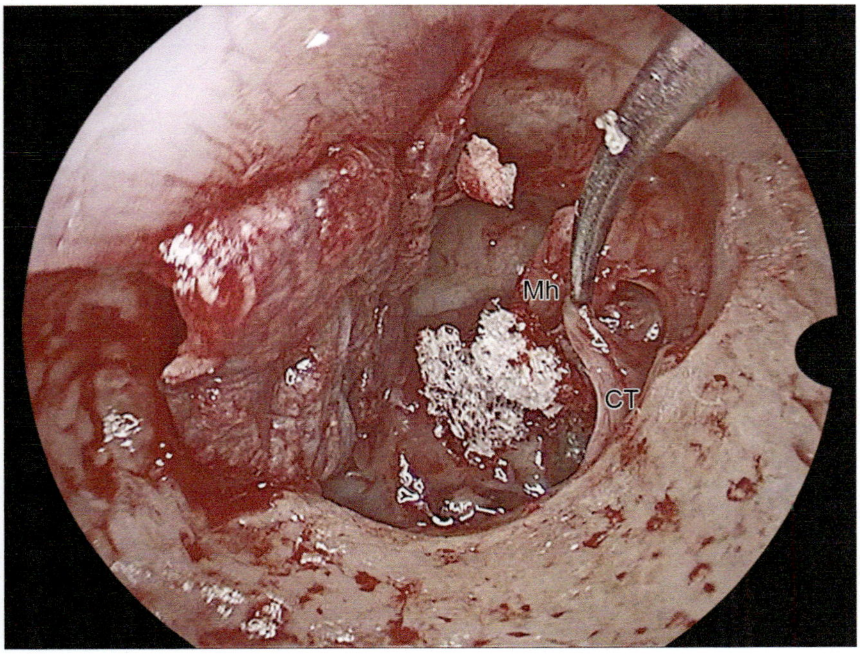

Fig. 8D: Methods of lateral attic bone removal: Chorda tympani nerve being dissected away inferiorly.
(Mh: malleus handle; CT: chorda tympani)

TIP **ATTIC BONE DRILLING**

- While drilling the scutum, the endoscope is placed on the cartilaginous external auditory canal, maintaining a safe distance between the endoscope tip and the rotating burr tip
- The speed of the rotating burr is kept at medium
- The tip of the scope should be kept free from soiling with bone dust by regular irrigations
- The rotating burr tip should never come in direct contact with the middle ear mucosa as it causes considerable bleeding, tissue loss and scarring
- Wilson bone punch should only be used after the incudostapedial joint has been dislocated to avoid iatrogenic ossicular chain trauma

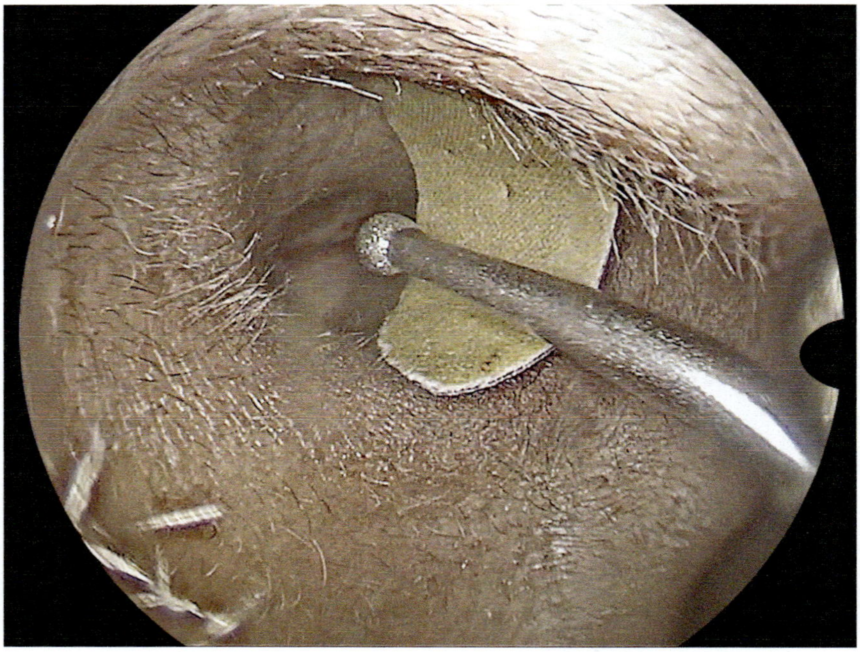

Fig. 9A: Protection of external auditory canal skin from shaft of rotating burr, using cut-out of suture pack (catgut).

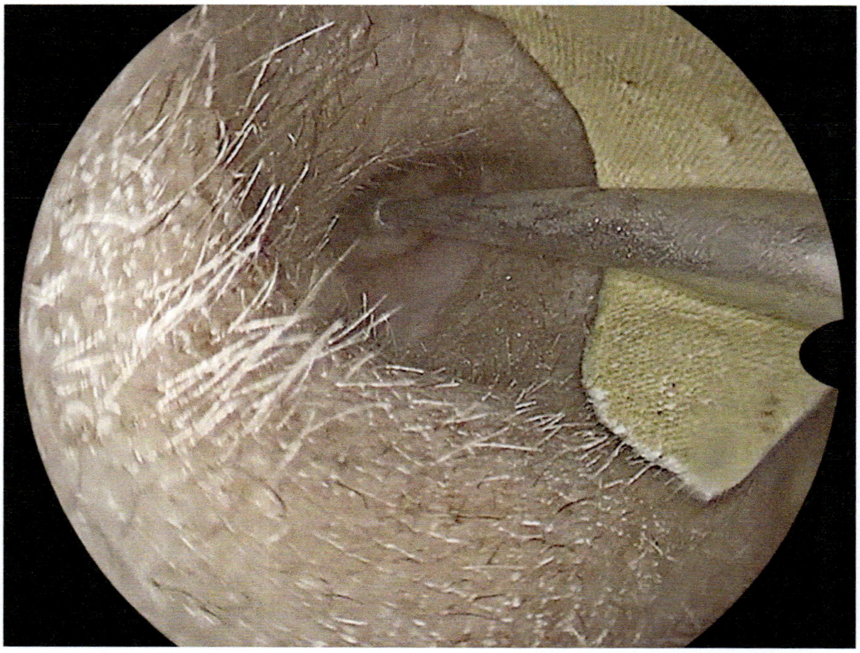

Fig. 9B: The rotating burr being advanced over the catgut foil to protect the skin.

PEARL **USE OF WILSON BONE PUNCH**

- Wilson bone punch is analogous to the commonly used Kerrison bone punch in functional endoscopic sinus surgery (FESS)
- It is used to punch out the bone of the outer attic wall
- The rough scalloped edges that remain after punching are smoothened out by drilling with a diamond burr
- Wilson punch helps in faster removal of a greater amount of bone in lesser time

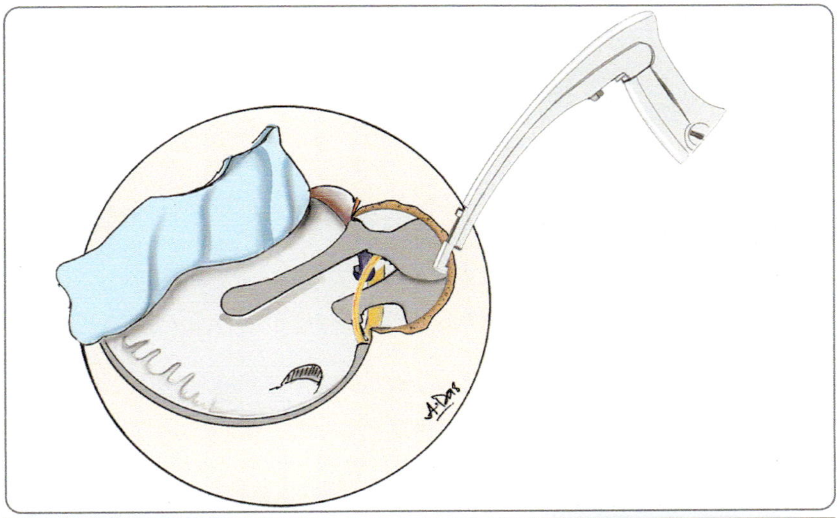

Fig. 10A: Pictorial depiction of use of Wilson bone punch to remove lateral attic wall bone.

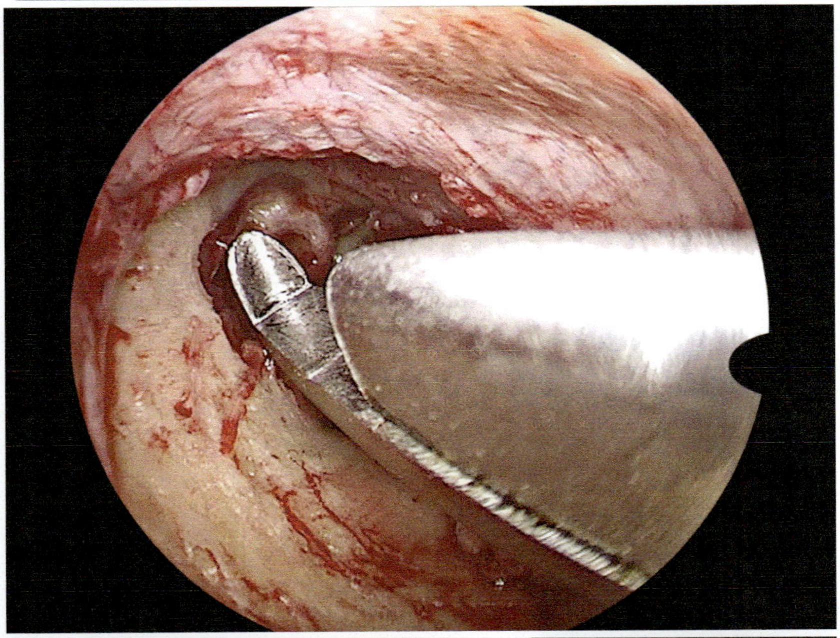

Fig. 10B: Method of introduction of the Wilson bone punch.

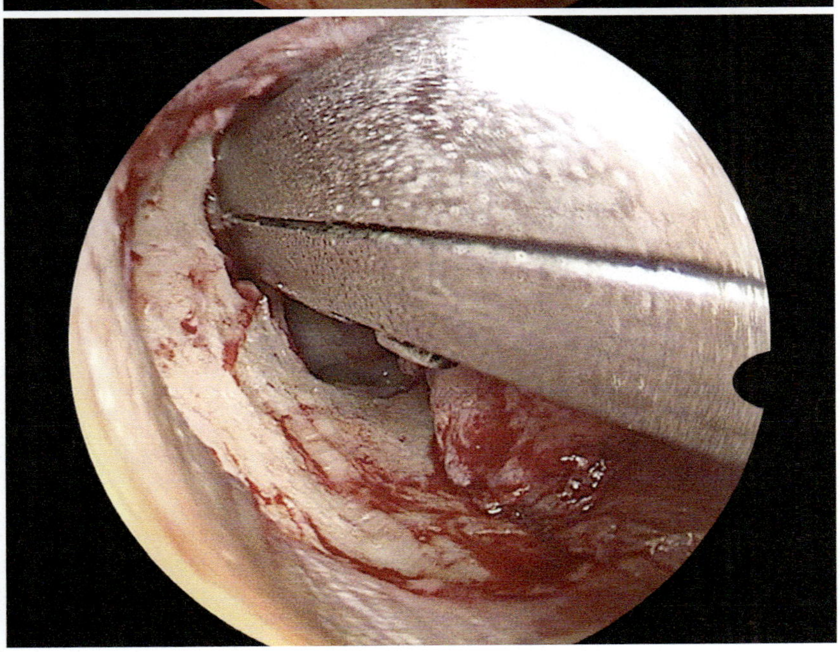

Fig. 10C: Method of engaging the instrument.

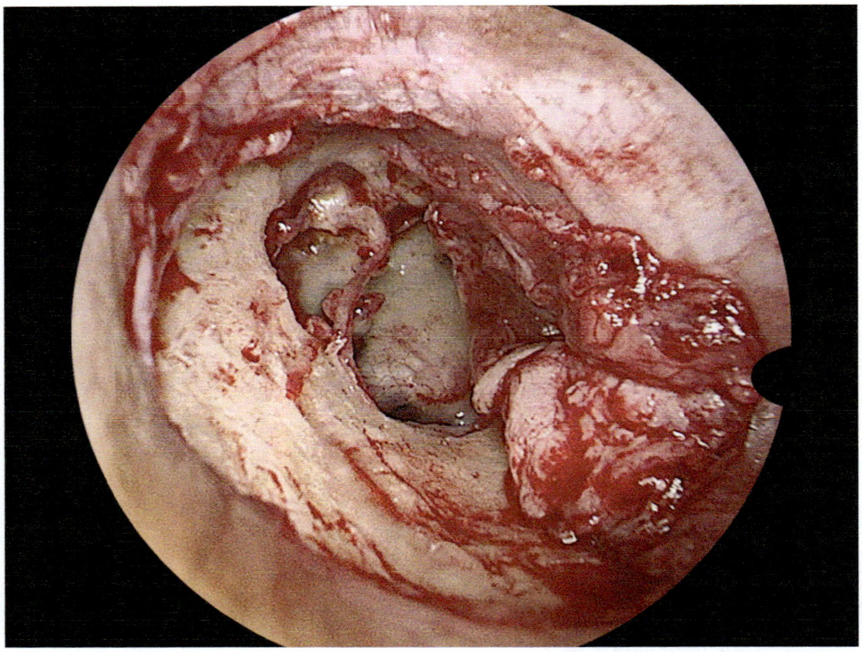

Fig. 10D: Bony defect after use of Wilson bone punch.

5. Ossicular Chain Management

- The incudostapedial joint is dislocated before commencement of substantial drilling/curette/bone punch use, depending on the disease process, for example, cholesteatoma extending medial to ossicles or planned ossicular chain reconstruction.
- Incudostapedial joint discontinuity is commonly seen as a result of the disease process itself.
- If intact, it has to be dislocated gently using a sharp pick or a joint knife in a posterior-to-anterior direction.
- Thereafter, the incudomalleolar joint is dislocated and incus is delivered out.
- The malleus head is nipped at its neck using a malleus nipper to expose the anterior epitympanic space.

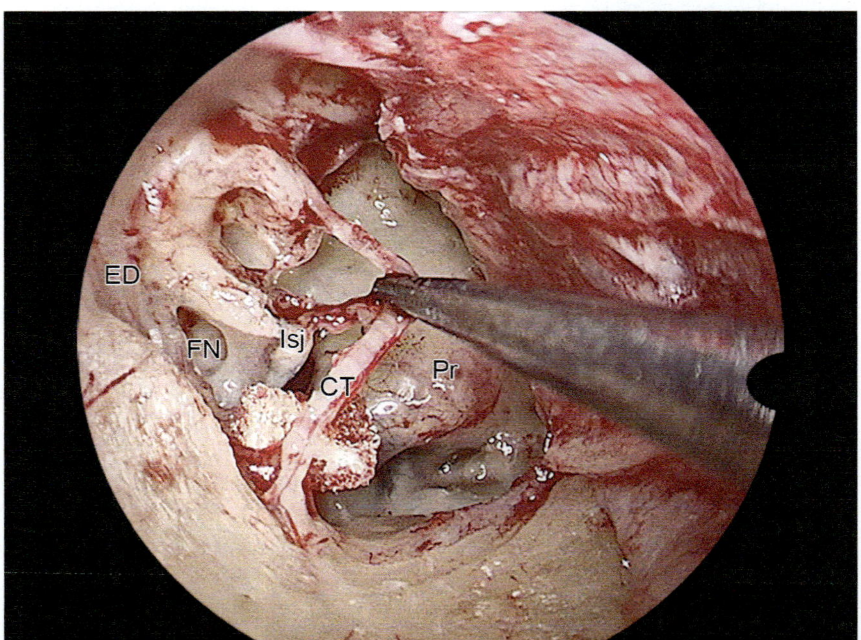

Fig. 11A: Dissection of chorda tympani. (CT: chorda tympani; ED: epitympanic diaphragm; FN: facial nerve; Isj: incudostapedial joint; Pr: promontory)

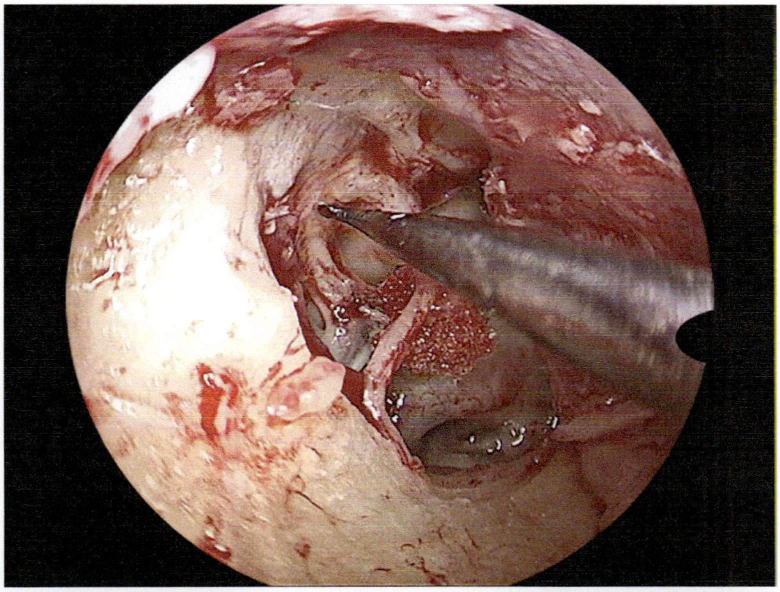

Fig. 11B: Disarticulation of incudomalleolar joint.

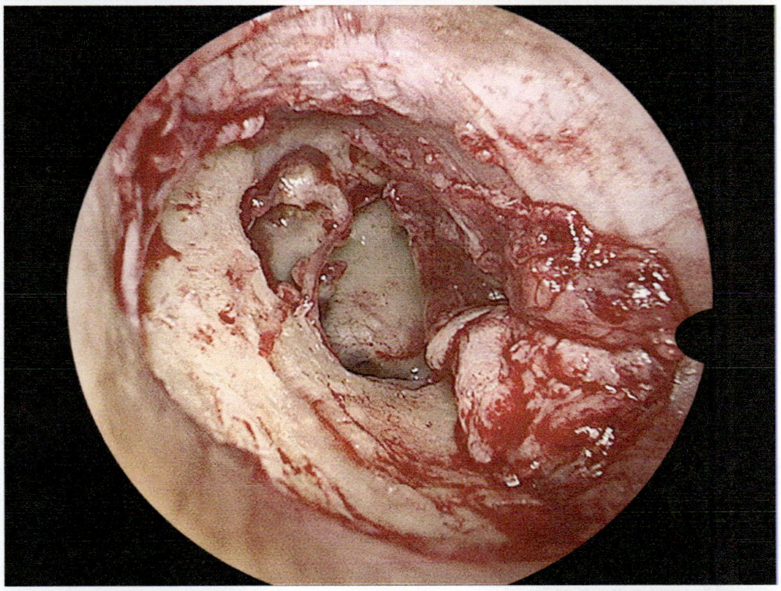

Fig. 11C: Incus removed.

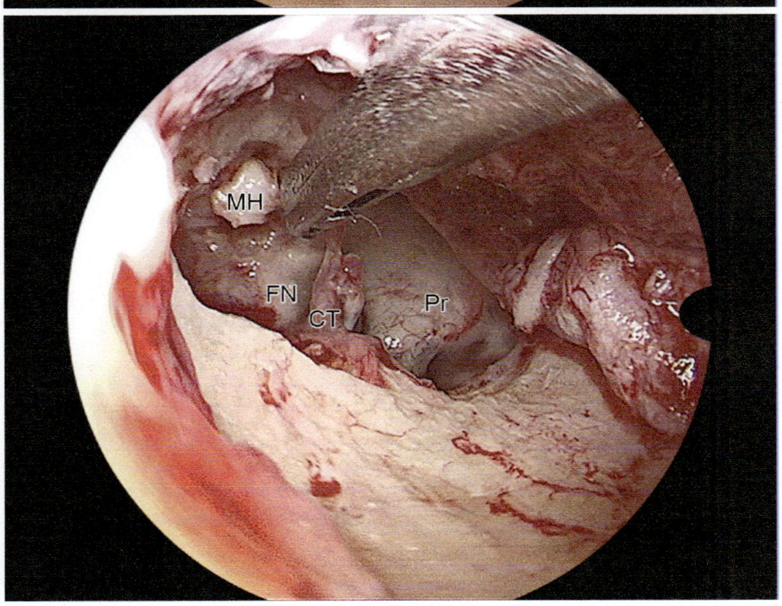

Fig. 11D: Nipping of malleus head.
(CT: chorda tympani; FN: facial nerve; MH: malleus head; Pr: promontory)

6. Dissection Continues

- Following initial steps of tympanomeatal flap elevation and dissection of retraction pocket, ossicular chain management (that is, removal of incus and nipping of head of malleus) is imperative to ensure adequate exposure of the entire epitympanum.
- Only after optimal exposure of the epitympanum (both anterior and posterior epitympanic spaces), complete resection of retraction pocket can be done.
- This prevents epithelial remnants being left behind and reduces the chances of recurrence.

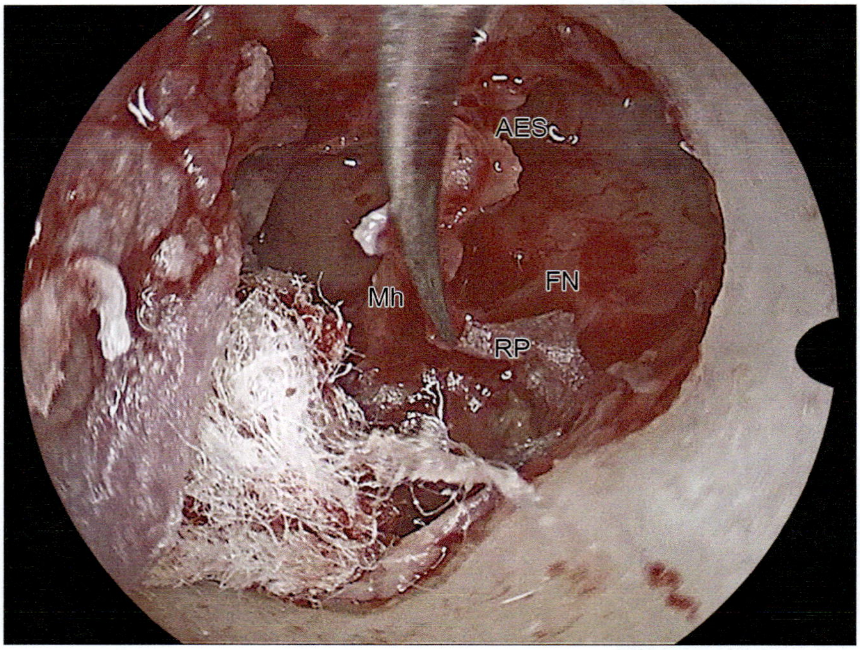

Fig. 12A: Dissection of retraction pocket from epitympanum.
(AES: anterior epitympanic space; FN: facial nerve; Mh: malleus handle; RP: retraction pocket)

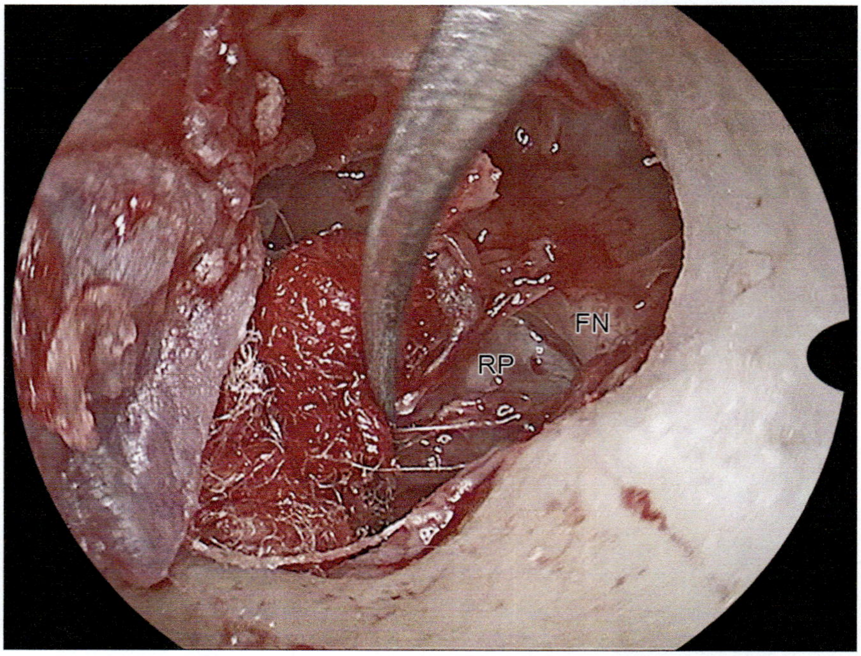

Fig. 12B: Dissection of retraction pocket from facial nerve and oval window.
(FN: facial nerve; RP: retraction pocket)

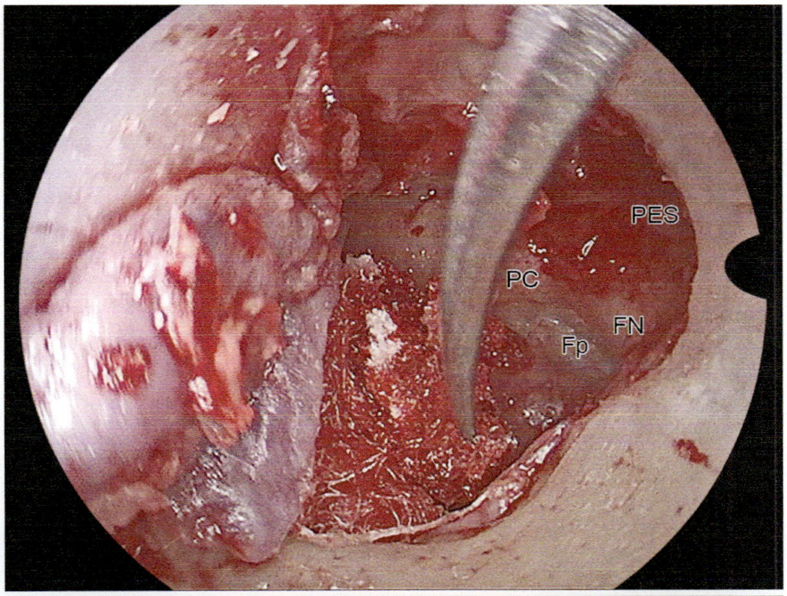

Fig. 12C: Dissection of retraction pocket from round window area.
(FN: facial nerve; Fp: footplate; PC: processus cochleariformis; PES: posterior epitympanic space)

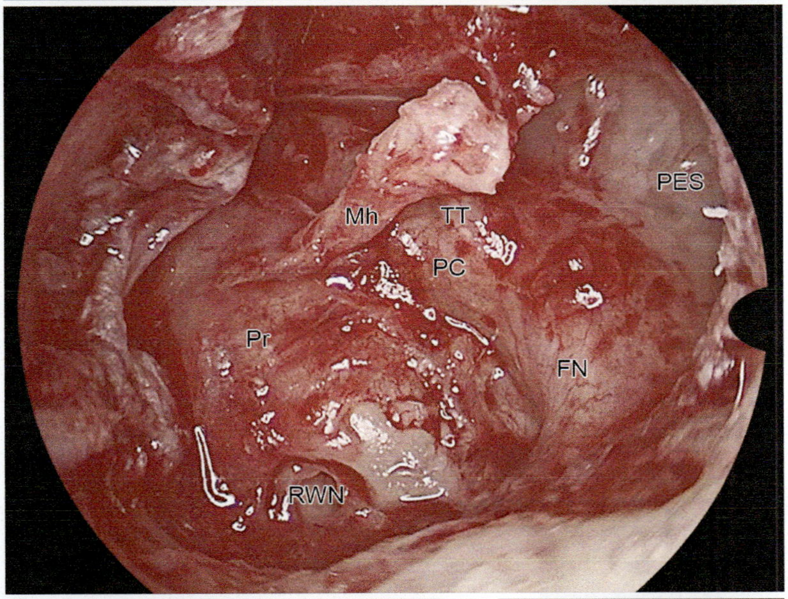

Fig. 12D: Identification of landmarks ofter dissection.
(FN: facial nerve; Mh: malleus handle; PC: processus cochleariformis; PES: posterior epitympanic space; Pr: promontory; RWN: round window niche; TT: tensor tympani tendon)

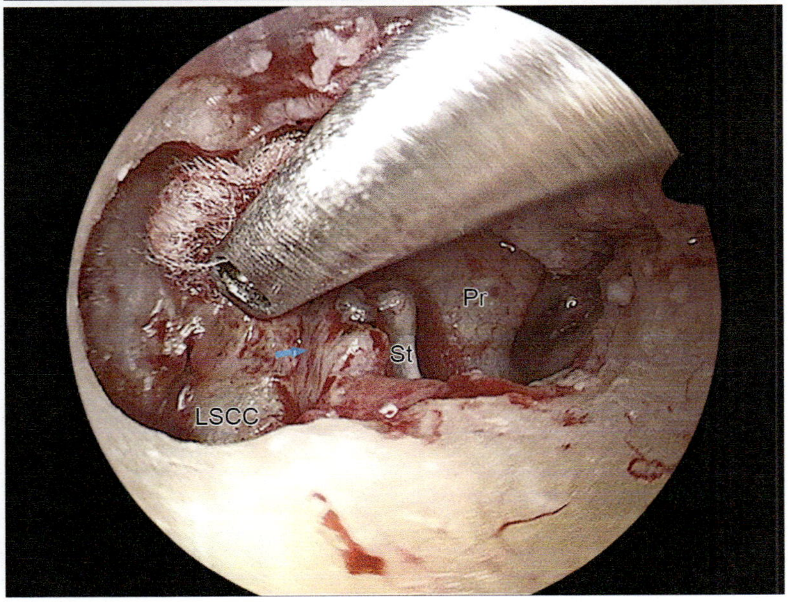

Fig. 13A: Clearance of hypertrophied mucosal folds from fallopian canal using suction middle ear dissector (blue arrow: retraction pocket).
(LSCC: lateral semicircular canal; Pr: promontory; St: stapedius tendon)

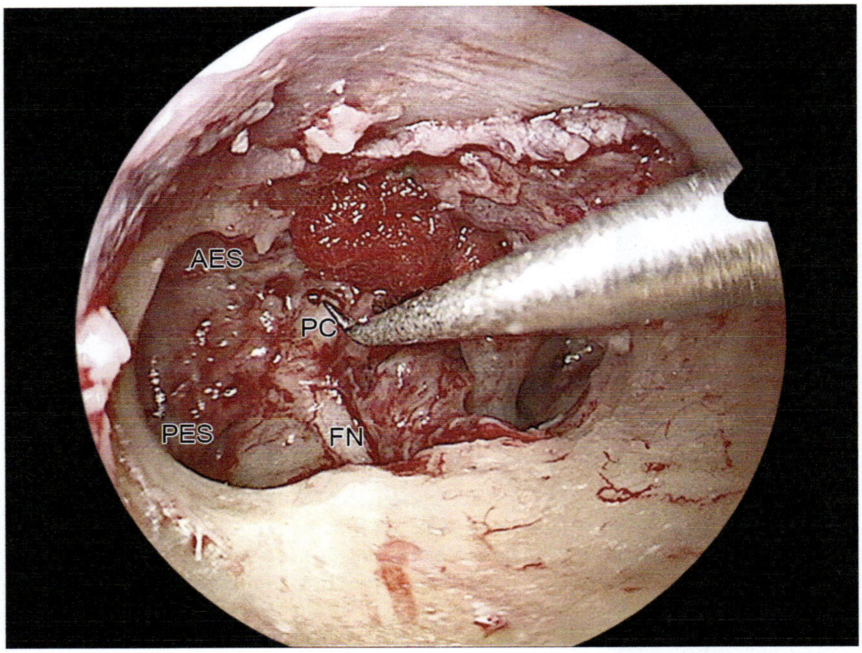

Fig. 13B: Clearance of hypertrophied mucosal folds around supratubal recess.
(AES: anterior epitympanic space; FN: facial nerve; PC: processus cochleariformis; PES: posterior epitympanic space)

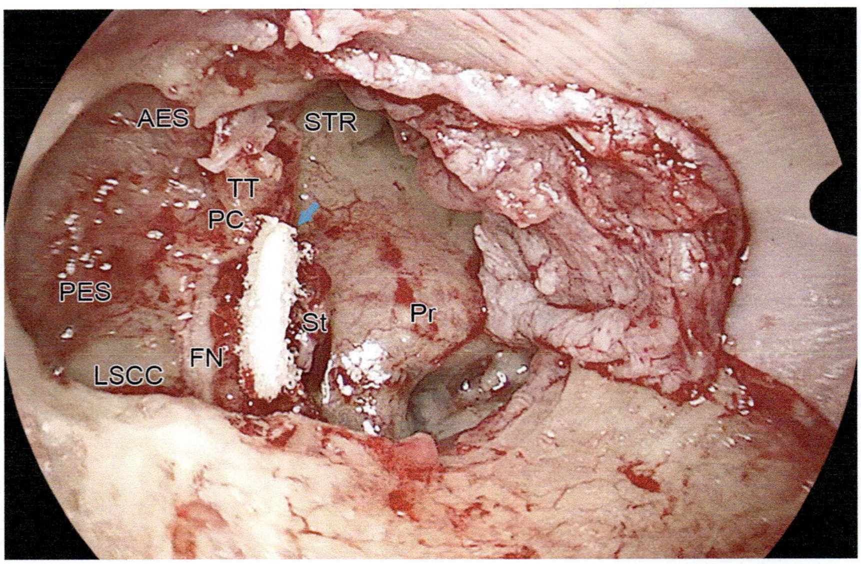

Fig. 13C: Clearance of hypertrophied mucosal folds around footplate area (epitympanum).
(Blue arrow: Gelfoam; AES: anterior epitympanic space; FN: facial nerve; LSCC: lateral semicircular canal; PC: processus cochleariformis; PES: posterior epitympanic space; Pr: promontory; St: stapedius tendon; STR: supratubal recess; TT: tensor tympani tendon)

7. Inspection of Anterior Epitympanic Space

- Anterior epitympanic space is the anterior most part of the attic.
- It is an important area often missed during surgery.
- In case of complete tensor fold, hindering the clearance of anterior epitympanic space, the tensor fold is opened using a ball-point probe or curved pick. The opening is then enlarged by passing a dry gelfoam. (For further details vide chapter "Endoscopic Epitympanic Exploration").

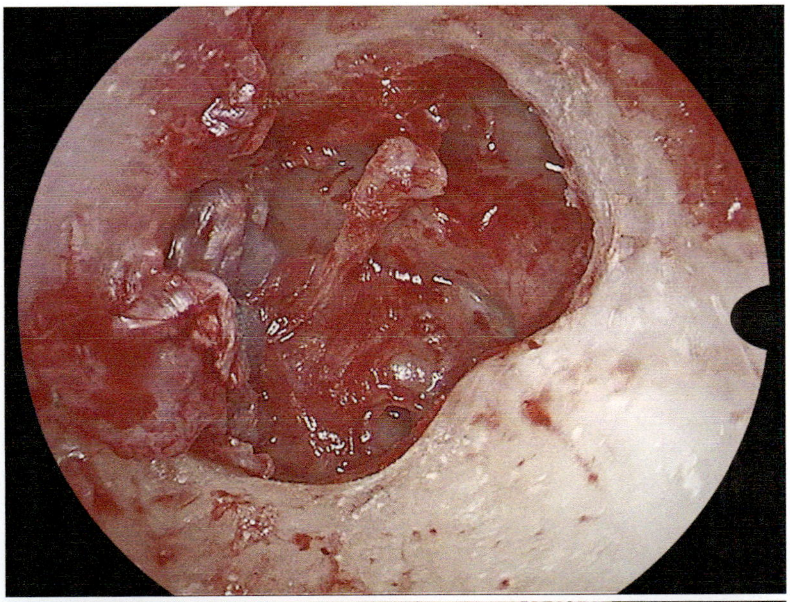

Fig. 14A: Inspection of anterior epitympanic space (AES).

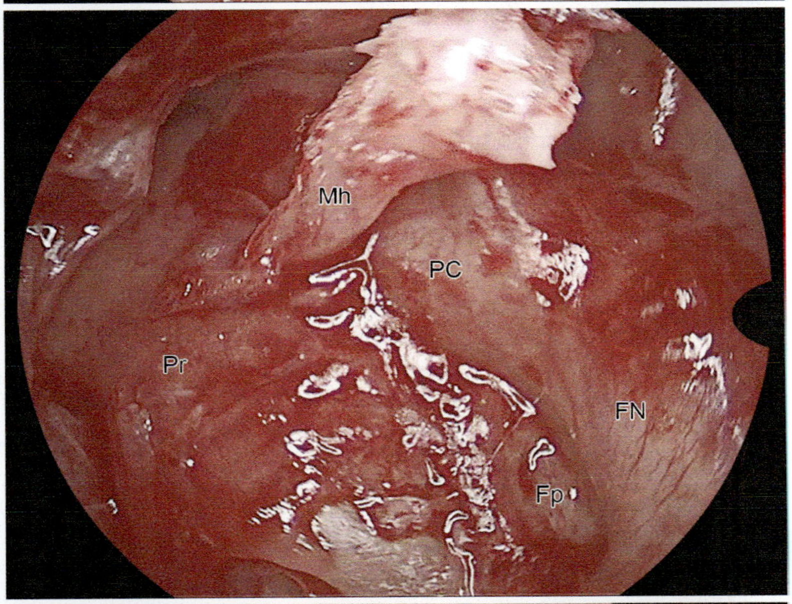

Fig. 14B: Close-up view.
(FN: facial nerve; Fp: foot plate; Mh: malleus handle; PC: processus cochleariformis; Pr: promontory)

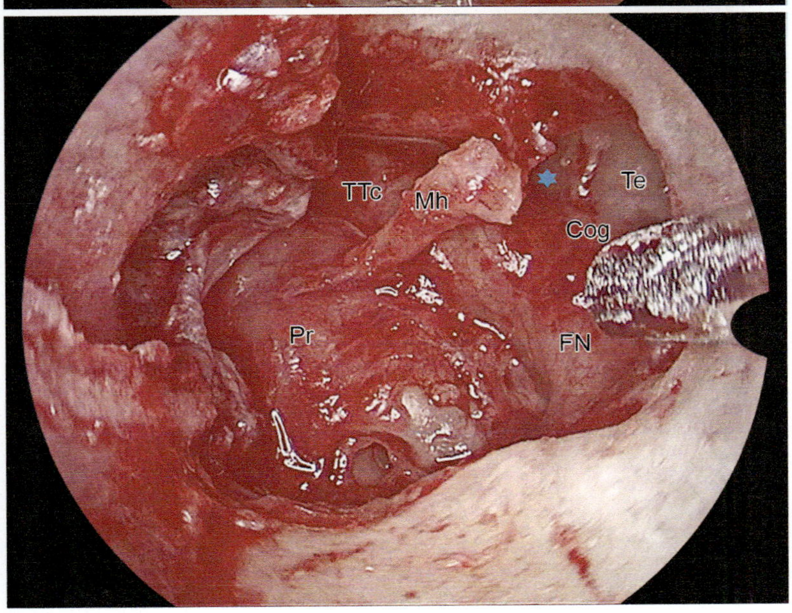

Fig. 14C: Final view after disease clearance showing important landmarks (star mark: AES).
(FN: facial nerve; Mh: malleus handle; Pr: promontory; Te: Tegmen tympani; TTc: canal for tensor tympani)

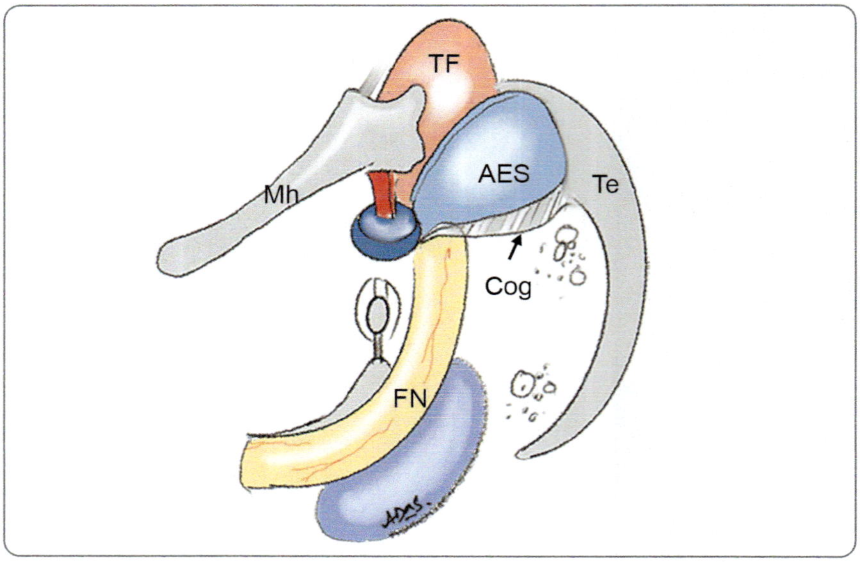

Fig. 14D: Schematic depiction of head-on view of epitympanum after disease clearance. (AES: anterior epitympanic space; FN: facial nerve; Mh: malleus handle; Te: Tegmen tympani; TF: tensor fold)

8. Final Reconstruction

- After completion of disease clearance, the size of the bony lateral attic wall defect is measured using our custom designed graduated dissector.
- For reconstruction, tragal cartilage is harvested.
- The harvested tragal cartilage is sliced into unequal two parts: the thicker part with attached perichondrium is used for attic reconstruction. The final size is again reconfirmed using our custom designed graduated dissector.
- Thinner slice is placed over alloplastic prosthesis used (Teflon PORP/TORP, as per the situation) to promote epithelialization and avoid extrusion.
- Appropriate ossicular chain reconstruction is done (vide Endoscopic Ossiculoplasty chapter).

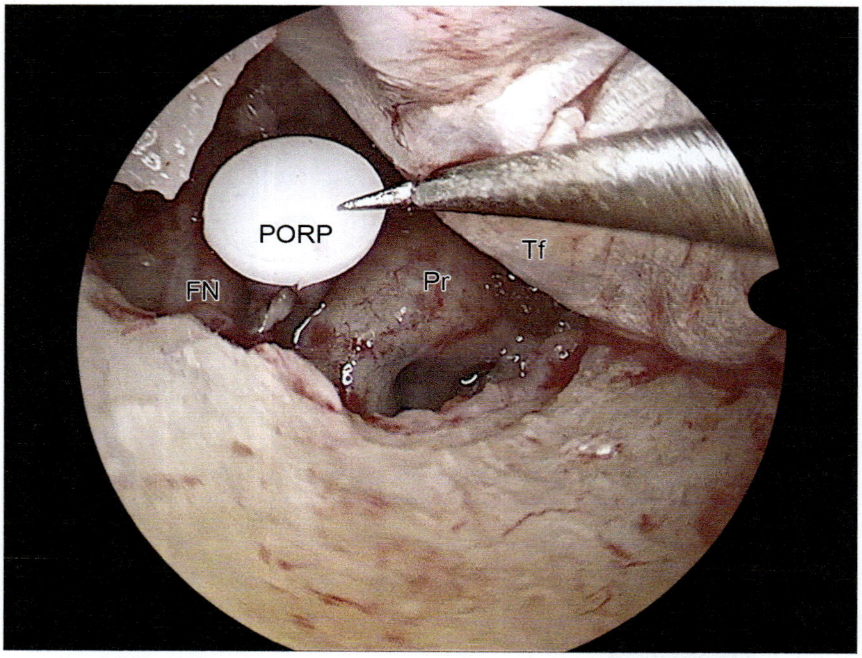

Fig. 15A: Partial ossicular replacement prosthesis (PORP) placed over stapes head.
(FN: facial nerve; Pr: promontory; Tf: tympanomeatal flap)

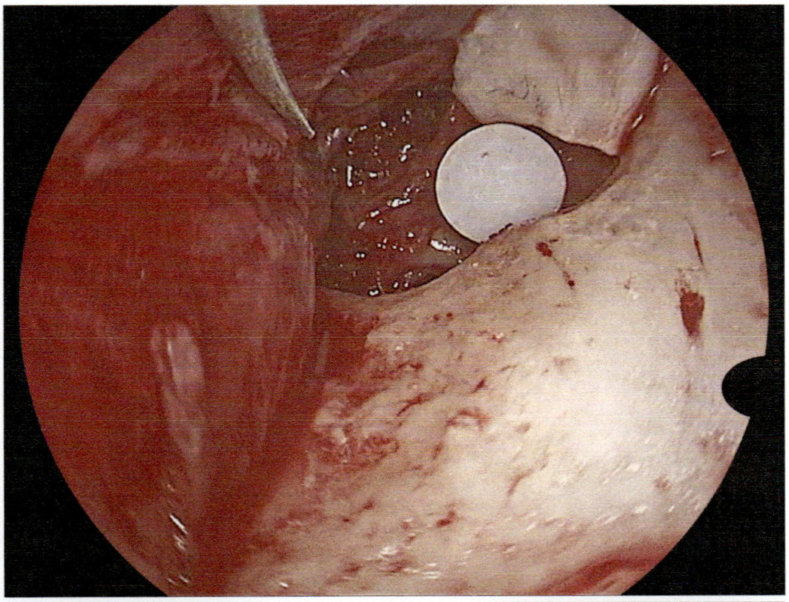

Fig. 15B: Final reconstruction: Placement of PORP.

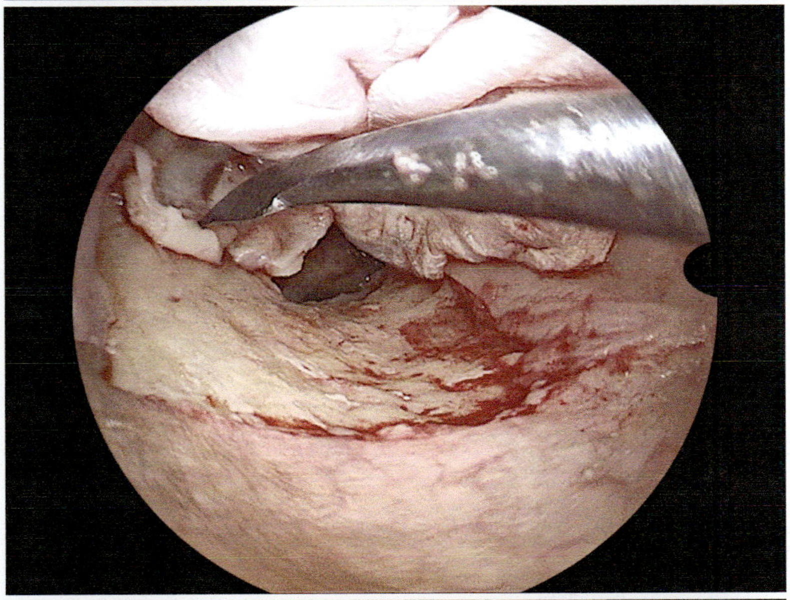

Fig. 15C: Final reconstruction: Attic reconstruction with tragal cartilage.

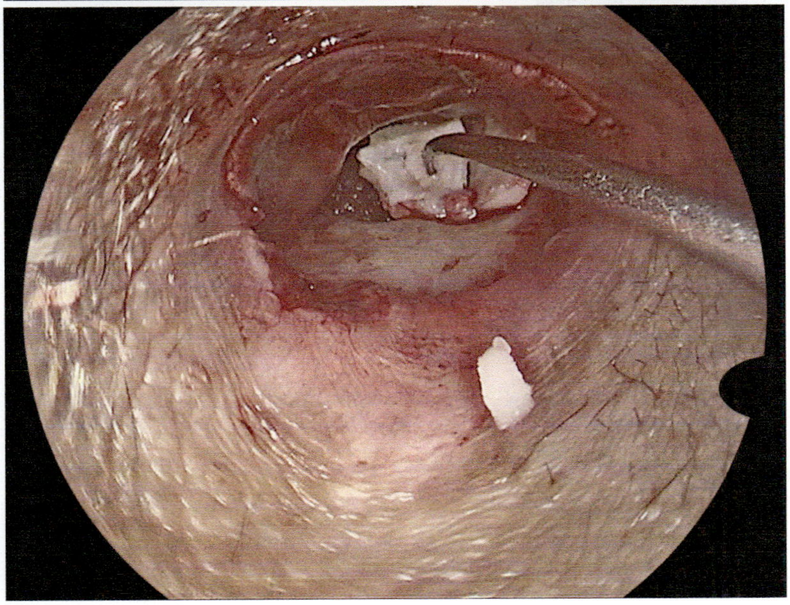

Fig. 15D: Final reconstruction: Placement of cartilage cap over prosthesis.

PEARL

Endoscopic atticotomy entails lesser bone removal. Hence, the resultant defect being smaller, the long-term complications such as retraction pocket formation or cartilage displacement are also less.

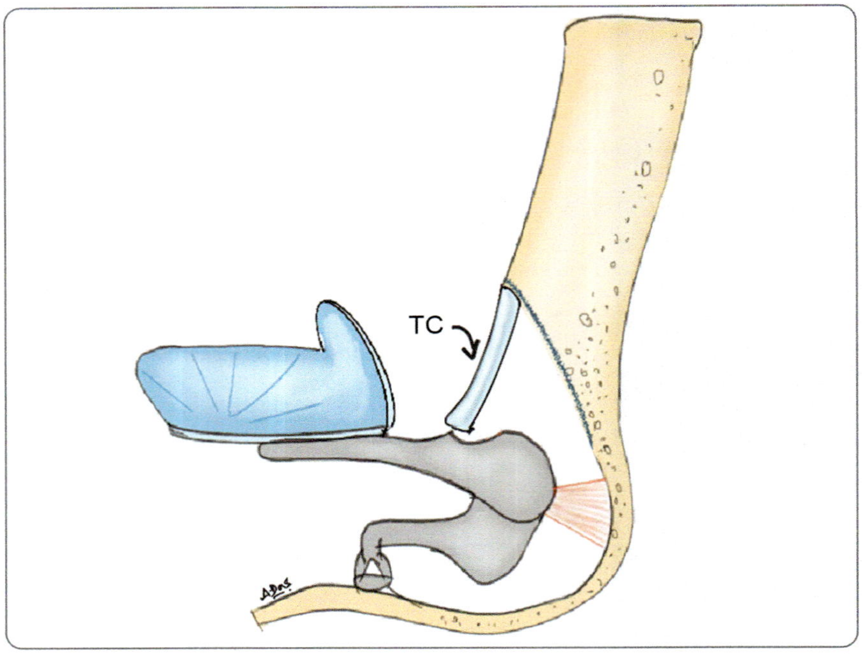

Fig. 16: Pictorial depiction: Tragal cartilage (TC) used to reconstruct resultant attic defect.

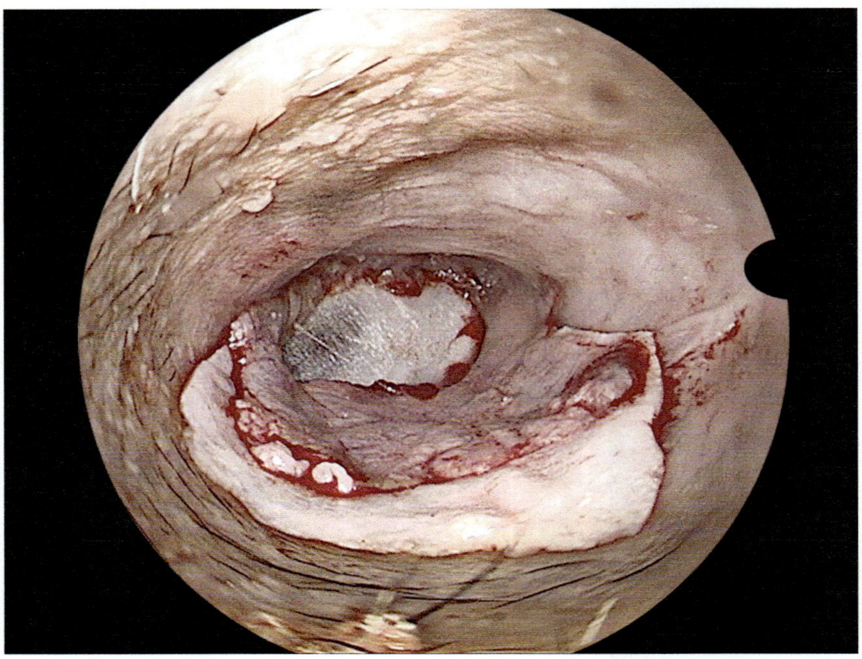

Fig. 17A: Final view after graft placement.

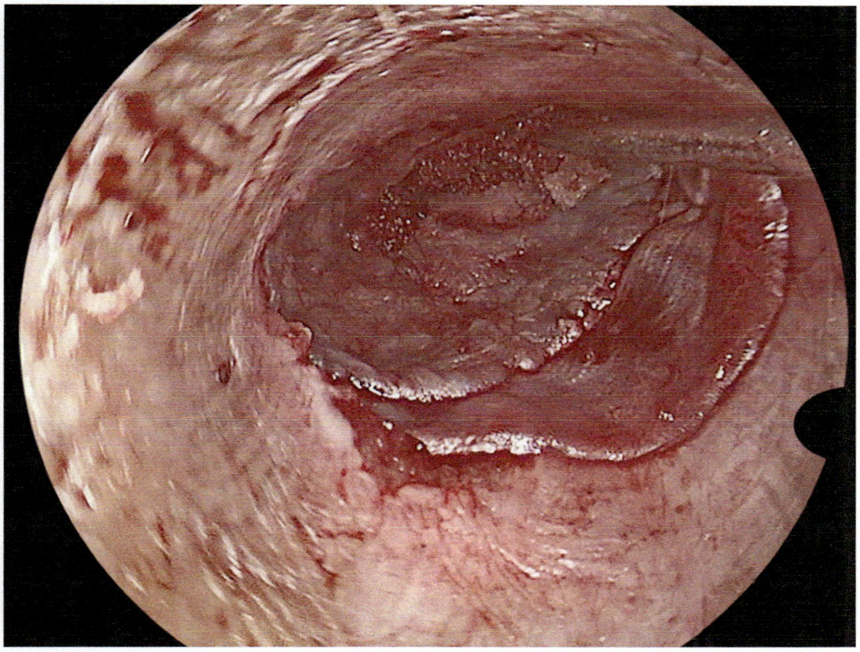

Fig. 17B: Gelfoam placement.

REFERENCE

1. Tarabichi M. Endoscopic management of limited attic cholesteatoma. Laryngoscope. 2004;114(7):1157-62.

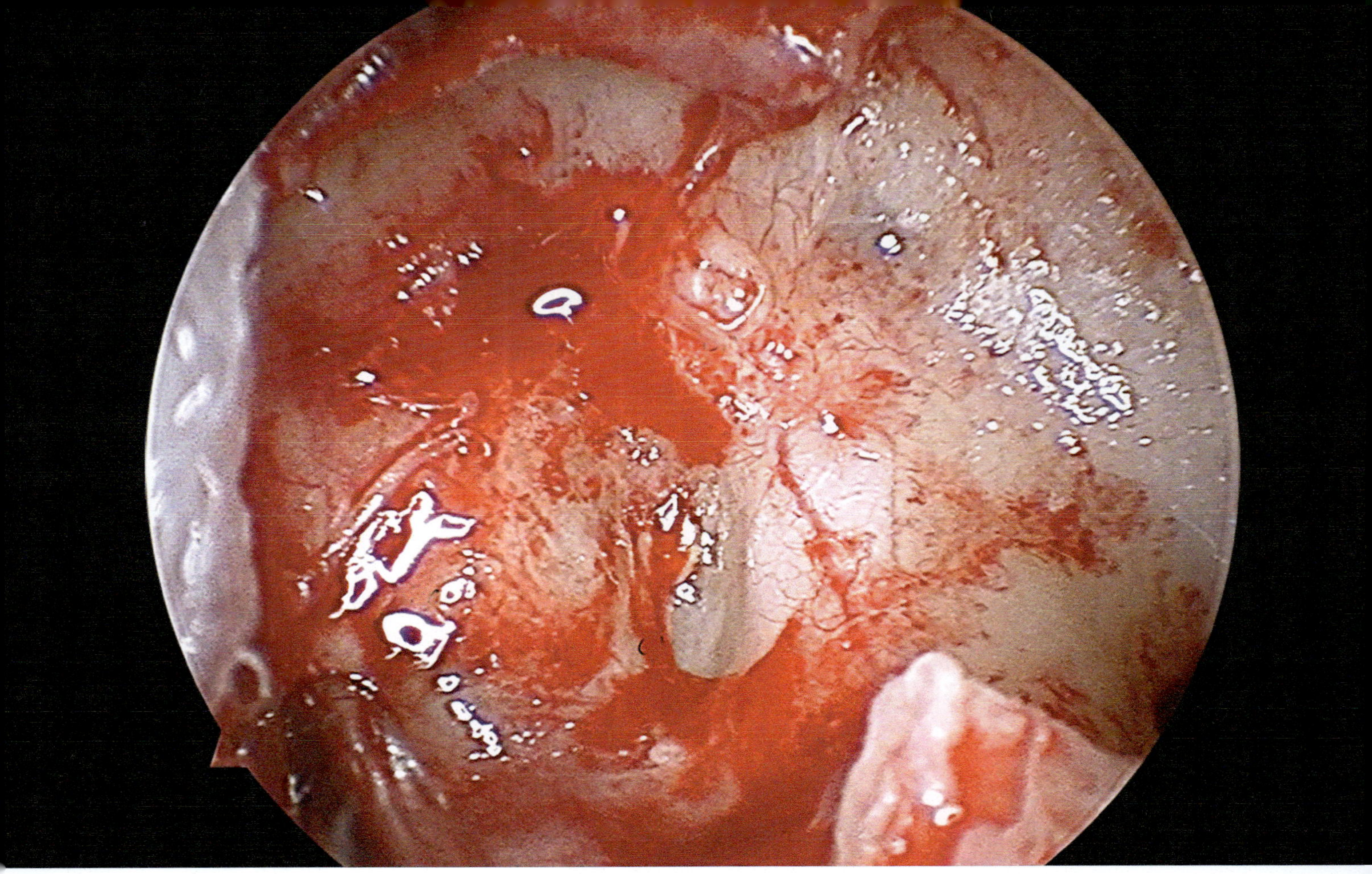

CHAPTER **11**

Minimally Invasive Endoscopic Mastoid Surgery

Arindam Das, Sandipta Mitra

Chapter Outline

INTRODUCTION

Mastoid exploration for cholesteatoma has been described in literature as the exenteration of the mastoid air cells, aimed at complete eradication of the disease.

Classically, mastoid exploration for squamosal disease has been done with the help of the operating microscope, via postaural approach. Depending on disease extent, mastoidectomy for cholesteatoma can be either a canal wall-up or canal wall-down mastoidectomy. For extensive disease, canal-wall down mastoidectomy has been advocated because of better disease clearance, less chances of residual or recurrent disease. Inside-out approach, a variant of canal wall down mastoidectomy includes atticotomy, atticoantrostomy or a complete canal wall-down mastoidectomy. The outside-in technique involves drilling of the outer cortical bone and then proceeding inwards. Cortical mastoidectomy is the classical example of such an approach.

Endoscopic mastoid exploration is nothing but an inside-out approach, following the disease along its natural course, with the help of endoscopes (straight and angled). Better visualization, magnified view and the ability to bypass the bony barriers and directly visualize the disease entails less soft tissue removal. However, when similar *selected limited disease* is approached via conventional microscopic mastoidectomy, it results in a considerable amount of bone removal, in order to gain access to the diseased areas for complete disease clearance and hence unnecessary disruption of normal tissues.

Principle of endoscopic mastoidectomy and its difference with microscopic mastoidectomy (inside-out CWD Technique)

Points of difference	*Microscopic mastoidectomy*	*Endoscopic mastoidectomy*
Anatomical site of bone drilling	Bone of root of the zygomatic arch drilled from lateral to medial to expose the entire attic (anterior and posterior epitympanic spaces), aditus, antrum	Medial aspect of scutum is drilled to expose the entire attic (anterior and posterior epitympanic spaces), extending into aditus and antrum
Amount of bone drilling	More	Less
Posterior canal wall	Entire canal wall lowered	Only posterosuperior aspect is drilled
Volume of defect to be reconstructed	More	Less
Lateral cortical bone	Drilled in order to exteriorize cavity	Intact
Resultant cavity	One single cavity in which mastoid communicates with tympanic cavity	Mastoid cavity remains separate from the tympanic cavity after reconstruction

Endoscopic mastoidectomy can be thought as a step ahead of endoscopic atticotomy which in turn is the next step of the least invasive, most conservative endoscopic epitympanic exploration. For differences between the three surgeries, vide "Endoscopic transcanal atticotomy" chapter.

INDICATIONS OF MINIMALLY INVASIVE ENDOSCOPIC MASTOID SURGERY

- Epitympanic or mesotympanic cholesteatoma with a contracted/sclerosed mastoid (diagnosed by imaging)
- No associated intracranial complications
- No extracranial intratemporal complications such as labyrinthitis, lateral semicircular canal fistula, facial nerve palsy, petrositis, etc.

CONTRAINDICATIONS OF MINIMALLY INVASIVE ENDOSCOPIC MASTOID SURGERY

- Disease extending posterior to (beyond) lateral semicircular canal
- Well-pneumatized mastoid, for example, in pediatric age group
- Narrow converging external auditory canal configuration (medial part is narrower than lateral)
- Cholesteatoma sac > 8 mm detected on non-echoplanar DW-MRI

RATIONALE OF MINIMALLY INVASIVE ENDOSCOPIC MASTOID SURGERY

With proper selection of cases, limited squamosal disease can be better treated with minimally invasive endoscopic mastoid surgery. The reasons are:

- Less bone drilling
- Magnified view
- Ability to look around corners to ensure complete disease clearance. Also, if more extensive disease is found on-table, one should be flexible enough to convert it into a more radical surgery keeping in mind complete extirpation of disease: the prime principle of cholesteatoma surgery.
- Greater chance of selectively preserving anterior mucosal folds and ligaments, if unaffected by disease. This results in lesser scarring of the anterior ventilation pathways postoperatively
- Greater tissue preservation results in more stable reconstruction

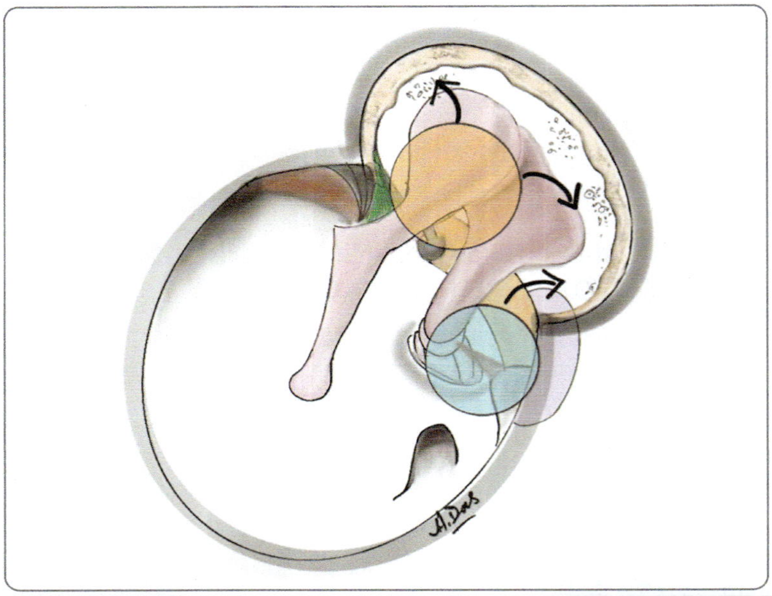

Fig. 1: Common types of cholesteatoma and their pattern of spread—Epitympanic cholesteatoma (orange zone) spreads both anteriorly as well as posteriorly—Mesotympanic cholesteatoma or posterior-superior retraction pocket (blue zone) spreads posteriorly toward mastoid antrum.

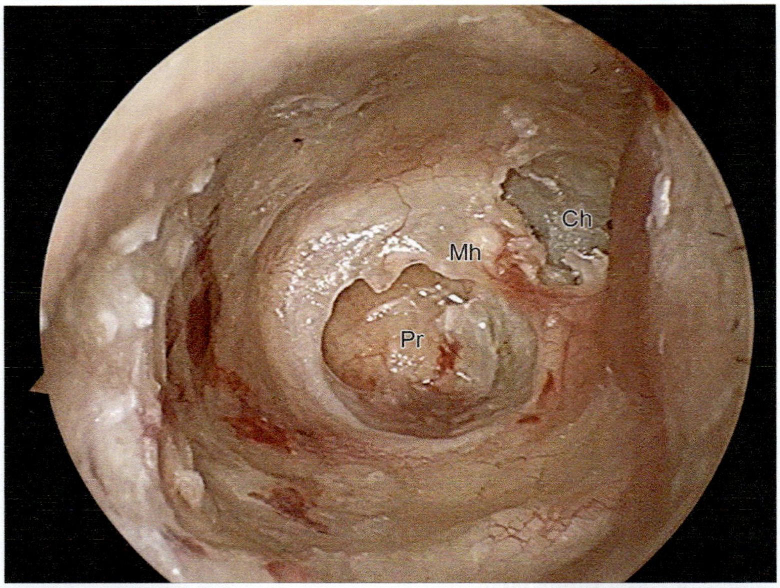

Fig. 2A: Intraoperative pictures showing epitympanic cholesteatoma.
(Ch: cholesteatoma; Mh: handle of malleus; Pr: promontory

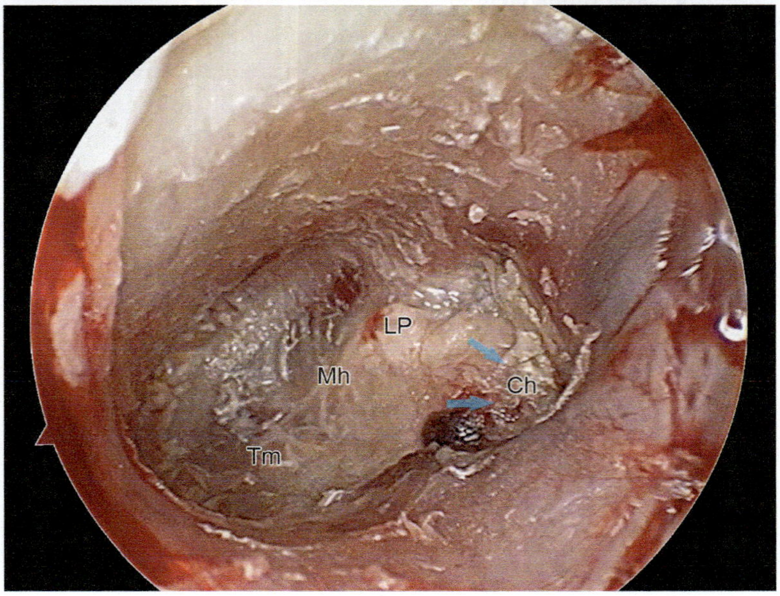

Fig. 2B: Intraoperative pictures showing mesotympanic cholesteatoma (blue arrow showing direction of spread).
(LP: lateral process of malleus; Mh: handle of malleus; Tm: tympanic membrane; Ch: cholesteatoma)

Steps of Surgery

- *Anesthesia:* Local anesthesia with four quadrant infiltration with 2% Lidocaine with Adrenaline (1:100,000), 0.5 mL each quadrant, is used for local infiltration. For pediatric age group and un-cooperative patients, general anesthesia is used.

TIP

When general anesthesia is used, hypotensive anesthesia with use of tranexamic acid as per protocol (vide "Principles of Endoscopic Ear Surgery" chapter) should be used to minimize intraoperative bleeding.

- *Incision:* Incision has three parts. A superior limb, an inferior limb and a horizontal limb connecting the two. The horizontal limb is fashioned proximal to the *bony-cartilaginous junction* of the external auditory canal. The inferior limb is positioned at 6 o' clock position, 1 mm away from the inferior annulus and joins the lower border of the horizontal limb. The superior incision is placed keeping a width of 1 mm and is extended further anteriorly upto the Eustachian tube.

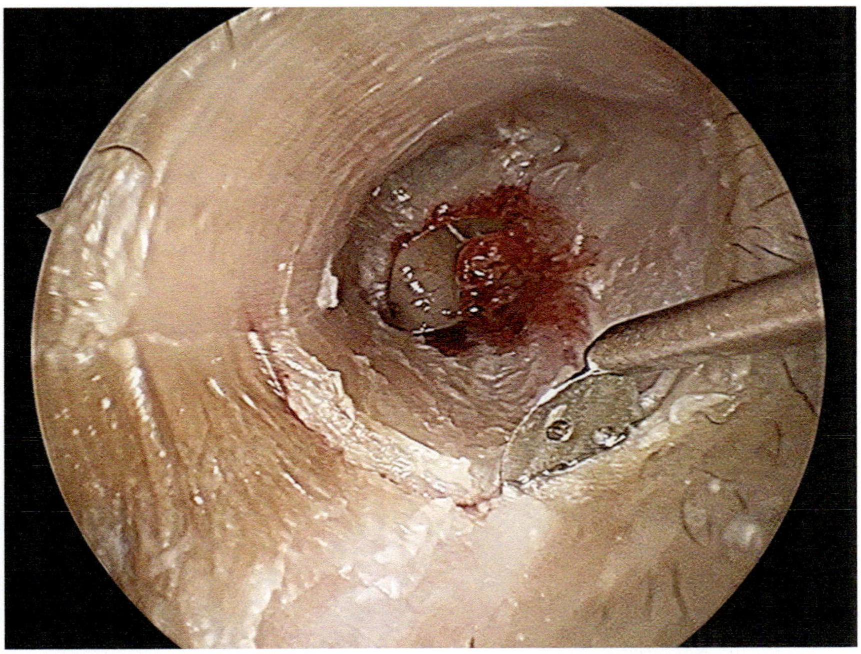

Fig. 3A: Steps of canal incision (left ear). Horizontal limb.

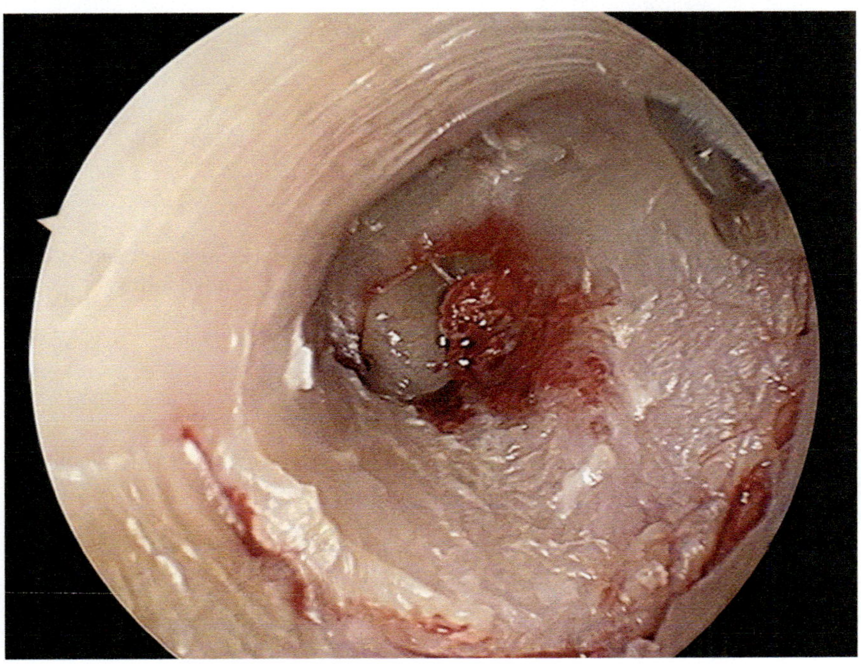

Fig. 3B: Steps of canal incision (left ear). Superior limb.

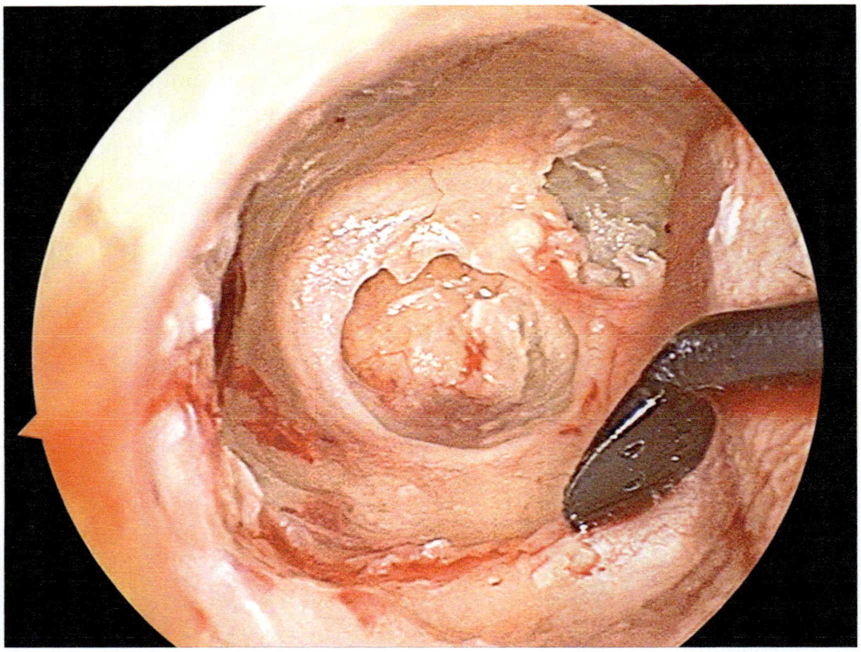

Fig. 3C: Steps of canal incision (left ear). Horizontal limb being extended superiorly.

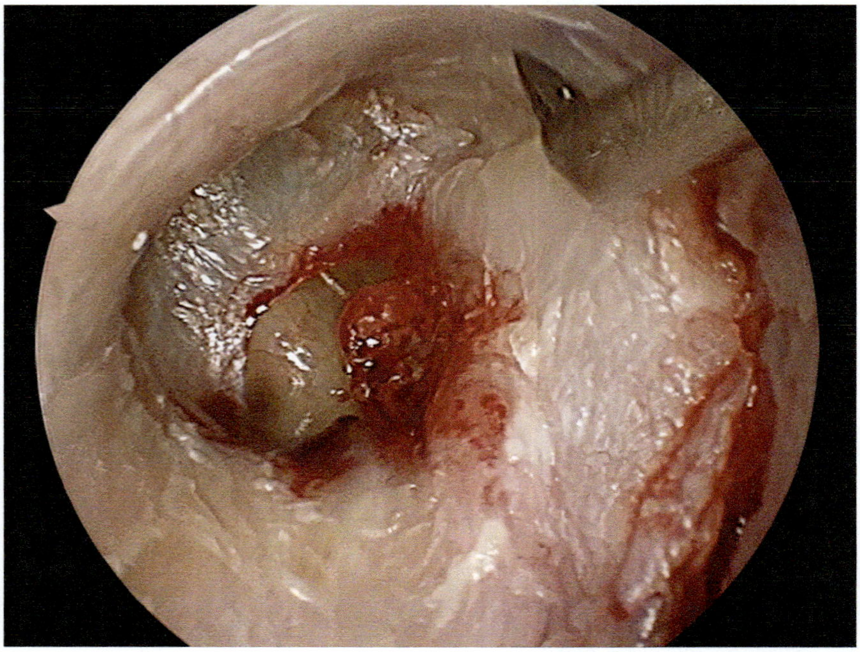

Fig. 3D: Steps of canal incision (left ear). Superior limb being extended further anteriorly.

TIP

The rationale of keeping a larger flap in this case is to completely cover the defect which is larger than that in an endoscopic atticotomy.

- *Flap elevation:* The resultant flap is then gently elevated upto the annulus with the help of cotton balls soaked in adrenaline.

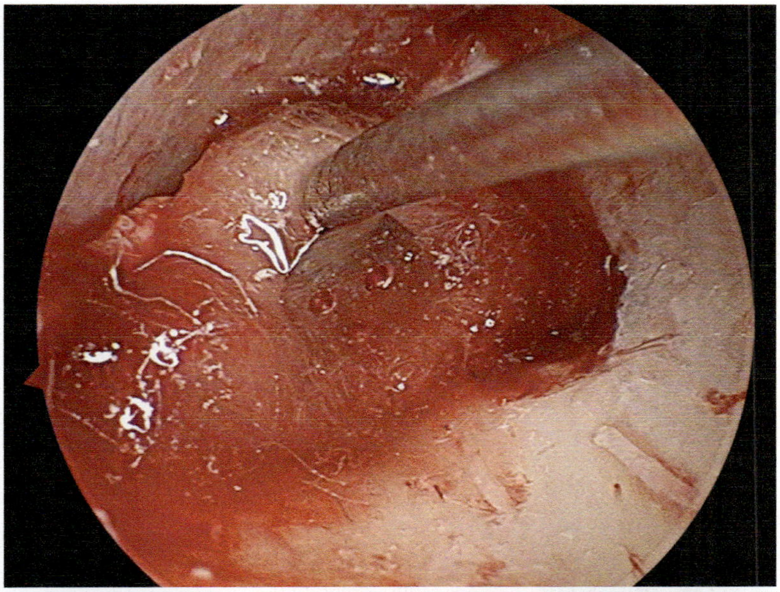

Fig. 4A: Steps of flap elevation: Use of adrenaline soaked cotton ball to elevate the tympanomeatal flap.

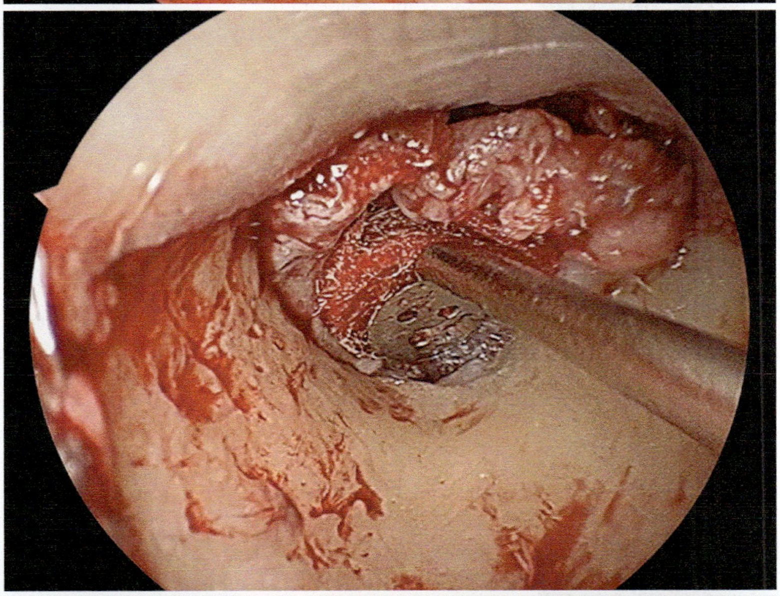

Fig. 4B: Steps of flap elevation: Round knife being used to delineate the annulus.

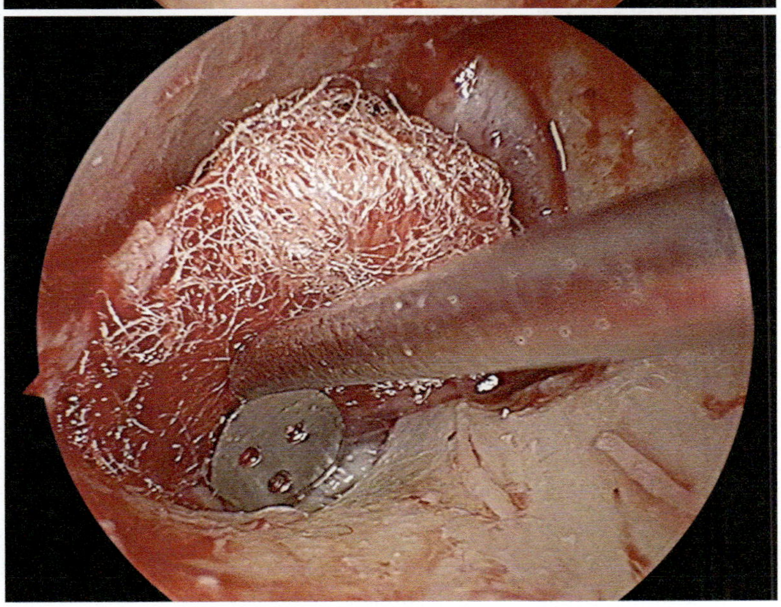

Fig. 4C: Steps of flap elevation: Round knife being used to delineate the chorda tympani nerve and lift off the annulus.

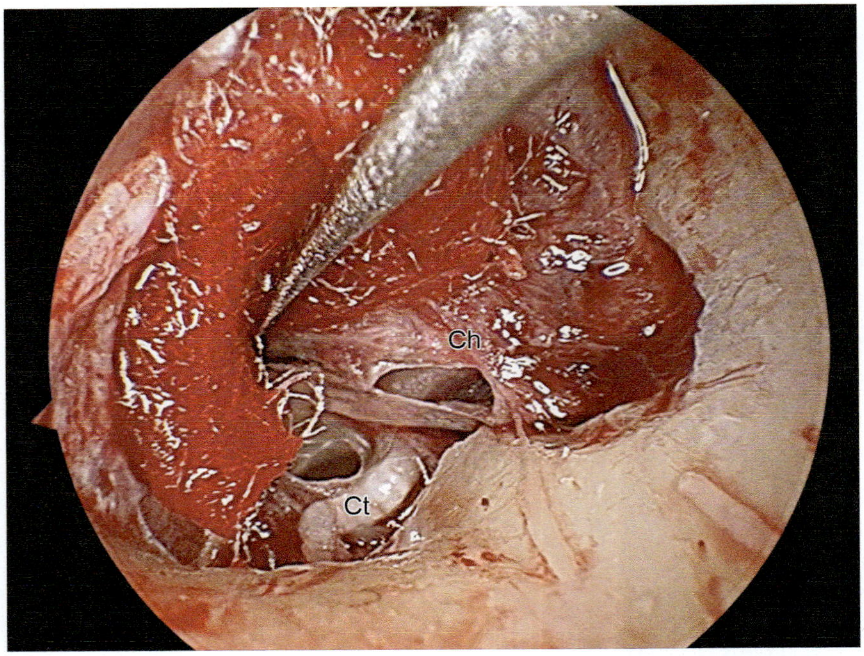

Fig. 4D: Steps of flap elevation: Cholesteatoma sac being delineated.
(CT: chorda tympani nerve; Ch: cholesteatoma sac)

> **TIP**
>
> The tympanomeatal flap needs to be elevated gently taking care not to cause tear. The cotton balls are placed against the flap and the pressure over the round knife is exerted grazing the bone of the canal, against the cotton ball. Once the flap has been raised, the anterosuperior part needs to be cut sharply with a curved iris scissors.

- *Separation of cholesteatoma sac from healthy flap:*
  - The flap has to be sharply cut at the junction of the diseased pocket and normal tympanic membrane.
  - After careful elevation of the flap, it is tucked inferiorly in the hypotympanum to protect it from the rotating burr and suction tip.

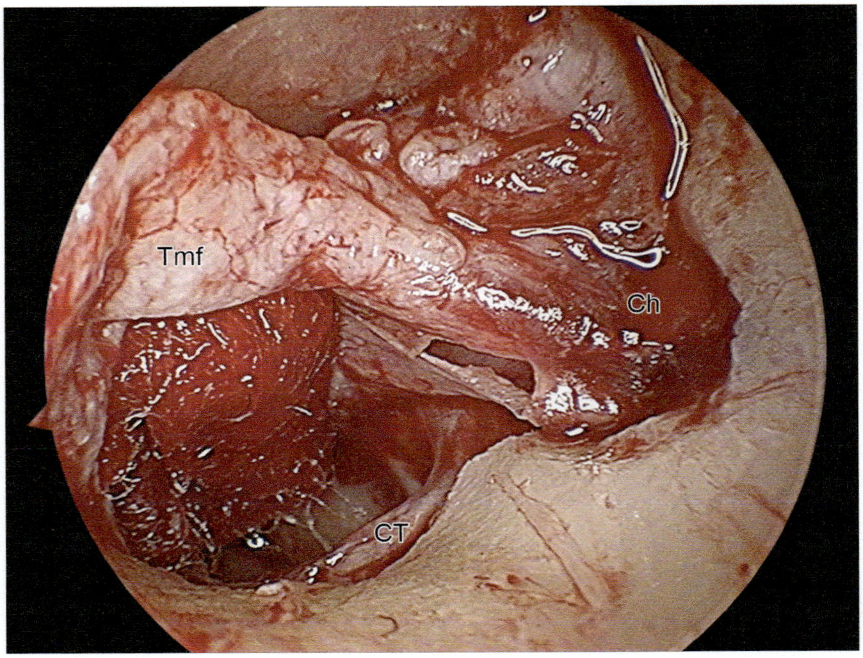

Fig. 5A: Steps of separation of cholesteatoma sac from healthy flap.
(Ch: Cholesteatoma sac; CT: chorda tympani; Tmf: tympanomeatal flap)

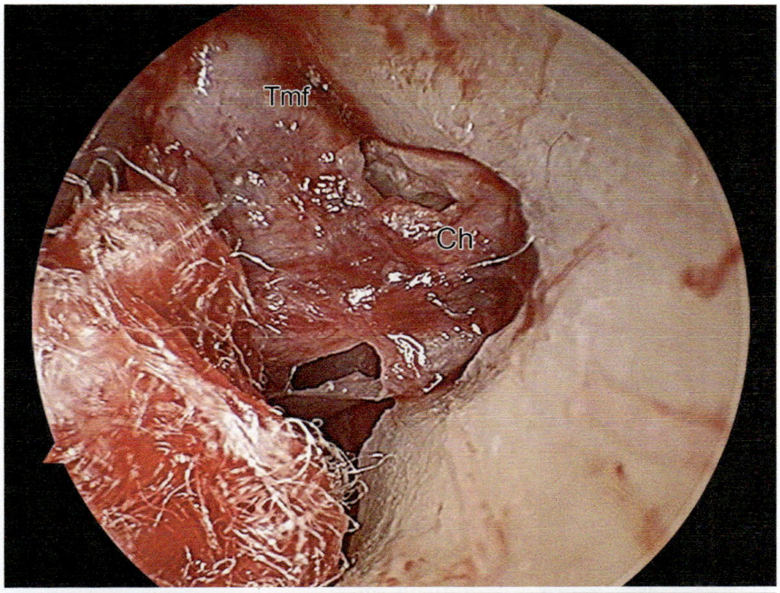

Fig. 5B: Steps of separation of cholesteatoma sac from healthy flap.
(Ch: Cholesteatoma sac; Tmf: tympanomeatal flap)

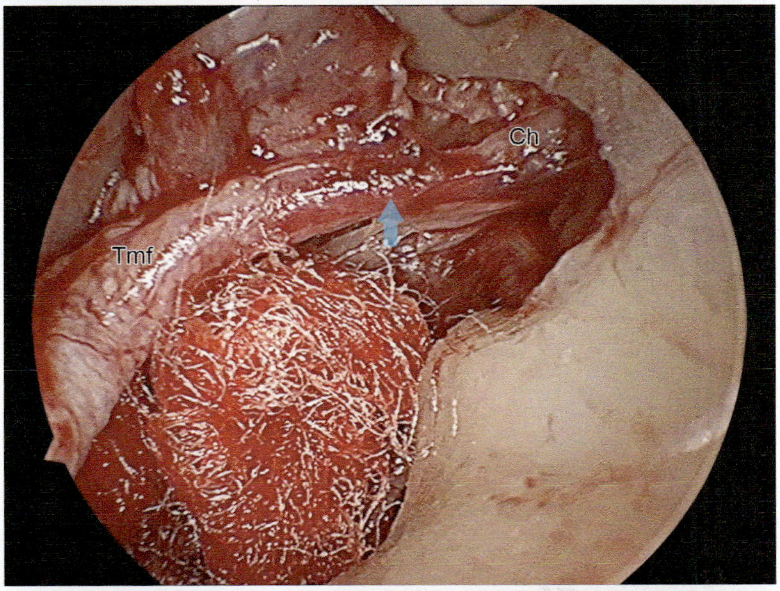

Fig. 5C: Steps of separation of cholesteatoma sac from healthy flap. Blue arrow: Demarcation between healthy flap and cholesteatoma sac.
(Ch: cholesteatoma sac; Tmf: tympanomeatal flap)

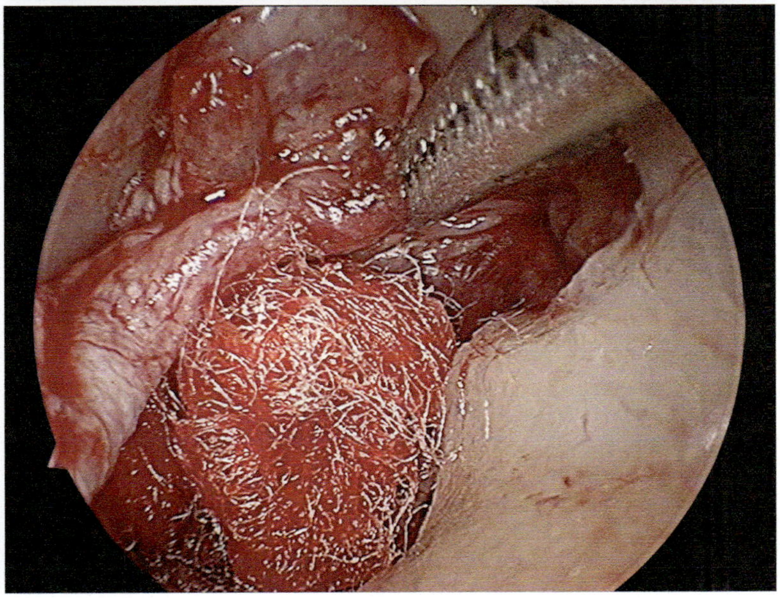

Fig. 5D: Steps of separation of cholesteatoma sac from healthy flap: Alligator forceps being used to tease off healthy flap from sac.

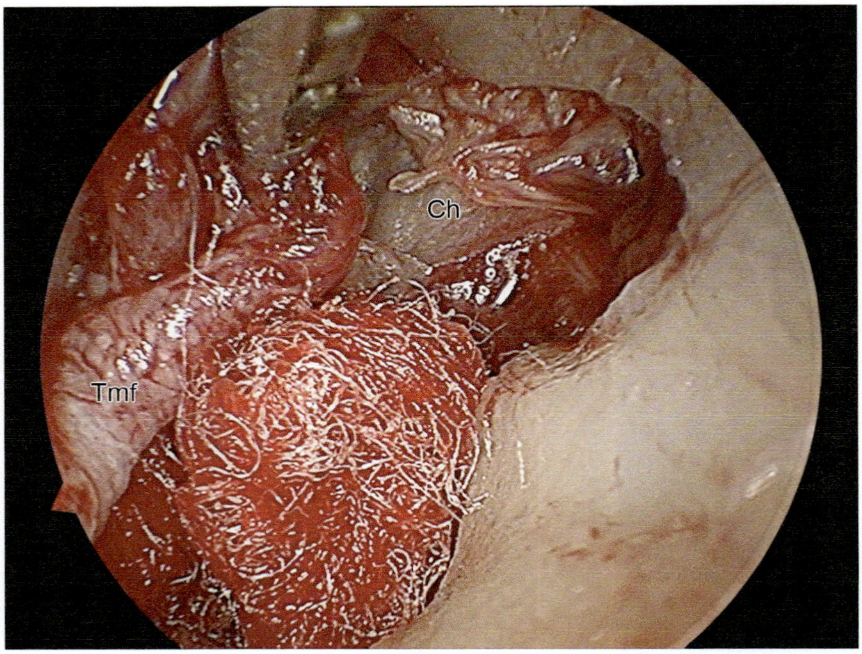

Fig. 5E: Steps of separation of cholesteatoma sac from healthy flap. Healthy flap separated from the sac.
(Ch: cholesteatoma sac; Tmf: tympanomeatal flap)

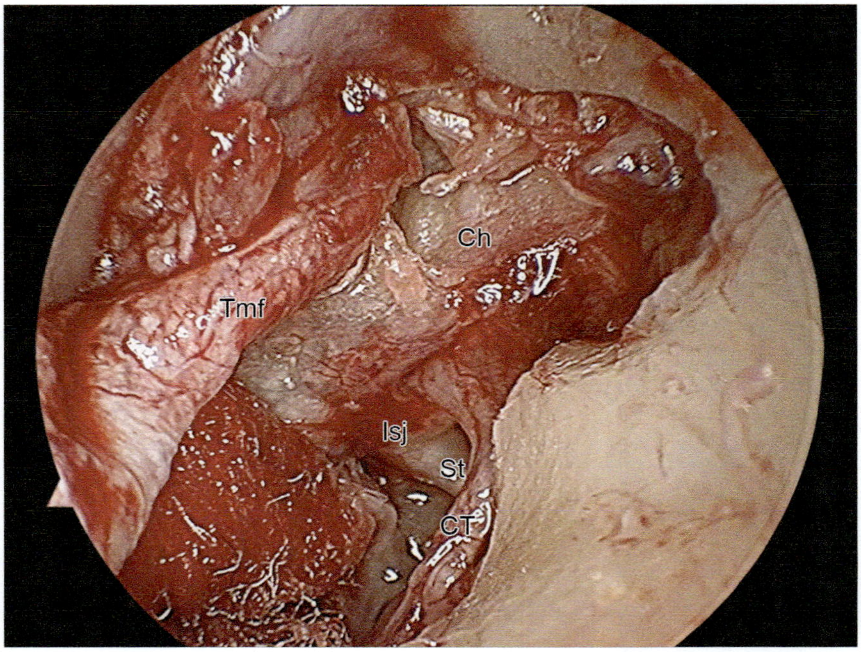

Fig. 5F: Steps of separation of cholesteatoma sac from healthy flap: Healthy flap separated and tucked inferiorly.
(Ch: Cholesteatoma sac; Isj: incudostapedial joint; CT: chorda tympani; Tmf: tympanomeatal flap; St: stapedial tendon)

- *Chorda tympani nerve management:* The chorda tympani nerve is identified, separated from its crest and reposited inferiorly.

TIP

It is aimed to preserve the chorda as far as practicable. However, if damaged due to disease involvement or during handling, it is advisable to section it close to its origin.

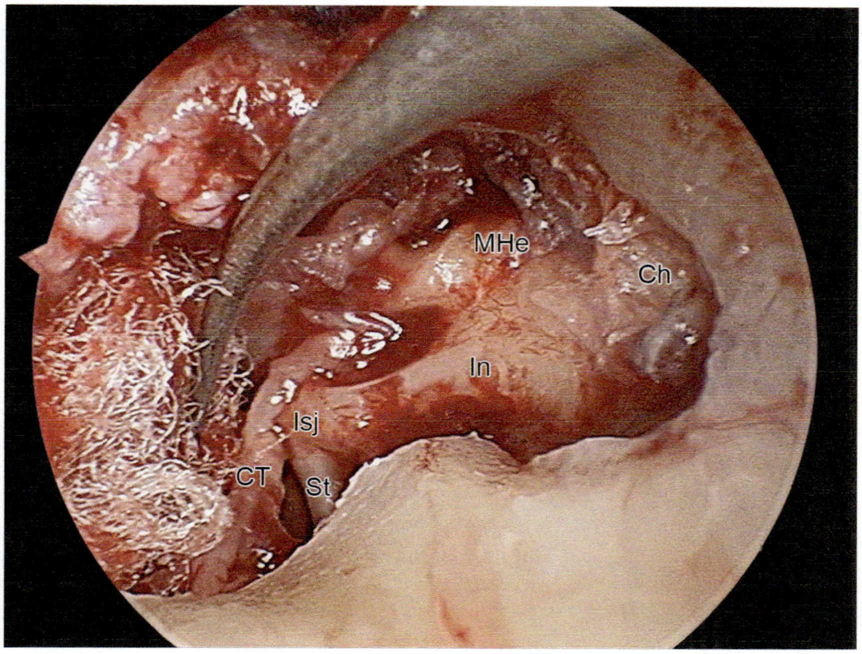

Fig. 6A: Dissection of chorda tympani (MHe: head of malleus; Ch: cholesteatoma sac; In: incus; Isj: incudostapedial joint; CT: chorda tympani; St: stapedial tendon)

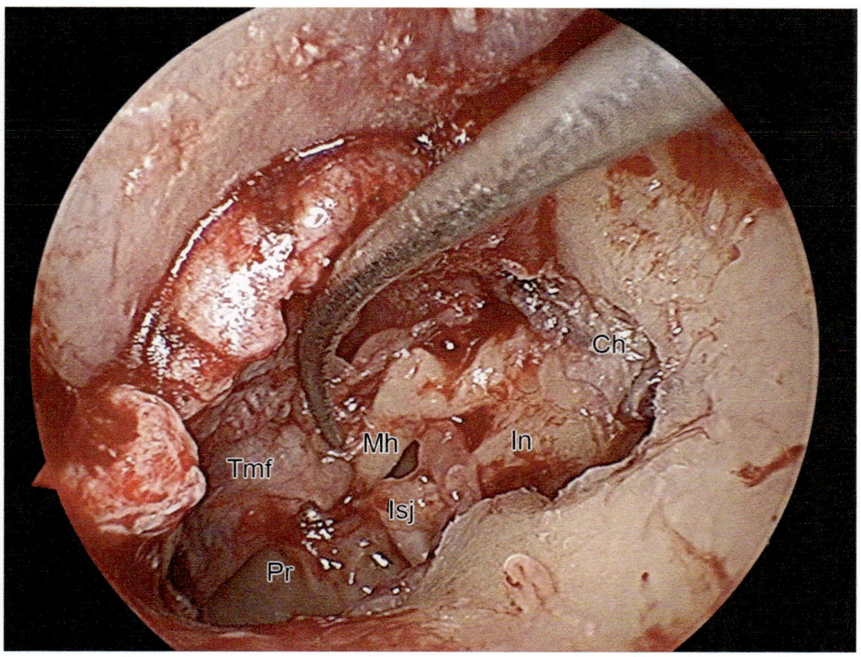

Fig. 6B: Dissection of chorda tympani: Smooth curved pick being used to separate flap from handle of malleus.
(Mh: malleus handle; Ch: cholesteatoma sac; In: incus; Isj: incudostapedial joint; Tmf: tympanomeatal flap; Pr: promontory)

- *Bone drilling:*
  - The exposed lateral attic wall and posterosuperior canal wall are drilled with a 2–2.3 mm diamond burr, layer by layer
  - The entire bone need not be drilled. It is only thinned such that the final egg-shell of bone can be removed using a House curette
  - Alternatively, a Wilson bone punch may be used (vide "Endoscopic transcanal atticotomy" chapter)
  - Drilling is continued in the posterosuperior direction over the aditus toward the antrum
  - The aim is to visualize the incus and the malleus completely
  - The ampullary end of the lateral semicircular canal has to be visualized clearly

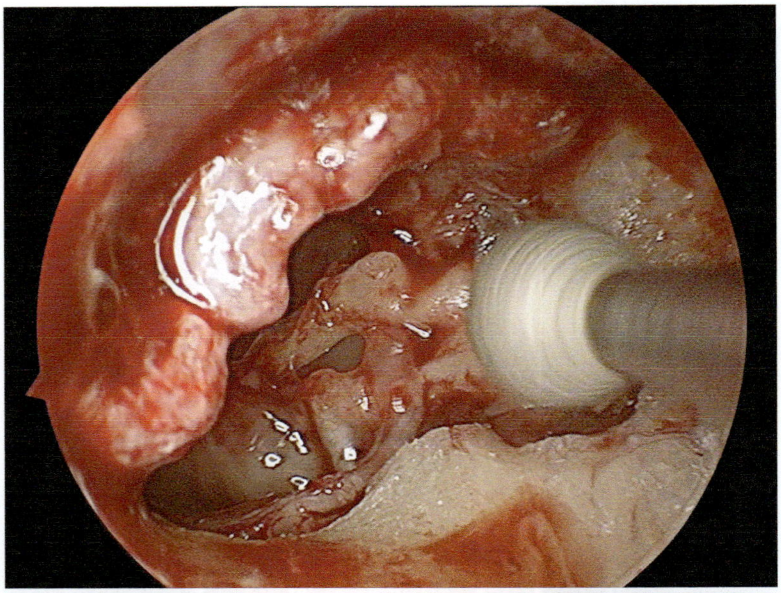

Fig. 7A: Steps of bone drilling: Starting from lateral attic wall.

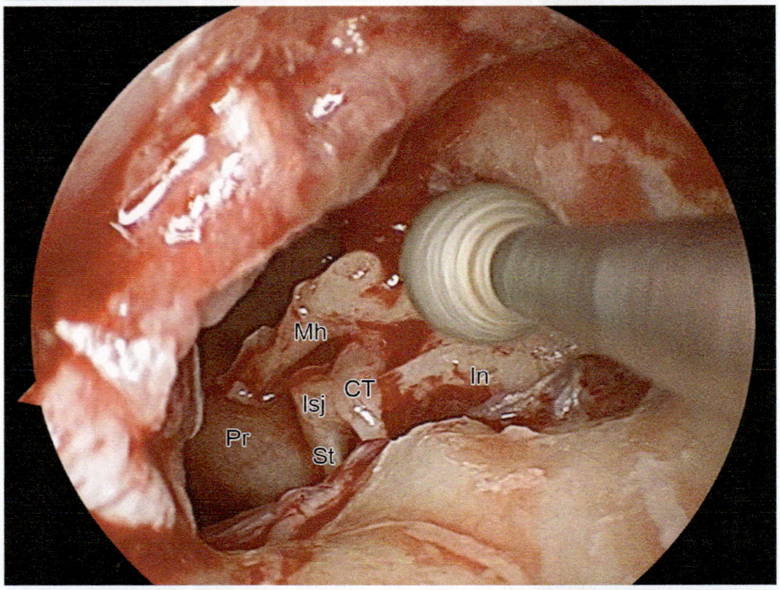

Fig. 7B: Steps of bone drilling: Extending superiorly up to tegmen tympani.
(Mh: malleus handle; In: incus; Isj: incudostapedial joint; CT: chorda tympani; Pr: promontory; St: stapedial tendon)

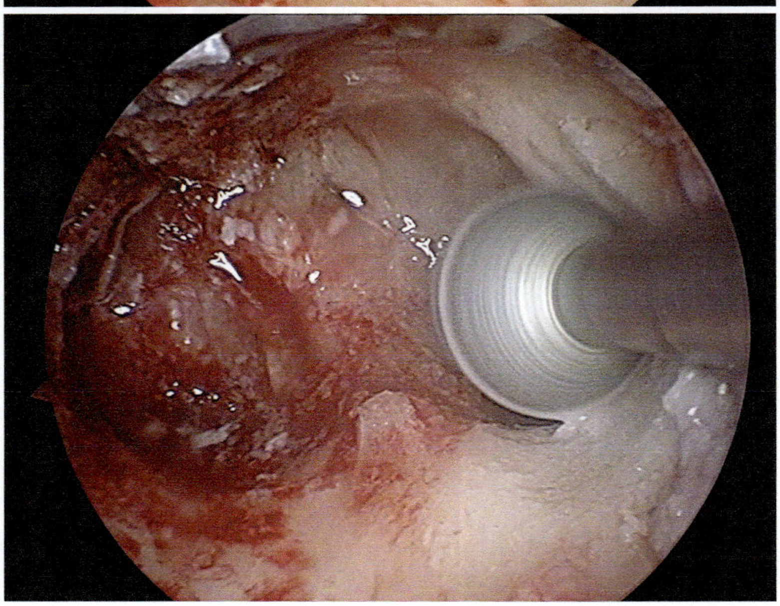

Fig. 7C: Steps of bone drilling: Proceeding posteriorly toward aditus.

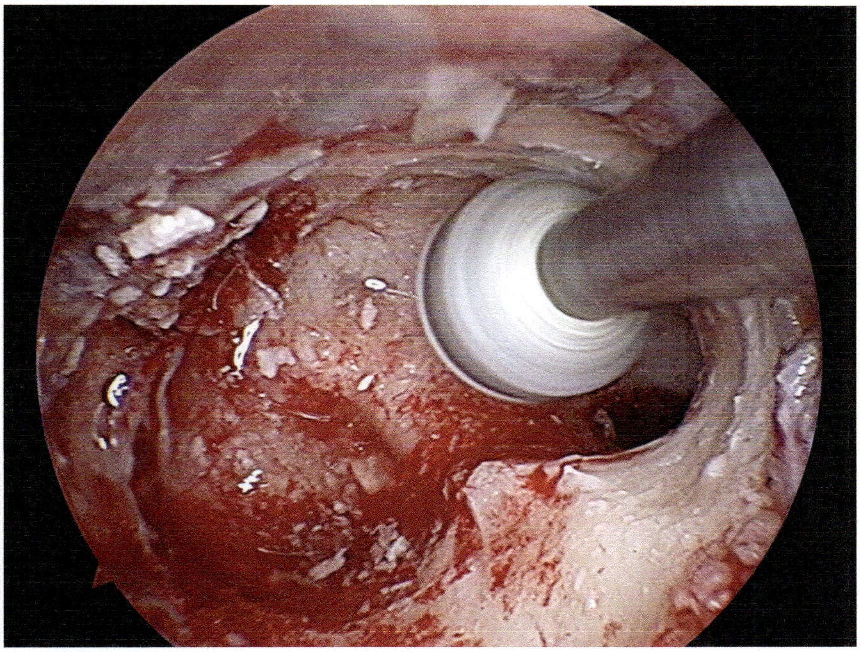

Fig. 7D: Steps of bone drilling: Aditus exposed completely.

PEARL

The bony lateral attic wall is often found eroded in epitympanic cholesteatoma due to disease process. Hence, the amount of bone drilling is actually less. The major bone that needs to be drilled is that of posterosuperior canal wall.

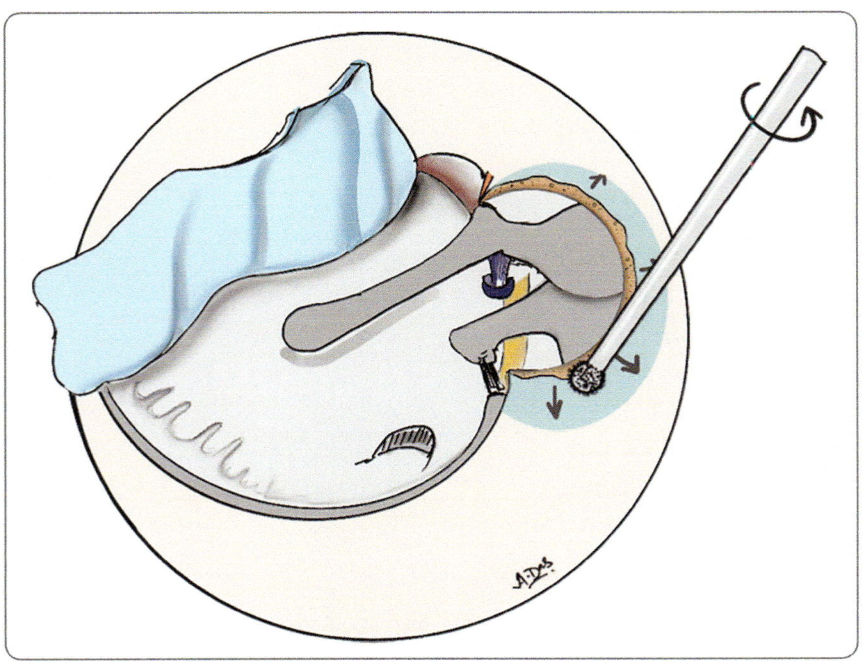

Fig. 8A: Schematic representation of extent of bone removal (blue shaded area represents the additional bone drilling over and above the routine atticotomy bone drilling).

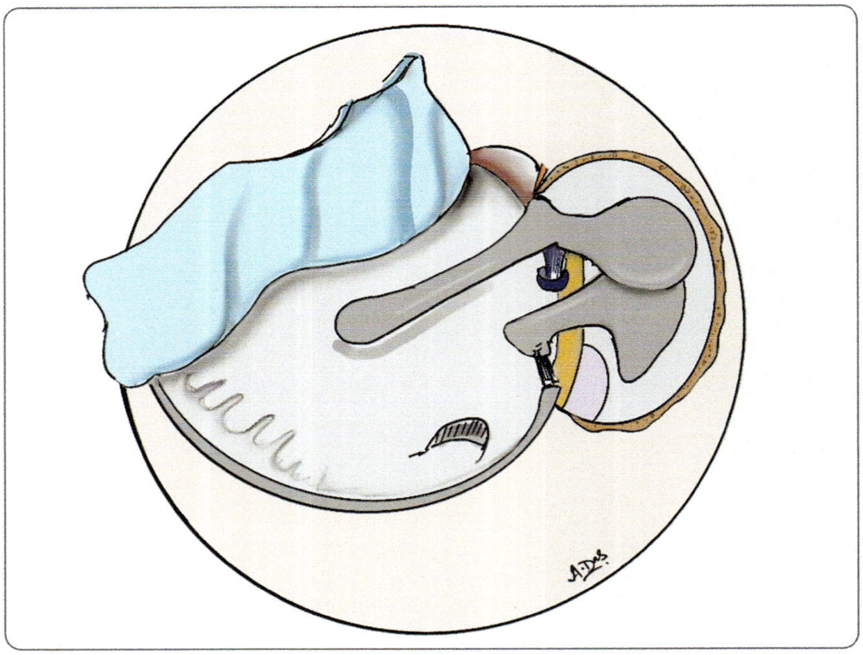

Fig. 8B: Final view following bone removal.

- Thereafter, the disease extent is confirmed with the help of angled scopes such as 30 or 45-degree endoscopes

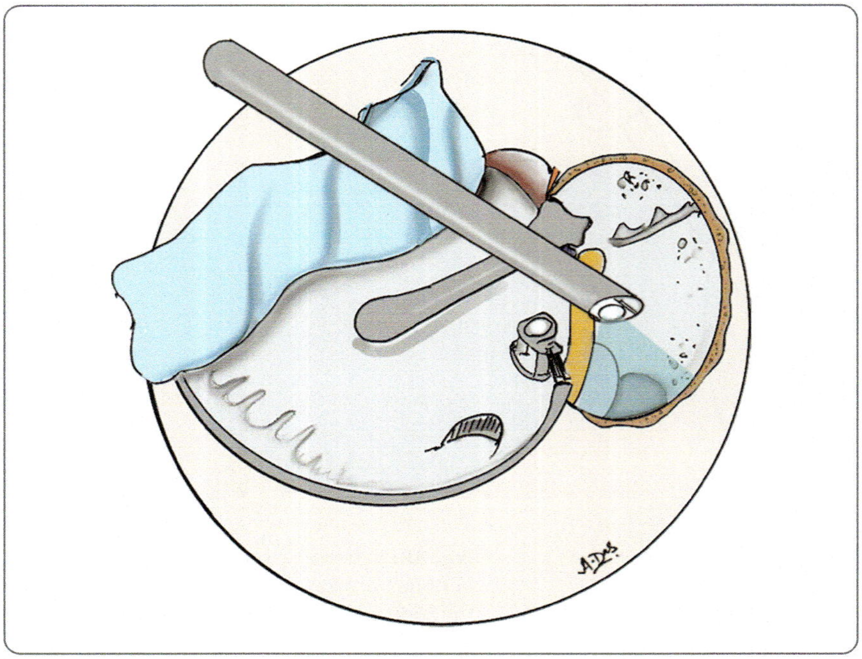

Fig. 9A: Use of 30 or 45-degree endoscopes to visualize disease extent in antrum.

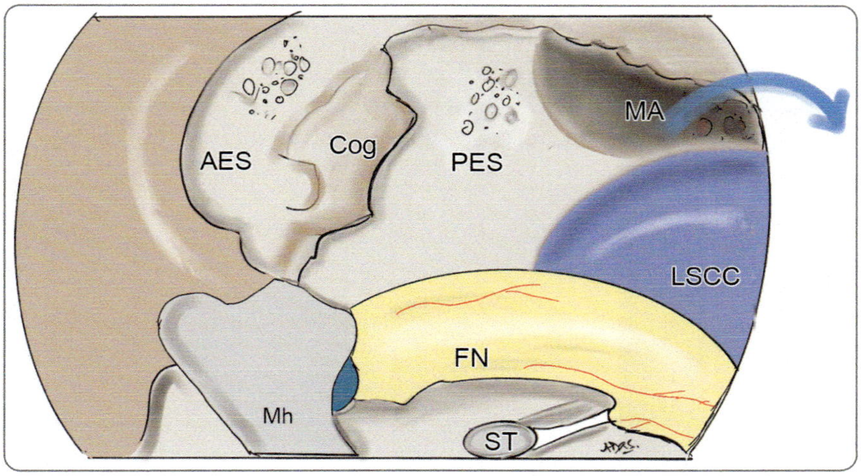

Fig. 9B: 30-degree view of aditus and antrum from middle ear.
(Mh: malleus handle; FN: facial nerve; ST: stapedius; LSCC: lateral semicircular canal; AES: anterior epitympanic space; PES: posterior epitympanic space; MA: mastoid antrum)

- *Ossicular chain management:*
  - Incudostapedial joint discontinuity is commonly seen as a result of the disease process itself
  - Incus (lenticular process > long process) happens to be the most common ossicle to get eroded by disease process followed by stapes superstructure and handle of malleus[1]
  - The management algorithm is as follows:

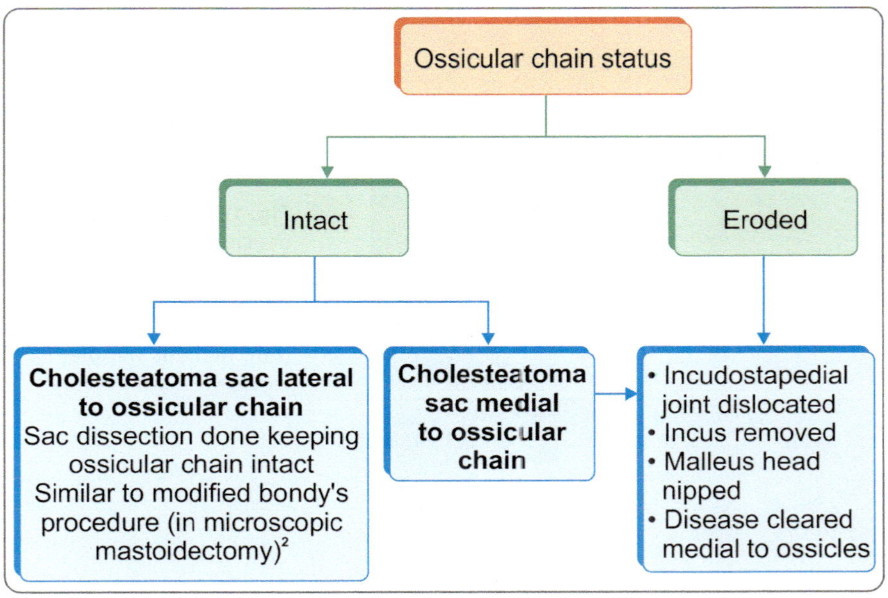

  - The incudostapedial joint is dislocated before commencement of significant drilling/curette/bone punch use, depending on the disease extent, for example, cholesteatoma extending medial to ossicles or planned ossicular chain reconstruction
  - Incudostapedial joint discontinuity is commonly seen as a result of the disease process itself
  - If intact, it has to be dislocated gently using a sharp pick or a joint knife in a posterior-to-anterior direction
  - Thereafter, the incudomalleolar joint is dislocated and incus is delivered out
  - The malleus head is nipped at its neck using a malleus nipper to expose the anterior epitympanic space
- The cholesteatoma sac is exposed entirely
- The sac is gently dissected off the bony crevices with the help of Plester's side knife

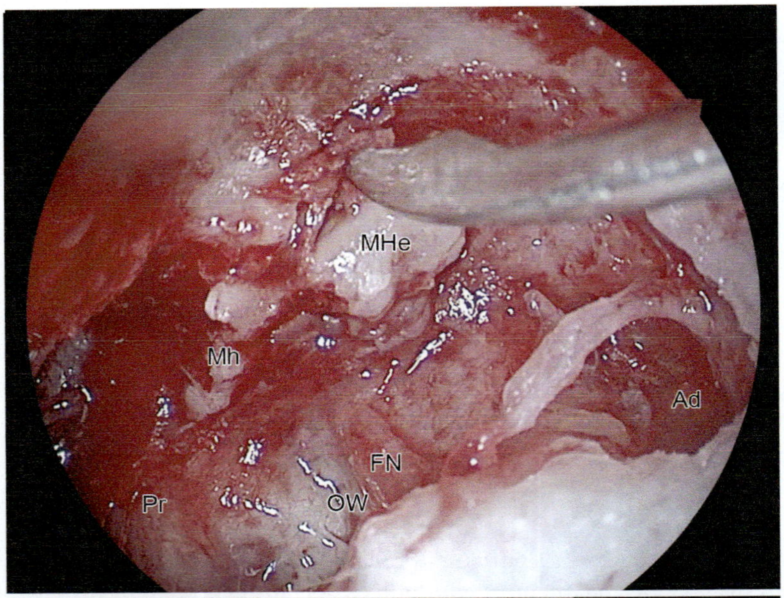

Fig. 10A: Cholesteatoma sac extending medial to ossicles/ossicular chain erosion: Disease medial to ossicles.
(MHe: malleus head; Mh: malleus handle; Ad: aditus; FN: facial nerve; Ow: Oval window; Pr: promontory)

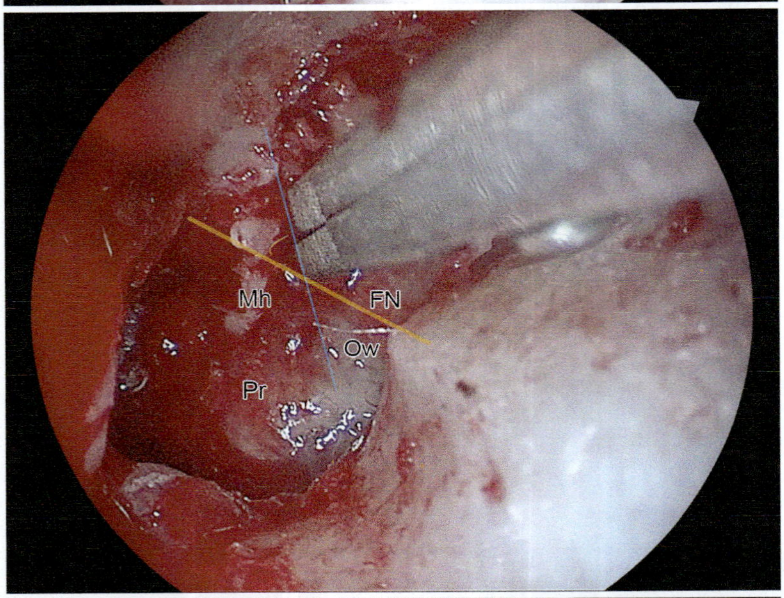

Fig. 10B: Cholesteatoma sac extending medial to ossicles/ossicular chain erosion: Position of malleus nipper while nipping head of malleus (blue line—nipper kept at an angle of 20–25 degrees to the axis of horizontal facial nerve—orange line).
(Mh: malleus handle; FN: facial nerve; Ow: Oval window; Pr: promontory)

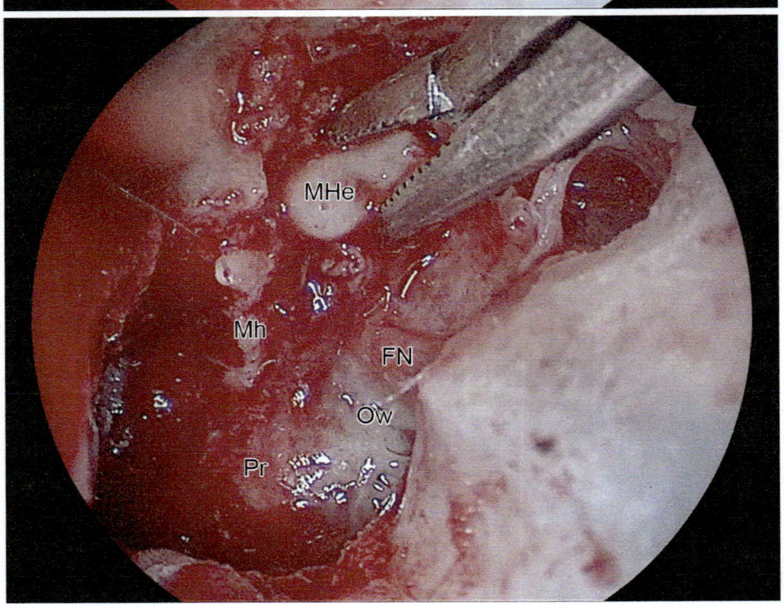

Fig. 10C: Cholesteatoma sac extending medial to ossicles/ossicular chain erosion: Malleus head nipped and delivered out.
(MHe: Malleus head; Mh: malleus handle; FN: facial nerve; Ow: Oval window; Pr: promontory)

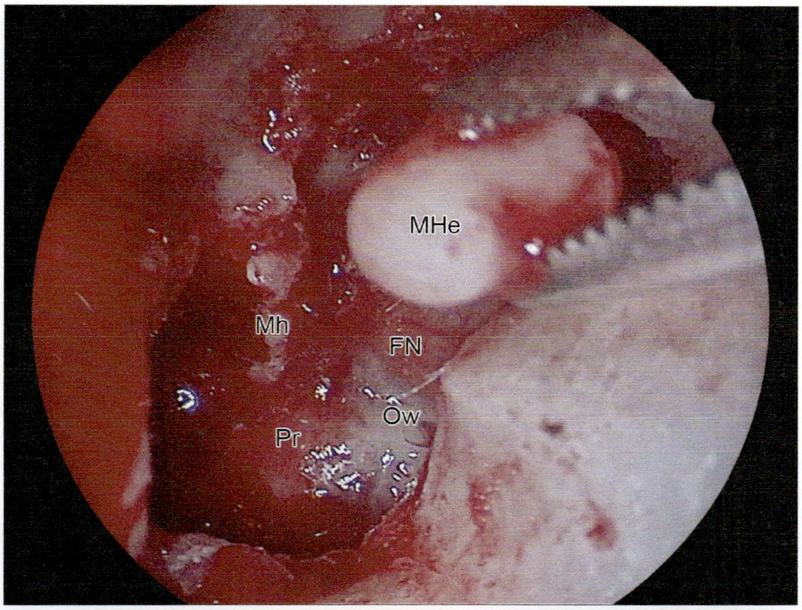

Fig. 10D: Cholesteatoma sac extending medial to ossicles/ossicular chain erosion: Malleus head nipped and delivered out (using alligator forceps).
(MHe: malleus head; Mh: malleus handle; FN: facial nerve; Ow: Oval window; Pr: promontory)

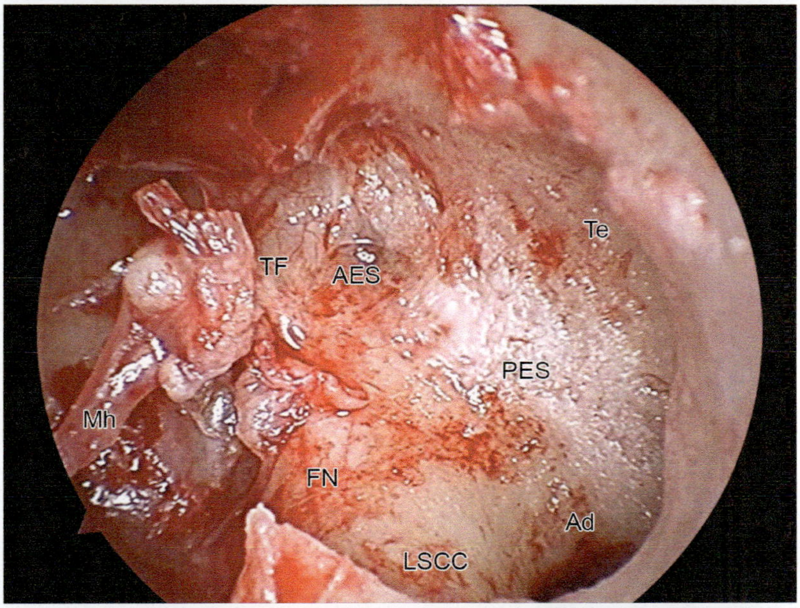

Fig. 10E: Cholesteatoma sac extending medial to ossicles/ossicular chain erosion. Final view following disease clearance.
(LSCC: lateral semicircular canal; Te: Tegmen; PES: posterior epitympanic space; Ad: aditus; FN: facial nerve; TF: tensor fold; AES: anterior epitympanic space ; Mh: malleus handle)

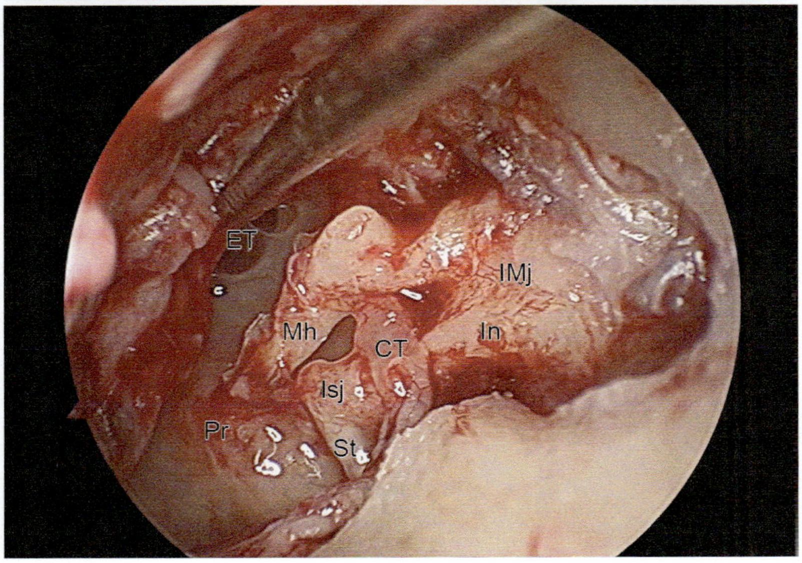

Fig. 11: Cholesteatoma sac lateral to intact ossicular chain.
(CT: chorda tympani; ET: eustachian tube; IMj: incudomalleolar joint; In: incus; Isj: incudostapedial joint; Mh: malleus handle; Pr: promontory; St: stapedial tendon)

- *Dissection of cholesteatoma sac:*
  - Certain specialized instruments are useful while performing one-handed cholesteatoma sac dissection
  - These include:
    - Panetti set-suction dissector
    - Double-curved Bill's elevator
    - Curved suction elevator cum dissector
  - The main principle is to provide adequate tension over the sac to create a dissection plane between the sac and underlying bone by suction with simultaneous dissection

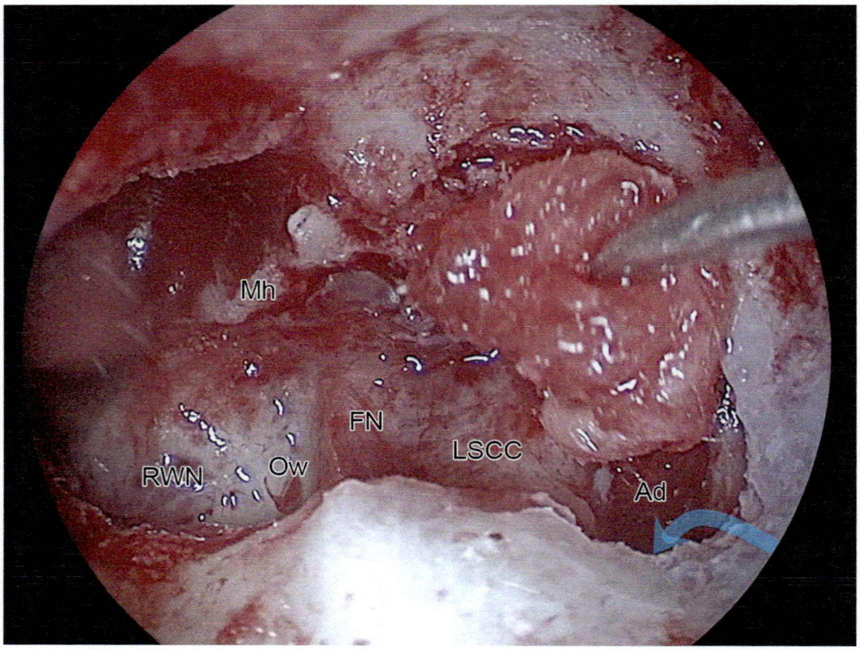

Fig. 12A: Steps of dissection of cholesteatoma sac (Note the use of curved elevator used to remove the cholesteatoma sac from mastoid antrum—blue arrow).
(Mh: malleus handle; FN: facial nerve; RWN: round window niche; Ow: Oval window; LSCC: lateral semicircular canal; Ad: aditus)

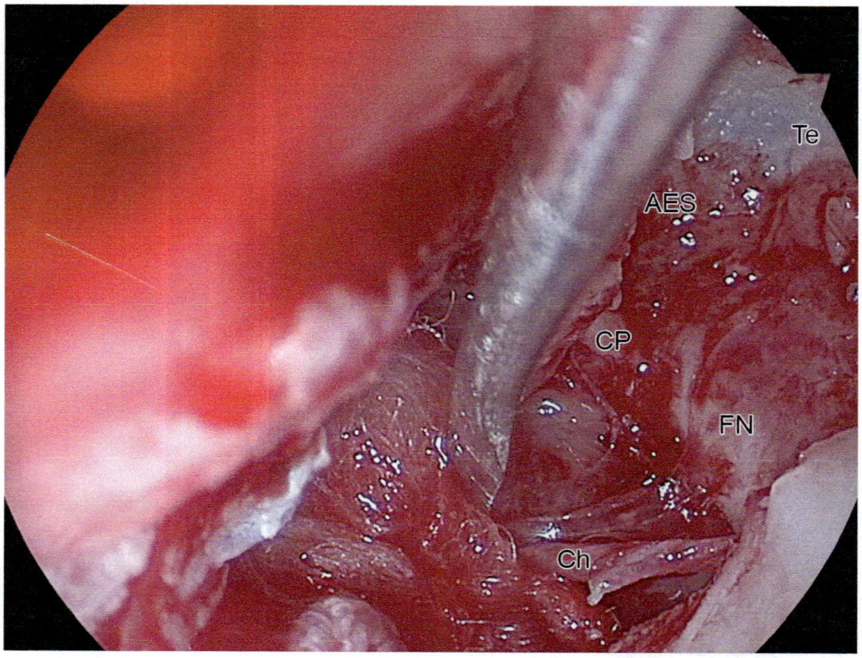

Fig. 12B: Steps of dissection of cholesteatoma sac.
(Te: tegmen; AES: anterior epitympanic space; CP: processus cochleariformis; FN: facial nerve; Ch: cholesteatoma sac)

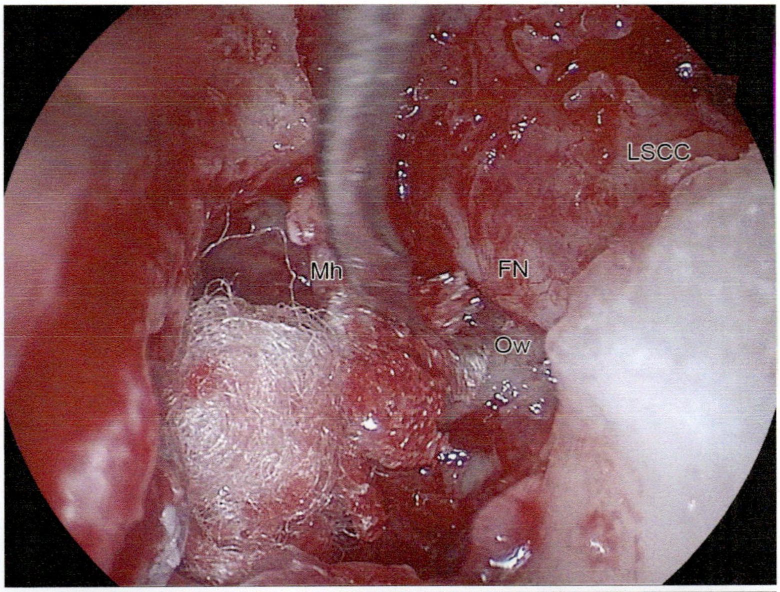

Fig. 12C: Steps of dissection of cholesteatoma sac. (FN: facial nerve; Mh: malleus handle; Ow: Oval window; LSCC: lateral semicircular canal)

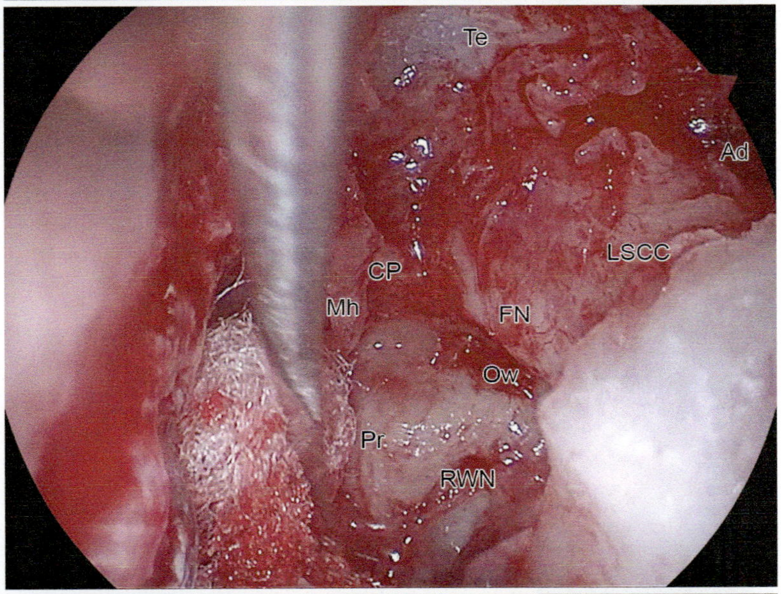

Fig. 12D: Steps of dissection of cholesteatoma sac. (CP: processus cochleariformis; FN: facial nerve; Mh: malleus handle; Ow: Oval window; LSCC: lateral semicircular canal; Ad: aditus; Te: tegmen; RWN: round window niche; Pr: promontory)

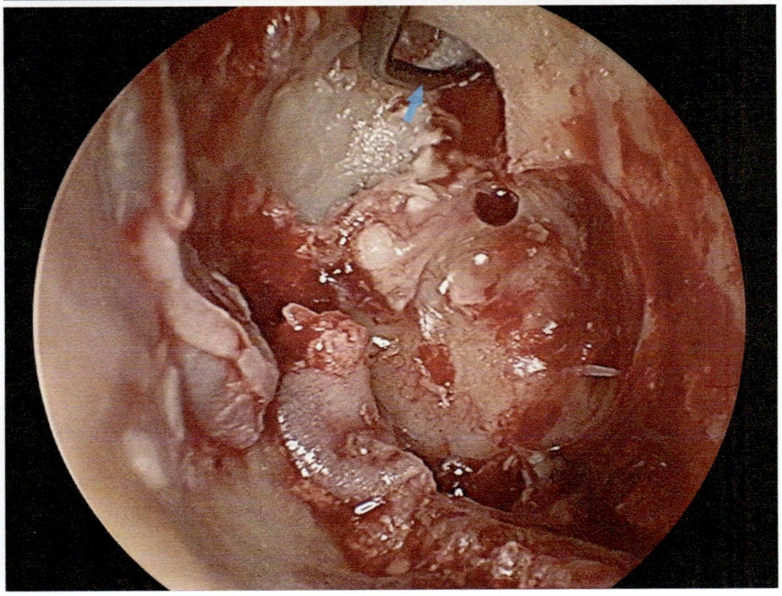

Fig. 12E: Steps of dissection of cholesteatoma sac (Note the use of double-curved Bill's instrument used to remove the cholesteatoma sac from mastoid antrum—blue arrow).

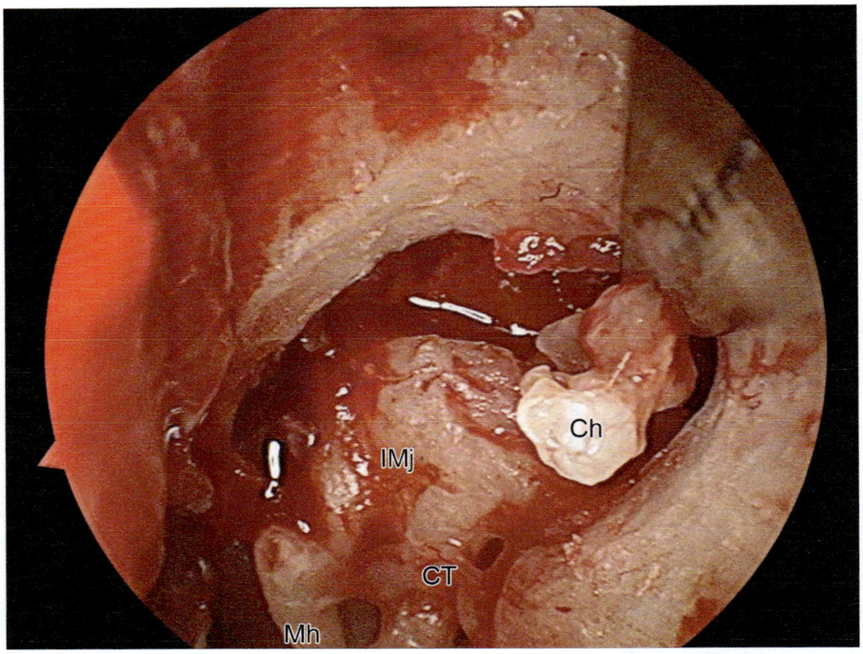

Fig. 12F: Steps of dissection of cholesteatoma sac: Cholesteatoma sac being removed using alligator forceps.
(Ch: cholesteatoma sac; IMj: incudomalleolar joint; CT: chorda tympani nerve; Mh: malleus handle)

TIP **DISSECTION OF CHOLESTEATOMA SAC OVER FACIAL NERVE**

- Cholesteatoma sac must be dissected in continuity with the middle ear mucosa while working over the tympanic segment of facial nerve.
- The sac is pushed inferiorly by blunt cotton dissection and then sharply cut free from the surface of the underlying nerve (or fallopian canal, if intact) with microscissors or iris scissors.
- Extreme caution must be exercised while performing sharp dissection over the nerve especially at the second genu (the most common site of iatrogenic facial nerve injury)

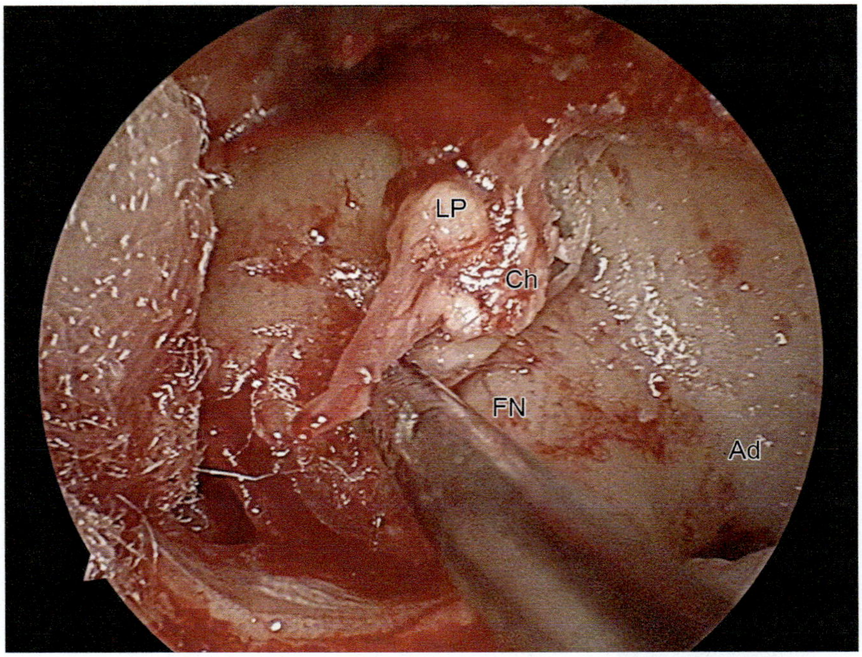

Fig. 13A: Disease clearance over facial nerve: Disease seen extending over facial nerve behind neck of malleus over processus cochleariformis.
(LP: lateral process of malleus; Ch: cholesteatoma; FN: facial nerve; Ad: aditus)

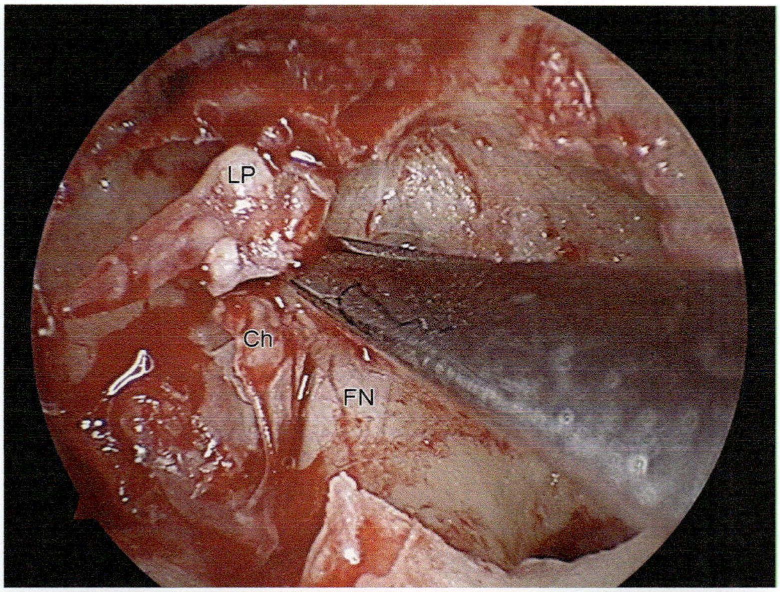

Fig. 13B: Disease clearance over facial nerve: Sectioning of tensor tympani tendon.
(LP: lateral process of malleus; Ch: cholesteatoma; FN: facial nerve)

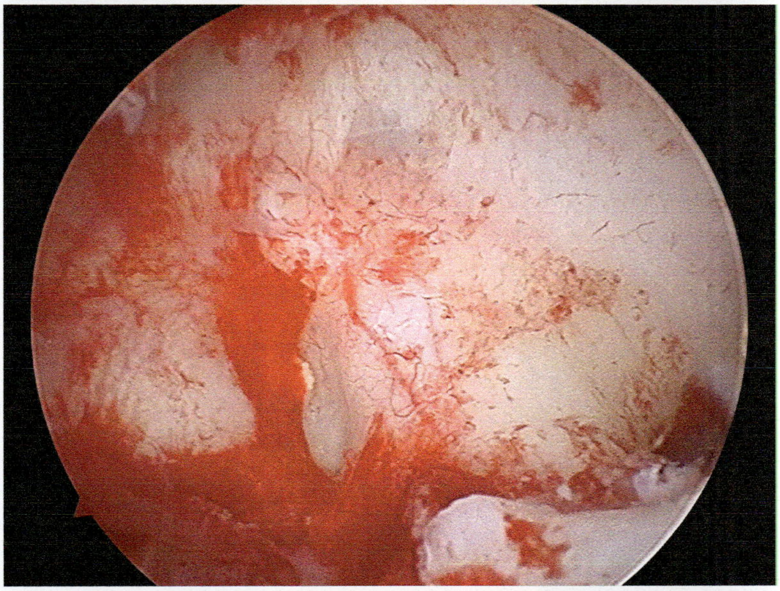

Fig. 13C: Disease clearance over facial nerve: Saline irrigation of the cavity after disease clearance.

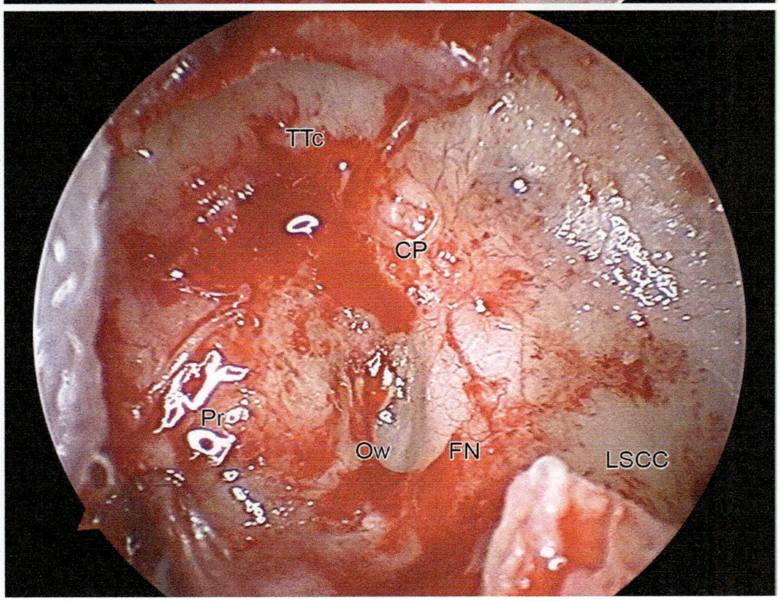

Fig. 13D: Disease clearance over facial nerve: View after disease clearance.
(FN: facial nerve; TTc: canal for tensor tympani; CP: processus cochleariformis; Ow: oval window; LSCC: lateral semicircular canal; Pr: promontory)

- The sac is excised in continuity, taking care not to leave any squamous epithelium behind
- After the disease has been completely removed, the resultant cavity is inspected

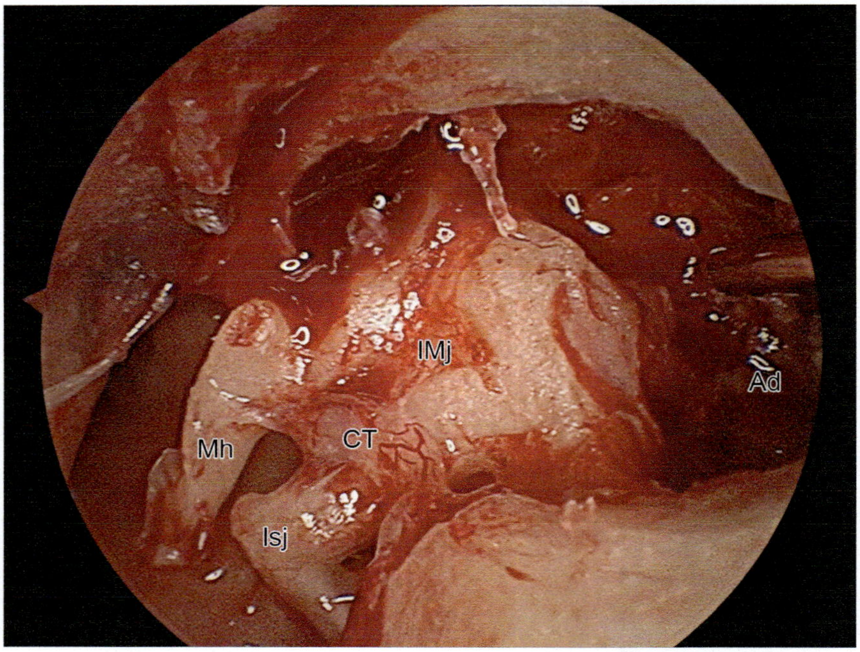

Fig. 14A: Disease clearance in intact ossicular chain: Zero-degree endoscopic view.
(Ad: aditus; IMj: incudomalleolar joint; CT: chorda tympani; Mh: malleus handle; Isj: incudostapedial joint)

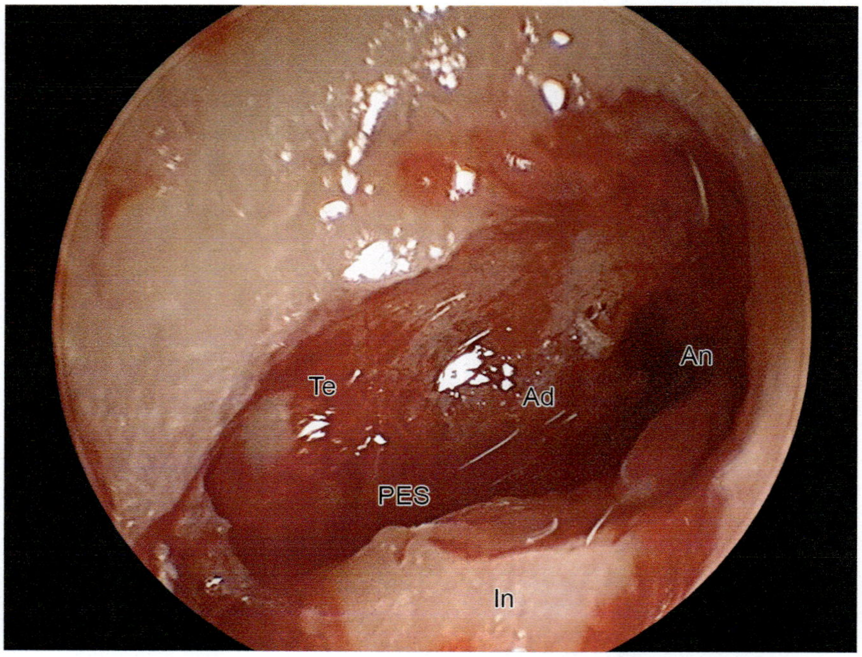

Fig. 14B: Disease clearance in intact ossicular chain: Final 30-degree endoscopic view to visualize the aditus and antrum.
(Te: Tegmen; PES: posterior epitympanic space; In: Incus; Ad: aditus; An: antrum)

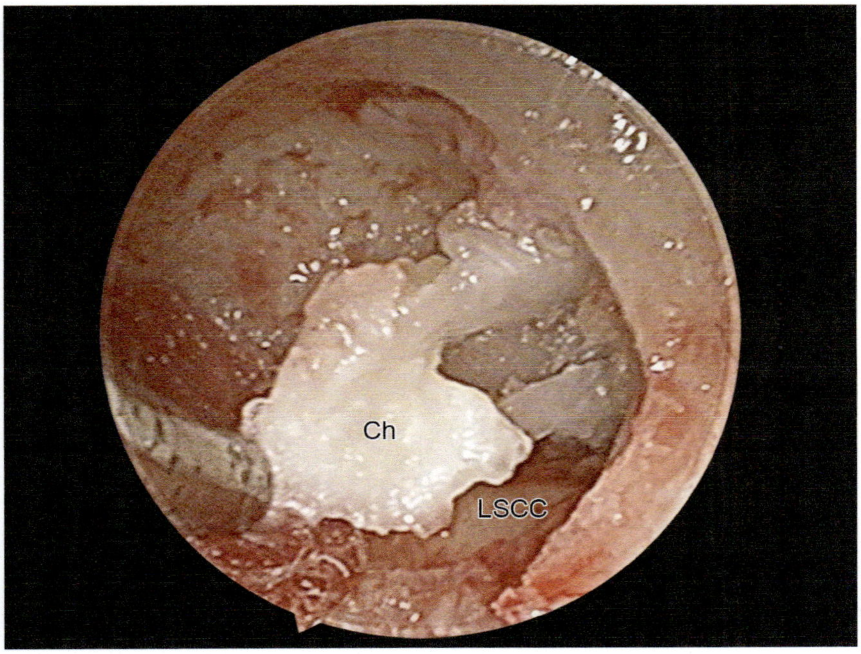

Fig. 15A: Disease clearance in ossicular chain necrosis/removal: Cholesteatoma sac being cleared out of aditus with the help of curved suction instrument.
(Ch: cholesteatoma sac; LSCC: lateral semicircular canal)

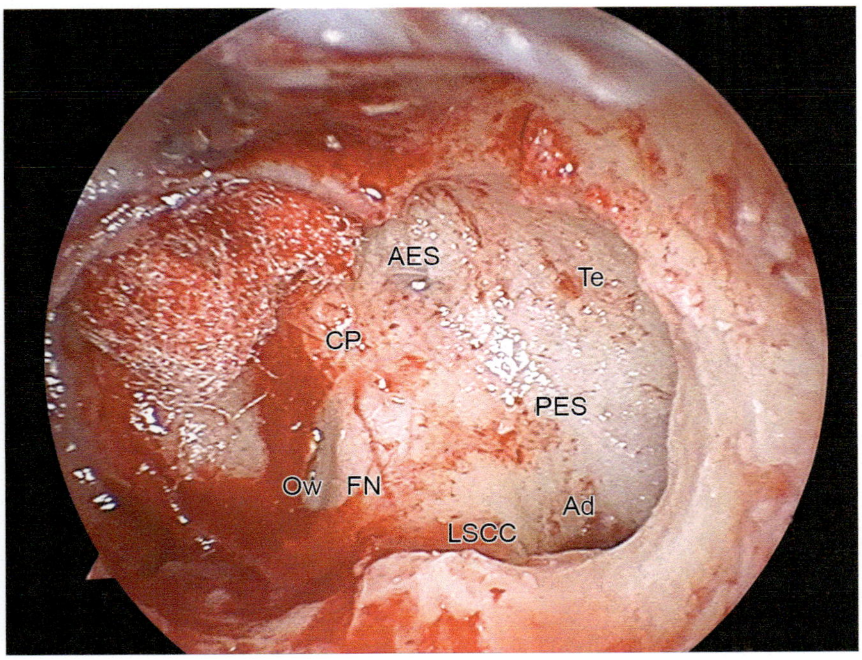

Fig. 15B: Disease clearance in ossicular chain necrosis/removal: Final view following disease clearance.
(Ad: aditus; AES: anterior epitympanic space; CP: processus cochleariformis; FN: facial nerve; LSCC: lateral semicircular canal; Ow: oval window; PES: posterior epitympanic space; Te: tegmen)

- *Cavity obliteration and reconstruction:*
  - *Obliteration:* The antrum and sinodural angle are obliterated with cartilage pieces (tragal) and perichondrium. This is done to reduce the volume of the resultant defect

TIP

Any obliteration should only be performed after ensuring complete disease has been cleared and no squamous epithelium is left behind that may get buried underneath the obliterating tissues.

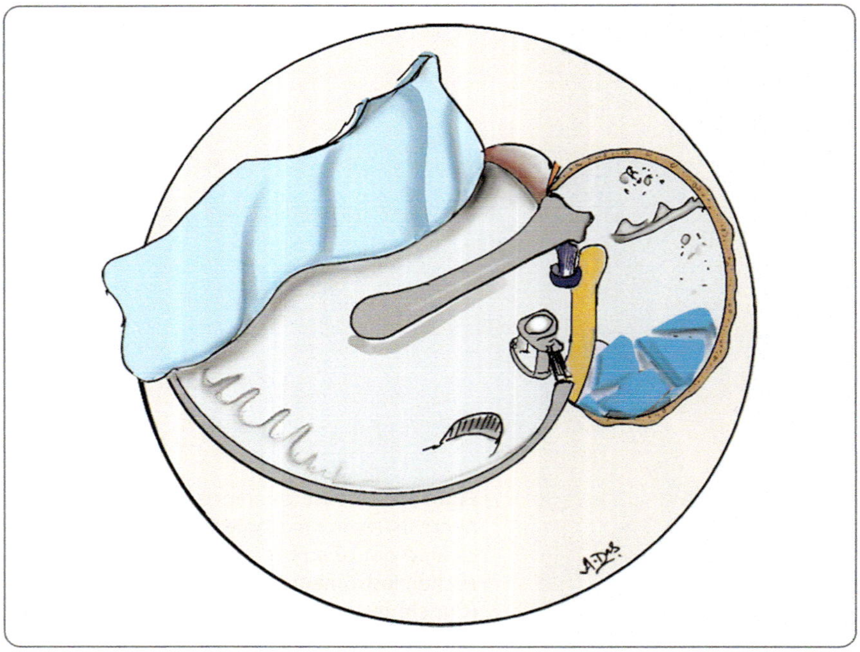

Fig. 16: Cavity obliteration: Obliteration of mastoid antrum with pieces of tragal cartilage and perichondrium.

- *Reconstruction:* The resultant defect of the lateral attic and posterosuperior canal wall is reconstructed using a tragal cartilage. This is done to avoid retraction pocket formation postoperatively, maintaining the middle ear space that is ventilated physiologically.

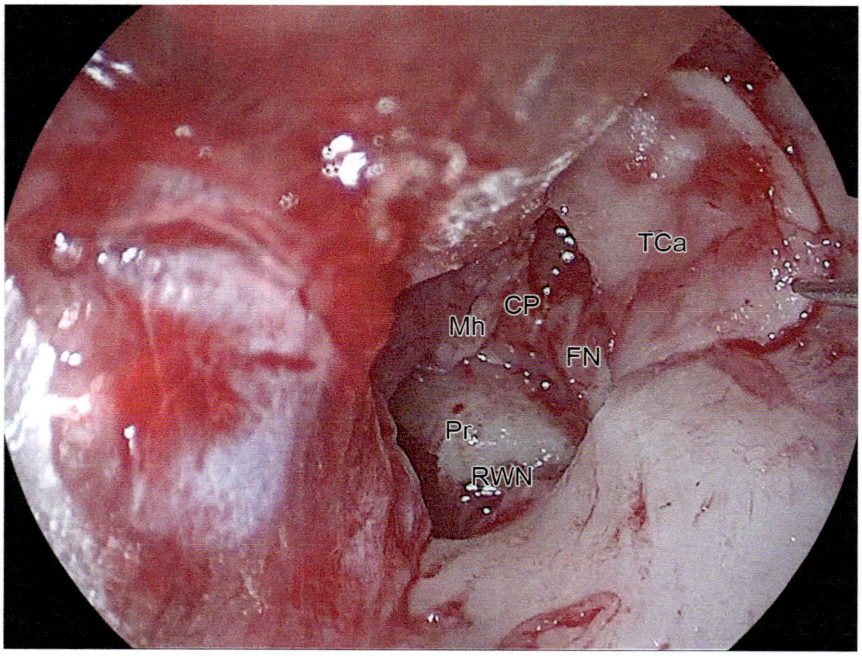

Fig. 17A: Reconstruction of resultant defect with tragal cartilage: Intraoperative view.
(CP: processus cochleariformis; FN: facial nerve; Mh: malleus handle; Pr: promontory; RWN: round window niche; TCa: tragal cartilage)

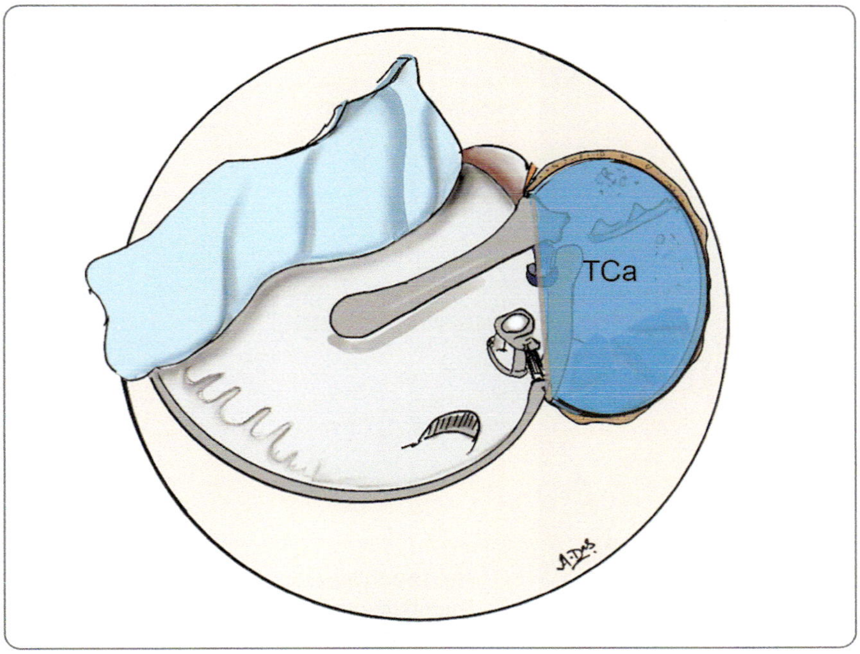

Fig. 17B: Reconstruction of resultant defect with tragal cartilage: Schematic representation. (TCa: tragal cartilage)

- *Tympanic membrane reconstruction*: Temporalis fascia graft harvested from a small posterosuperior scalp incision is used for tympanic membrane reconstruction.

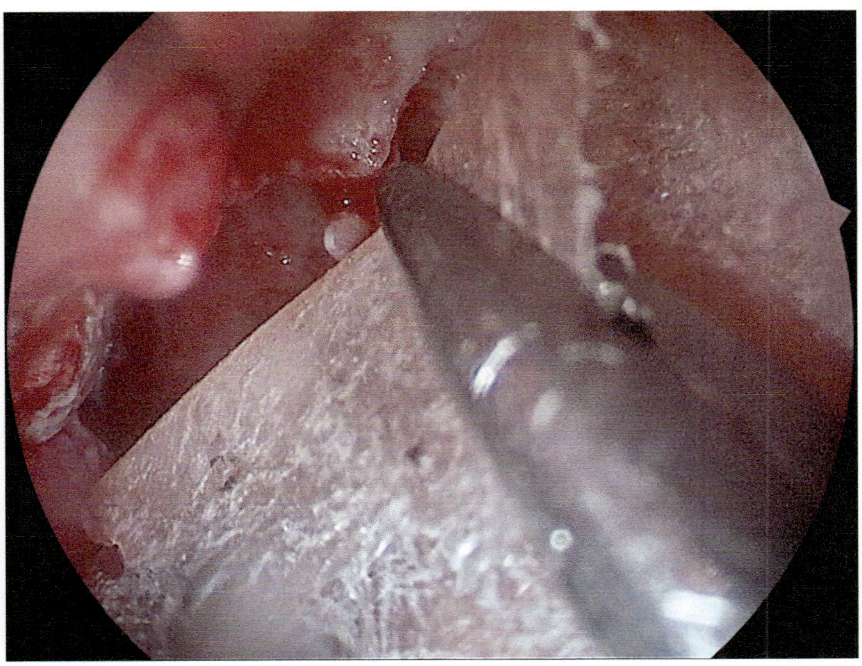

Fig. 18A: Tympanic membrane reconstruction. Temporalis fascia graft being introduced using alligator forceps.

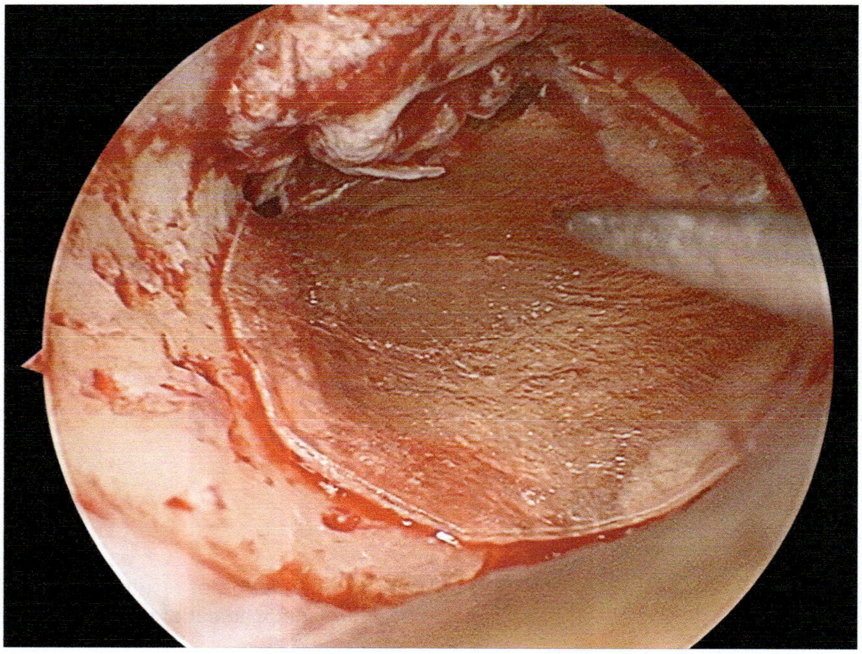

Fig. 18B: Tympanic membrane reconstruction. Smooth curved pick being used to spread the graft.

- *Ossicular chain reconstruction:* Appropriate ossicular chain reconstruction is done (vide endoscopic ossiculoplasty chapter). In the presence of stapes superstructure, a partial ossicular replacement prosthesis (PORP) is used. A total ossicular replacement prosthesis (TORP) is used in the absence of stapes superstructure.
- Gelfoam is placed around the reconstructed ossicular assembly to stabilize it and in the external canal around the margins of the flap.

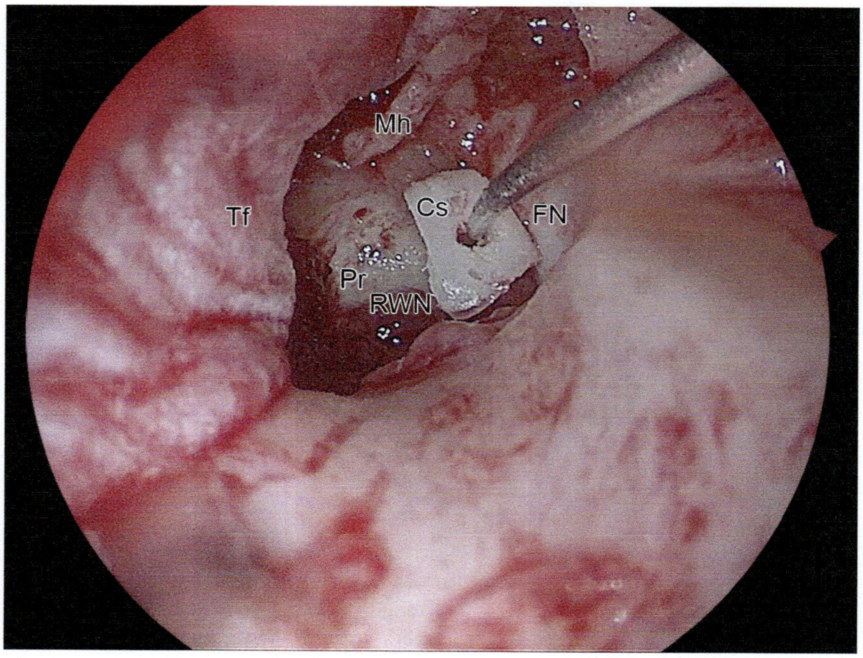

Fig. 19A: Ossicular chain reconstruction. Cartilage shoe being placed over mobile footplate. (Cs: cartilage shoe; FN: facial nerve; Mh: malleus handle; Pr: promontory; RWN: round window niche; Tf: temporalis fascia)

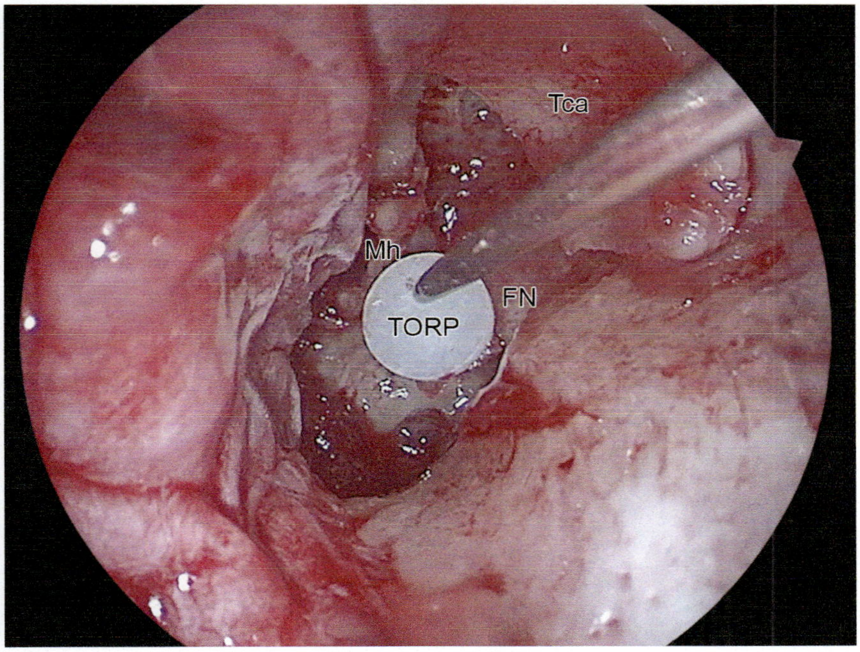

Fig. 19B: Ossicular chain reconstruction. TORP being placed over cartilage shoe.
(FN: facial nerve; Mh: malleus handle; Tca: tragal cartilage; TORP: total ossicular replacement prosthesis)

SPECIAL POINTS

- Role of endoscope in mastoid surgery is nascent and evolving, with new evidence coming into light every day, regarding its use
- Definite demarcation between indications and contraindications of endoscopic mastoid surgery are yet to be defined. Hence, the final judgment to use exclusive endoscopic approach for mastoid surgery is based on the clinical scenario and discretion of the operating surgeon
- One should never hesitate to convert to open microscopic approach whenever there is a doubt regarding the disease extent
- Combined endoscopic and microscopic technique is a novel technique which has its own advantages. However, its discussion is beyond the scope of this book
- Piezoelectric device in mastoid surgery is a unique invention which may change the course of endoscopic mastoid surgery in future. For further details vide chapter on "Recent Advances in Endoscopic Ear Surgery"

REFERENCES

1. Varshney S, Nangia A, Bist SS, Singh RK, Gupta N, Bhagat S. Ossicular chain status in chronic suppurative otitis media in adults. Indian J Otolaryngol Head Neck Surg. 2010;62(4): 421-6.
2. Shaan M, Landolfi M, Taibah A, Russo A, Szymanski M, Sanna M. Modified Bondy technique. Am J Otol. 1995;16(5):695-7.

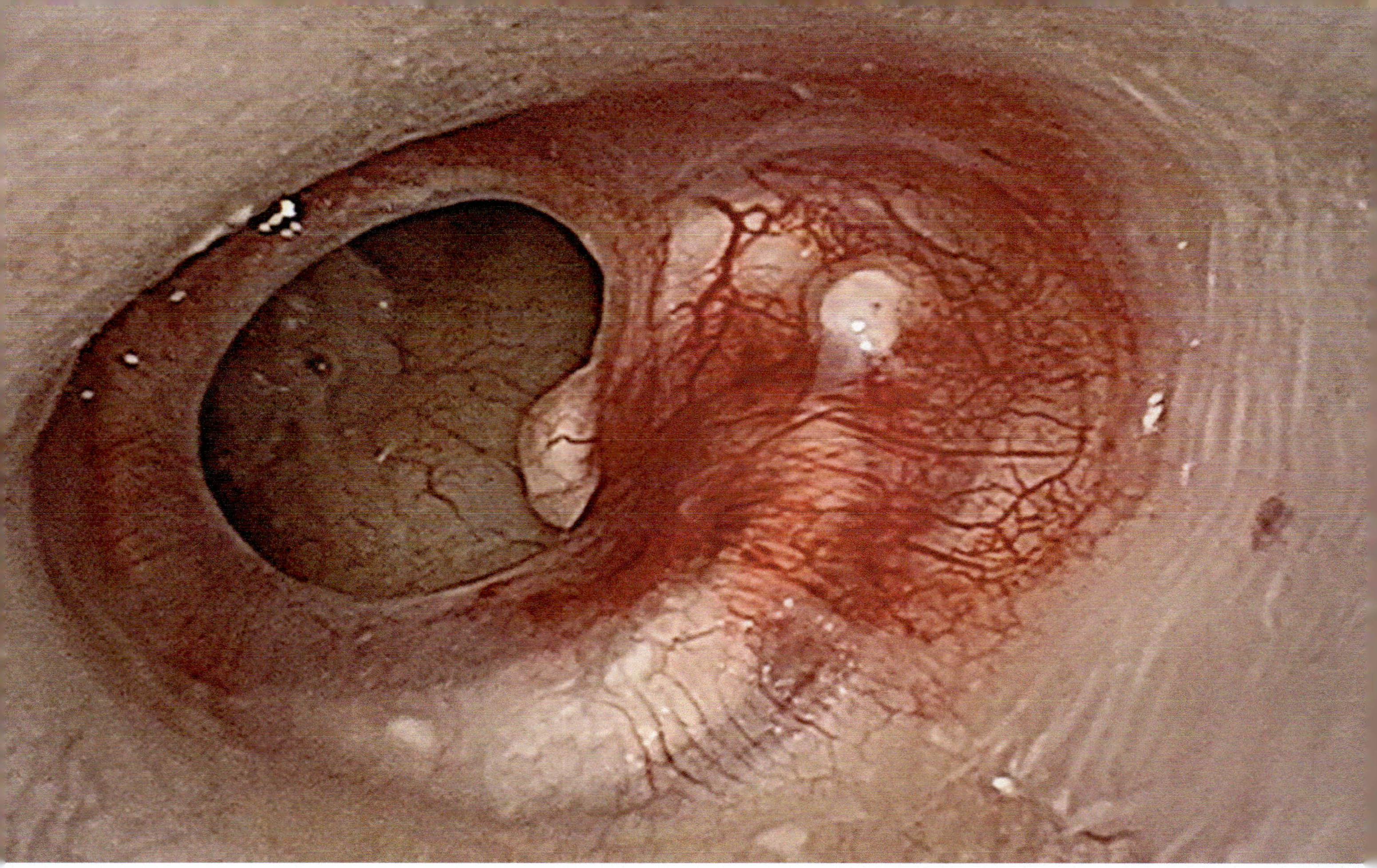

CHAPTER **12**

Endoscopic Management of Tympanosclerosis

Arindam Das, Sayan Hazra

Chapter Outline

INTRODUCTION

Tympanosclerosis is an abnormal yet common clinicopathological entity of the middle ear cleft, which typically presents as white plaque or chalk-like lesions, involving discrete regions of the tympanic membrane and/or middle ear.

ETIOPATHOGENESIS

Lamina propria (submucosa) of the tympanic membrane and/or basement membrane of the middle ear mucosa when exposed to long standing inflammatory infiltrates, results in increased fibroblast activity followed by degeneration of fibrous skeleton and abnormal fibrils formation. Subsequently, hyalinization of this layer sets in, giving way to the final stage of plaque maturation with/without calcification or even ossification.

Macroscopically two types of tympanosclerotic plaques can be described based on certain features:

1. *Chalk type*: Soft on palpation, easily removable and having chances of new sclerotic lesion even after complete resection due to continuance of underlying process.
2. *Rock type:* Hard white plaque, associated with inactive disease and usually does not progress or recur after removal.

SITES OF INVOLVEMENT AND ITS EFFECTS

The presence of well-organized thick layer of fibrous tissue within the pars tensa favors the formation of sclerotic plaques within it. In contrast, mucosa of middle ear cavity has loose subepithelial space accounting for lower incidence of tympanosclerosis. In the middle ear, it has predilection for certain cul-de-sac areas and ligaments having minimal glandular activity of mucosal cells with diminished cellular activity.[1]

Sites of involvement in order of frequency:
- 50% tympanic membrane (*myringosclerosis*)
- 30% middle ear cavity
- 20% both TM and ME cavity

TIP

Look for tympanosclerosis and ossicular discontinuity/fixation in any case of chronic otitis media having preoperative air-bone gap out of proportion to the size of perforation.

Tympanic Membrane

Sites of predilection of tympanic membrane: Tympanosclerosis[2]
- 80% with perforation
- 20% without perforation
- *Zones of predilection*: Anterior malleolar ligament
  - Posteroinferior quadrant
  - Diffuse involvement
  - The pars flaccida is never involved

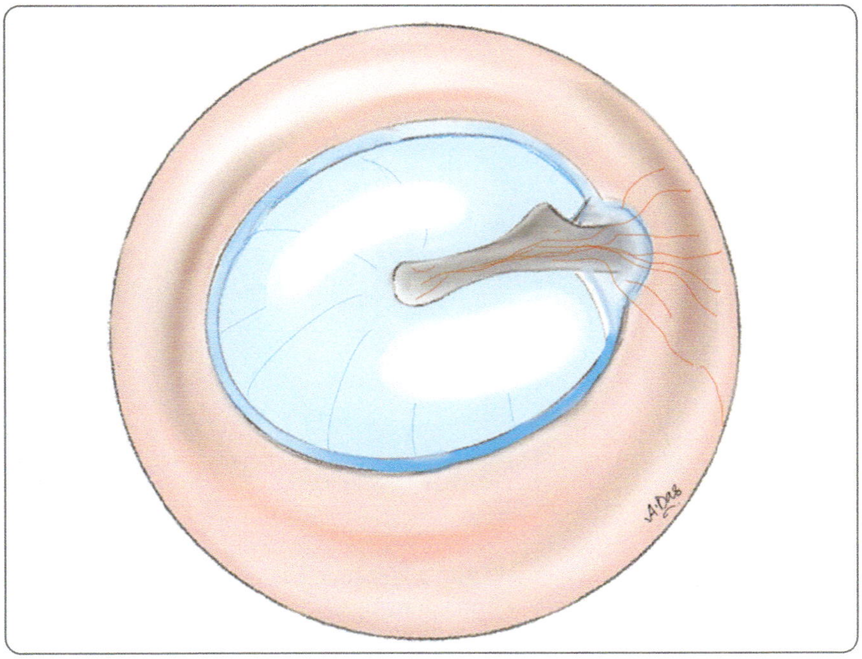

Fig. 1A: Tympanosclerosis with intact tympanic membrane.

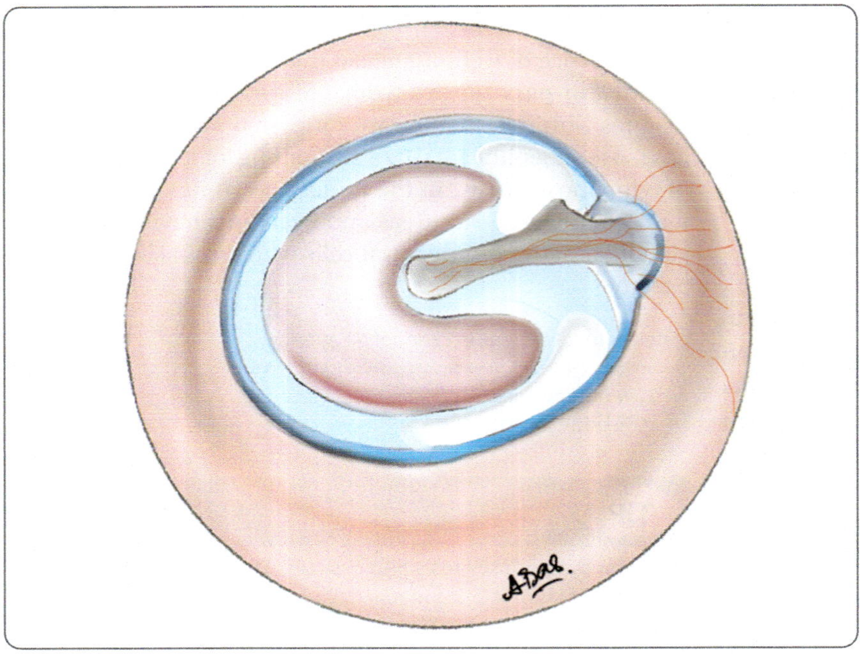

Fig. 1B: Tympanosclerosis with perforation.

Middle Ear Cavity

The common areas being anterior epitympanic space (AES), incudomalleal joint (IMJ), posterior epitympanic space (PES), oval window niche (OWN), stapes complex, and round window niche (RWN).[3]

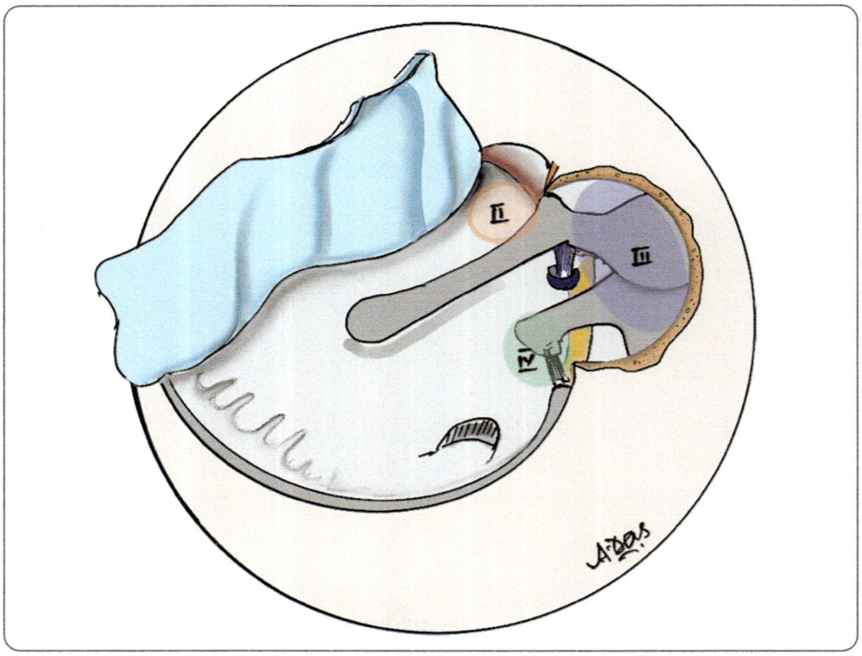

Fig. 2: Schematic depiction of various types of intratympanic tympanosclerosis depending on subsites of middle ear that are involved.

> **TIP**
>
> RWR is not a reliable parameter to check ossicular integrity and mobility. In recent times, preoperative CT scan with MIP and 3D reconstruction along with intraoperative palpation of individual ossicles provide more accurate results.

Type	*Diagrammatic representation*	*Middle ear cleft involved*	*Ossicular mobility*	*Management protocol*
I	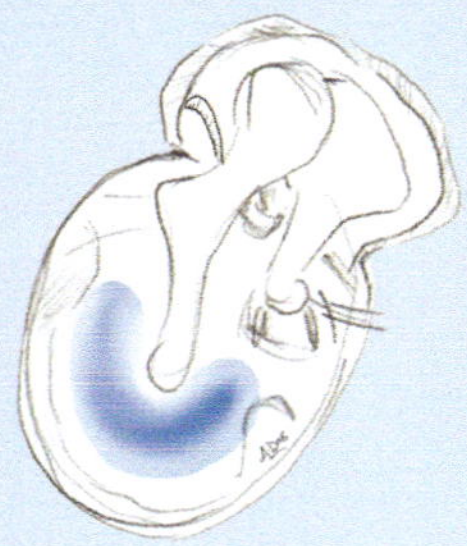	TM only (myringosclerosis)	Mobile RWR +	Endoscopic-tympanoplasty (Type 1)
II	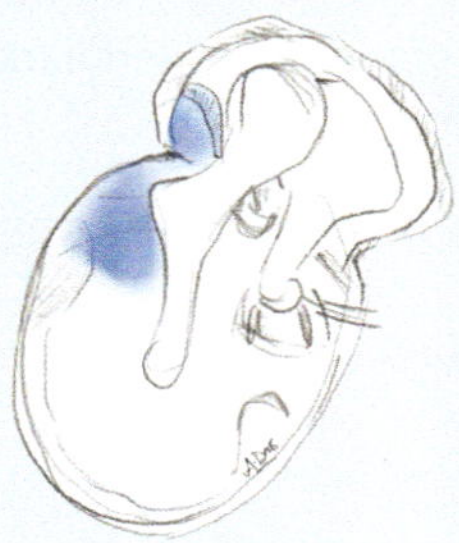	TM + Protympanum	Mobility restricted RWR +	Endoscopic-Tympanoplasty → Plaque removal and mobilization
III	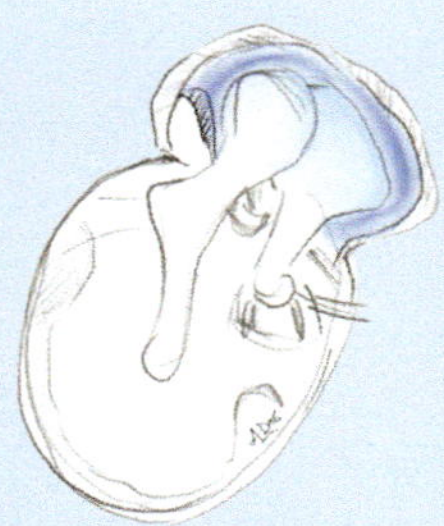	Epitympanum (AES + PES) IM joint involved	Immobile RWR –	Endo-atticotomy → Incus + malleus head removed → Ossiculoplasty (PORP)
IV	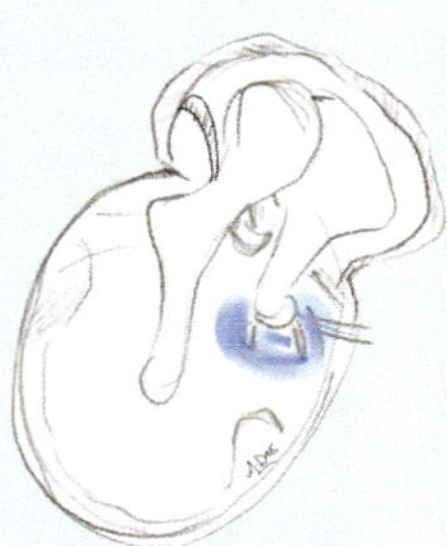	Any type + stapes involved	Immobile RWR –	Mobilization or 2nd stage stapedotomy

(AES: anterior epitympanic space; IM: incudomalleal; PORP: partial ossicular replacement prosthesis; PES: posterior epitympanic space; RWR: round window reflex; TM: tympanic membrane)

MANAGEMENT PROTOCOLS

Tympanic Membrane only viz. Myringosclerosis (Type I)

- This is by far the most common variety.
- Asymptomatic cases (incidental finding on otoscopy) do not need any operative management.
- In case of perforation with tympanosclerotic plaque, endoscopic type 1 tympanoplasty is done.

Surgical Steps

1. Margin of the perforation is freshened in the usual manner.

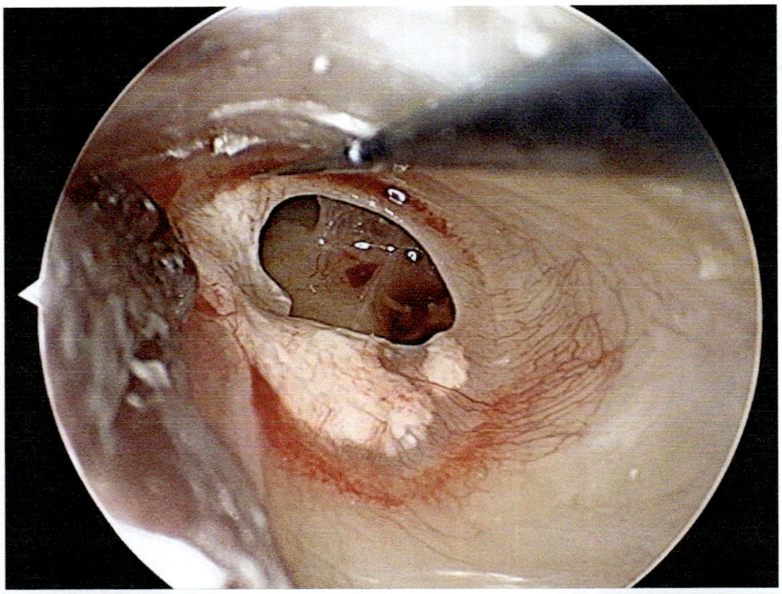

Fig. 3A: Freshening of margin of perforation along with plaque anteriorly.

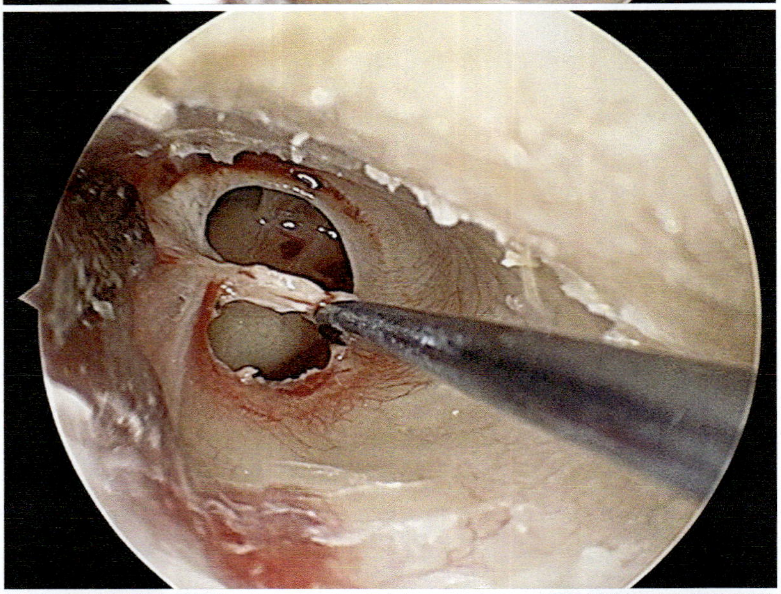

Fig. 3B: Freshening of margin of perforation along with plaque posteriorly.

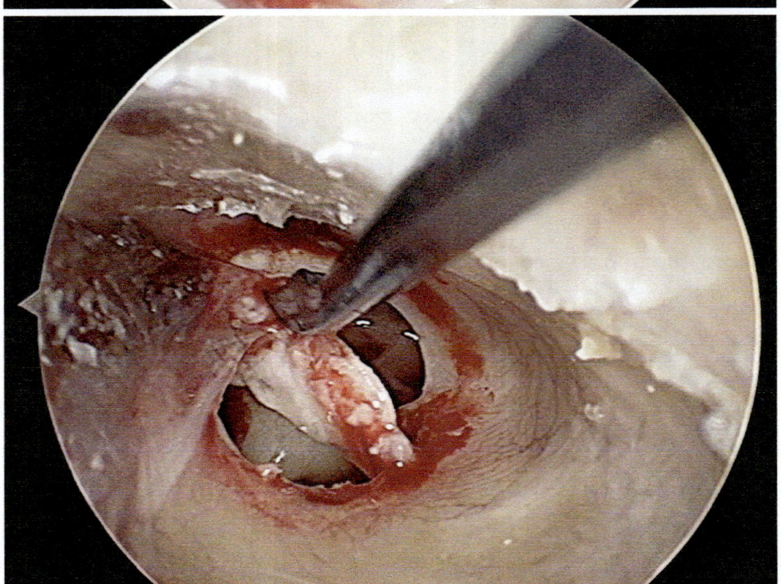

Fig. 3C: Freshening of margin of perforation along with plaque near malleus handle.

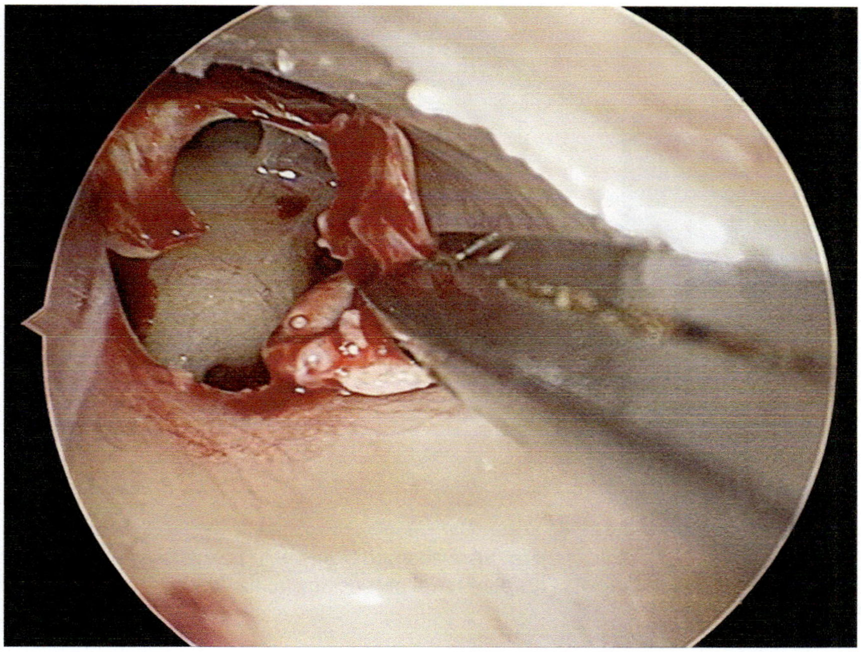

Fig. 3D: Entire plaque being removed with crocodile forceps.

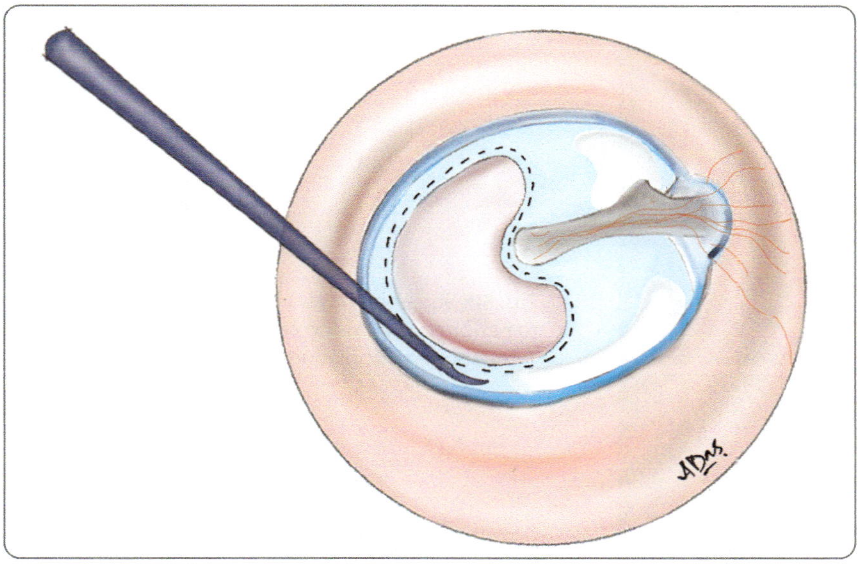

Fig. 4: Margin freshening using angulated pick or sickle knife.

2. Squamous layer is elevated from center to peripheral part using circular knife or Duckbill elevator.
3. A small tunnel is made with angled pick or flag knife between the plaque and lateral epithelium, thereby gradually undermining the whole plaque which is then removed with a crocodile forceps.

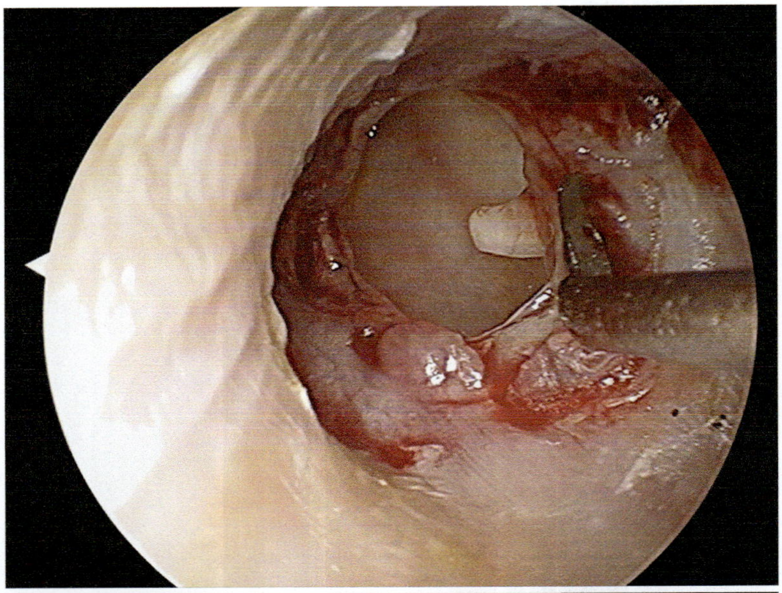

Fig. 5A: Squamous layer being elevated from center to peripheral part using circular knife.

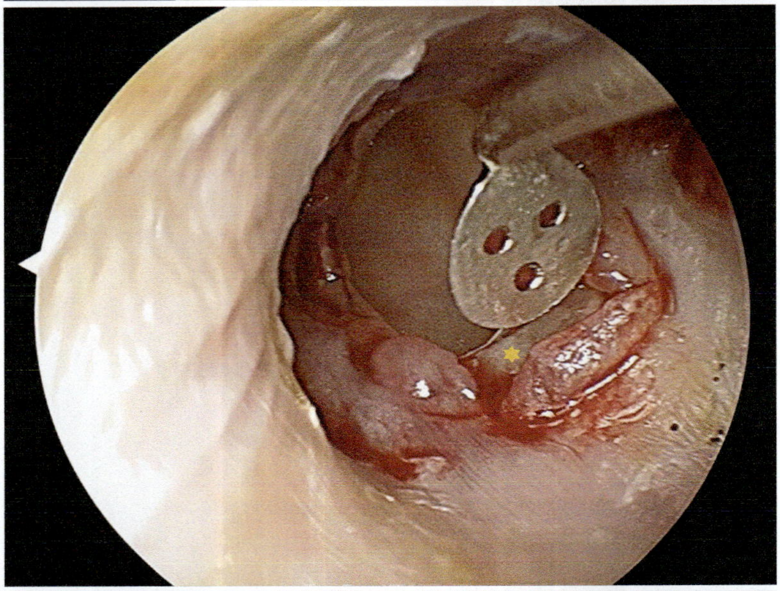

Fig. 5B: Squamous layer being elevated from center to peripheral part using circular knife. Yellow star: Tympanosclerotic plaque.

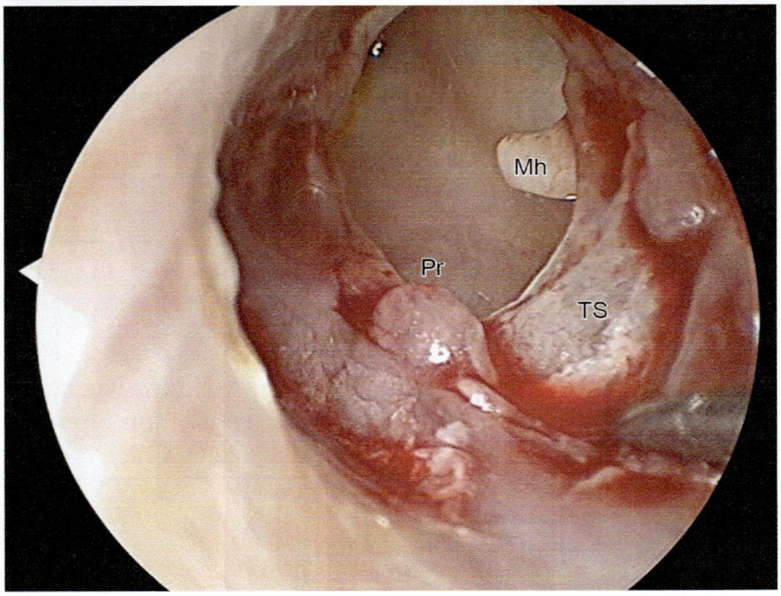

Fig. 5C: Tympanosclerotic plaque (TS) delineated posterior to malleus handle (Mh).
(Pr: promontory)

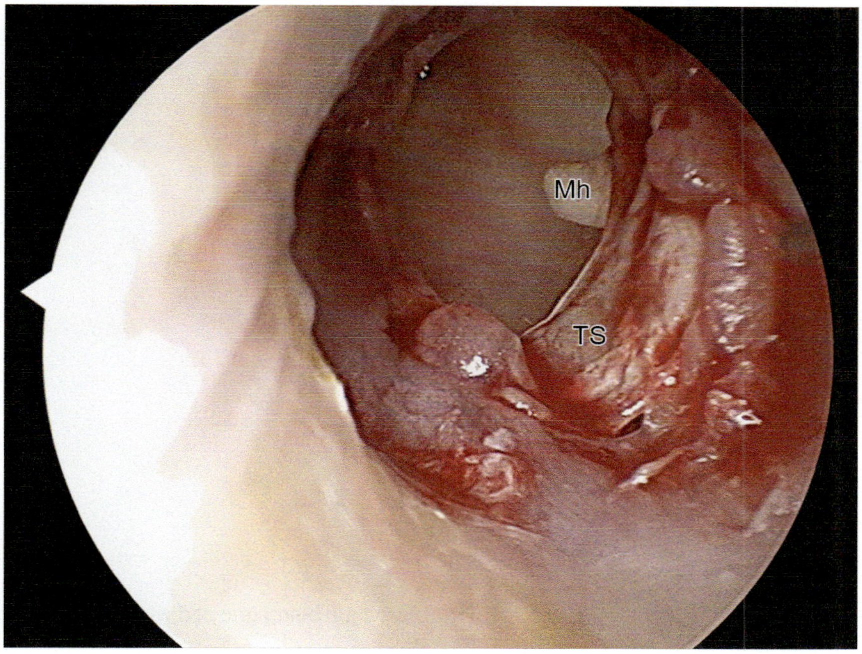

Fig. 5D: Tympanosclerotic plaque separated from fibrous annulus.
(Mh: Malleus handle; TS: Tympanosclerotic plaque)

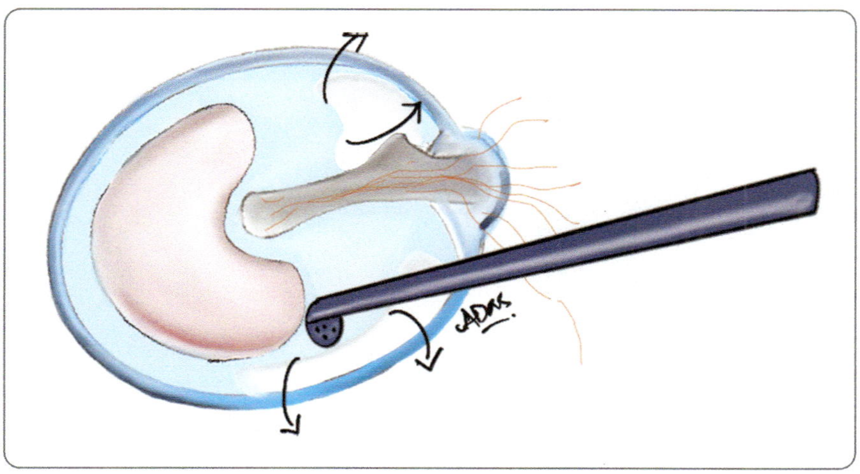

Fig. 6A: Direction of elevation of lateral squamous epithelium in center-to-periphery manner in order to expose the plaques using round knife.

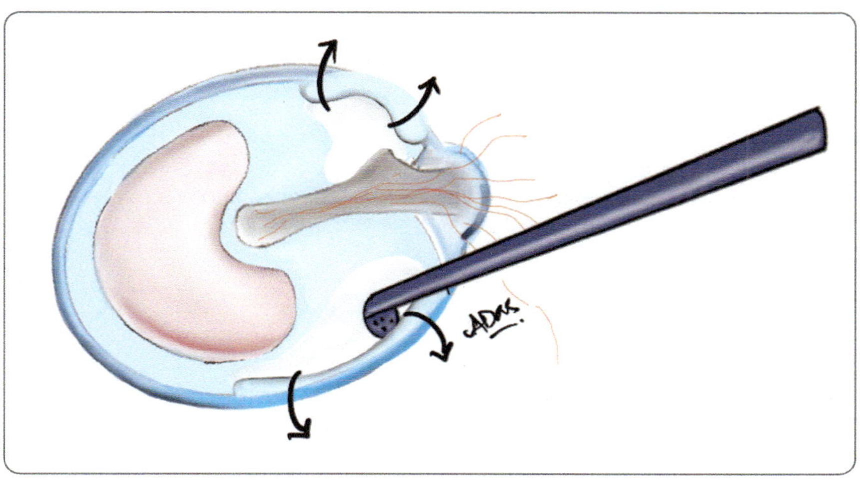

Figs. 6B: Direction of elevation of lateral squamous epithelium in center-to-periphery manner in order to expose the plaques using round knife: Entire plaque delineated after scraping off squamous layer.

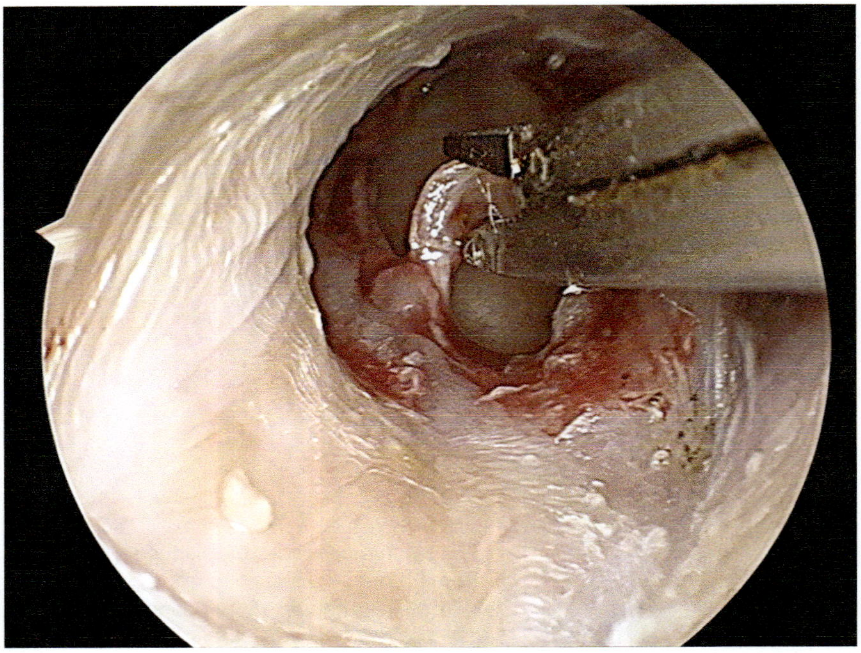

Fig. 7A: Plaque being grasped with crocodile forceps.

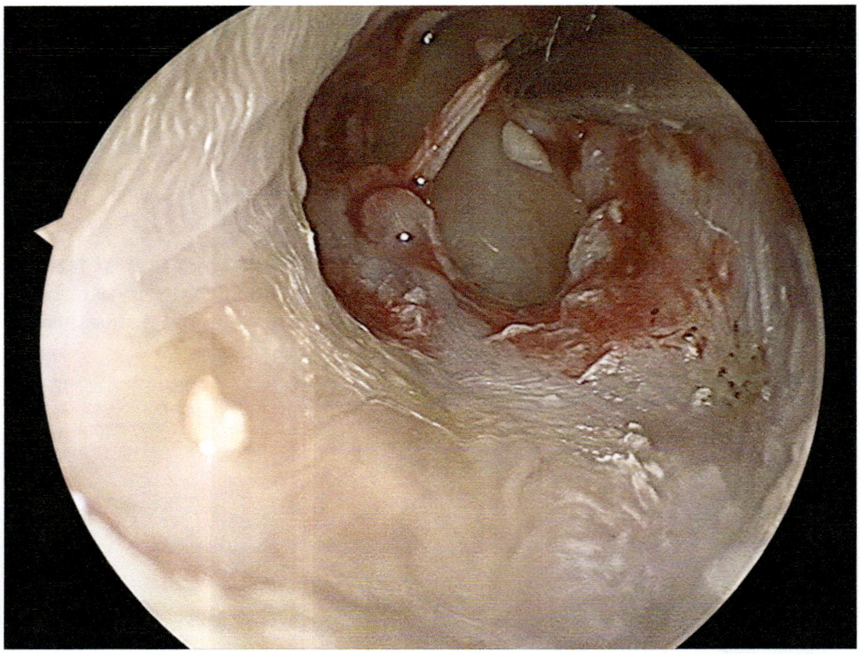

Fig. 7B: View after clearance.

4. Round window niche (RWN) needs to be inspected for tympanosclerotic plaques as obliterative tympanosclerosis can block the RWN completely which leads to unexplained hearing loss in the postoperative period due to the loss of phase difference.

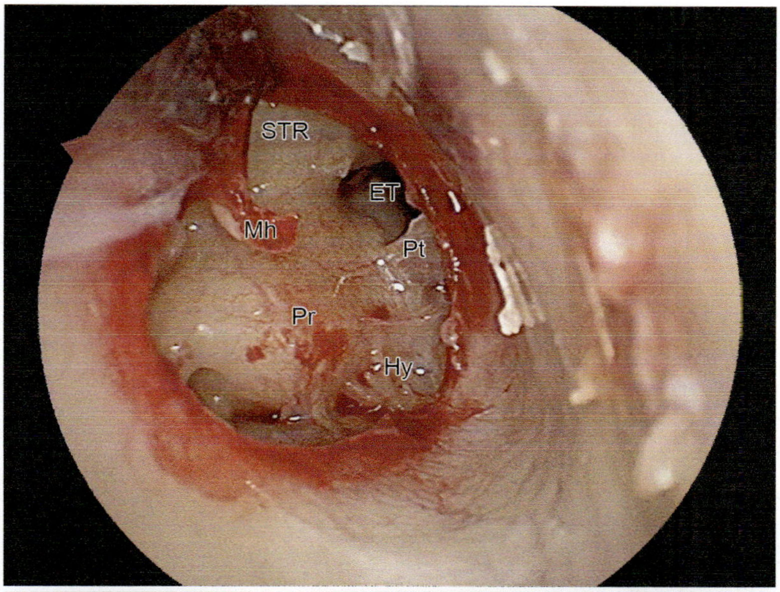

Fig. 8A: Inspection of middle ear cavity (right ear). (ET: Eustachian tube; Hy: hypotympanum; Mh: malleus handle; Pr: promontory; Pt: protiniculum, STR: supratubal recess)

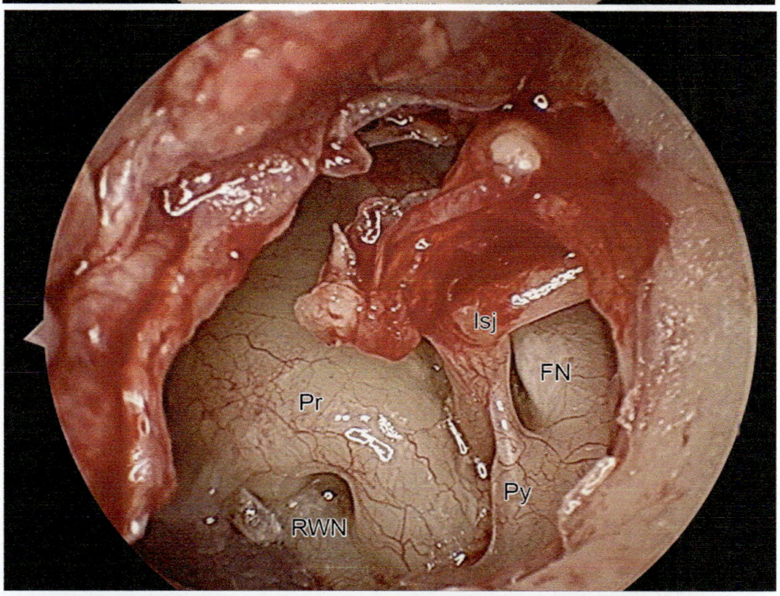

Fig. 8B: Inspection of middle ear cavity (left ear): Close-up view.
(FN: facial nerve; Isj: incudostapedial joint; Pr: promontory; Py: pyramid; RWN: round window niche)

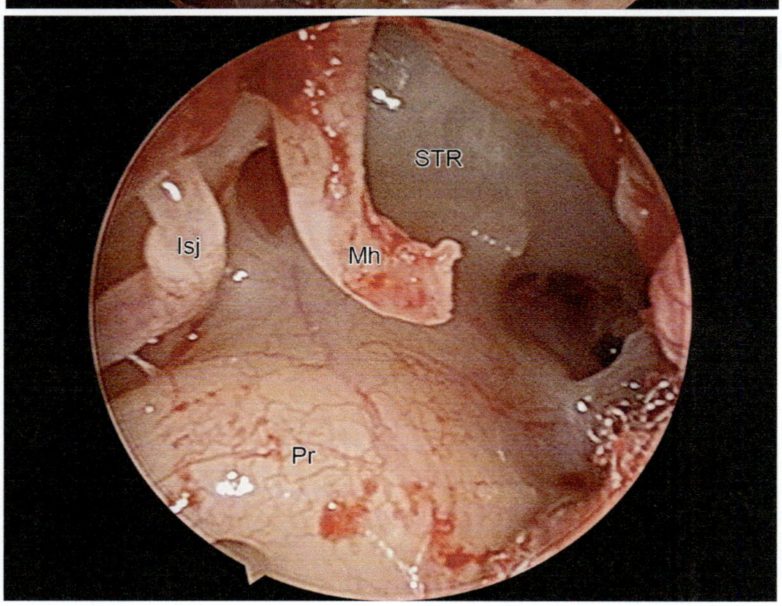

Fig. 8C: Inspection of middle ear cavity (right ear)—30 degree angled view.
(Isj: incudostapedial joint; Mh: malleus handle; Pr: promontory; STR: supratubal recess)

TIP

- The lateral squamous epithelium is spared as much as possible since it helps in the re-epithelialization for the graft placed underneath as well as keeps the size of remnant membrane bigger which is very essential.
- At times, plaques are firmly attached to the annular ligament. In such scenario it is advisable to resect part of the ligament along with the plaque. This promotes free mobility of the neotympanum.

PEARL

Tympanosclerotic plaques are devitalized and avascular tissue. So, it is advisable to remove every bit of plaque from the margins of the perforated drum to promote better graft take up.

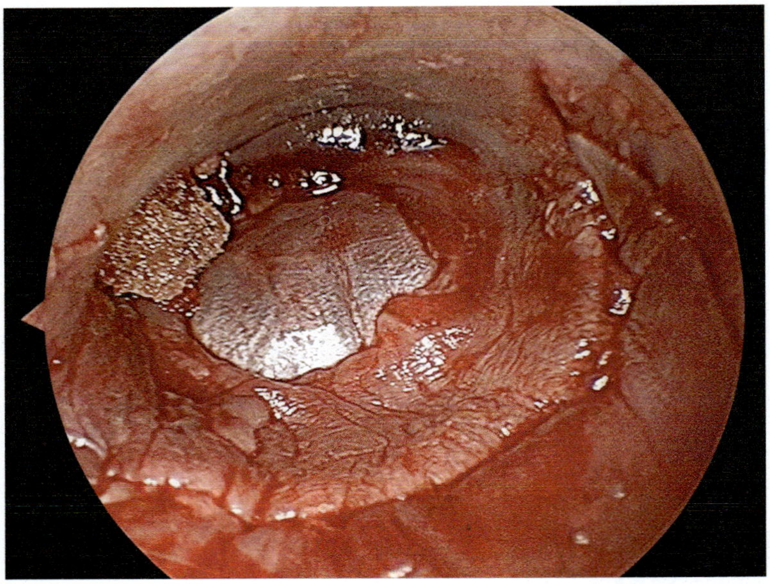

Fig. 9: Final view after grafting using temporalis fascia.

Tympanic Membrane + Protympanum Plaque (Type II)

- This encompasses the tympanic membrane along with protympanic space of the middle ear cleft. Anterior malleolar ligament (AML), Supratubal recess (STR) and tensor fold (TF) usually involved with tympanosclerotic plaque in this type.

Surgical Steps

1. Margin of the perforation is freshened in the usual manner.

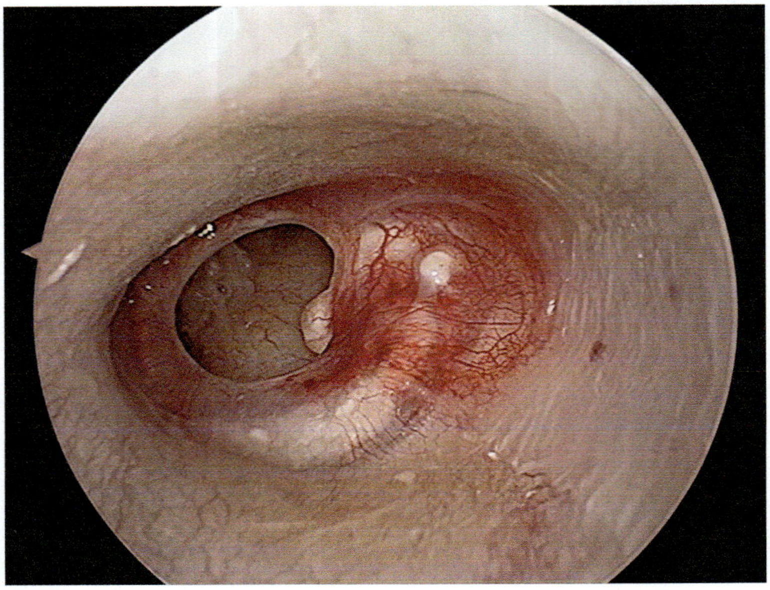

Fig. 10A: Sclerotic plaque as seen on initial inspection.

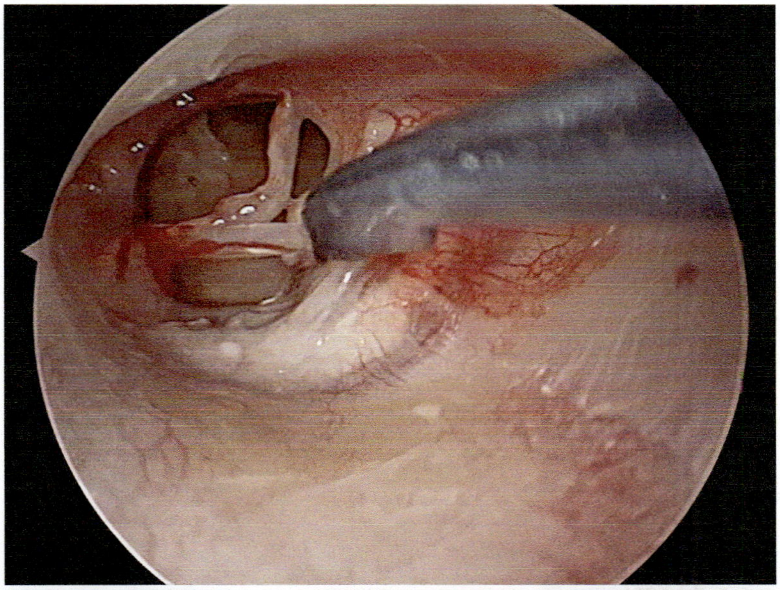

Fig. 10B: Margin of perforation being freshened.

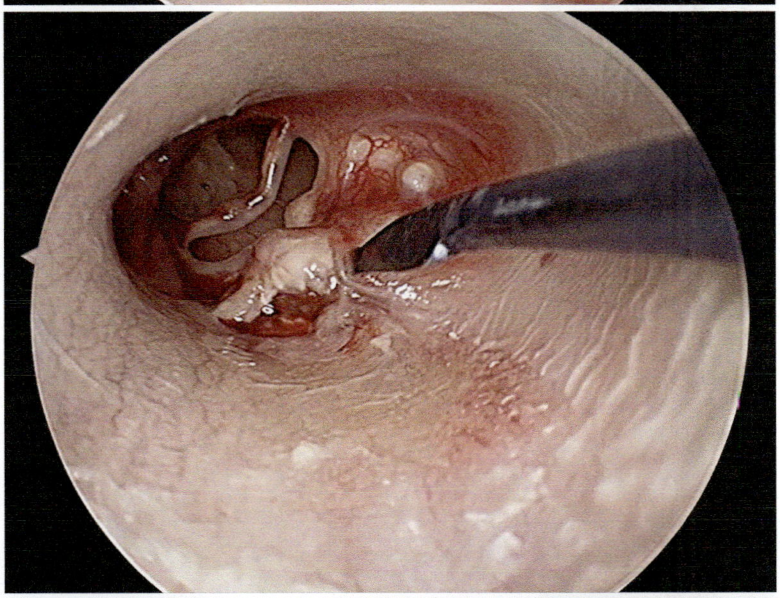

Fig. 10C: Plaque being delineated using sickle knife.

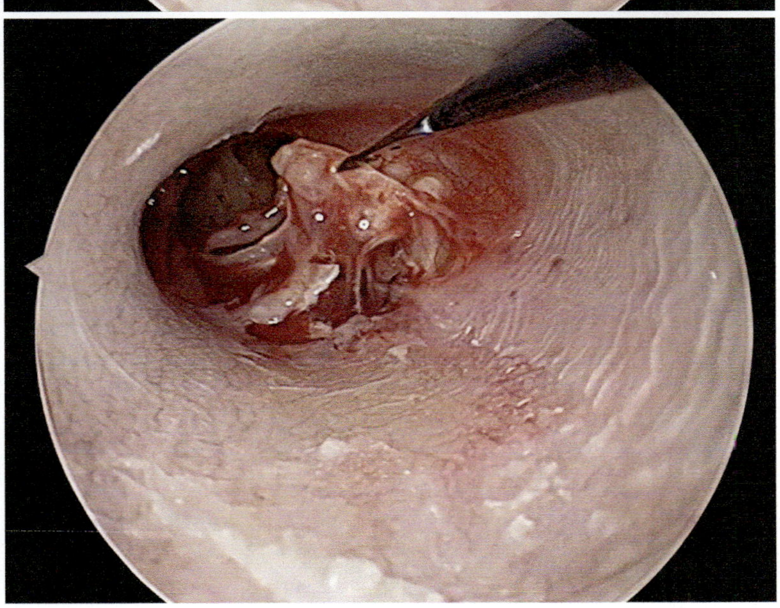

Fig. 10D: Plaque being lifted off squamous layer.

2. Flap is elevated up to posterosuperior aspect of Eustachian tube opening (protympanum).
3. Malleus fixation can occur due to tympanosclerosis which commonly takes place in the anterior annulus. In case this is found, it should be dissected carefully, preventing injury to the anterior malleal ligament (AML) and tensor tympani (TT) muscle. Failure to do so, often leads to persistent hearing loss even after successful grafting.

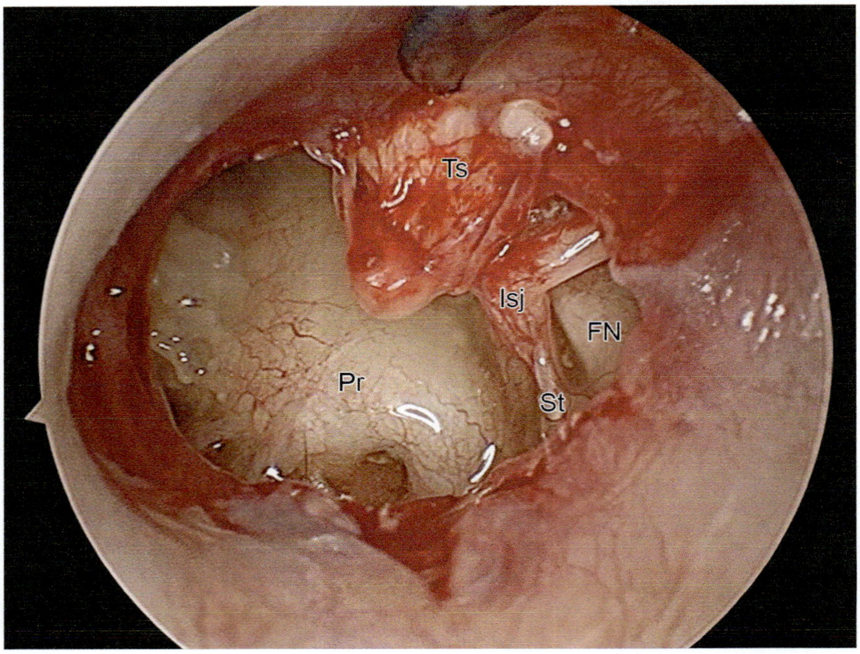

Fig. 11A: Protympanic tympanosclerotic plaques being removed.
(Ts: tympanosclerotic plaque; Isj: incudo-stapedial joint; FN: facial nerve; St: stapedial tendon; Pr: promontory)

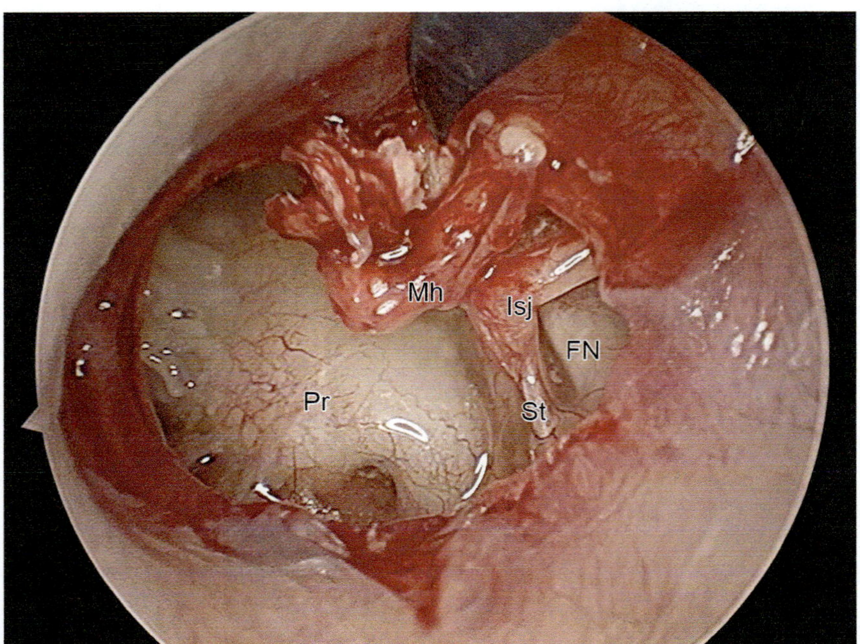

Fig. 11B: Protympanic tympanosclerotic plaques being removed: Sickle knife being used to delineate the plaque.
(Isj: incudostapedial joint; FN: facial nerve; Mh: malleus handle; St: stapedial tendon; Pr: promontory)

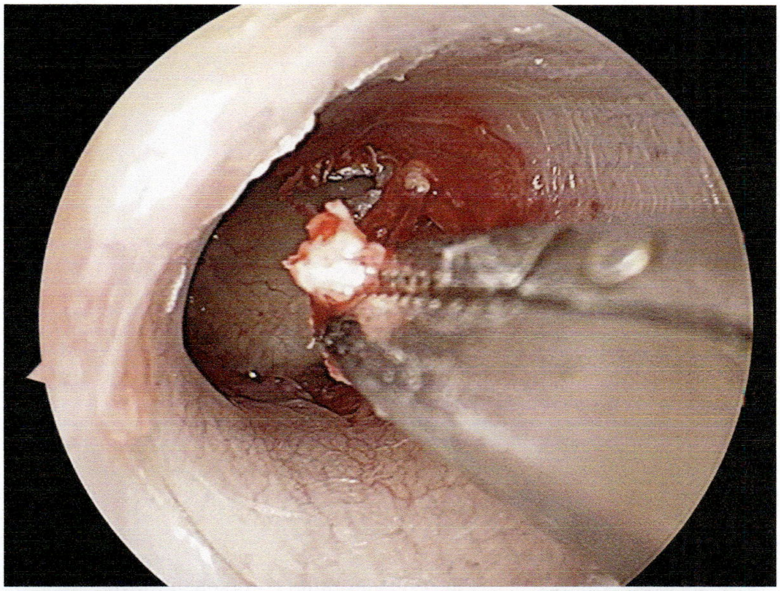

Fig. 11C: Protympanic tympanosclerotic plaques being removed using alligator forceps.

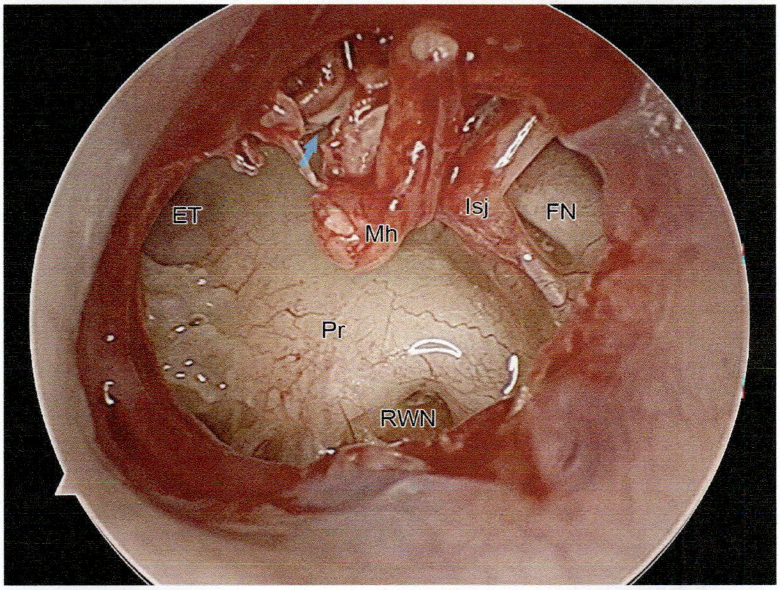

Fig. 11D: Plaque involving supratubal recess (blue arrow).
(Isj: incudostapedial joint; ET: Eustachian tube; FN: facial nerve; Mh: malleus handle; Pr: promontory; RWN: round window niche)

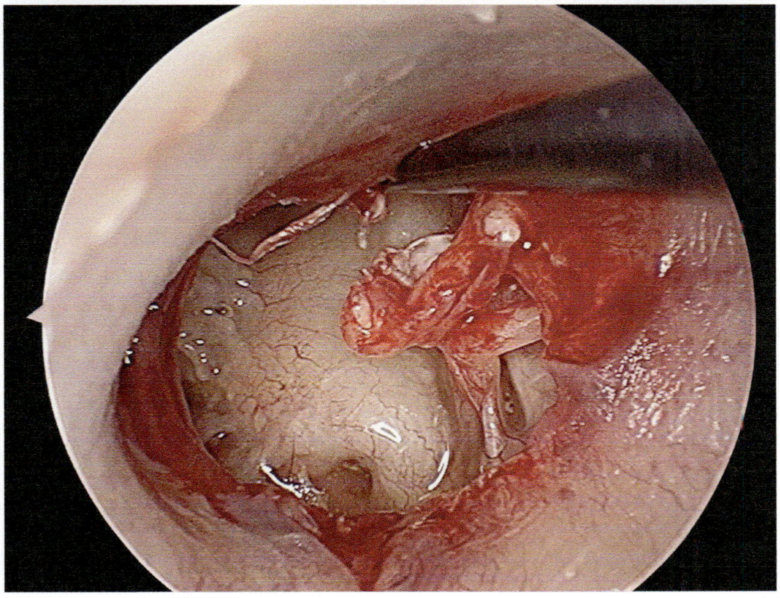

Fig. 11E: Dissection from protympanum.

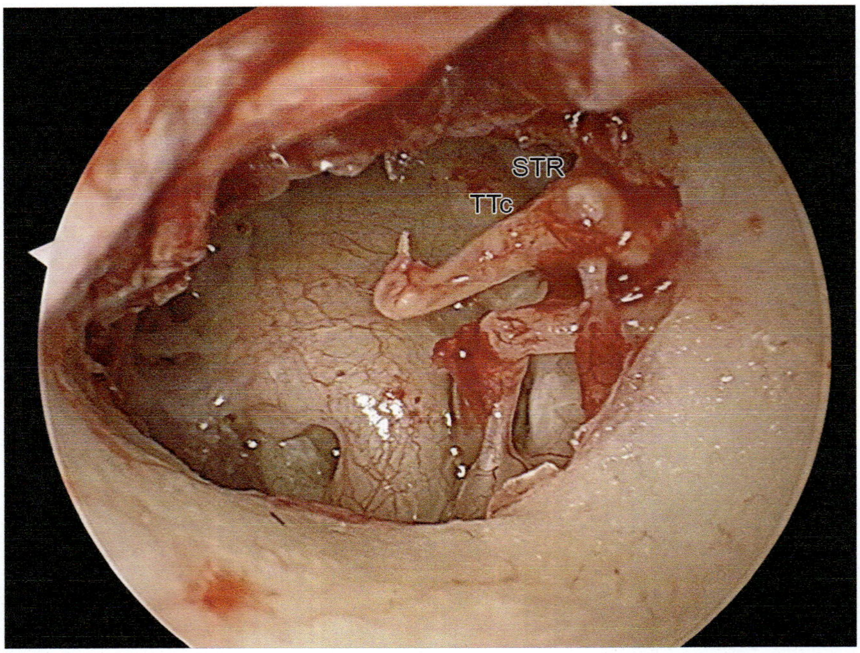

Fig. 11F: View after complete removal.
(STR: supratubal recess; TTc: canal for tensor tympani)

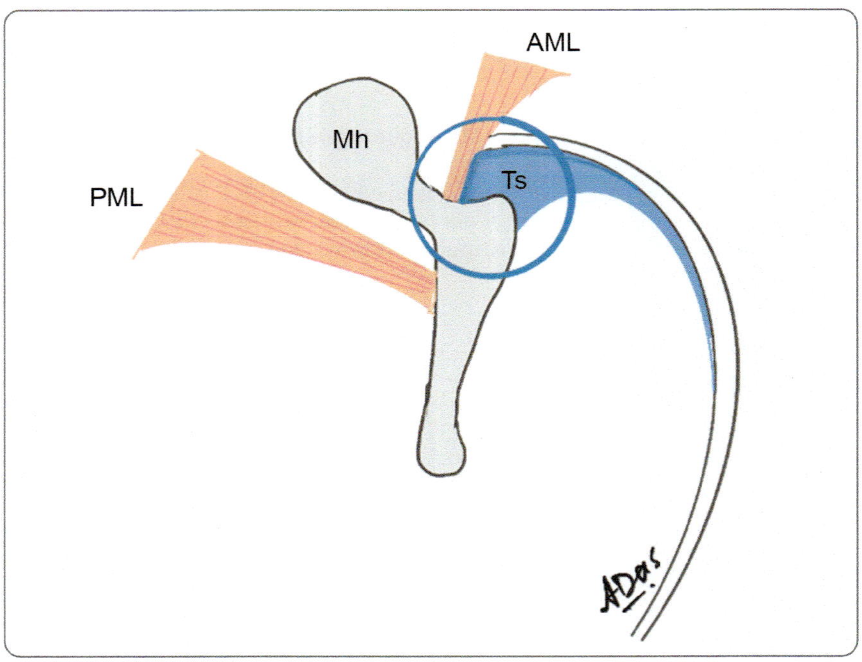

Fig. 12A: Schematic representation of disease around malleus.
(AML: anterior malleolar ligamental; Mh: malleus handle; Ts: tympanosclerotic plaques; PML; posterior malleolar ligamental)

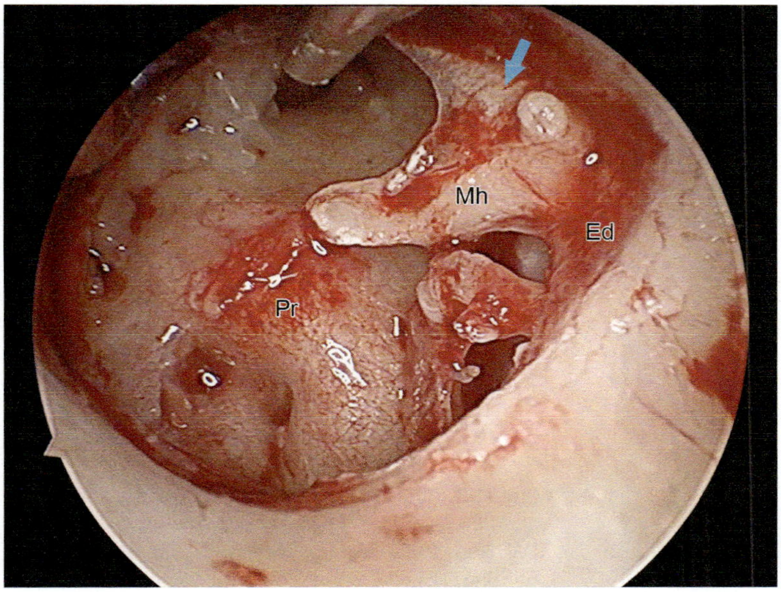

Fig. 12B: Surgical correlation of disease around malleus. Anterior malleal ligament (blue arrow) being depicted.
(Ed: epitympanic diaphragm; Mh: malleus handle; Pr: promontory)

4. Endoscopic atticotomy may be required in cases where malleus is not found to be mobile even after dissection of the plaques. Anterior epitympanic space is opened, with the extent of bone removal varying from case to case. Use of angled endoscope (30° Karl Storz 2.7 mm diameter), provides a clear view of the working area that includes the Eustachian tube opening, tensor tympani, anterior malleal fold, Tegmen tympani, cog, malleus head and horizontal portion of facial nerve, minimizing the need of bone work involving the posterosuperior canal wall.
5. Excision of the tympanosclerosis block fixing the malleus head to the tensor tympani, Tegmen or malleal fold can be achieved allowing adequate mobility of the malleus.
6. Mobility of individual ossicles is checked in the usual manner once Malleus is made free.
7. Tragal cartilage is used to fill the attic defect and underlay grafting is done to close off the perforation.

TIP

Always dissect the Tensor Fold (TF). Open this mucosal fold to establish anterior ventilation pathway. This is called *tensor tenoplasty*.

AES + PES, IM Joint Involved (Type III)

- Here, incudomalleal fixation occurs especially encasing the lateral side of the incudomalleal chain, fixing it to the lateral and anterior attic.

Surgical Steps

1. After freshening perforation margin and meatal flap elevation, wide endoscopic atticotomy is done to adequately expose the malleus head (MH) and incus body (IB).

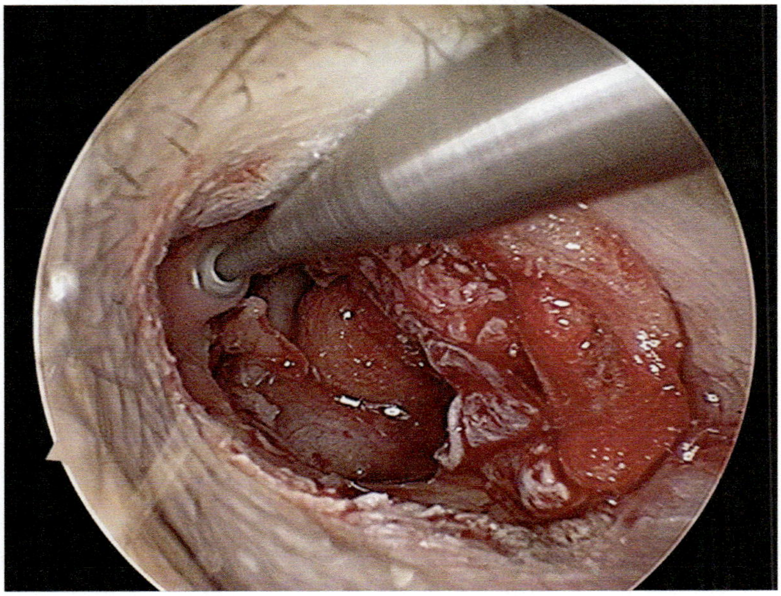

Fig. 13A: Atticotomy using diamond burr.

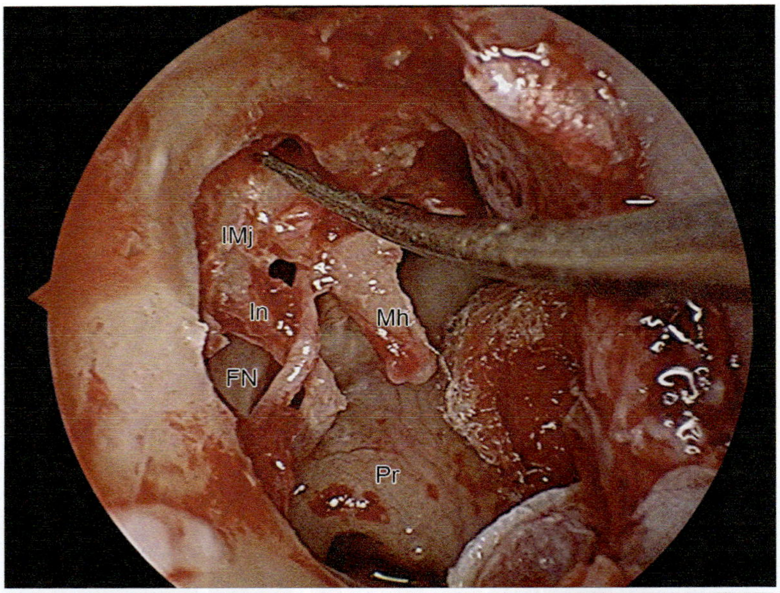

Fig. 13B: Angled pick used to clear disease from AES and PES.
IMj: incudomalleolar joint; In: incus; Mh: malleus handle; FN: facial nerve; Pr: promontory)

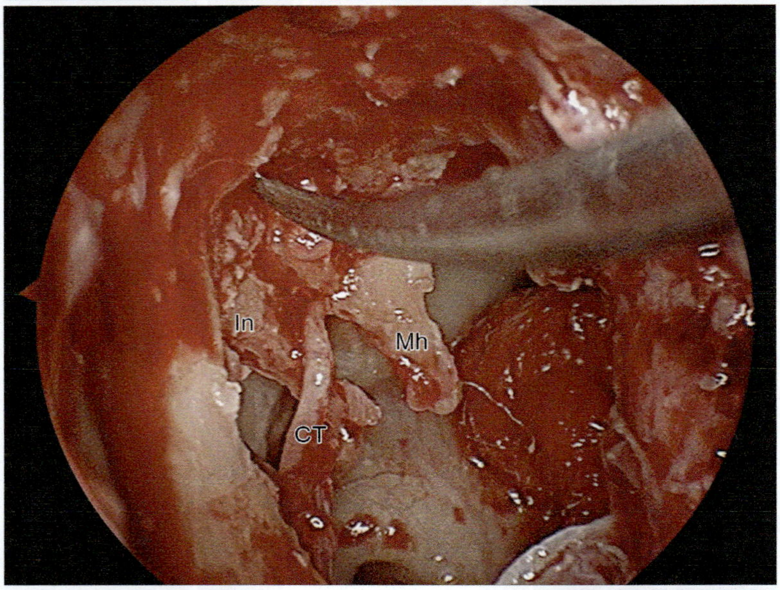

Fig. 13C: Angled pick used to clear disease from AES and PES.
(In: incus; Mh: malleus handle; CT: chorda tympani)

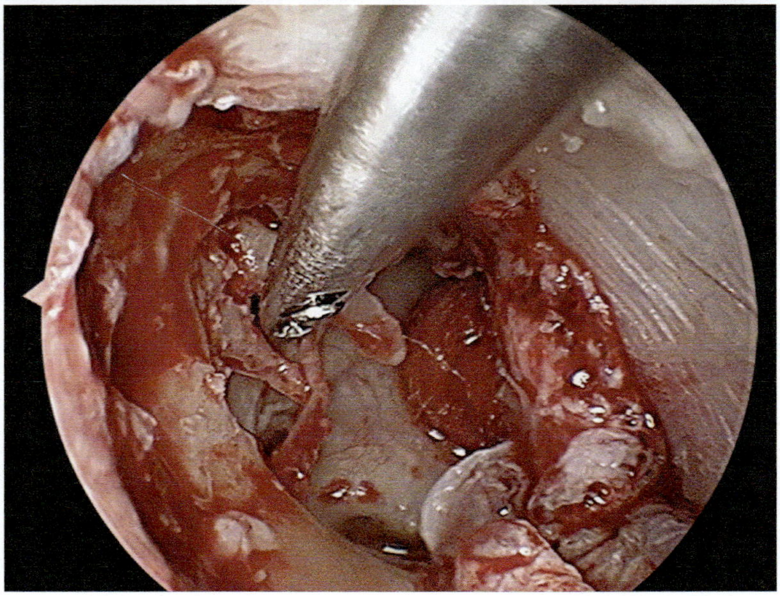

Fig. 13D: Malleus head being nipped.

2. In *Chalk type plaques*, angled/curved pick is used to remove the plaques meticulously from the malleus, especially anteriorly and around the joint. Heavy manipulation is discouraged to prevent sensorineural deficit.
3. In far extensive disease where this simple mobilization does not suffice, bypass technique has to be done wherein the incudostapedial joint is dislocated followed by removal of the incus from the incus-malleus assembly.
4. At times the sclerosis is so severe that the incus cannot be separated from the malleus, as it is almost fused to each other. In such cases, body of incus along with head of malleus is nipped away.

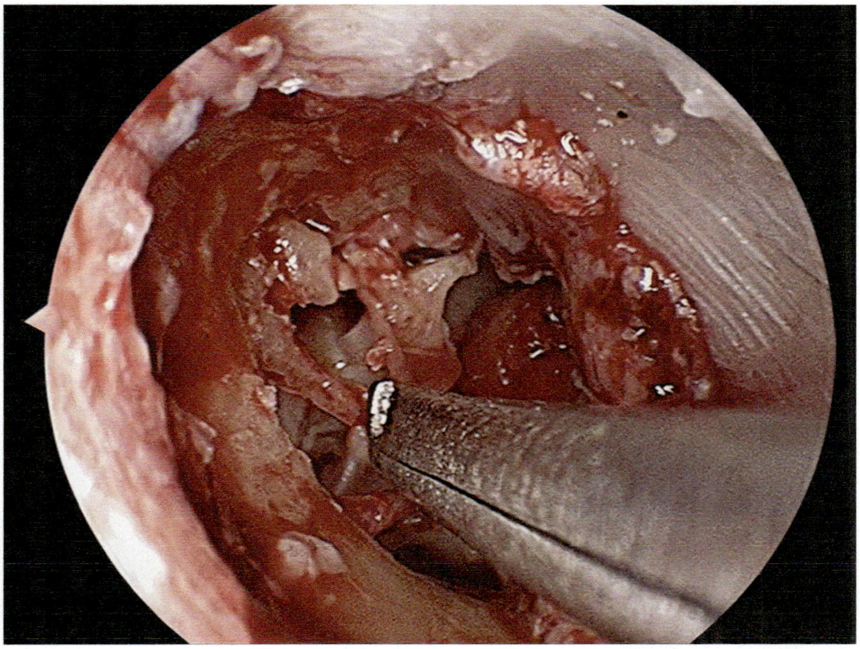

Fig. 14A: Nipping malleus head with a sharp nipper.

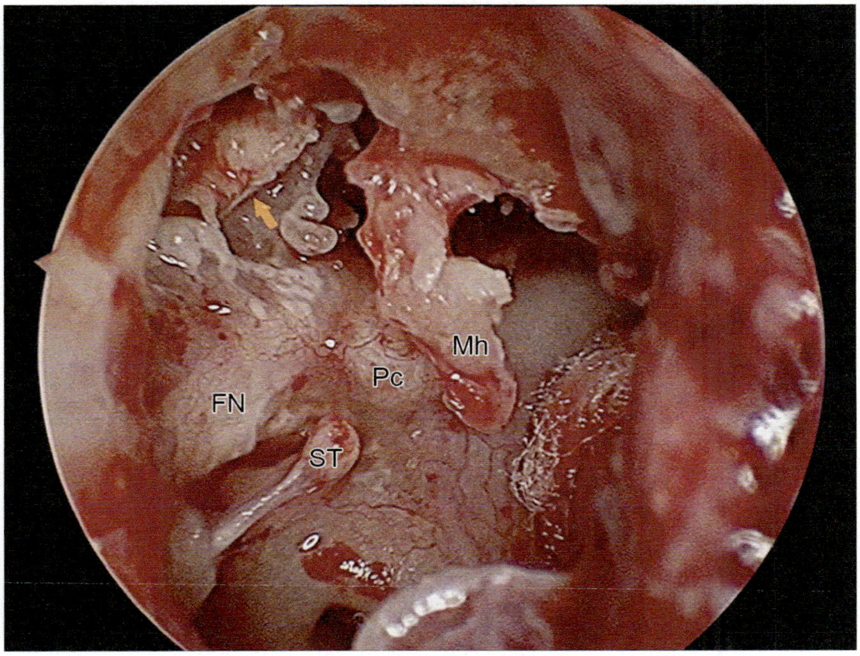

Fig. 14B: Sclerotic plaque in epitympanum (orange arrow).
(Mh: malleus handle; Pc: processus cochleariformis; FN: facial nerve; ST: stapes)

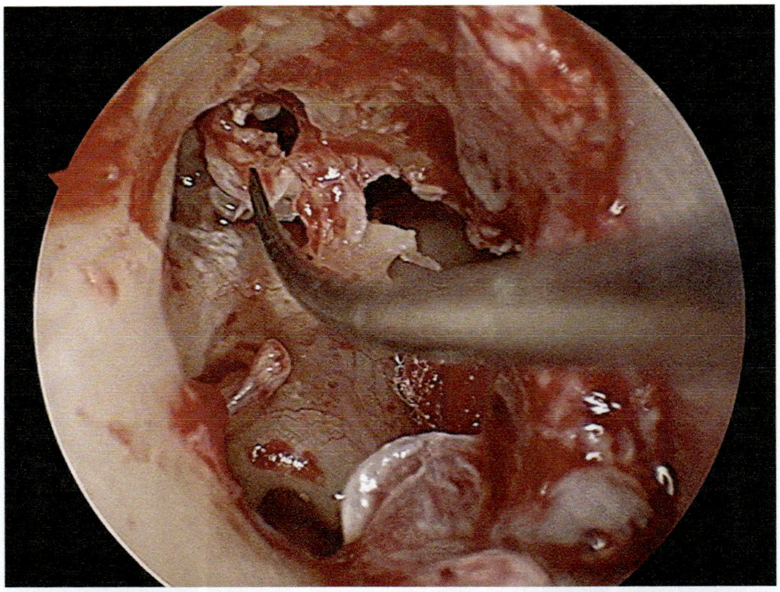

Fig. 14C: Dissection of plaque using smooth curved pick.

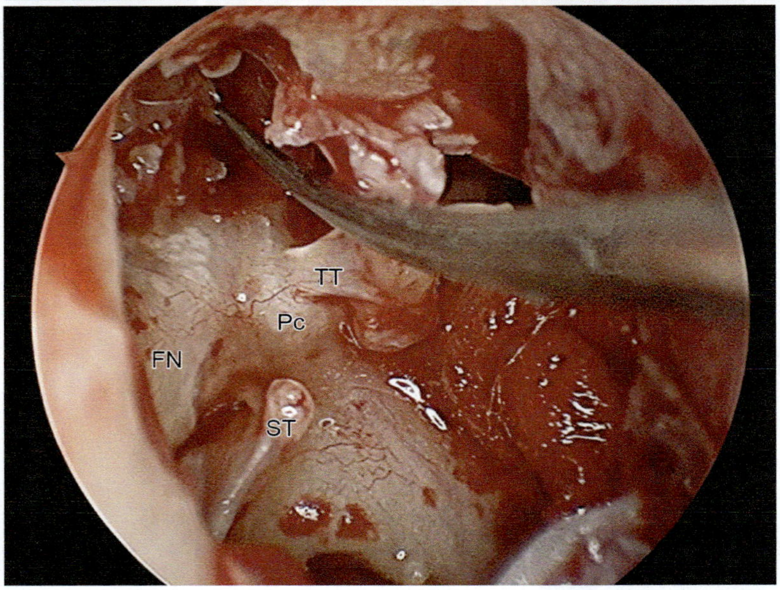

Fig. 14D: Final view after complete clearance. (ST: scala tympani; TT: tensor tympani; Pc: processus cochleariformis; FN: facial nerve)

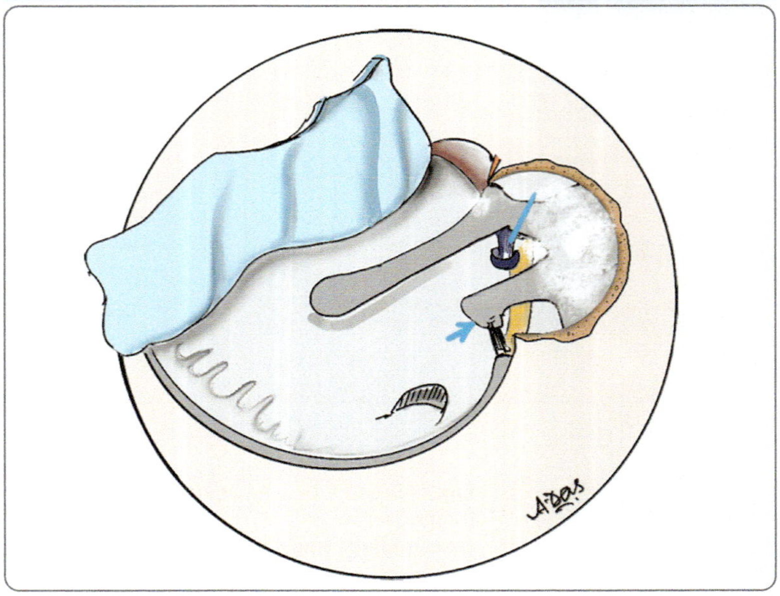

Fig. 15A: IS joint is separated followed by removal of incus and nipping of malleus handle.

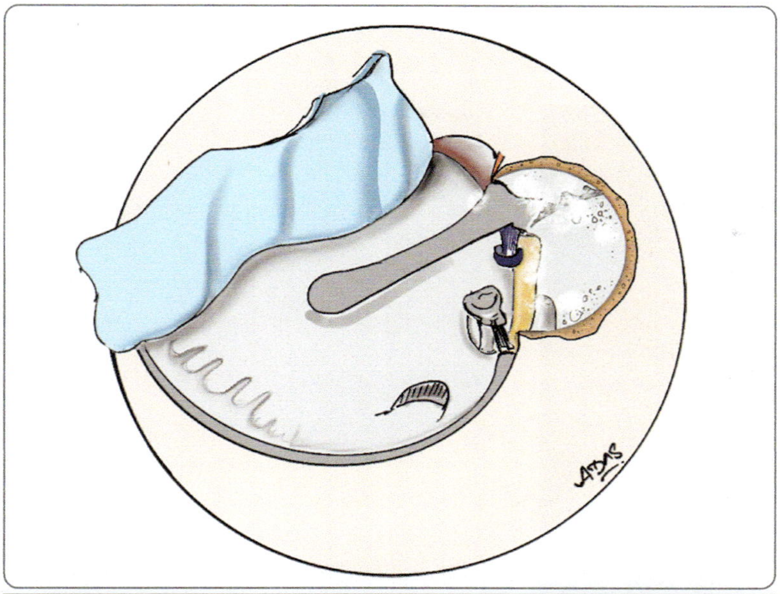

Fig. 15B: Exposure of area of interest.

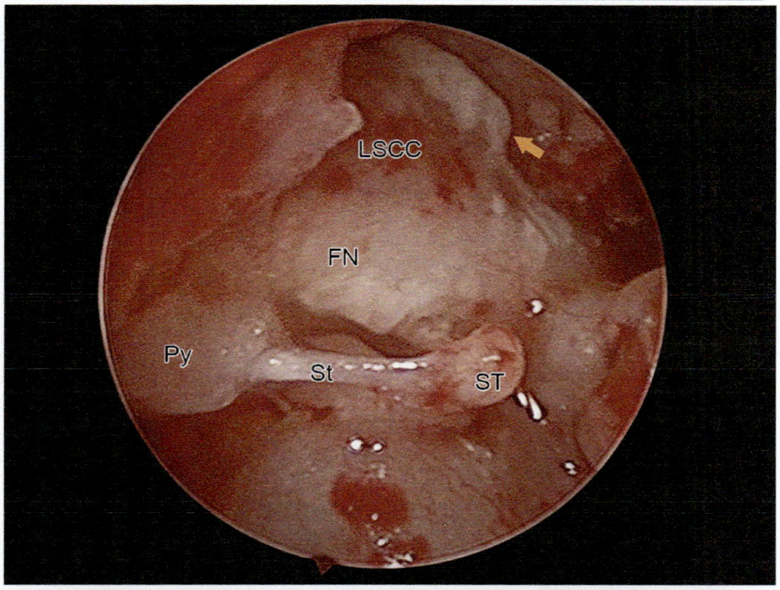

Fig. 16A: Angled scope being used to visualize extensive tympanosclerosis (orange arrow) involving fallopian canal and lateral semicircular canal (LSCC). (LSCC: lateral semicircular canal; FN: facial nerve; Py: processus pyramidalis; ST: stapes; St: stapedial tendon)

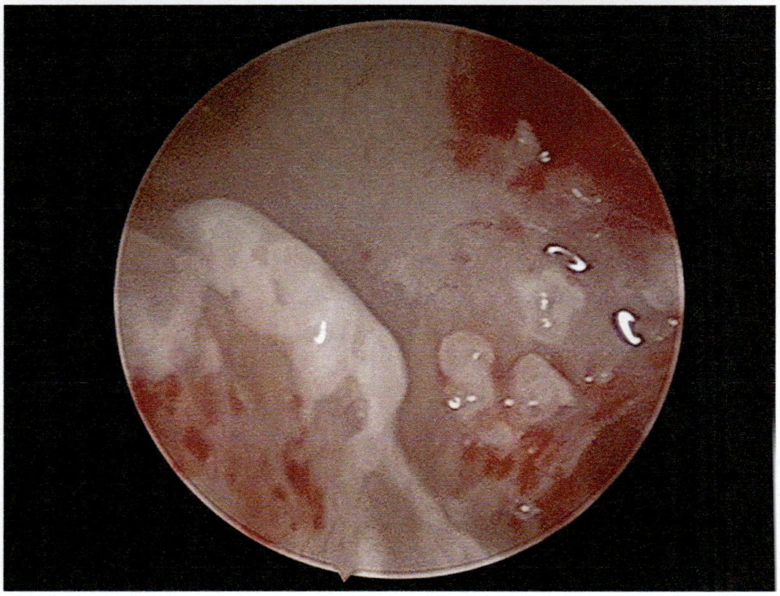

Fig. 16B: Closer view of the same as figure A.

5. Ossiculoplasty is done with Teflon PORP (short columella) in either of these scenarios, in the same sitting.

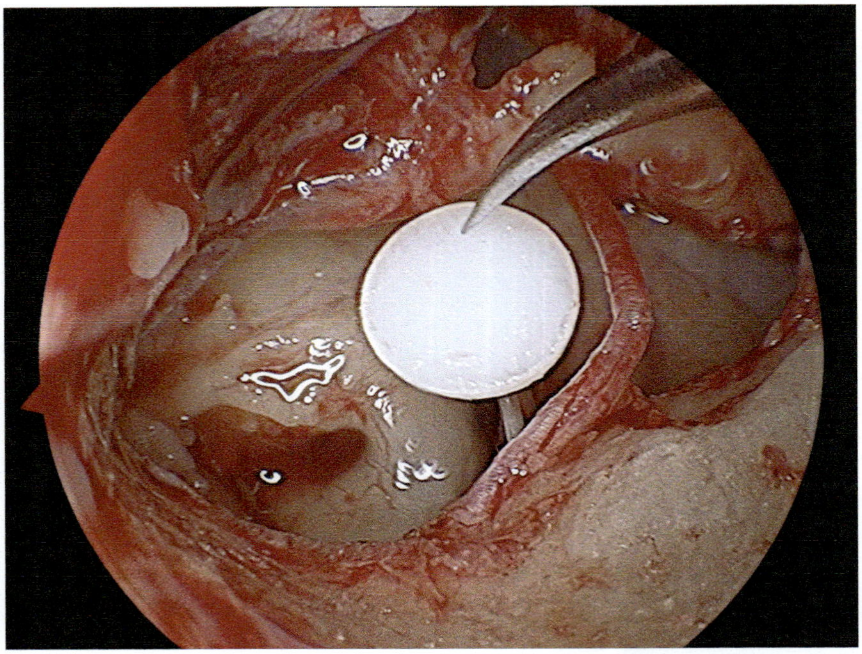

Fig. 17A: Ossiculoplasty using Teflon PORP.

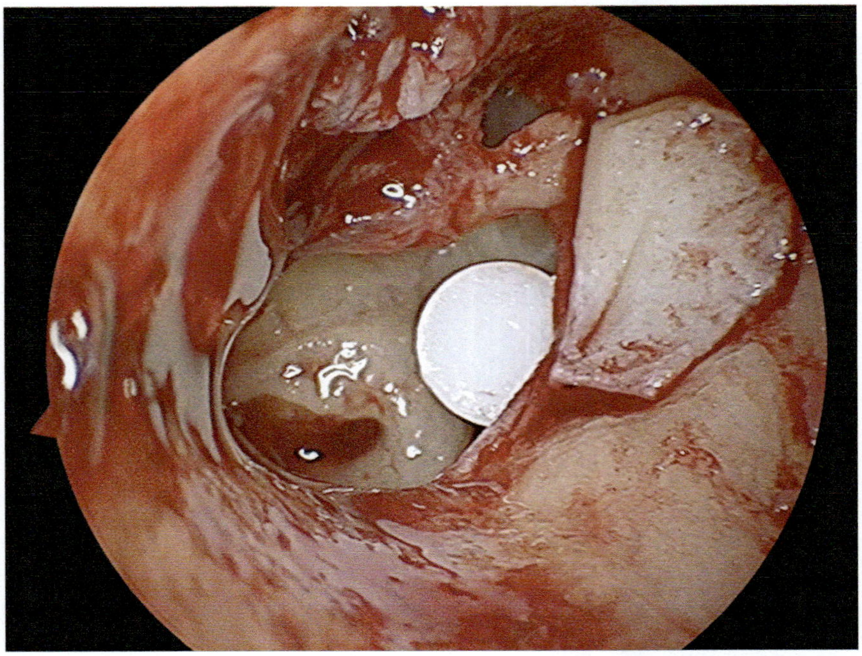

Fig. 17B: Attic defect being covered with sliced cartilage.

TIP

Incudostapedial joint should be dislocated prior to nipping the malleus head.

Any Type + Stapes Involved (Type IV)

- Common areas of involvement include—Incudostapedial joint (ISJ), stapes crura (AC and PC), footplate (Fp) and annular ligament.

Surgical Steps

1. Margin of perforation is freshened in the usual manner along with tympanomeatal flap elevation. Middle ear inspection and ossicular mobility is checked for individual ossicles along with stapes footplate as in any stapes surgery.
2. In case of limited disease, plaques are removed from around the stapes using sharp pick.
3. In advance cases, endoscopic atticotomy is done for proper exposure and mobilization of TS plaque, as it is done in Type III.

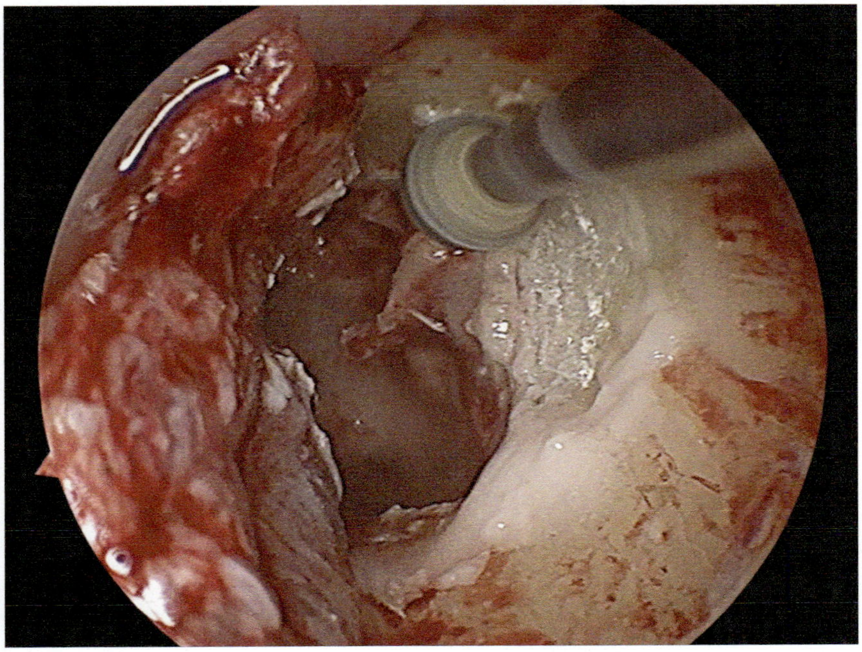

Fig. 18A: Atticotomy

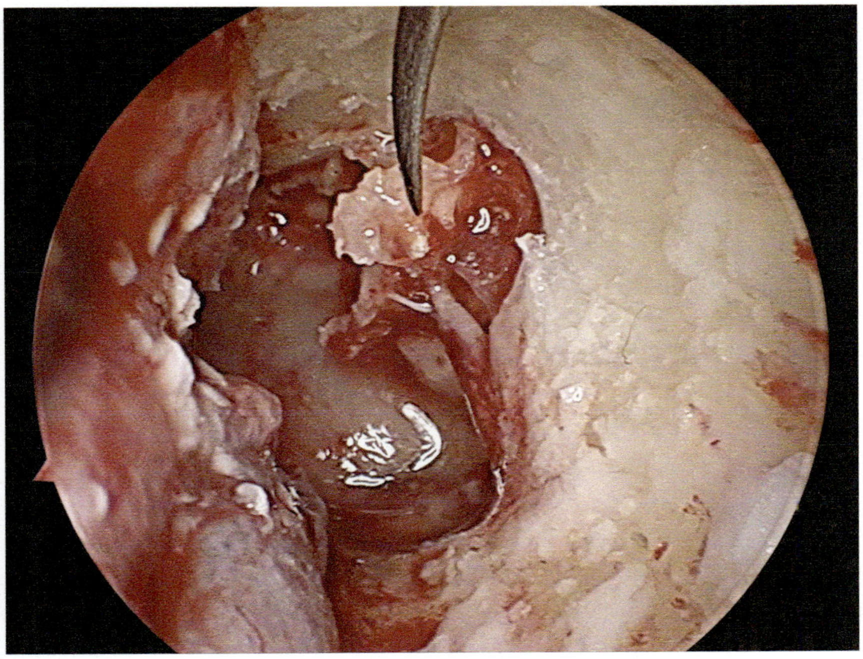

Fig. 18B: Dissection using sharp smooth curved pick.

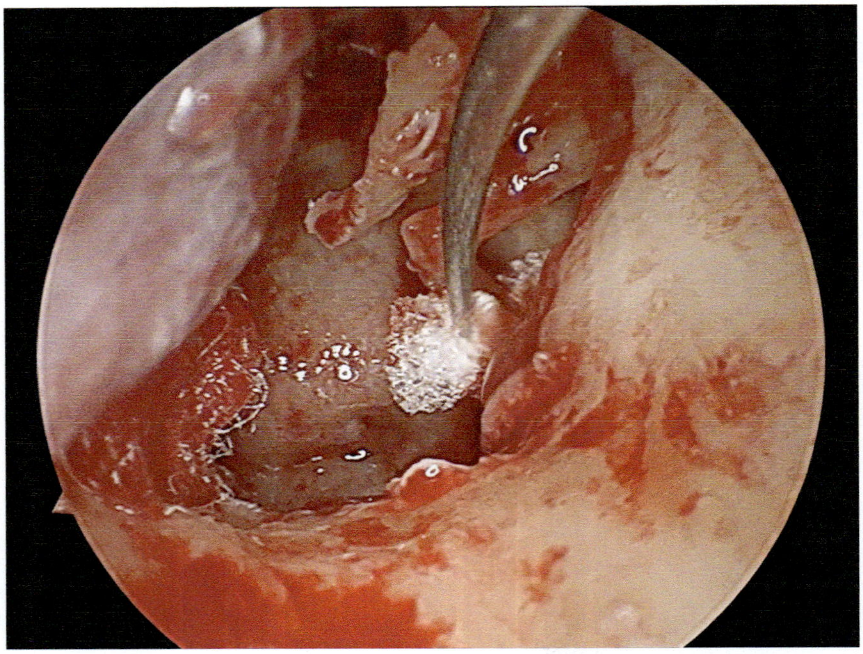

Fig. 18C: Gelfoam dissection around ossicles.

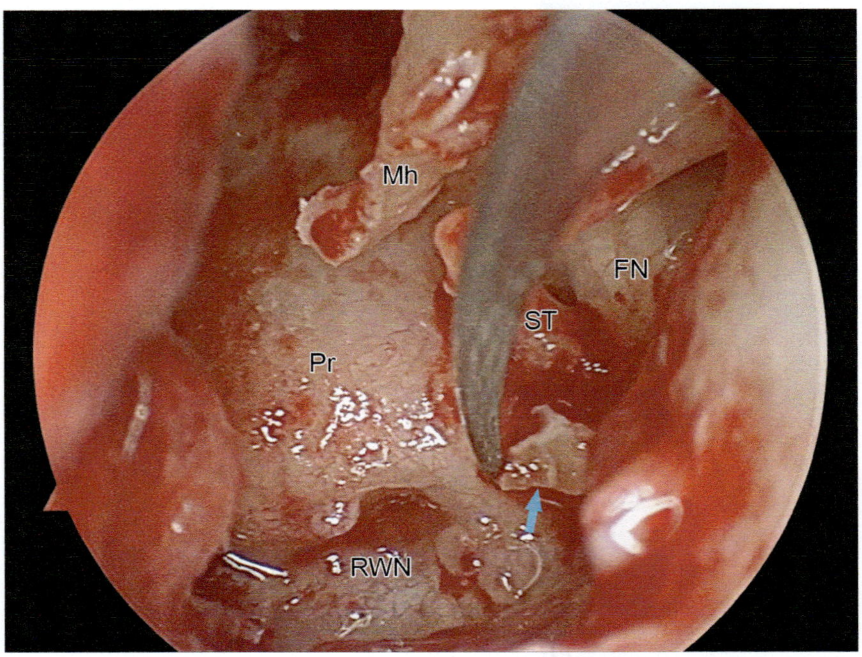

Fig. 18D: Plaque (blue arrow) being removed from around stapes (ST).
(Mh: malleus handle; FN: facial nerve; Pr: promontory; RWN: round window niche)

4. Extensive disease wherein the annular ligament of footplate is fixed (obliterative tympanosclerosis), warrants bypass technique or staged surgery in which the primary surgery is aimed at closure of tympanic membrane perforation with a graft and subsequently second stage surgery is performed after at least 3 months to restore hearing by stapedotomy. *(Endoscopic stapedotomy[4] has been described in respective chapter in this book.)*

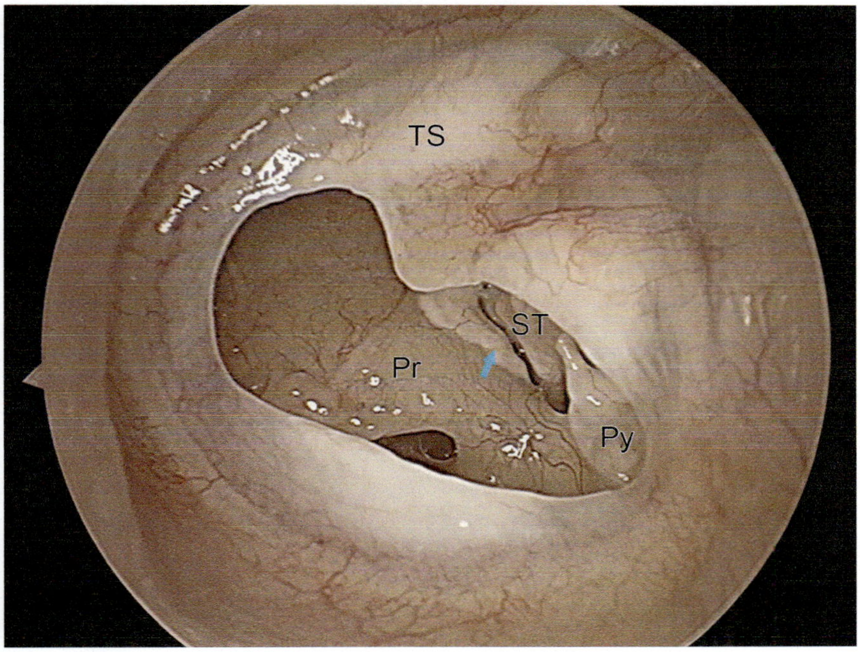

Fig. 19A: Type IV tympanosclerosis (TS): Involving stapes (ST).
(Pr: promontory; Py: processus pyramidalis)

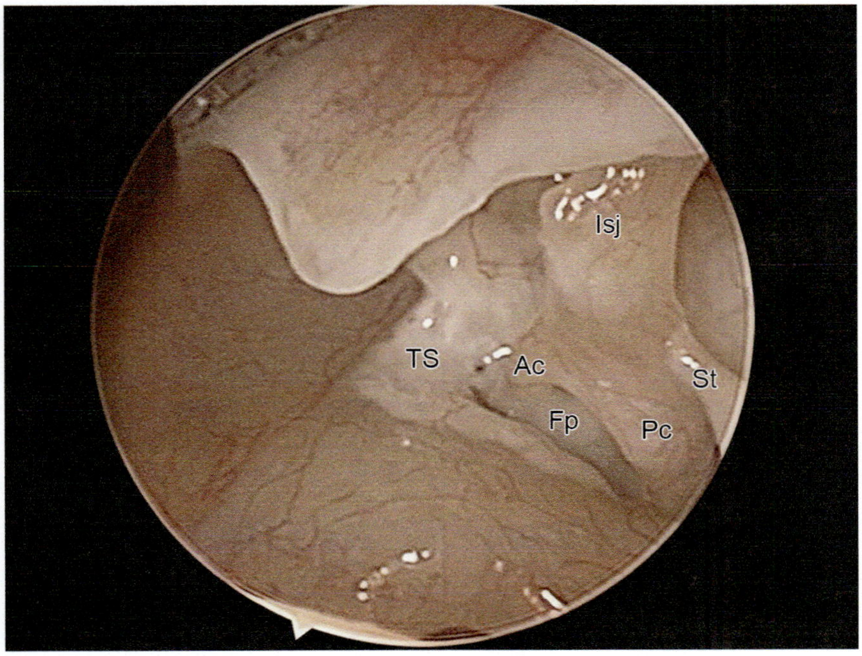

Fig. 19B: Type IV tympanosclerosis (TS): View through perforation showing TS on anterior crus (Ac), posterior crus (Pc), foot plate (Fp). Incudostapedial joint (Isj) and stapedius muscle (St) also shown here.

PEARL

- Chances of SNHL in management of type IV tympanosclerosis due to the need for stapes mobilization. Thus, excessive manipulation is to be avoided.
- Always look for perilymph fistula[5]

- *N.B*: Tympanic membrane defect is closed with temporalis fascia graft in all the cases by underlay technique. Gelfoam is used to support the tympanomeatal flap and the attic defect created to gain exposure is repaired with ipsilateral tragal cartilage.

REFERENCES

1. Mckee GJ, Karr AG. Tympanosclerosis: a scanning electron microscopic study. Clin Otol. 1989;14:11-6.
2. Bhaya MH, Schachern PA, Morizono T, Paparella MM. Pathogenesis of tympanosclerosis. Otolaryngol Head Neck Surg. 1993;109(3 Pt 1):413–20. (ISSN: 0194-5998)
3. Pal I, Sengupta A. Clinicopathological and audiological study of tympanosclerrosis. Indian J Otolaryngol Head Neck Surg. 2005;57:235-9.
4. Kamal, S. Surgery of tympanosclerosis. J Laryngol Otol. 1997;111(10):917-23.
5. GDL S. Tympanomastoid disease. In: Gibb AG, MFW S, editors. Otology. London: Butterworths; 1982. pp. 3-18.

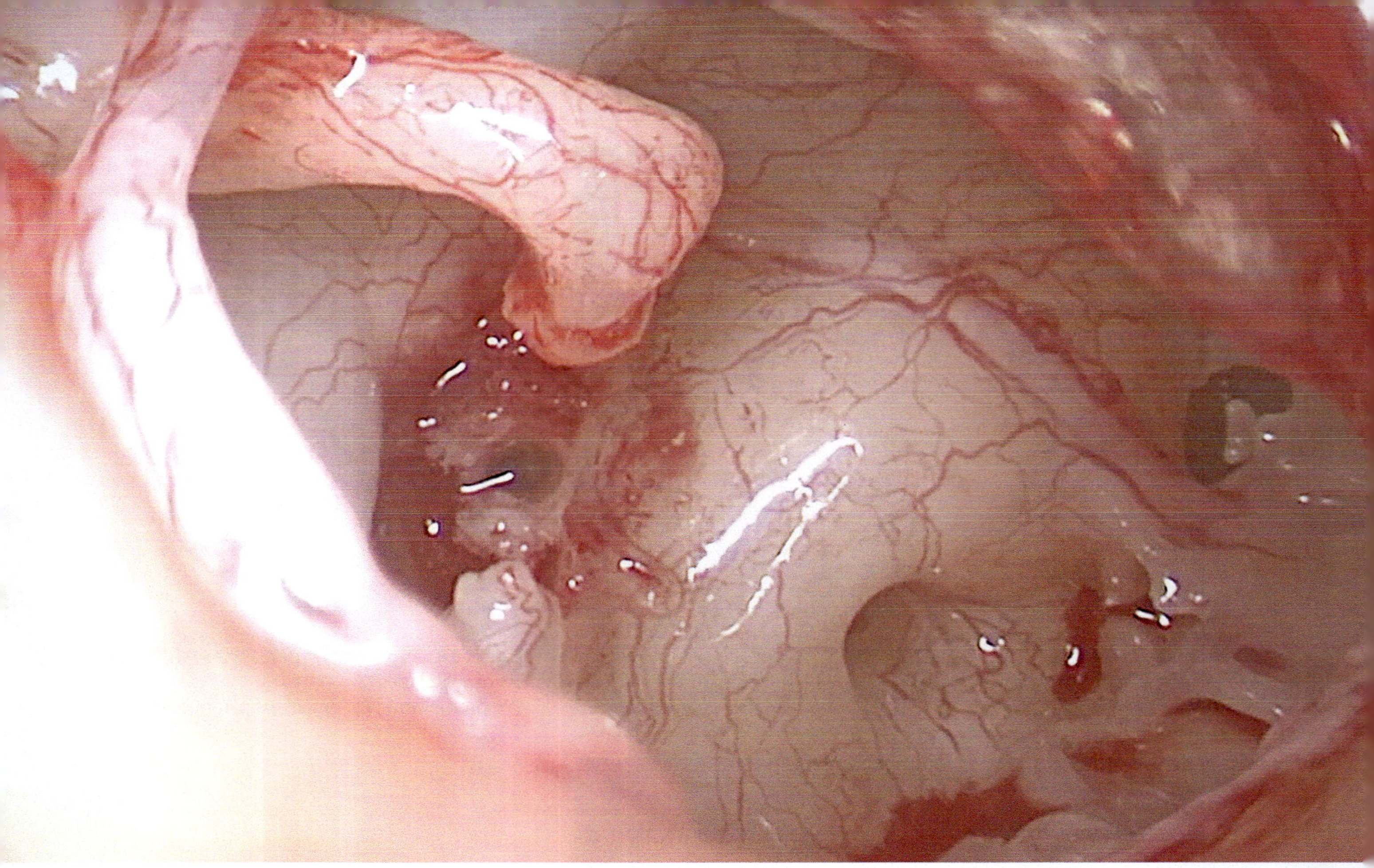

CHAPTER 13

Endoscopic Stapes Surgery

Arindam Das, Sandipta Mitra

Chapter Outline

INTRODUCTION

Otosclerosis has been defined as a localized hereditary disorder of metabolism of otic capsule enchondral bone that is characterized by disordered resorption and deposition of bone.[1]

A number of surgical approaches for treatment of otosclerosis have been described in literature, of which the most noteworthy are stapedotomy and stapedectomy. Stapedotomy is the creation of an opening in the footplate of stapes followed by placement of a stapes prosthesis. Shea performed the first stapedectomy in the year 1956. He is regarded as the pioneer of the modern surgical treatment of otosclerosis.[2]

Endoscopes offer a wider panoramic and magnified view of the working area without sacrifice of any soft tissue lying ahead. In contrast, in microscopic stapedotomy, it is often required to curette the posterosuperior canal wall in order to visualize the incudostapedial complex with considerable amount of chorda tympani manipulation.

It has been found that endoscopic stapedotomy entails lesser bone removal, chorda tympani handling, better visibility of the footplate area, lesser operating time, less postoperative pain, and minimal postoperative taste alteration when compared to microscopic stapedotomy.[3]

SPECIAL PREOPERATIVE CONSIDERATIONS

- *Preoperative diagnostic otoendoscopy*: This can be useful to know the gross anatomical dimension and slant of the external auditory canal, presence of any major canal humps, etc. These factors, especially for beginners have significant impact as it enables careful planning before surgery
- *Preoperative imaging*: In clinically suspicious or revision cases, imaging can give valuable clues regarding anatomical variations such as wide vestibular aqueduct which may give rise to an intraoperative gusher. In such cases, sole endoscopic approach may not turn out to be successful and that a back-up microscope should be kept at hand.

SPECIAL INSTRUMENTS FOR ENDOSCOPIC STAPES SURGERY

- Annulus elevator
- 2 mm angled pick
- Angled curette
- Curved microscissors
- Angled measuring rod (Fisch)
- Perforators of different sizes
- Hand burrs
- Skeeter drill

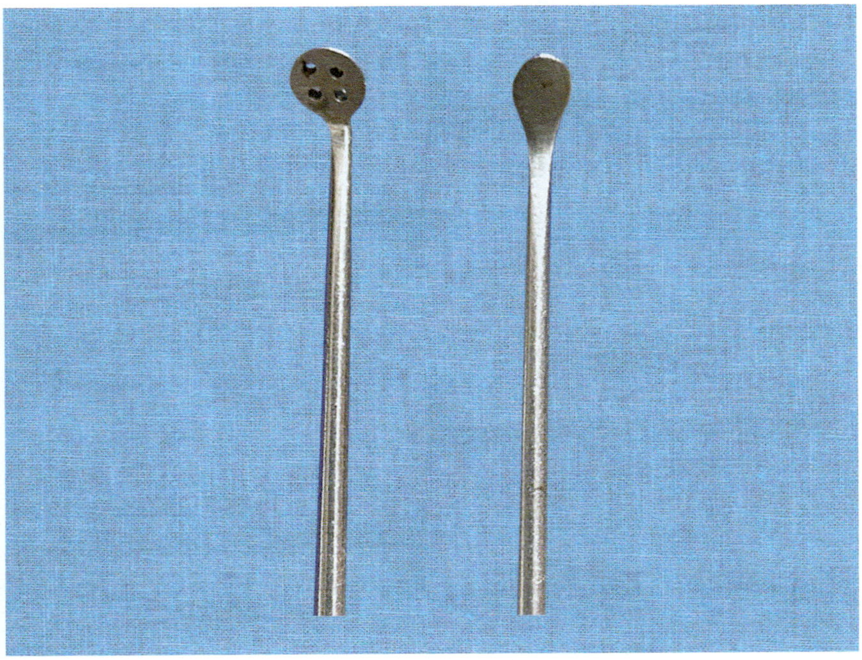

Fig. 1: Round knife and annulus elevator.

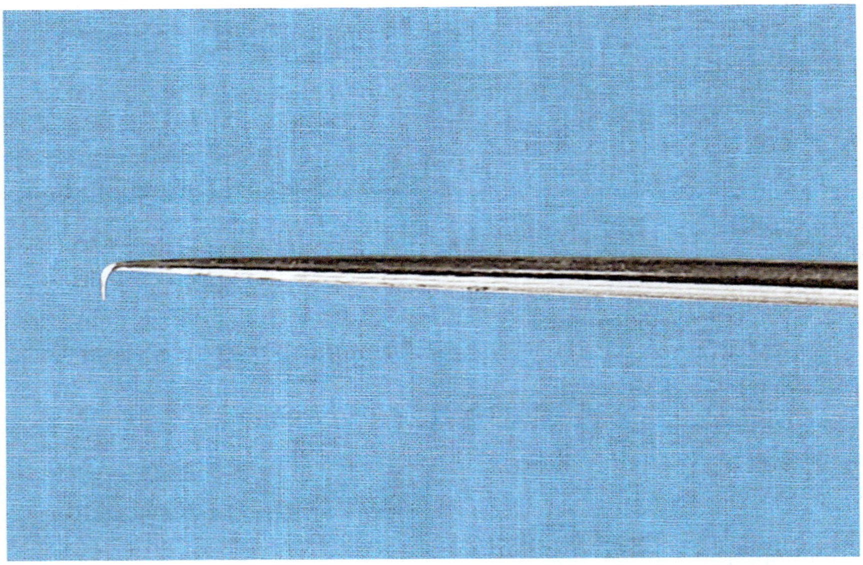

Fig. 2: 2 mm angled pick.

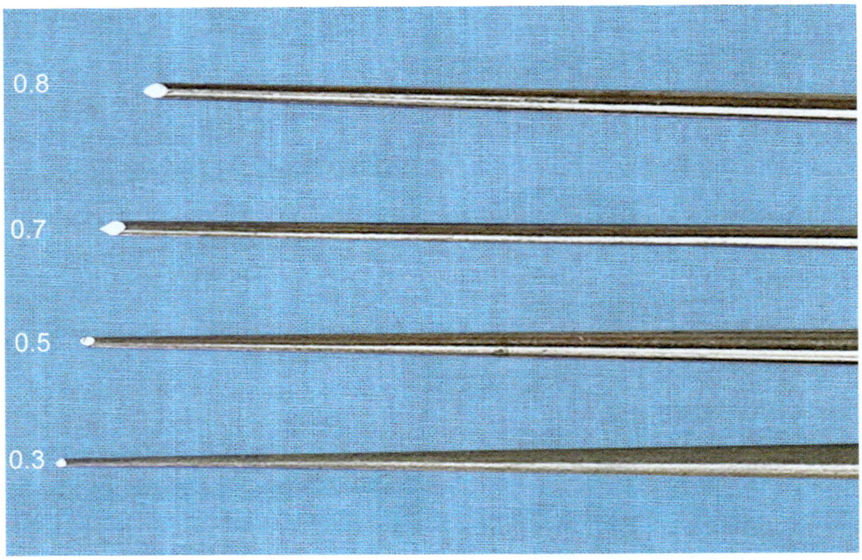

Fig. 3: Perforators of different sizes.

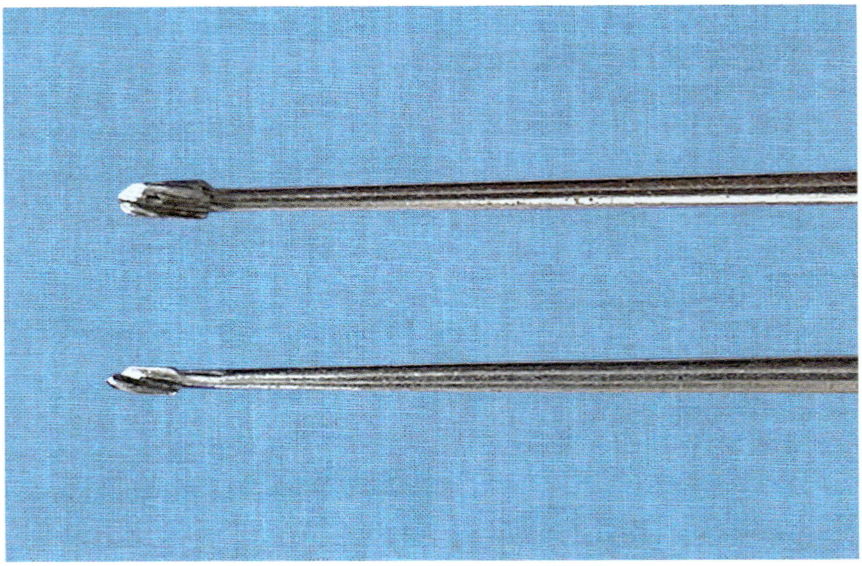

Fig. 4: 0.8 and 0.9 mm hand burrs.

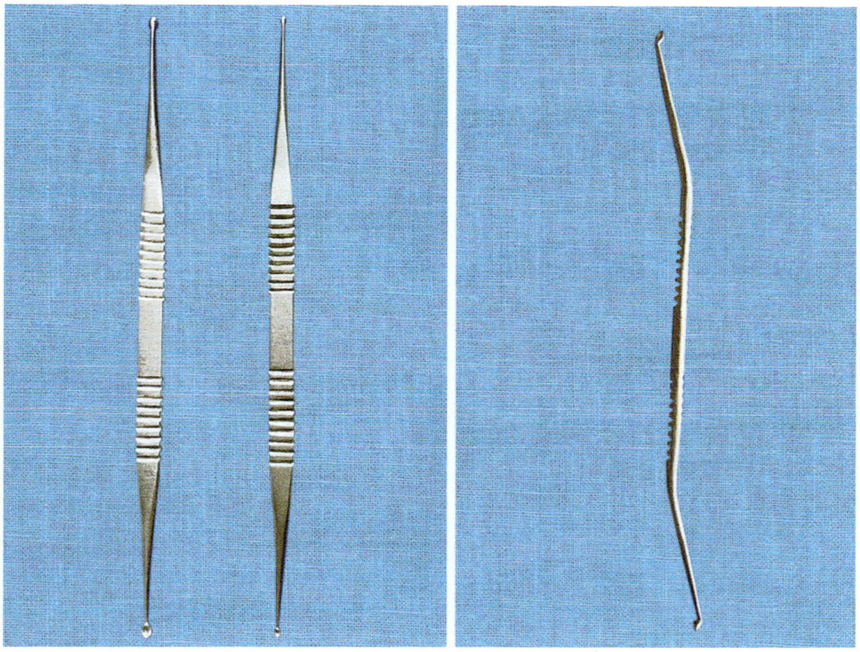

Fig. 5: Angled curette of different sizes.

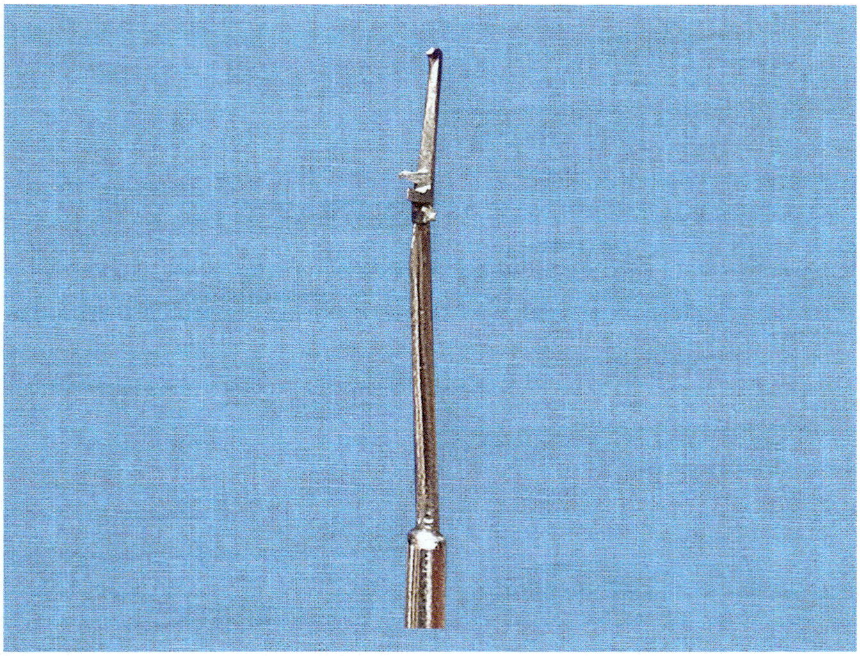

Fig. 6: Angled measuring rod (Fisch).

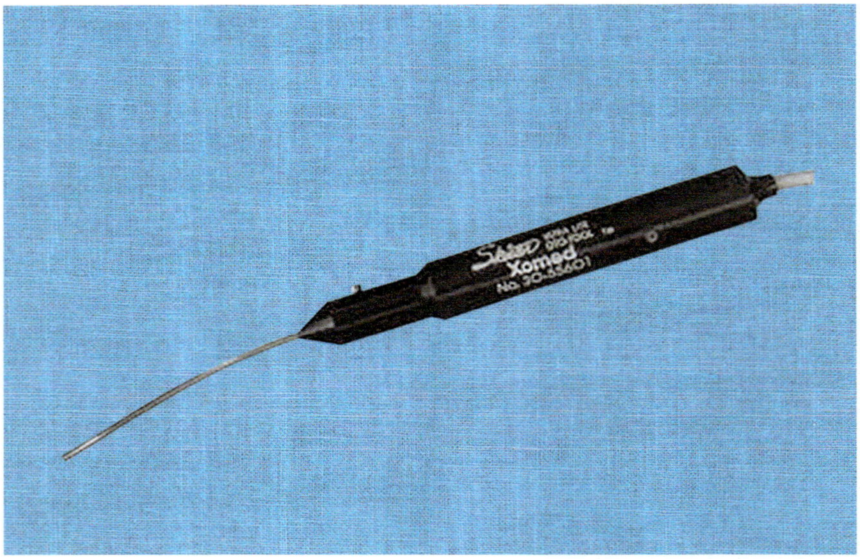

Fig. 7: Skeeter drill.

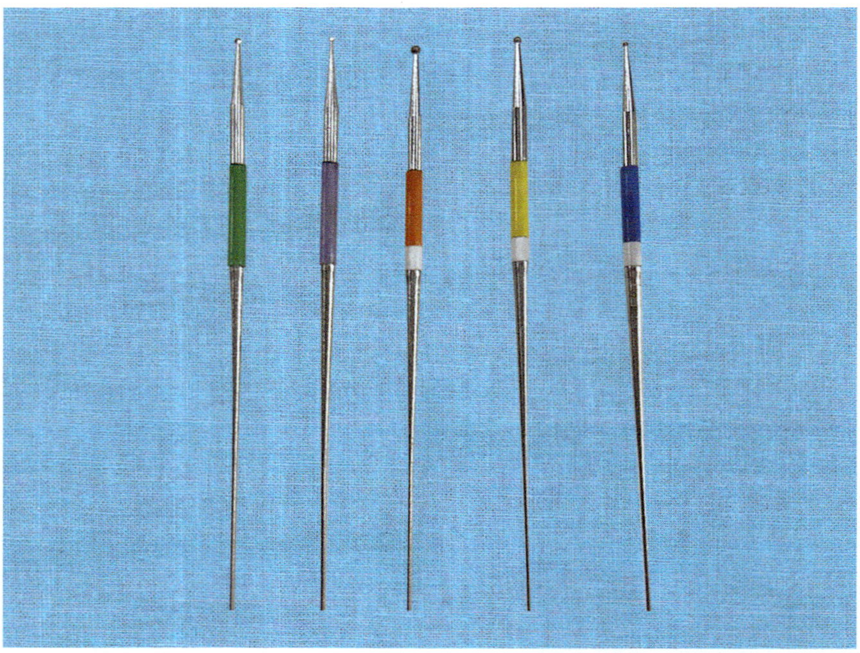

Fig. 8: Burrs for skeeter drill; single color—cutting burr, dual colored—diamond burr.

ENDOSCOPIC STAPEDOTOMY

Endoscopic stapedotomy	*Microscopic stapedotomy*
• Chorda tympani nerve is identified • The nerve is dissected minimally to obtain a ledge of bone to engage the curette • Minimal bone curettage • Nerve transposed back into its neocanal superiorly • Better visualization of incudostapedial complex	• Greater volume of bone has to be removed in order to attain a similar view of incudostapedial complex

- *Anesthesia:* Four quadrant infiltration with 2% Lidocaine with Adrenaline (1:1 00,000).

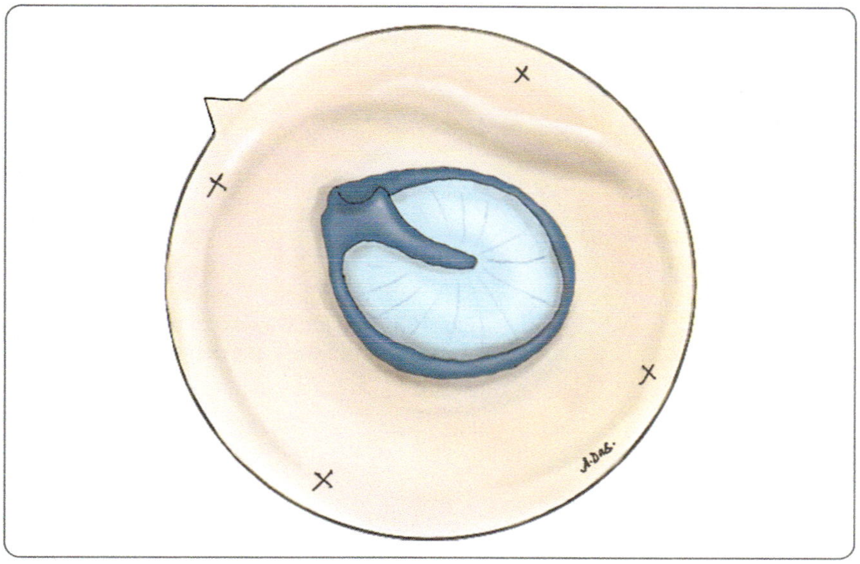

Fig. 9: Sites of four quadrant infiltration of local anesthesia (marked with x).

TIP

For anesthesia, needle of a finer gauge is of choice, to minimize trauma. Insulin syringe of 1cc capacity is the most appropriate for four quadrant infiltration.

PEARL

Lower gauge needles may cause trauma to canal skin and lead to bleb or hematoma formation. This again may impede visualization and pose difficulty during surgery. In case of such a situation, the bleb or hematoma may be punctured with a fine tipped angled pick followed by application of pressure with cotton ball soaked in adrenaline.

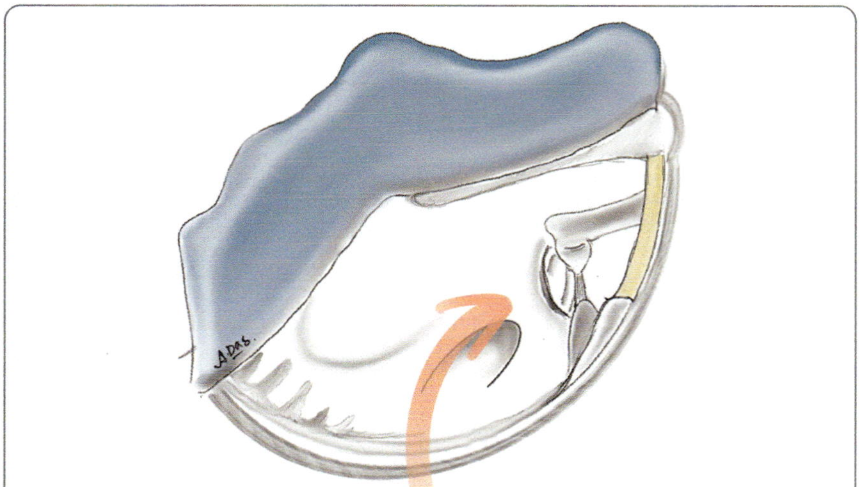

Fig. 10A: Working window of endoscopic stapedotomy. Schematic depiction.

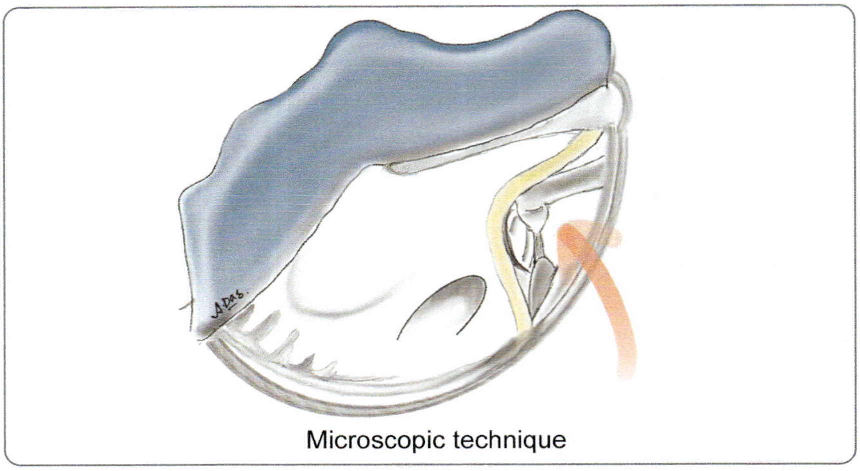

Fig. 10B: Working window of microscopic stapedotomy. Schematic depiction.

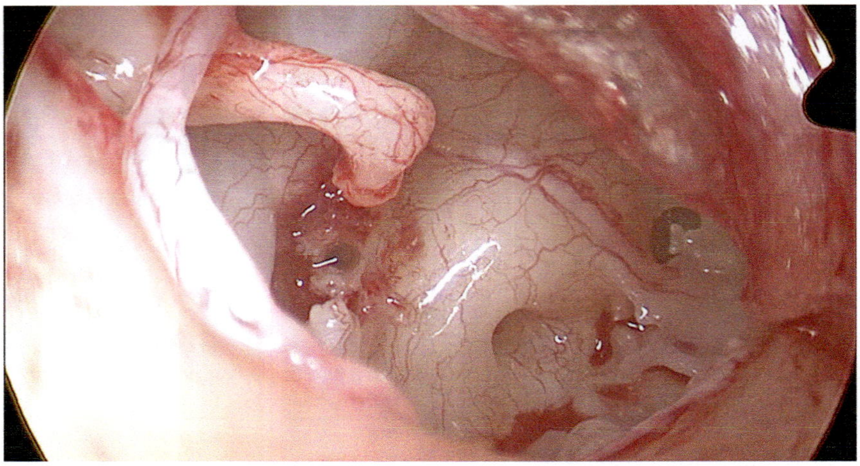

Fig. 10C: Working window of endoscopic stapedotomy.

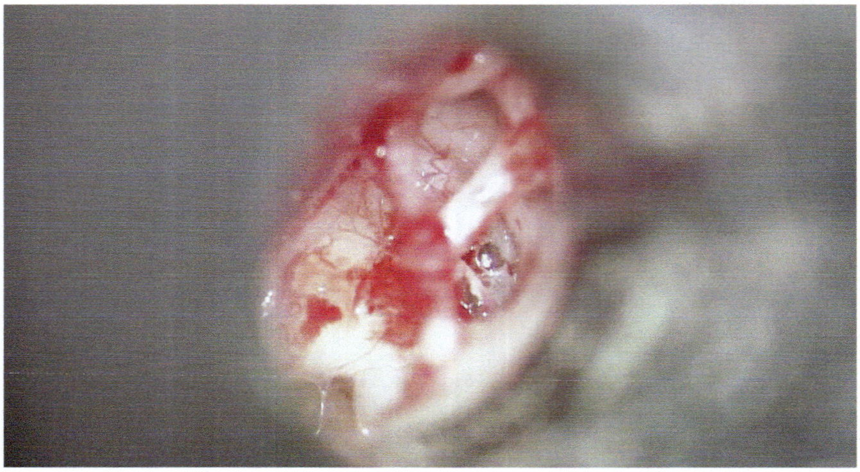

Fig. 10D: Working window of microscopic stapedotomy (transcanal technique using aural speculum).

Incision

- Incision is made 4–6 mm lateral to the annulus and curved superiorly just anterior to the lateral process of malleus.

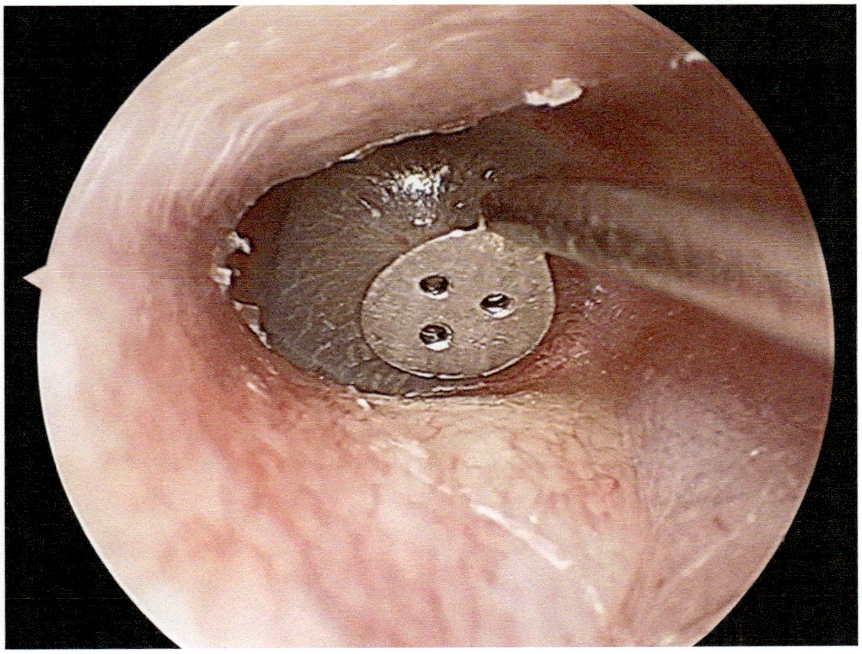

Fig. 11: Palpation of annulus with the help of round knife to correctly identify the site of incision.

> **TIP**
>
> Always palpate the position of the annulus prior to fashioning of the incision. The incision is then fashioned with respect to the position of the annulus.

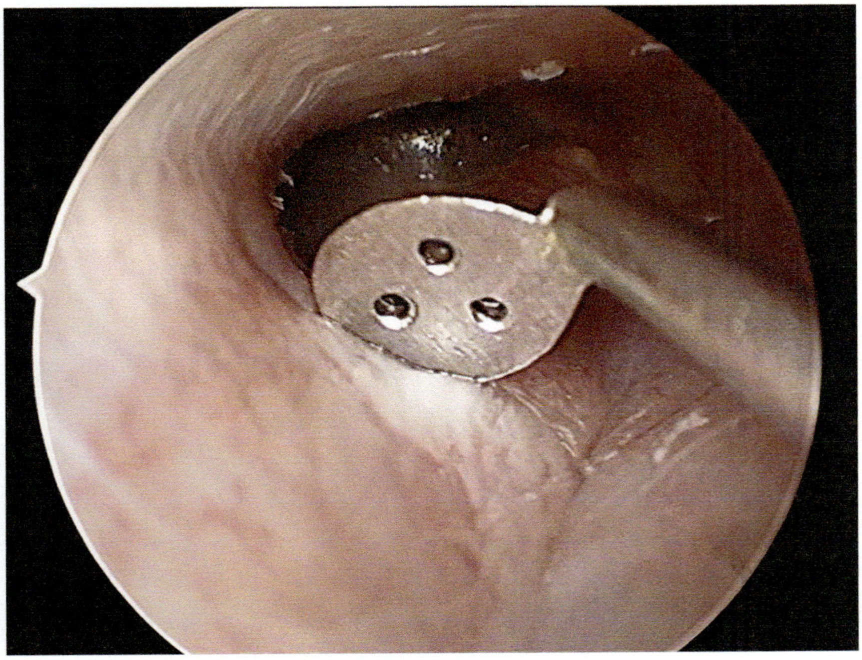

Fig. 12A: Horizontal limb of incision being placed 4–6 mm lateral to the annulus (left ear).

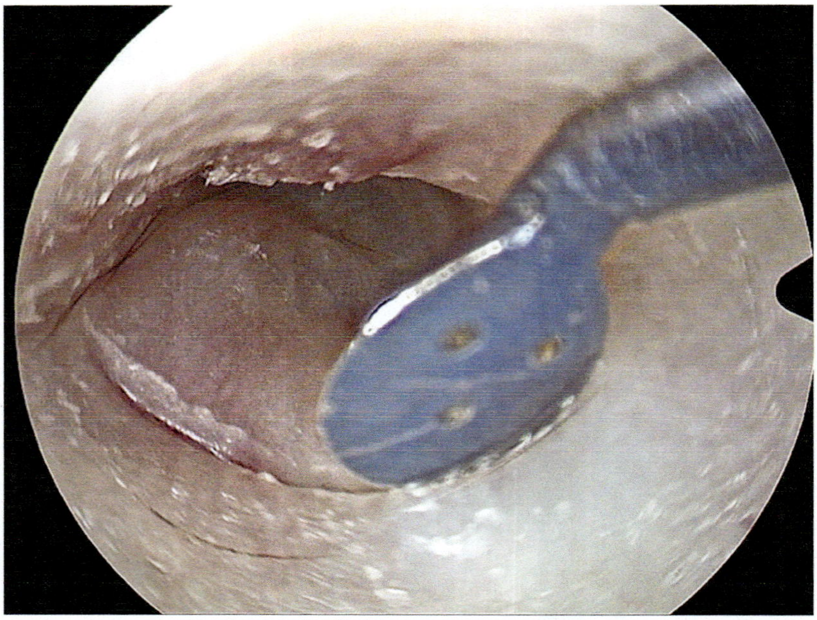

Fig. 12B: Horizontal limb of incision being placed 4–6 mm lateral to the annulus (right ear).

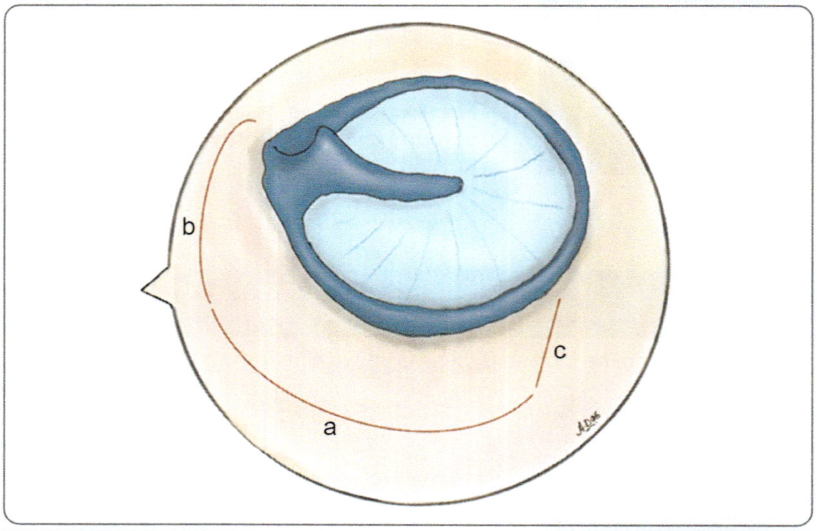

Fig. 13A: Schematic depiction of the three limbs of incision in right ear marked as a—horizontal limb, b—superior limb, c—inferior limb.

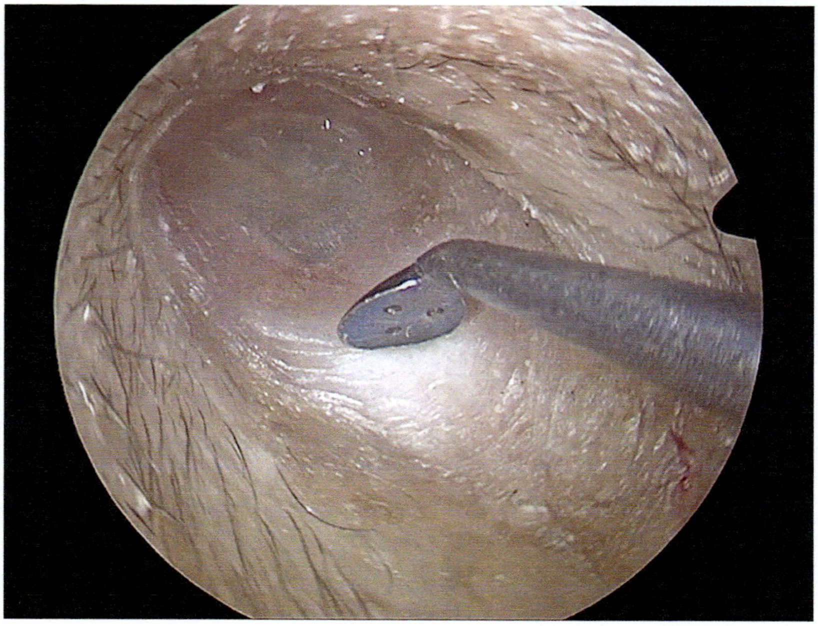

Fig. 13B: Horizontal limb of incision being placed with a sharp circular knife.

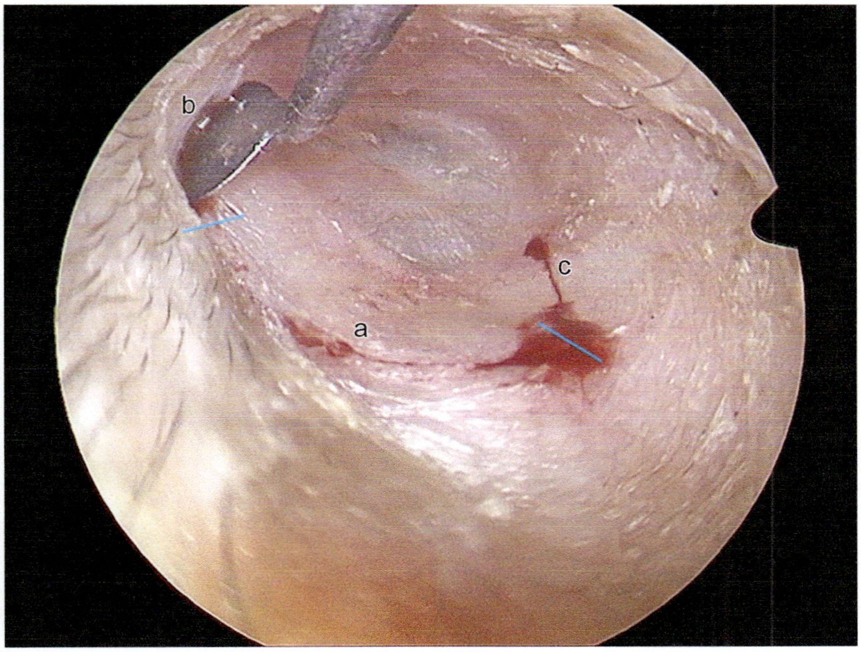

Fig. 13C: Superior limb of the incision being placed with circular knife.
(a—horizontal limb, b—superior limb, c—inferior limb)

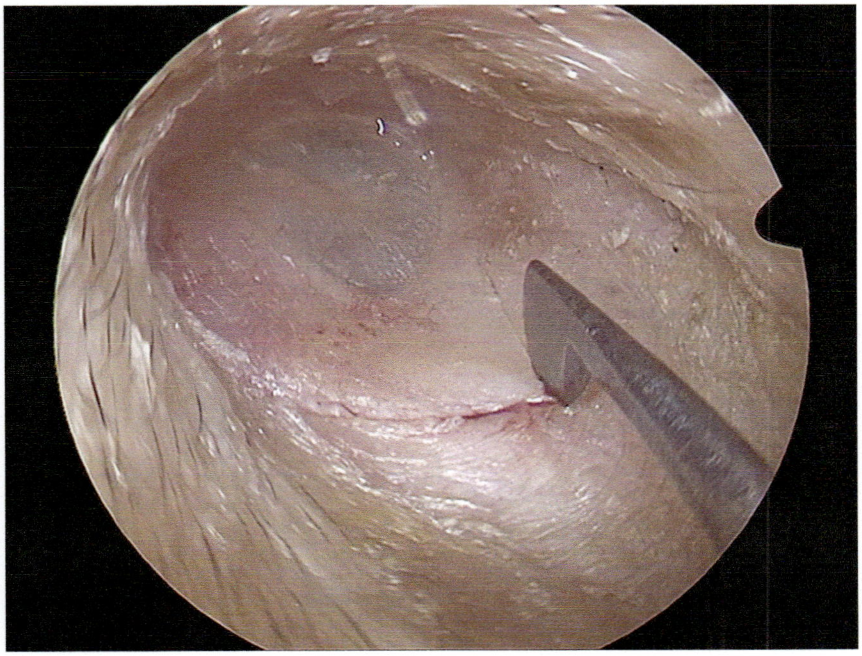

Fig. 13D: Inferior limb of incision being placed a side knife.

- The incision is extended inferiorly up to 6-O' clock position.
- Superiorly, the incision is extended just anterior to the lateral process of the malleus.

TIP

Anterior edge of the superior incision is cut sharply with angled micro or spring scissors

TIP

Sharpest available round knife is to be used for incision to avoid crush injury to canal wall soft tissue and subsequent tissue loss

Flap Elevation

- Tympanomeatal flap is gently raised till the level of the annulus.

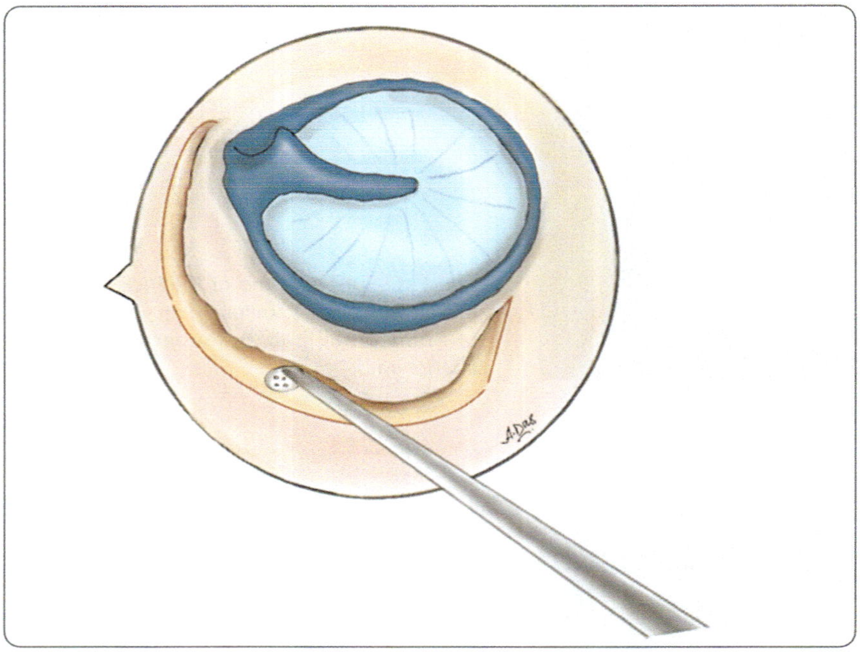

Fig. 14A: Schematic depiction of elevation of tympanomeatal flap.

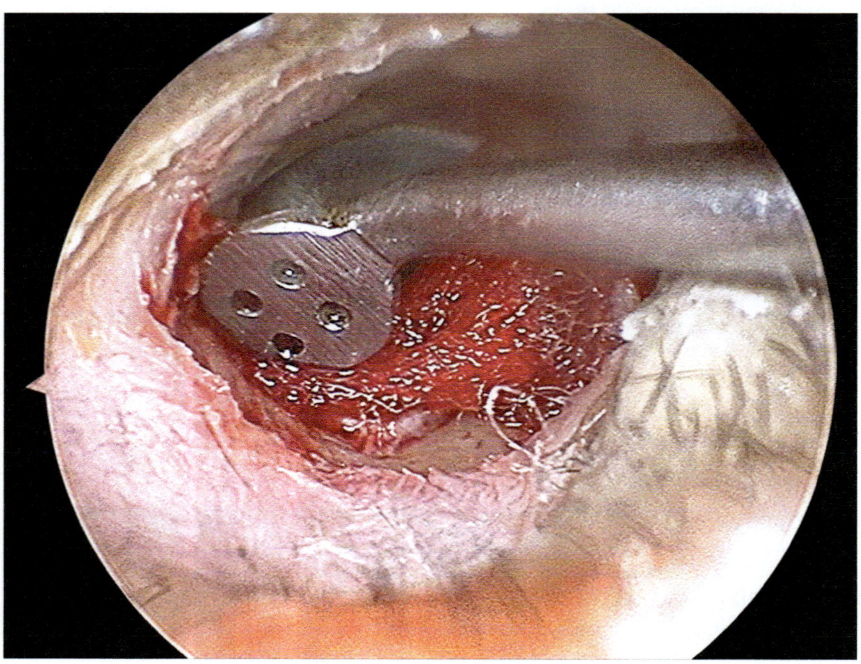

Fig. 14B: Flap elevation using adrenaline-soaked cotton pledgets.

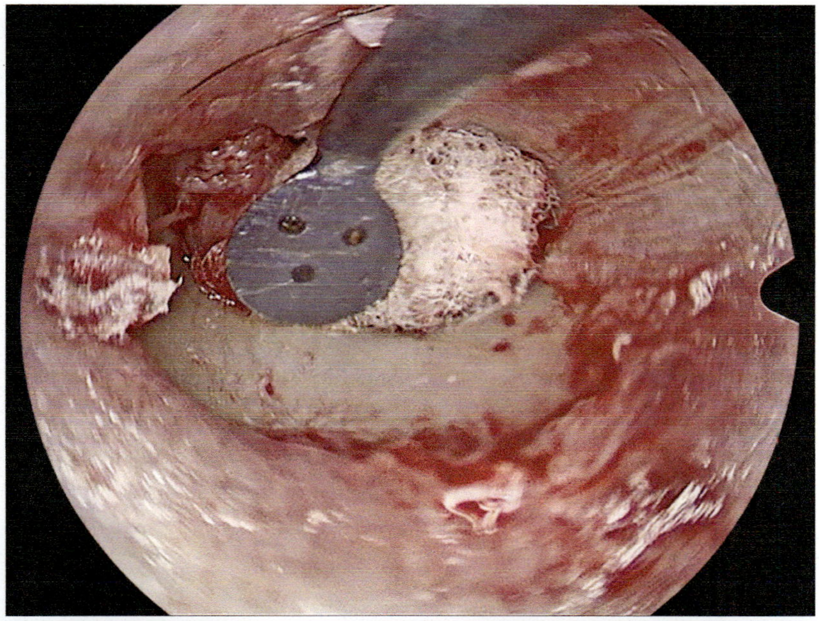

Fig. 14C: Flap elevation using adrenaline-soaked cotton pledgets: Note the direction of exertion of pressure over the bone, not over the pledget.

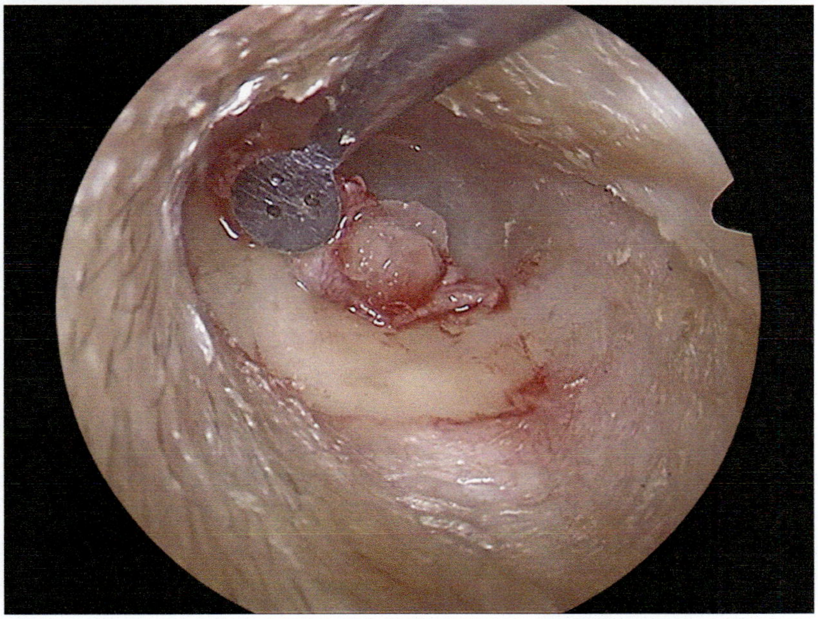

Fig. 14D: Flap elevation using adrenaline-soaked cotton pledgets; Note the bloodless field maintained using adrenaline soaked pledgets.

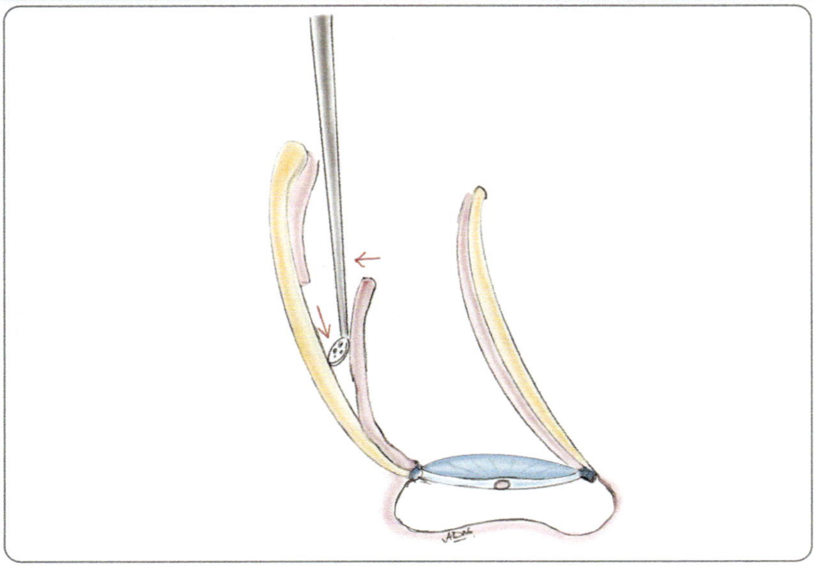

Fig. 15A: The correct direction of force during flap elevation grazing the bone of the external auditory canal to ensure flap integrity.

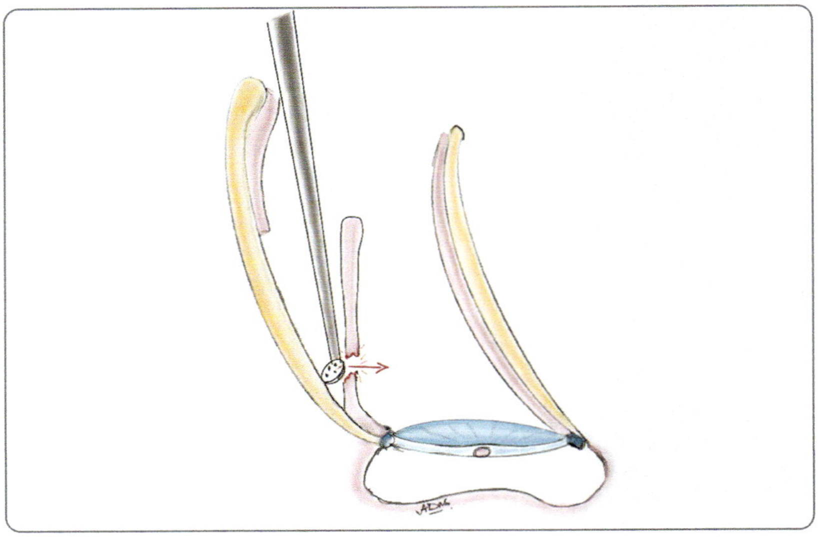

Fig. 15B: Misdirection of the force toward the flap may cause flap tear

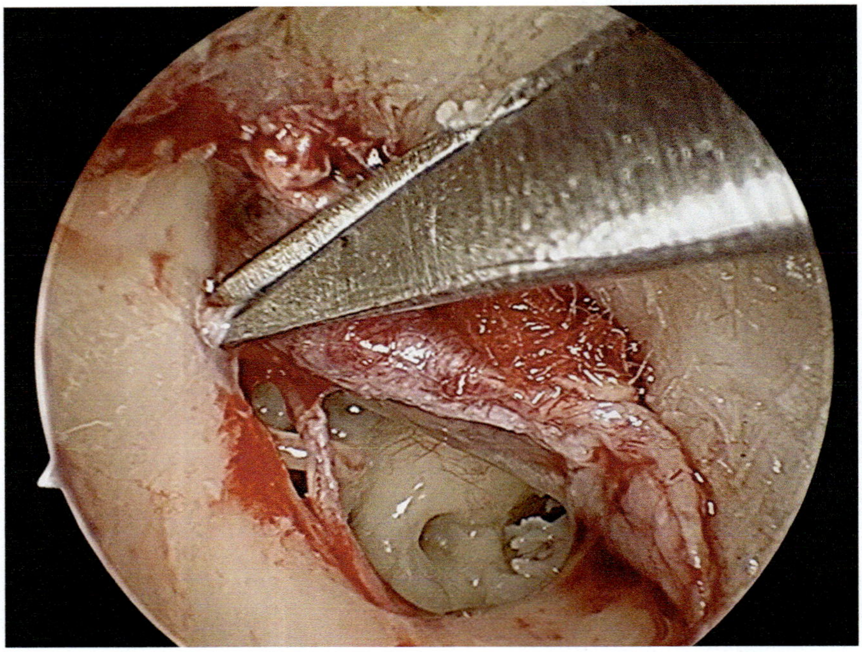

Fig. 16: Anterosuperior part of the flap fibres being tougher are sharply cut using an iris or microscissors.

TIP

- Use of cotton balls soaked in undiluted adrenaline at this stage helps in flap elevation, ensures flap protection from suction damage, and minimizes bleeding and soiling of the scope. Any bleeding point must be addressed promptly prior to entry into middle ear.

TIP

- Depending on the extent of bleeding, a stepwise approach must be followed that includes adrenaline soaked cotton balls, insulated monopolar ball point cautery and tranexamic acid according to protocol described previously.

Chorda Tympani Dissection

- Upon reaching the annulus, careful dissection is done so as to identify and preserve the chorda tympani nerve.

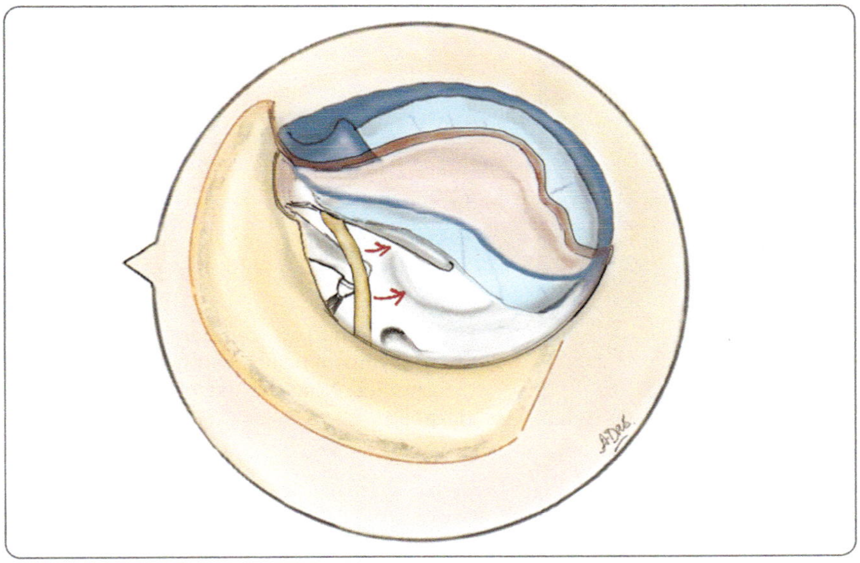

Fig. 17A: Method of chorda tympani dissection: Schematic depiction.

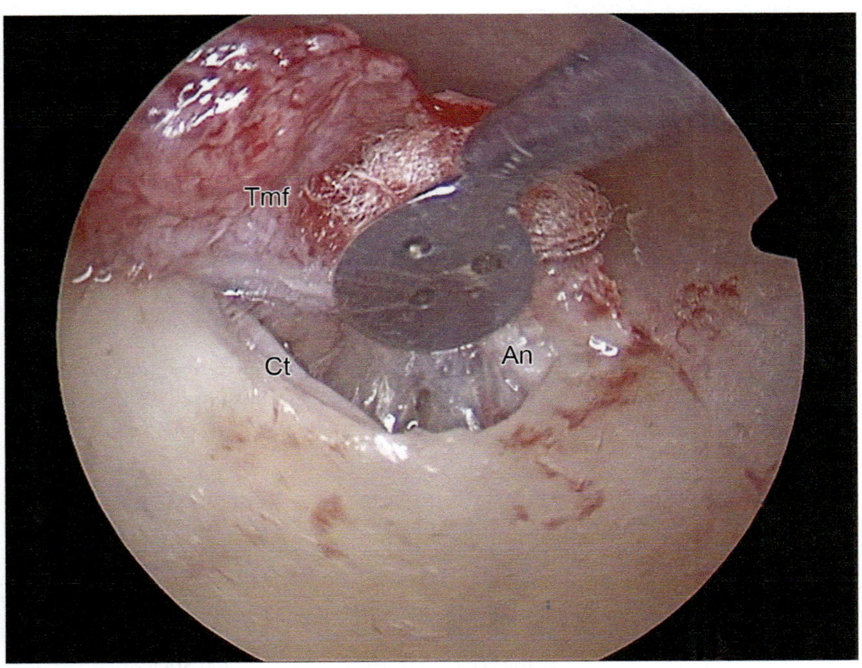

Fig. 17B: Method of chorda tympani dissection: Landmarks identified.
(Ct: chorda tympani nerve; An: annulus; Tmf: tympanomeatal flap)

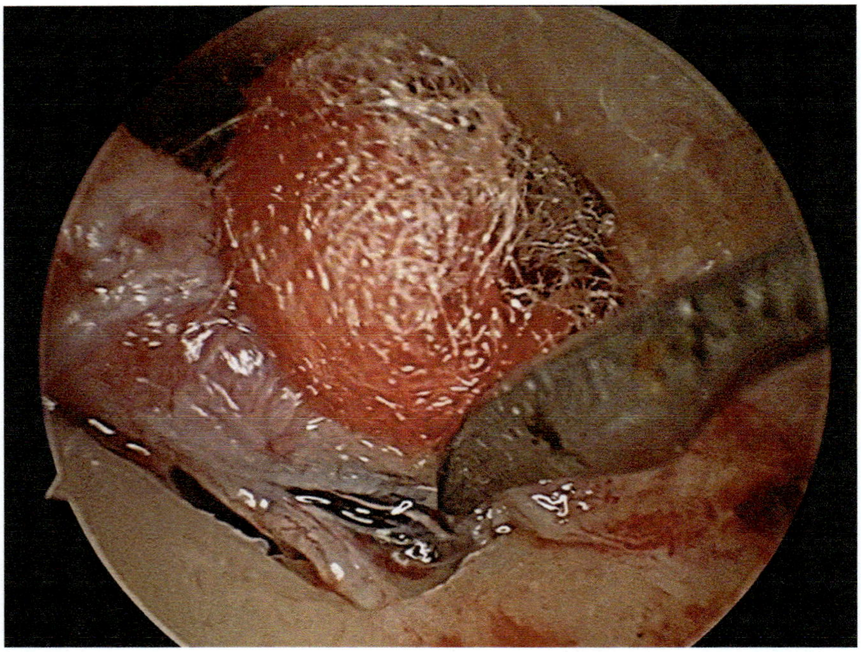

Fig. 17C: Method of chorda tympani dissection: Chorda tympani being sharply dissected from the annulus. Note the use of sickle knife for elevation.

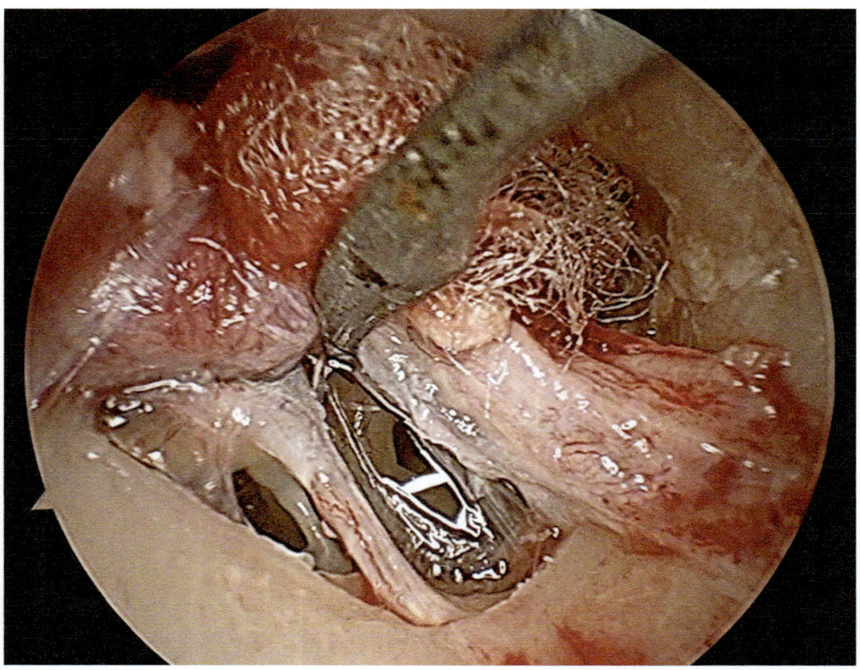

Fig. 17D: Method of chorda tympani dissection: Chorda tympani being sharply dissected from the annulus in the superior direction.

TIP

- Posterior tympanic spine serves as a valuable landmark as the starting point of annulus elevation. A curved instrument is negotiated in the space between the annulus and the chorda to separate the two followed by elevation of the annulus till 6 o'clock position.

TIP

- Minimal manipulation of chorda tympani should be done as far as practicable.

Tympanotomy

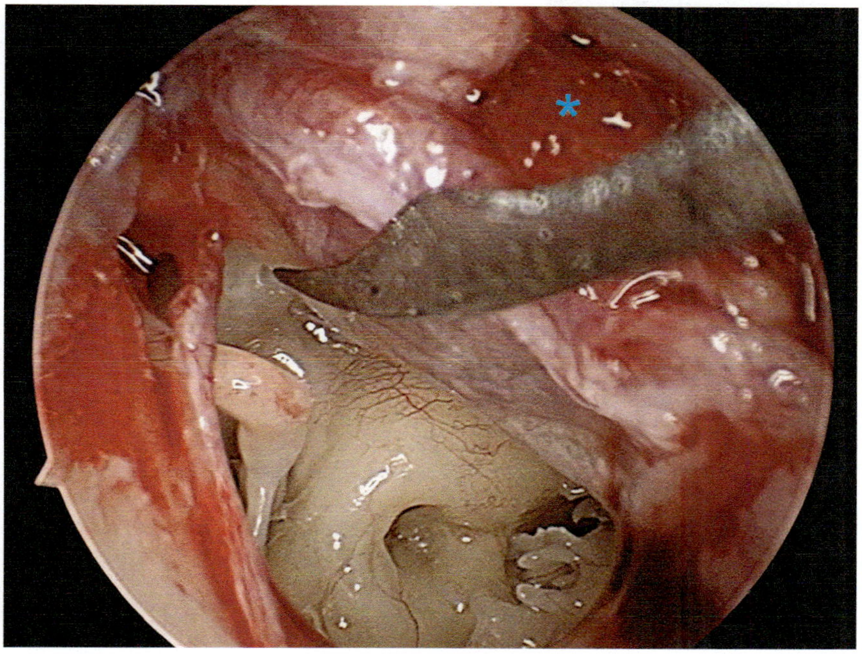

Fig. 18: Flap being stabilized anteriorly with a piece of gelfoam soaked in saline (blue asterisk).

- Once the flap has been elevated anteriorly, it is kept stable, away from the working field with a gelfoam soaked in normal saline which, at the same time, keeps the flap hydrated.

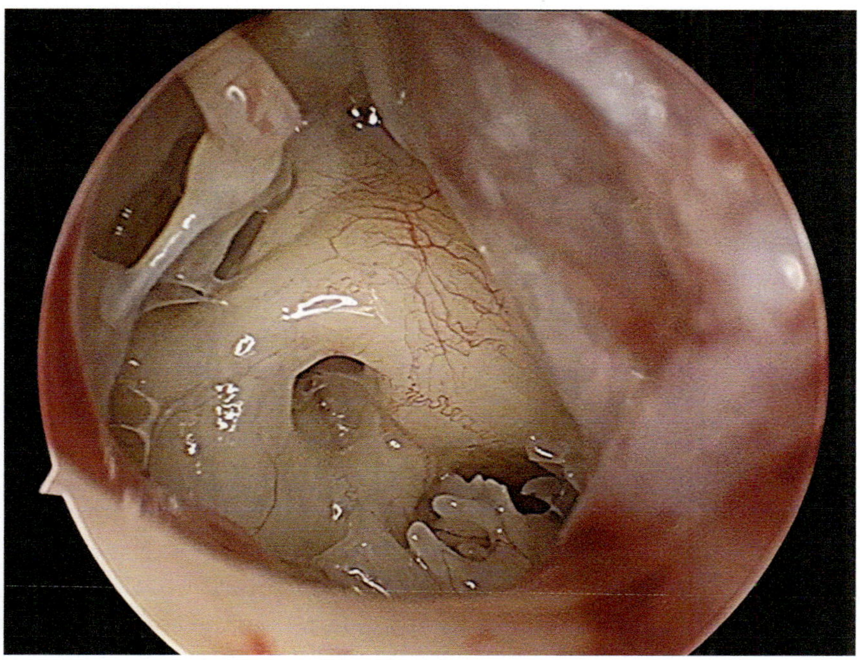

Fig. 19A: Complete exposure of the working corridor seen by positioning the scope in an inferior-to-superior direction.

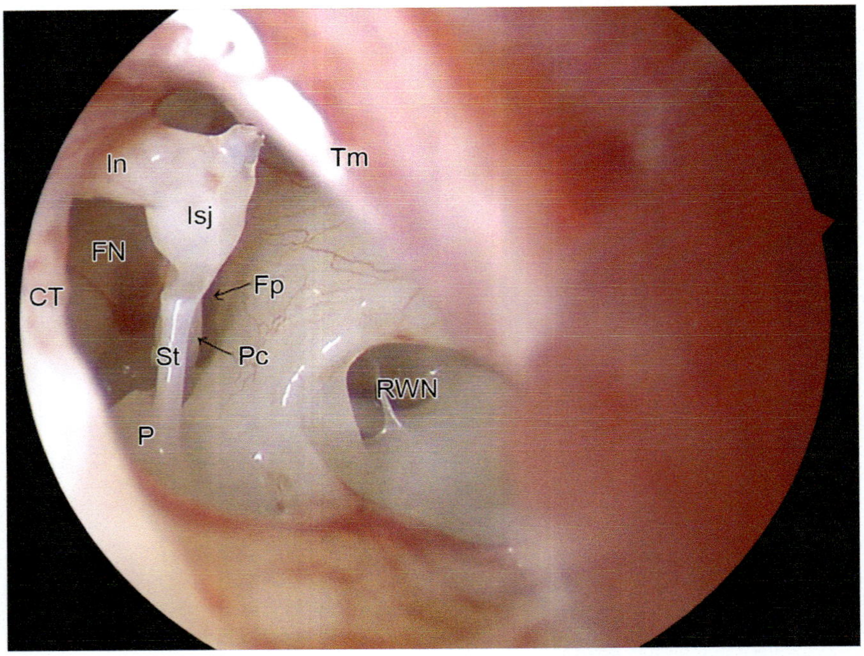

Fig. 19B: Complete exposure of the working corridor showing important landmarks. (CT: chorda tympani; FN: facial nerve, In: incus; Isj: incudostapedial joint; St: stapedius tendon; P: pyramid; Pc: posterior crura; Fp: footplate; RWN: round window niche; Tm: tympanic membrane)

PEARL

Endoscopes, especially 30° (Karl Storz 2.7 mm diameter, 18 cm length), at this stage, provide a clear view of the working area that includes the pyramidal eminence, stapedius tendon, incudostapedial joint, footplate area, and horizontal portion of facial nerve, *minimizing the need of bone work involving the posterosuperior canal wall. The visibility of the incudostapedial complex is to be assessed at this stage. One must be able to pass a straight instrument up to the level of footplate once the exposure is adequate.*

Incudostapedial Complex Visibility

We classified the view of incudostapedial complex from the margin of the annulus into four groups:[3]

1. Grade I = Only I-S joint is visible
2. Grade II = I-S joint + Stapedius (partial) visible
3. Grade III = I-S joint + Stapedius (complete) + Tip of Pyramid visible
4. Grade IV = I-S joint + Stapedius (complete) + Pyramid till base visible

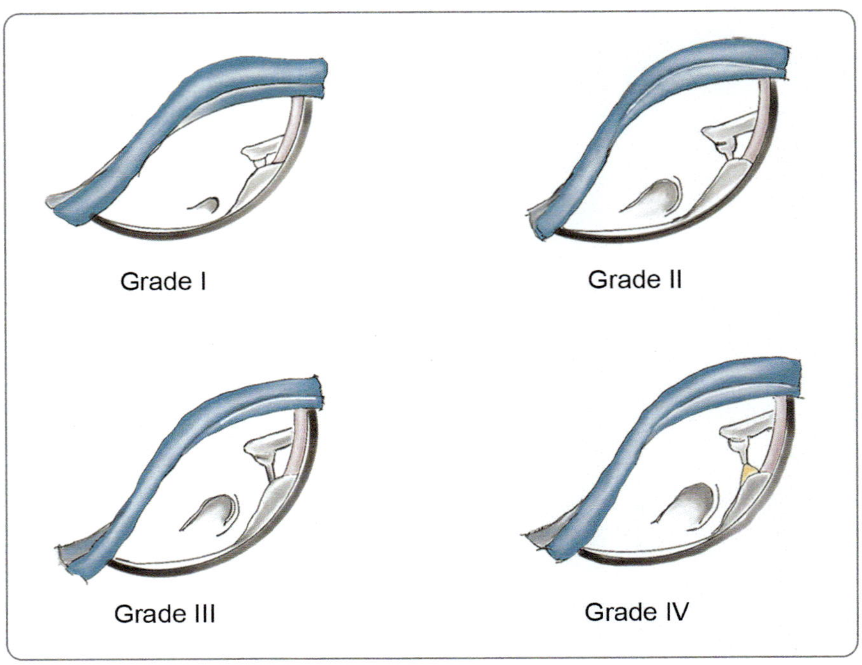

Fig. 20A: Grades of visibility of incudostapedial complex: Schematic depiction.

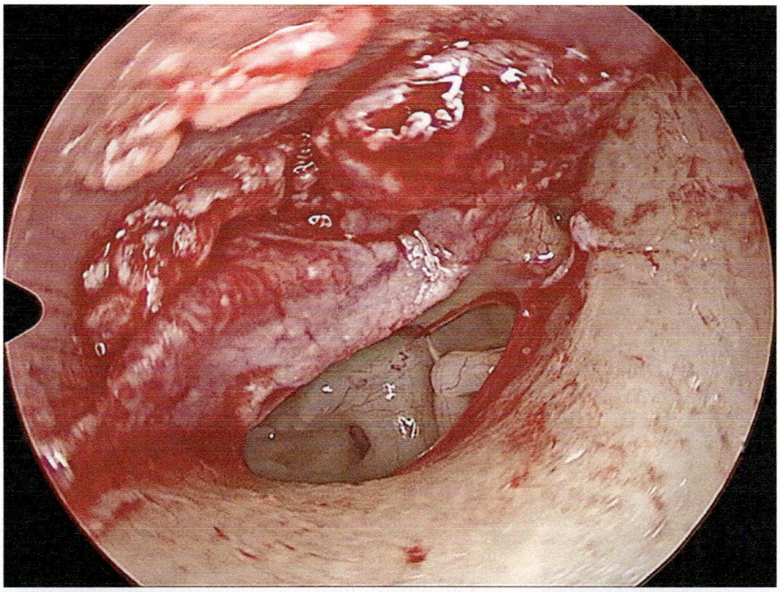

Fig. 20B: Grades of visibility of incudostapedial complex—Grade-I: Only I-S joint is visible.

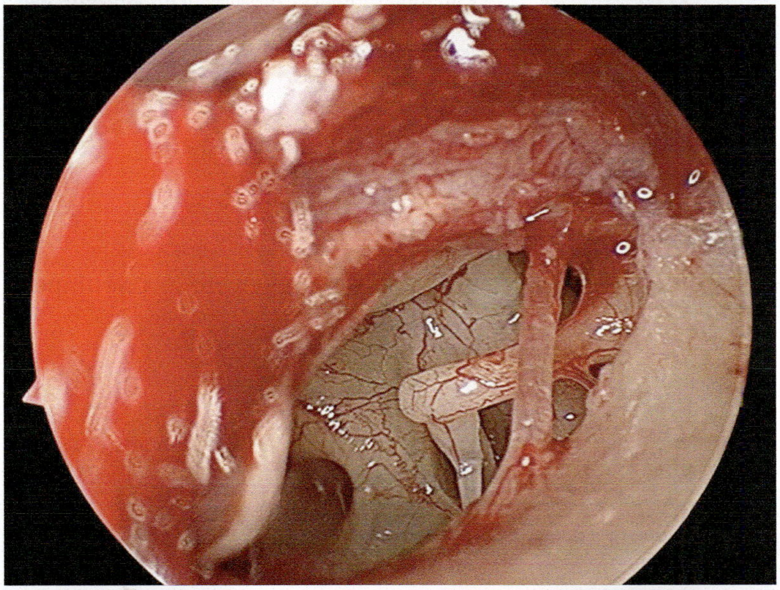

Fig. 20C: Grades of visibility of incudostapedial complex—Grade-II: I-S joint + Stapedius (partial) visible.

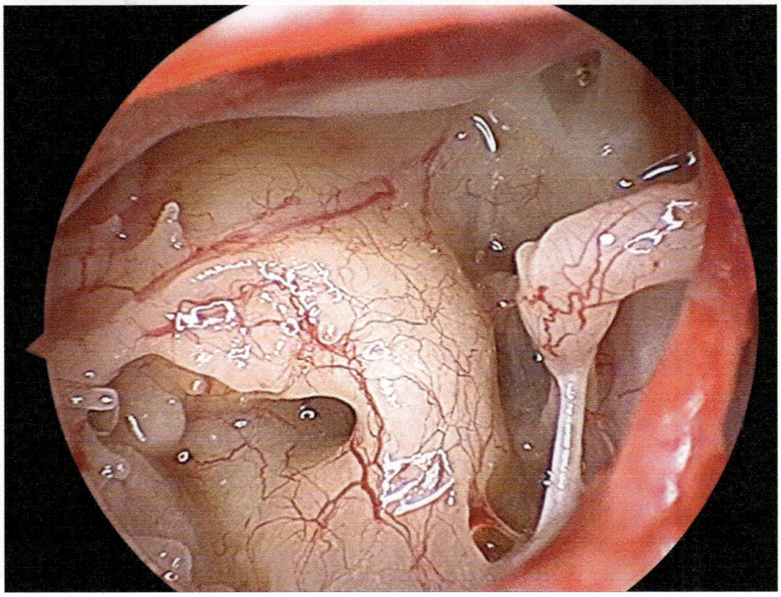

Fig. 20D: Grades of visibility of incudostapedial complex—Grade-III: I-S joint + Stapedius (complete) + Tip of Pyramid visible.

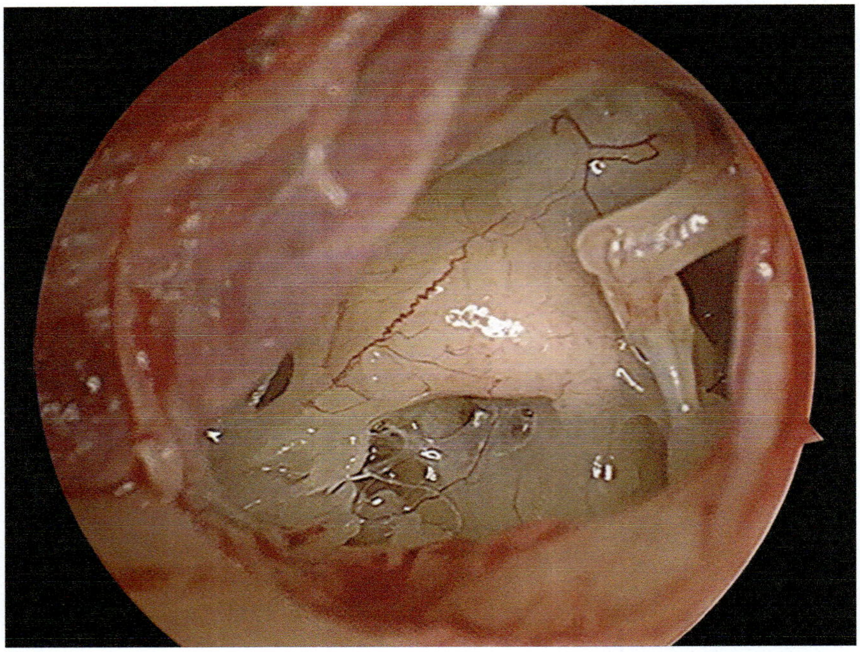

Fig. 20E: Grades of visibility of incudostapedial complex—Grade-IV: I-S joint + Stapedius (complete) + Pyramid till base visible.

Confirmation of Diagnosis

- Diagnosis is to be confirmed intraoperatively by gentle palpation of each ossicle separately with a fine-tipped microinstrument.

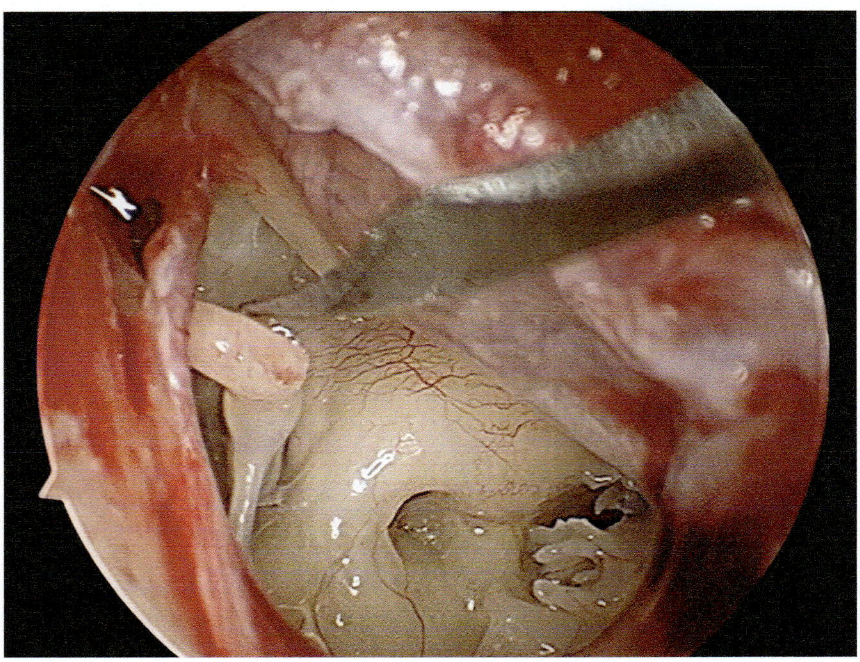

Fig. 21: Confirmation of diagnosis by palpation of individual ossicles. Note the direction of instrument (anterior-to-posterior) while palpating mobility of incus.

TIP

During palpation, it is imperative to follow the correct axis/direction to avoid iatrogenic ossicular dislocation. *Malleus is palpated in medial-lateral direction, incus in anterior-posterior and stapes in superior-inferior directions.*

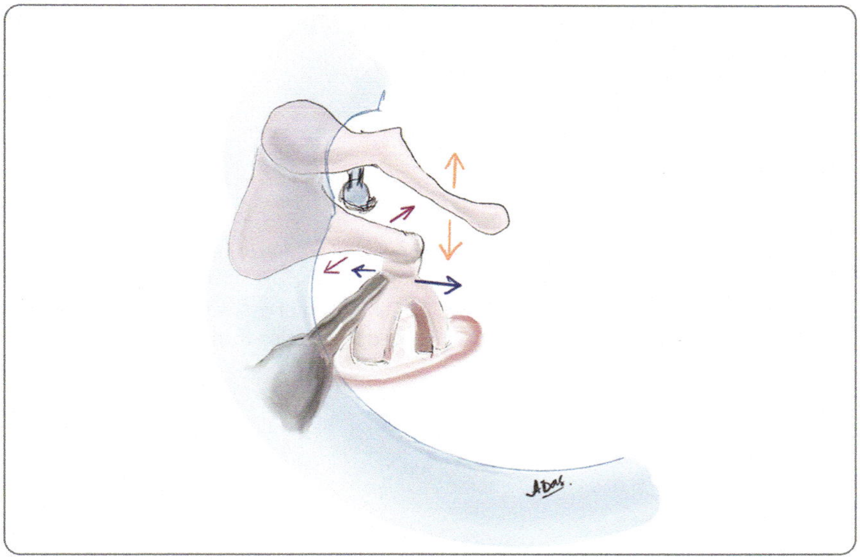

Fig. 22A: Schematic depiction of direction of palpation of ossicles to check mobility.

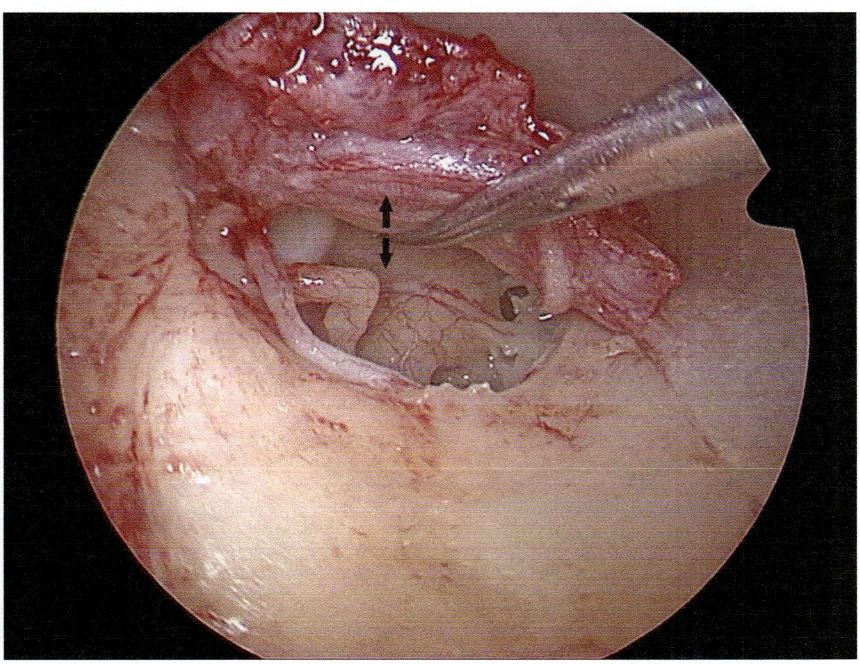

Fig. 22B: Method of ossicular palpation: Malleus is palpated in medial-to-lateral direction.

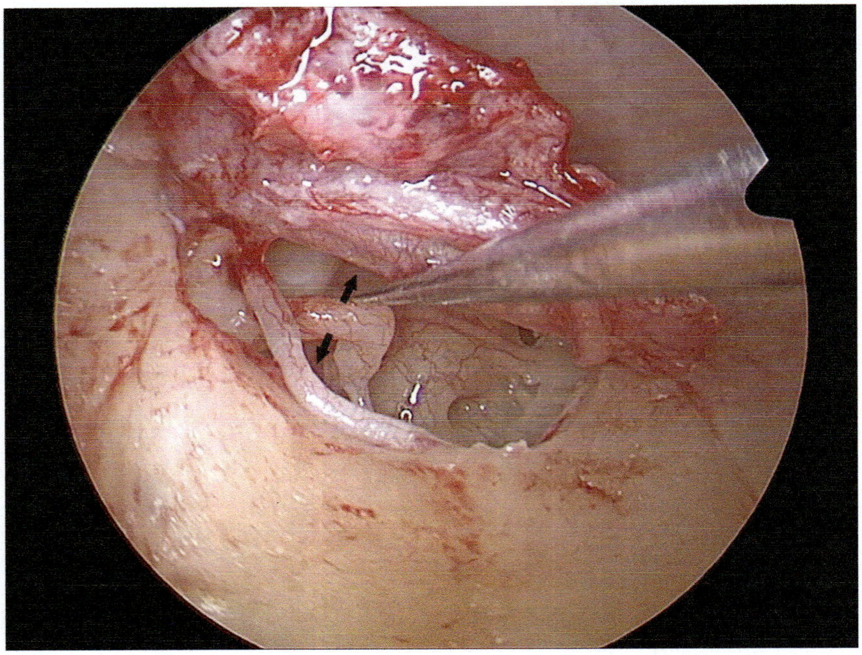

Fig. 22C: Method of ossicular palpation: Incus is palpated in anterior-to-posterior direction.

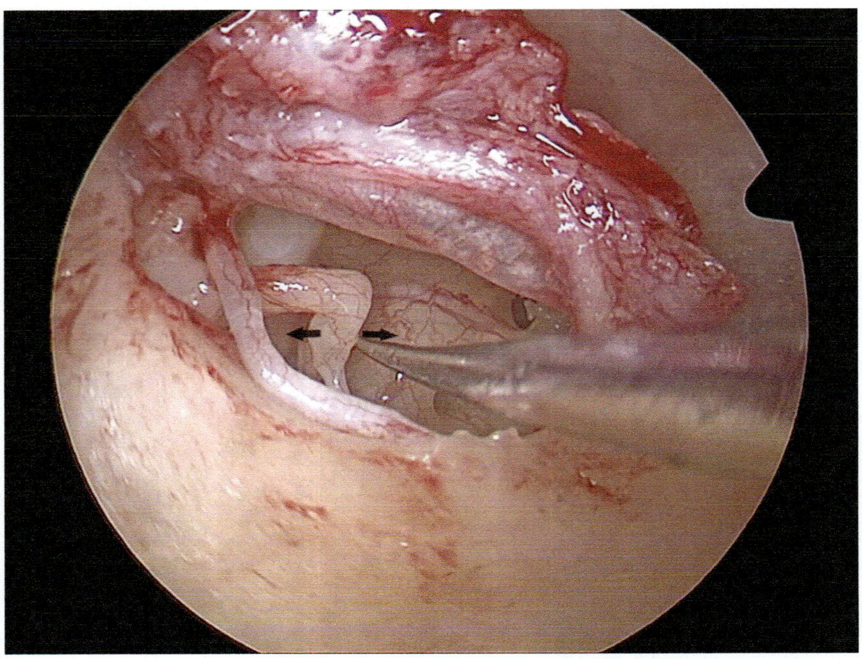

Fig. 22D: Method of ossicular palpation: Stapes is palpated in superior-to-inferior direction.

Bone Removal

- Posterosuperior canal wall may have to be curetted for adequate exposure. An angled curette is used to curette the canal wall, away from the ossicles, in order to optimally expose the incudostapedial complex.

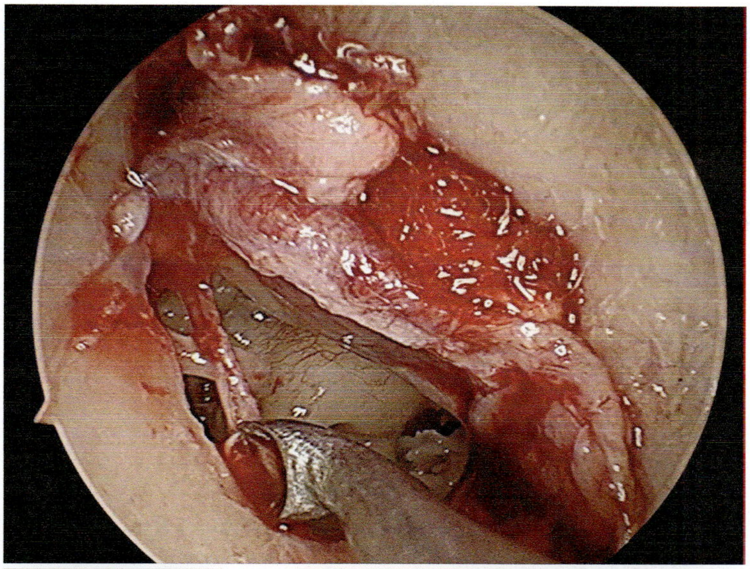

Fig. 23A: Posterosuperior canal wall curettage (Note the direction of curette is away from the ossicles) (right ear).

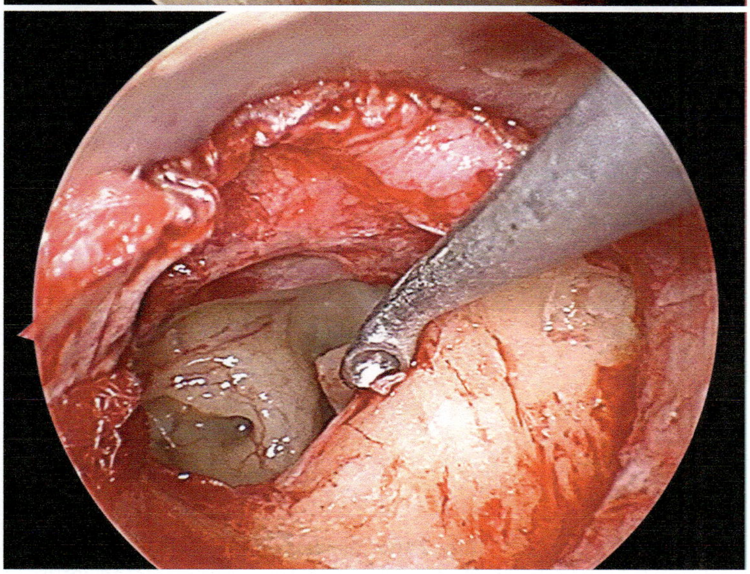

Fig. 23B: Posterosuperior canal wall curettage (Note the direction of curette is away from the ossicles) (left ear).

Final Exposure

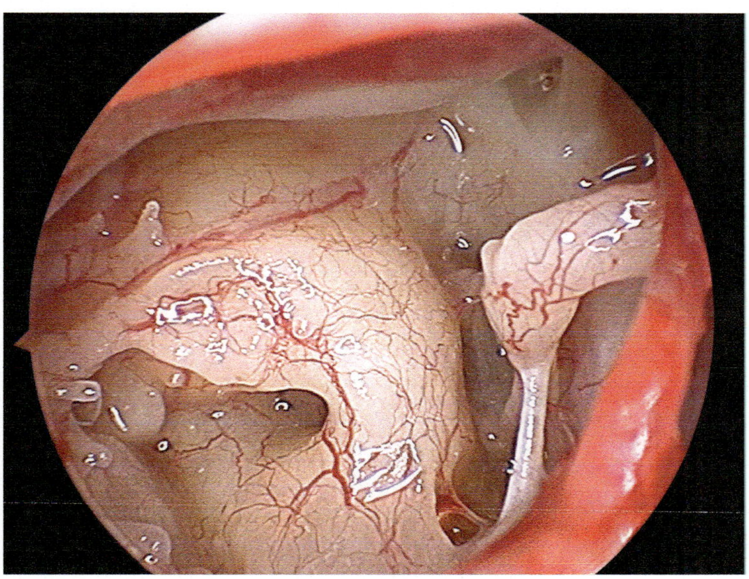

Fig. 24: Adequate exposure in stapes surgery; incudostapedial joint complex completely visible along with facial nerve (horizontal segment) superiorly and base of processus pyramidalis posteriorly.

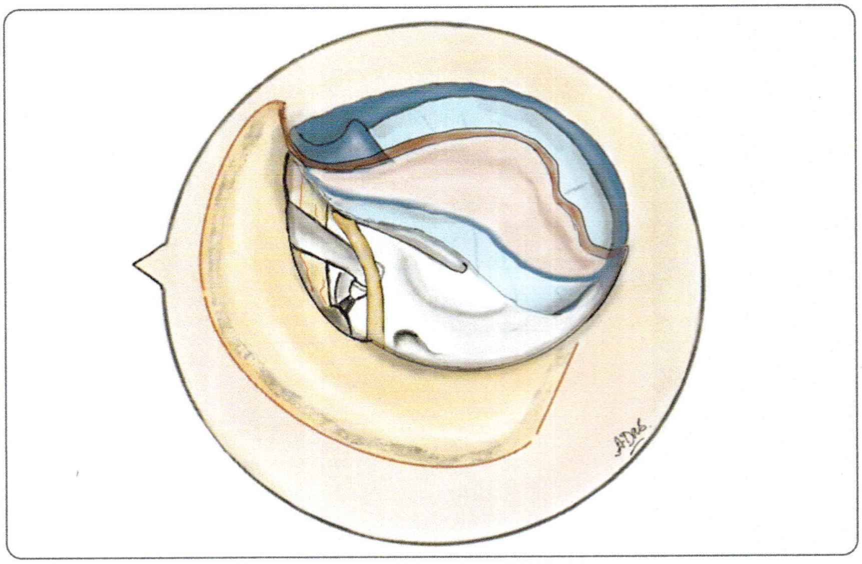

Fig. 25A: Chorda tympani reflected inferiorly during posterior canal wall bone curettage.

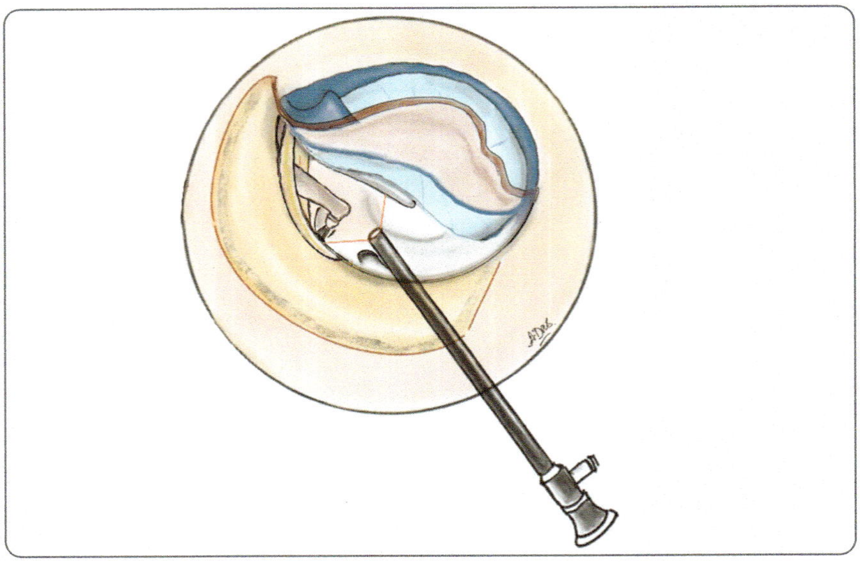

Fig. 25B: Chorda tympani repositioned in its neo-canal and endoscope directed infero-superiorly to visualize the working corridor.

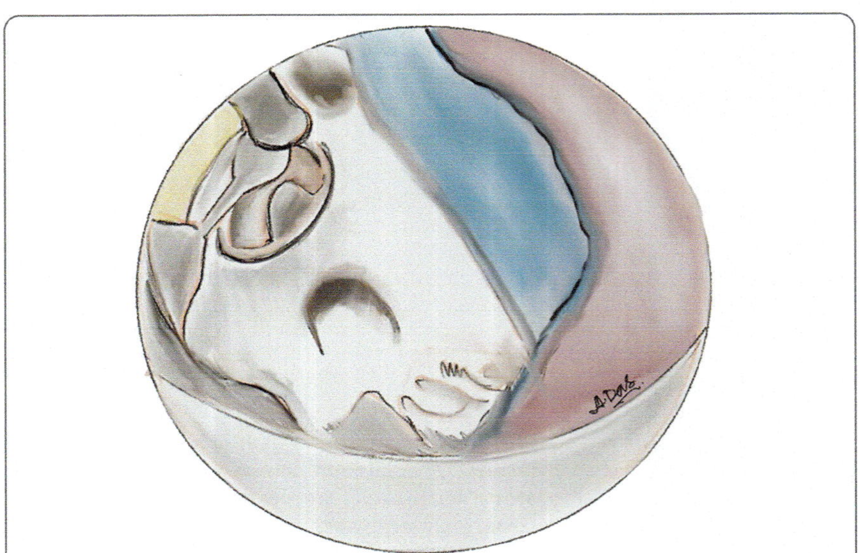

Fig. 26A: View of working corridor in an inferosuperior direction with the help of endoscope (Note the visibility of anterior and posterior crura with footplate): Schematic depiction.

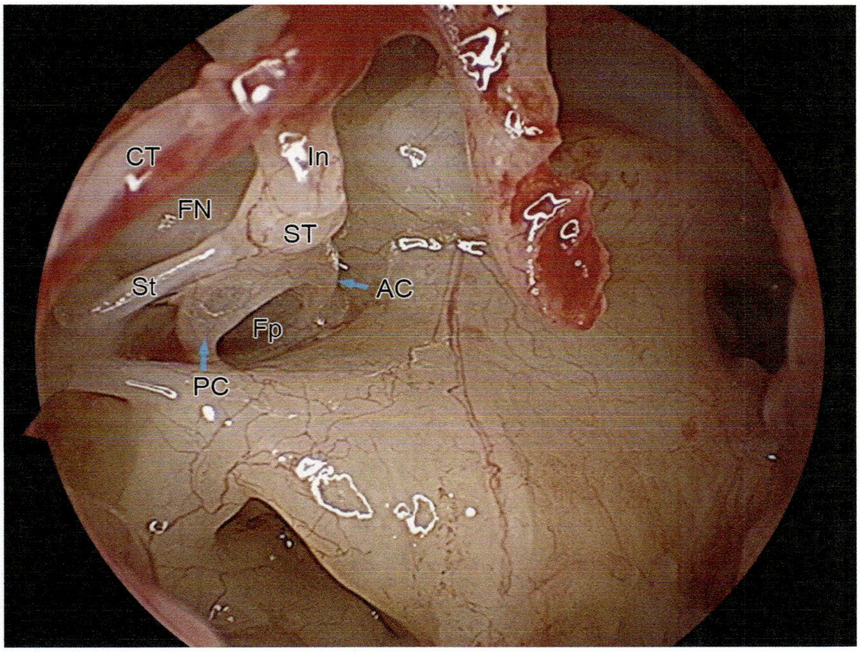

Fig. 26B: View of working corridor in an inferosuperior direction with the help of endoscope (Note the visibility of anterior and posterior crura with footplate): Intraoperative picture.
(CT: chorda tympani; FN: facial nerve, In: incus; St: stapedius tendon; ST: stapes PC: posterior crura; AC: Anterior crura; Fp: Footplate).

Incudostapedial Joint Disarticulation

- Incudostapedial joint is to be disarticulated from posterior-to-anterior direction using a joint knife or a fine-tipped angled pick
- The instrument should be introduced between the head of the stapes and lenticular process and care should be taken not to fracture the lenticular process

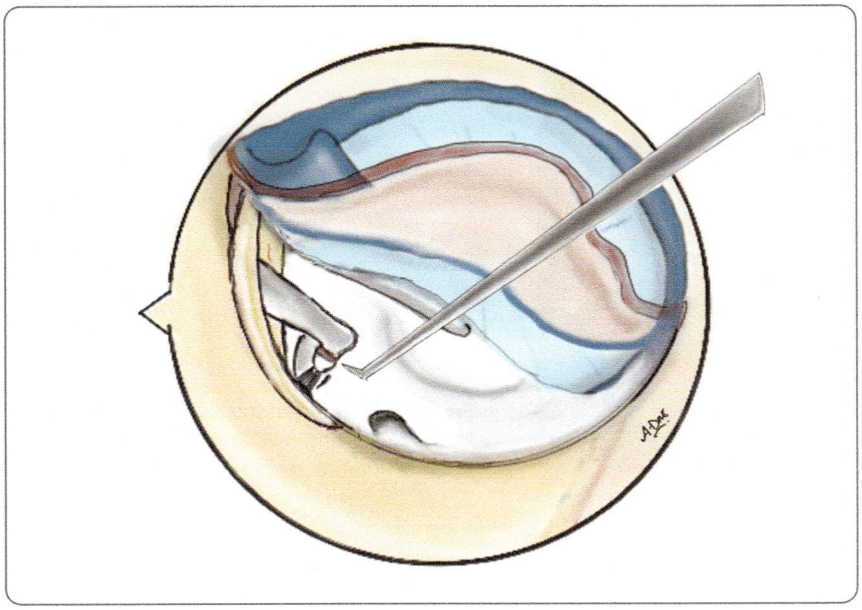

Fig. 27A: Incudostapedial joint disarticulation: Note the direction of movement of instrument from posterior-to-anterior: Schematic depiction (endoscopic view).

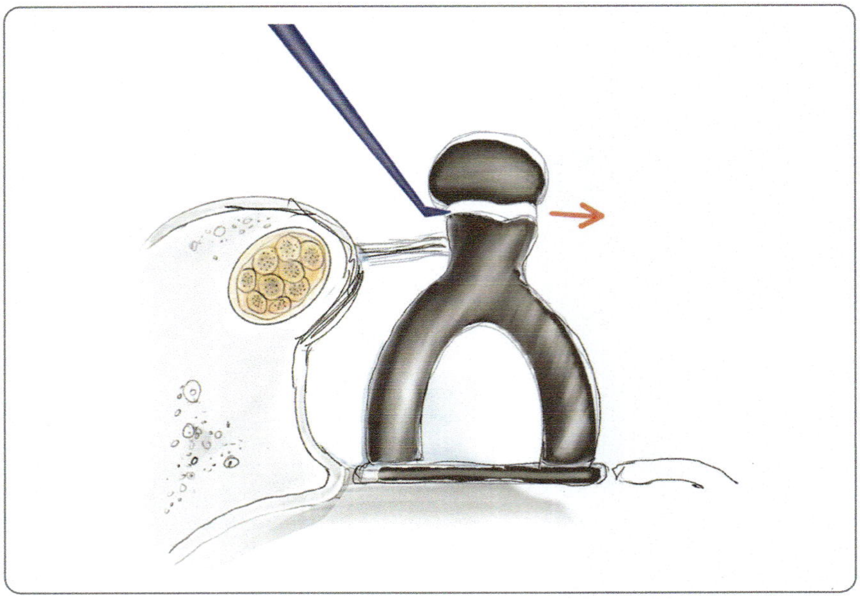

Fig. 27B: Direction of force exerted for disarticulation of incudostapedial joint.

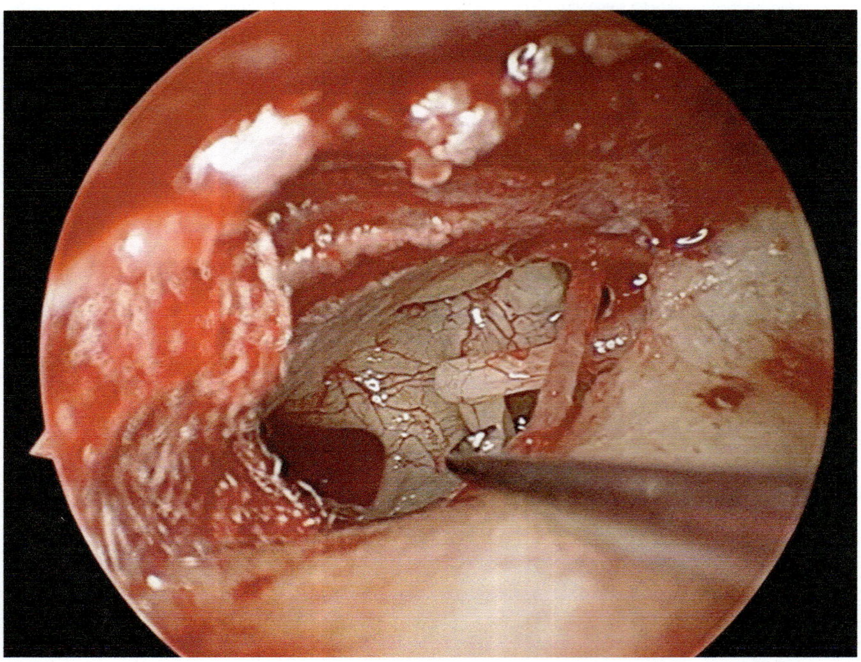

Fig. 27C: Incudostapedial joint disarticulation: Note the starting position of the sharp pick at the beginning of the disarticulation (left ear).

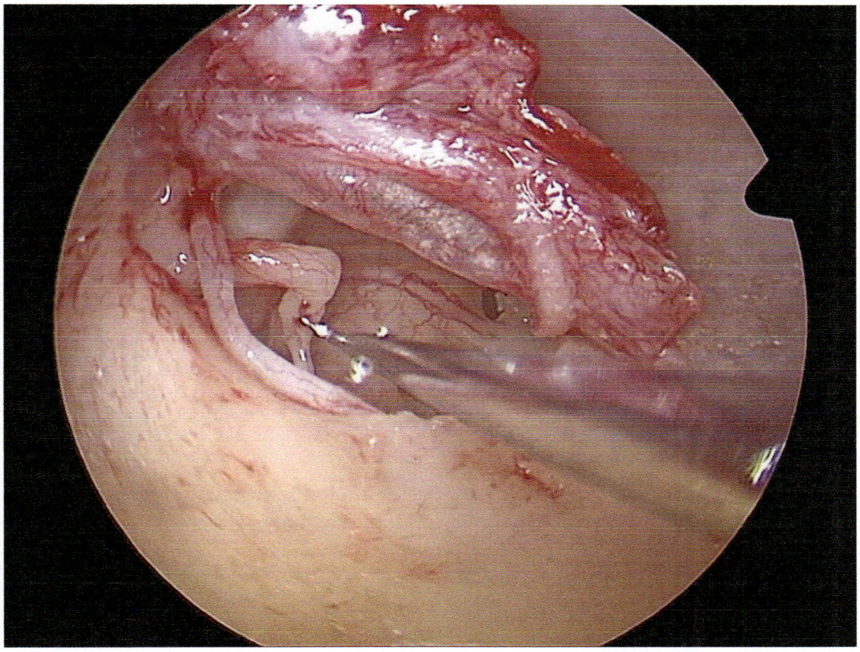

Fig. 27D: Incudostapedial joint disarticulation: Note the starting position of the sharp pick at the beginning of the disarticulation (right ear).

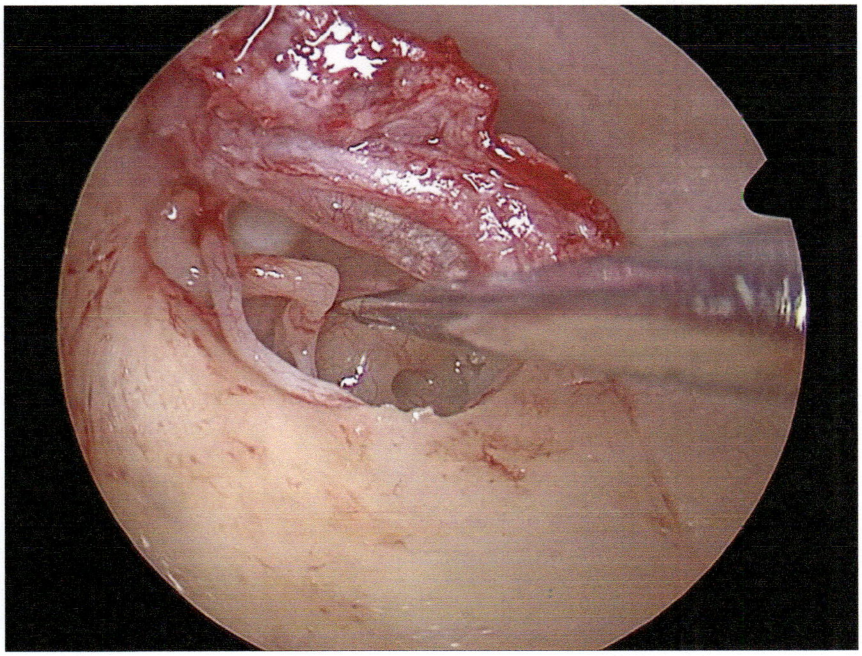

Fig. 27E: Incudostapedial joint disarticulation: Note the direction of movement of instrument from posterior-to-anterior: Intraoperative view.

Division of Stapedius Tendon

- Stapedius tendon is to be sharply cut with a 45° curved micro scissors negotiated from an inferior-to-superior axis from the hypotympanum area, staying close to the pyramid.

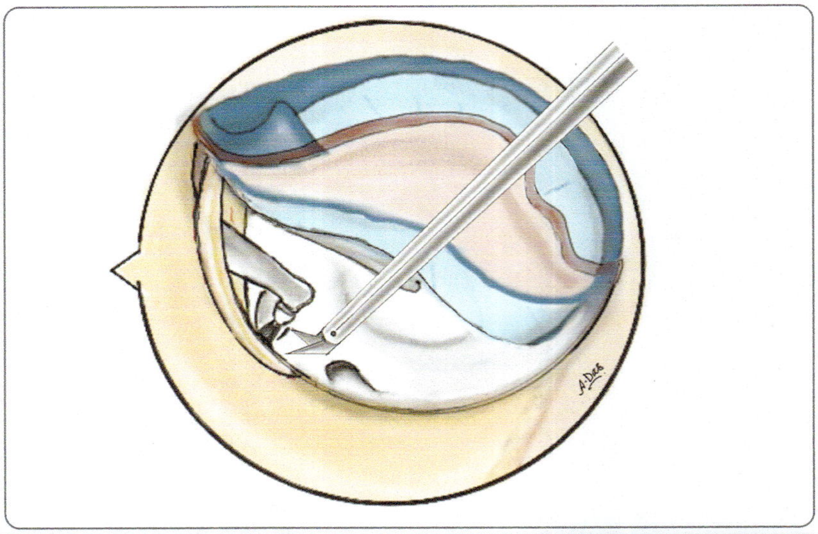

Fig. 28A: Use of angled microscissors for division of stapedius tendon (schematic depiction).

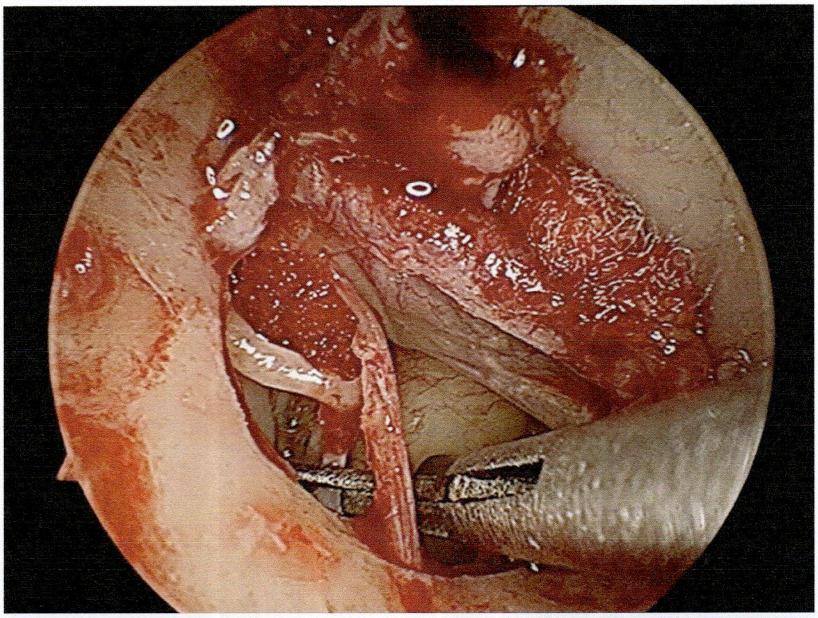

Fig. 28B: Division of stapedius tendon as close to the pyramid as possible: Intraoperative view—Division with angled microscissors.

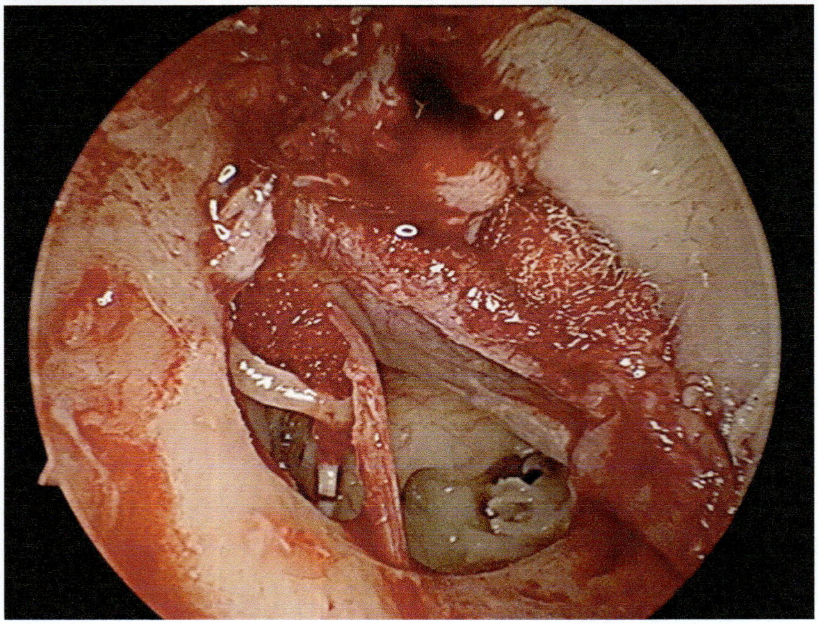

Fig. 28C: Division of stapedius tendon as close to the pyramid as possible: Intraoperative view—Note the cut end of stapedius tendon close to pyramid.

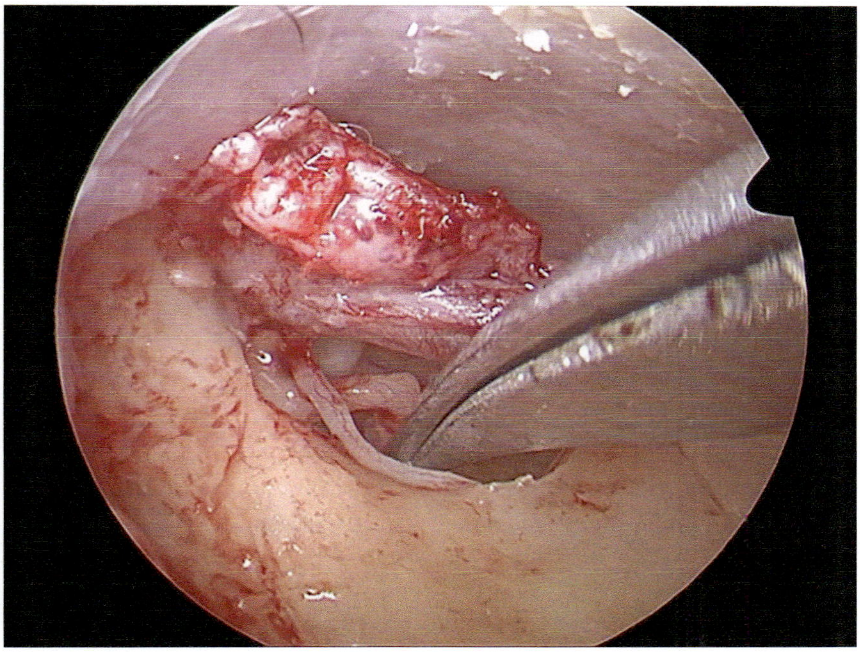

Fig. 28D: Alternate technique of stapedius tendon division with curved iris scissors.

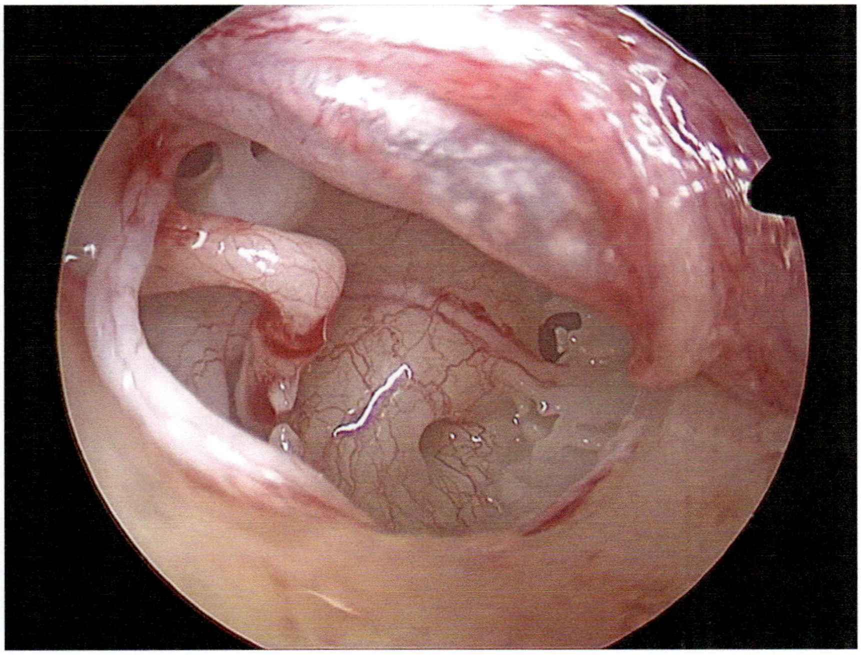

Fig. 28E: Division of stapedius tendon: Note the precisely cut ends of the tendon.

Crurotomy

- Posterior crura is then sharply drilled with skeeter drill or gently scratched at the base using a pick to break it. Thereafter, the thinner anterior crus is gently fractured towards the promontory to deliver out the stapes.

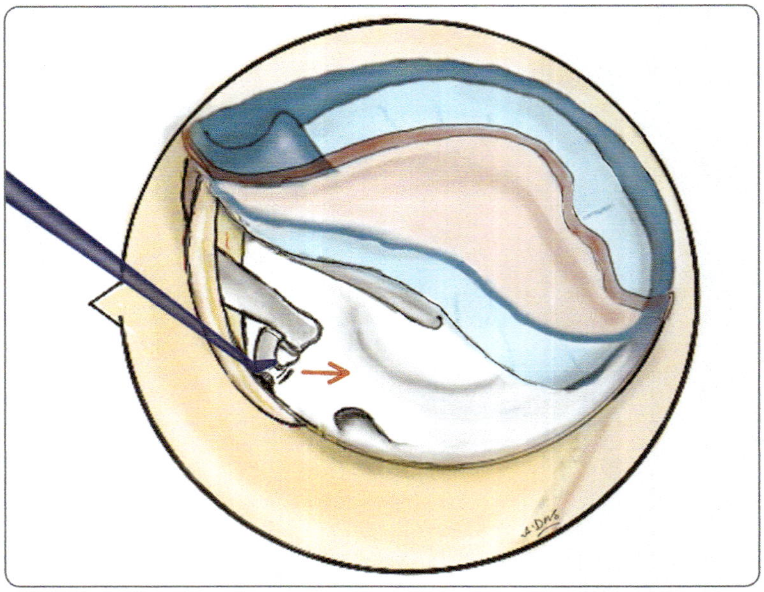

Fig. 29A: Schematic depiction of crurotomy: Posterior crura being fractured from superior-to-inferior direction.

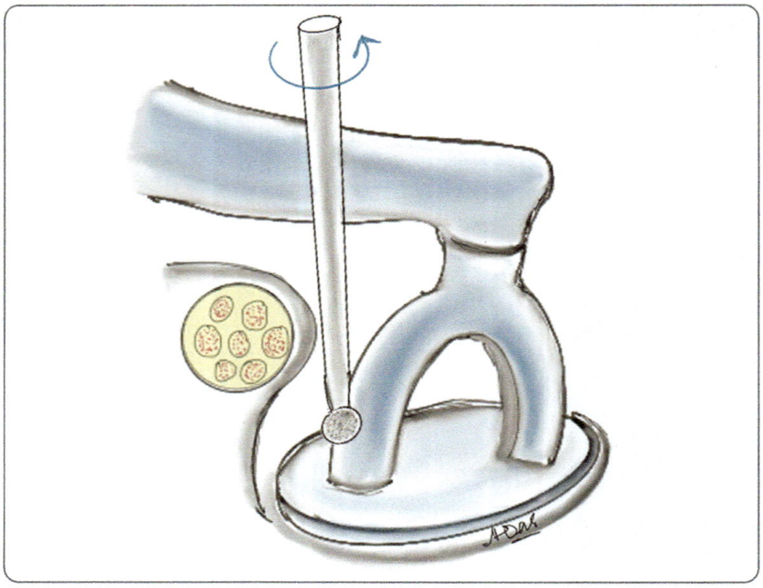

Fig. 29B: Schematic depiction of alternate technique of crurotomy: Use of skeeter drill to thin the posterior crura.

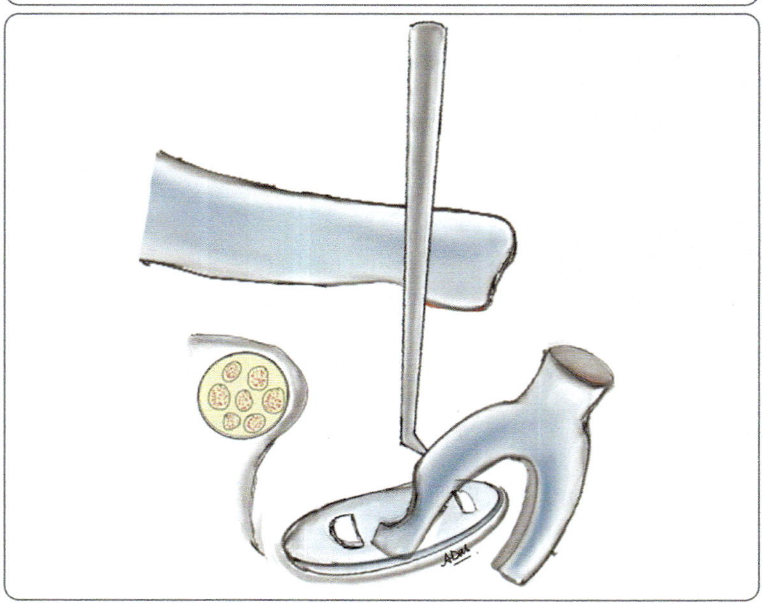

Fig. 29C: Schematic depiction of alternate technique of crurotomy: Anterior crura fractured downwards towards promontory.

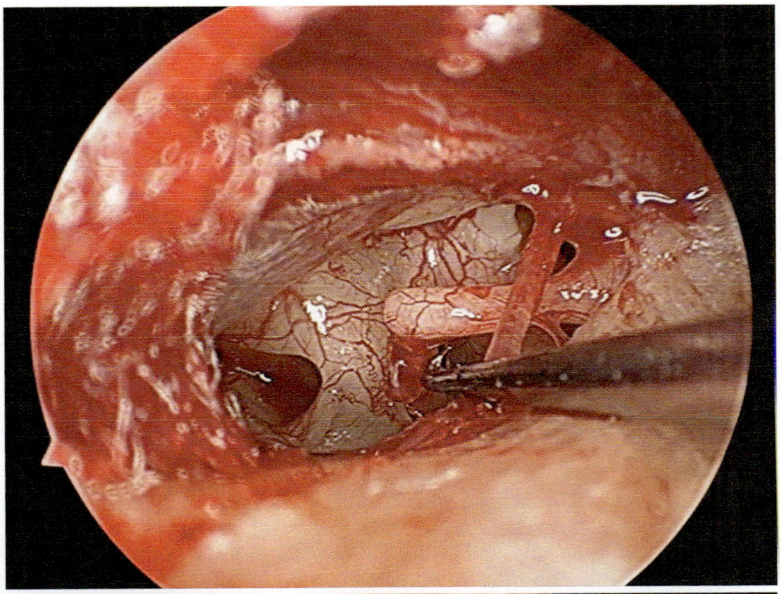

Fig. 30A: Intraoperative view of crurotomy: Note the position of the pick behind the head of stapes (left ear).

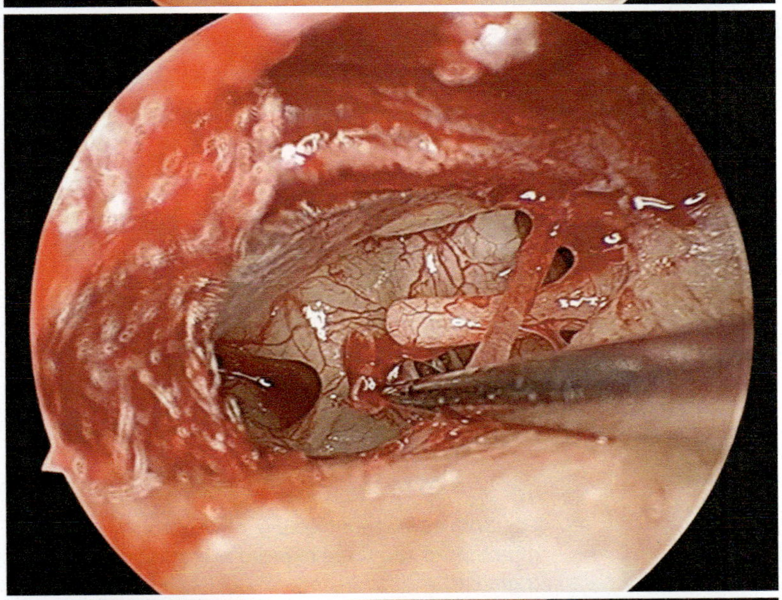

Fig. 30B: Intraoperative view of crurotomy: Note the direction of the force exerted towards promontory (left ear).

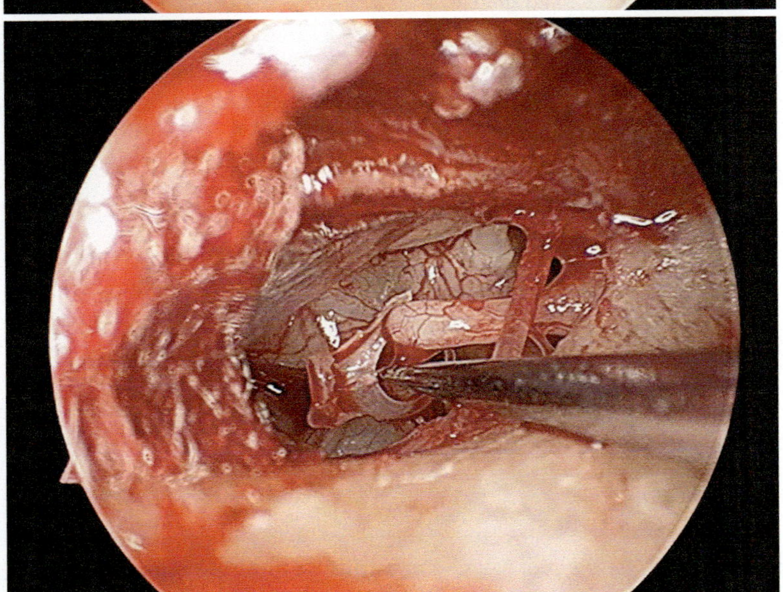

Fig. 30C: Intraoperative view of crurotomy: complete fracture of stapes suprastructure (left ear).

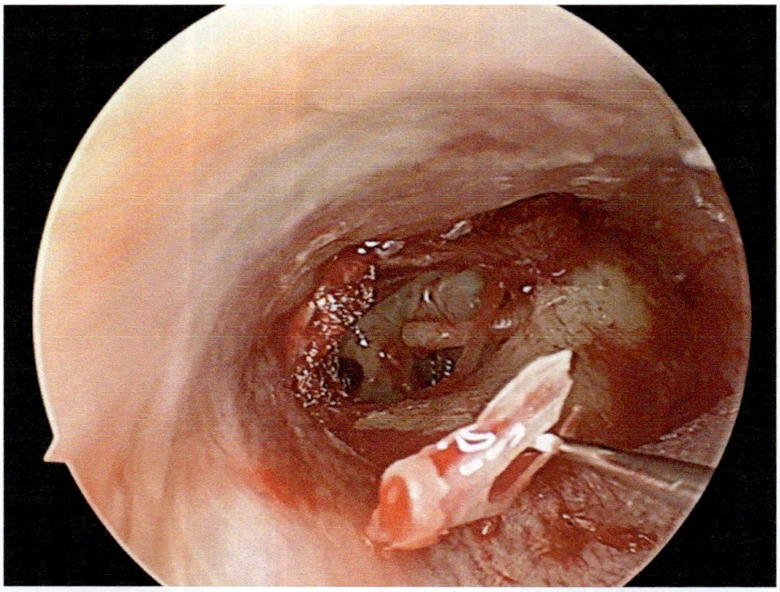

Fig. 30D: Intraoperative view of crurotomy: suprastructure being delivered out (left ear).

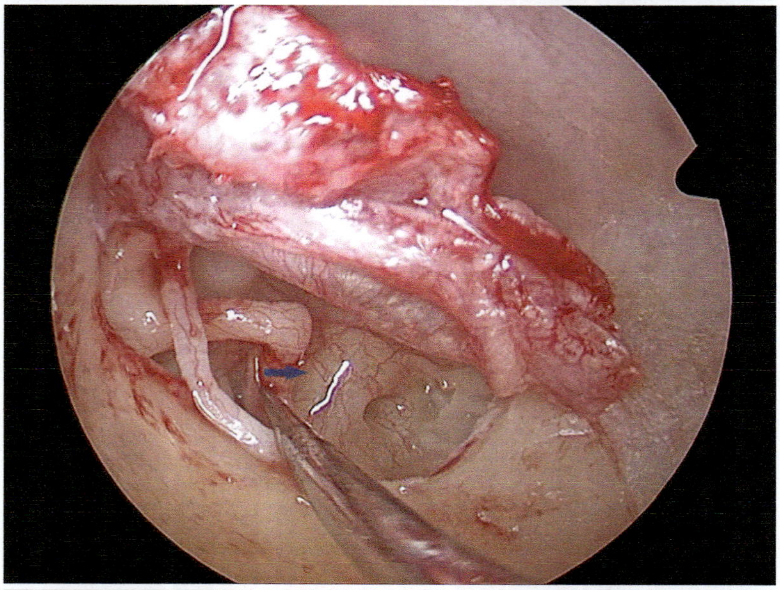

Fig. 30E: Intraoperative view of crurotomy: Note the direction of the force exerted towards promontory (right ear).

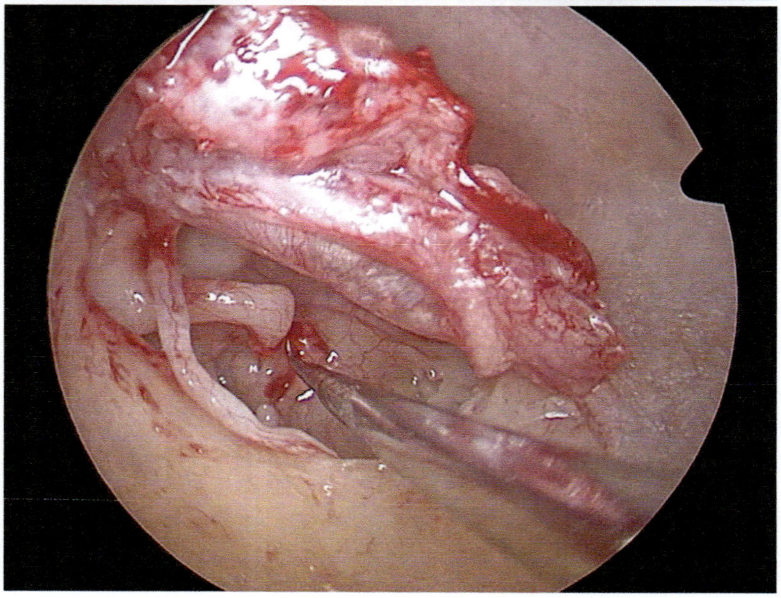

Fig. 30F: Intraoperative view of crurotomy: fracture of stapes suprastructure towards promontory (right ear).

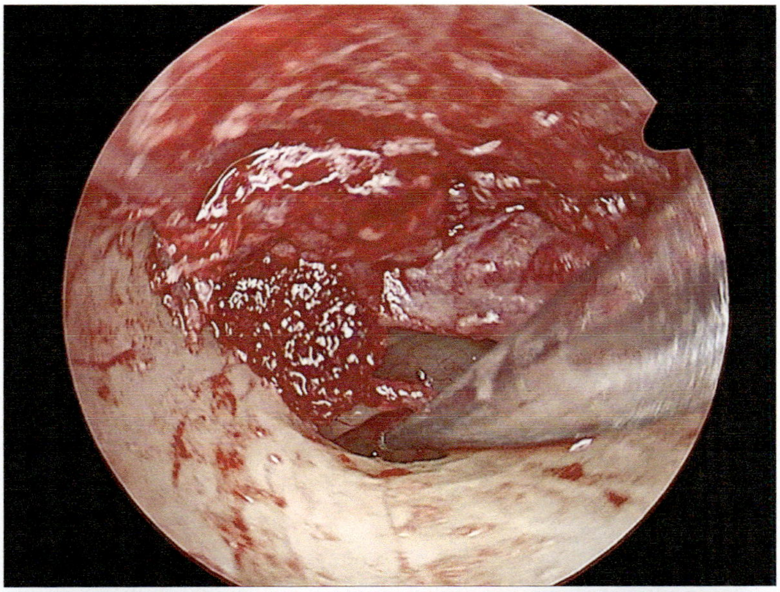

Fig. 31A: Intraoperative view of alternate technique of crurotomy: Use of skeeter drill to thin the posterior crura (right ear).

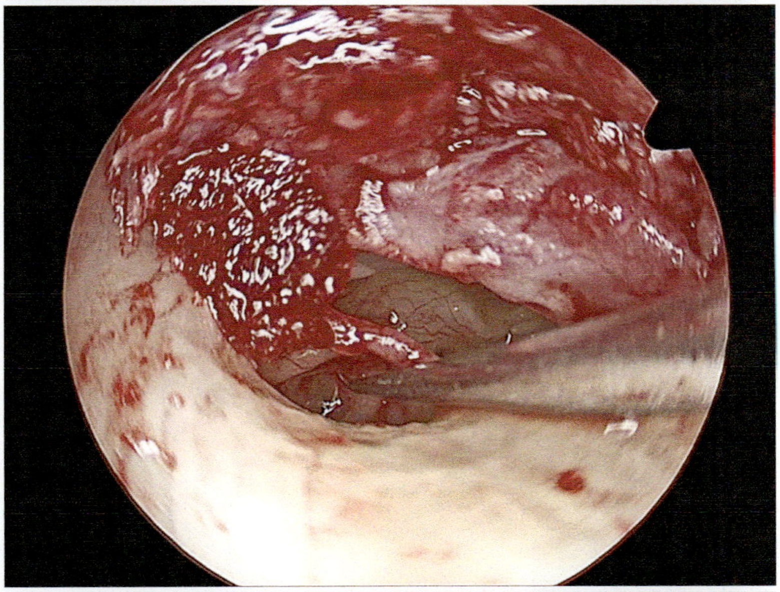

Fig. 31B: Intraoperative view of alternate technique of crurotomy: Suprastructure being fractured using 45° pick (right ear).

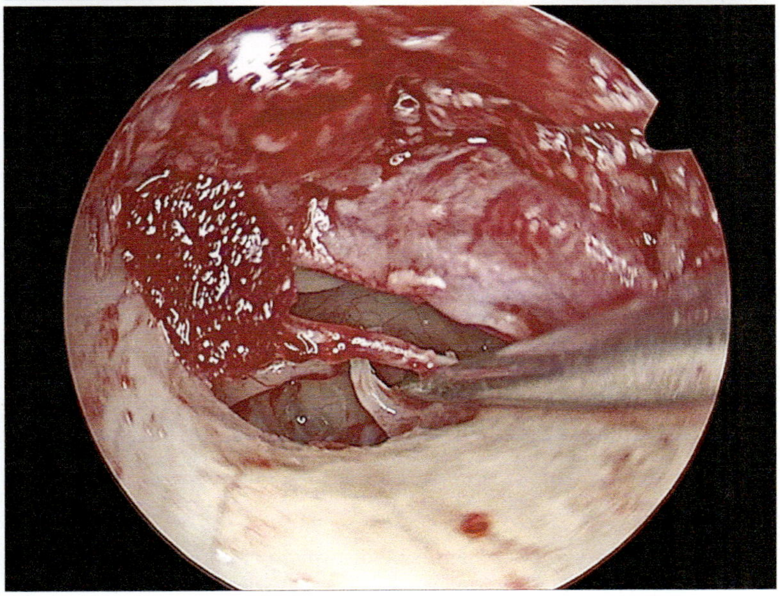

Fig. 31C: Intraoperative view of alternate technique of crurotomy: Suprastructure being delivered out of middle ear using a pick (right ear).

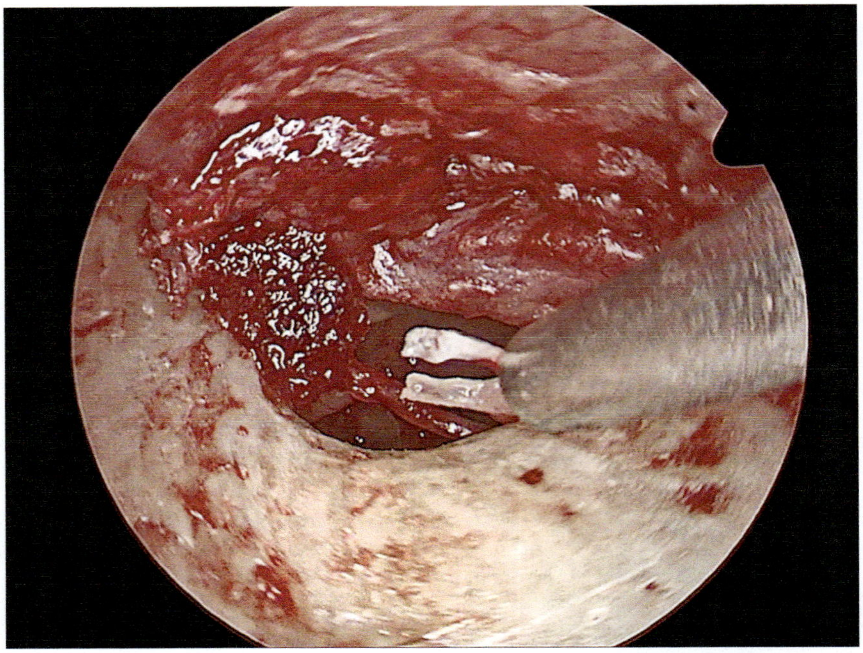

Fig. 31D: Intraoperative view of alternate technique of crurotomy: Suprastructure being delivered out of external auditory canal using a suction tip (right ear).

PEARL

These difficult areas can be easily accessed using long, curved pick, even when the posterosuperior canal is completely intact.

Footplate Inspection

Inspection of the footplate area is a critical step and it helps to understand the thickness, position and relative anatomy of this structure.

PEARL

Endoscope by virtue of its magnification, allows the surgeon to inspect the finer anatomical details of the footplate, its orientation and any additional anatomical structure visible on or near it.

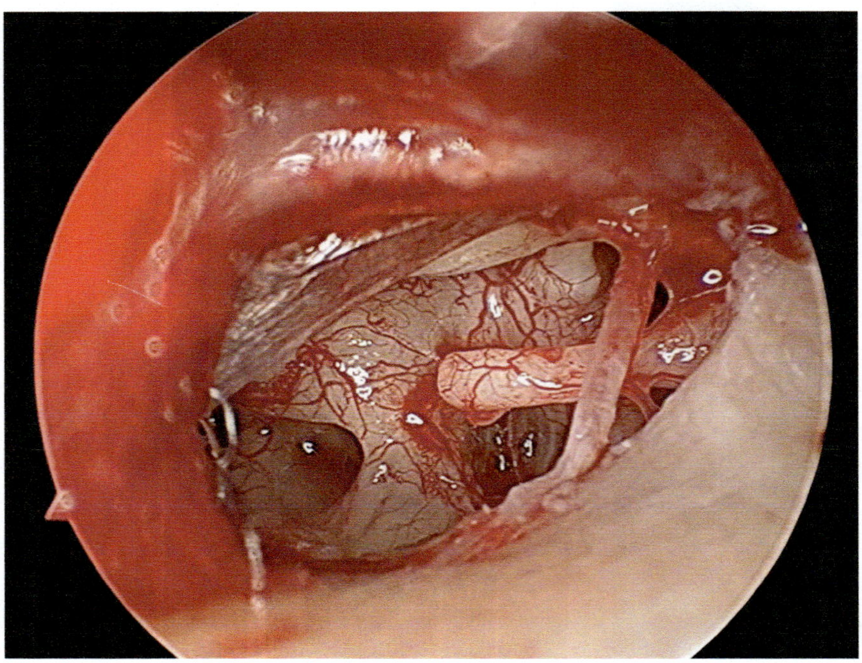

Fig. 32A: Inspection of stapes footplate (left ear).

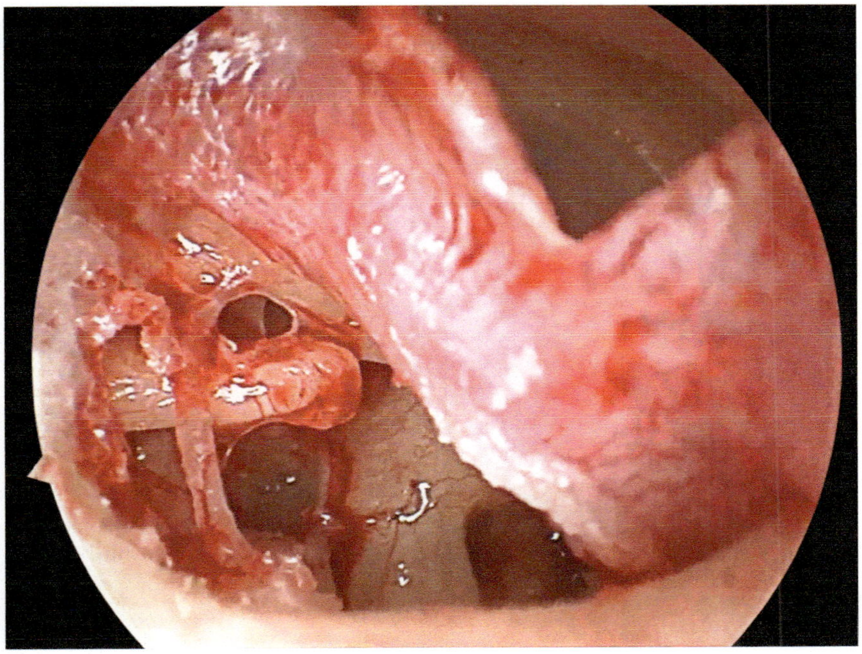

Fig. 32B: Inspection of stapes footplate (right ear).

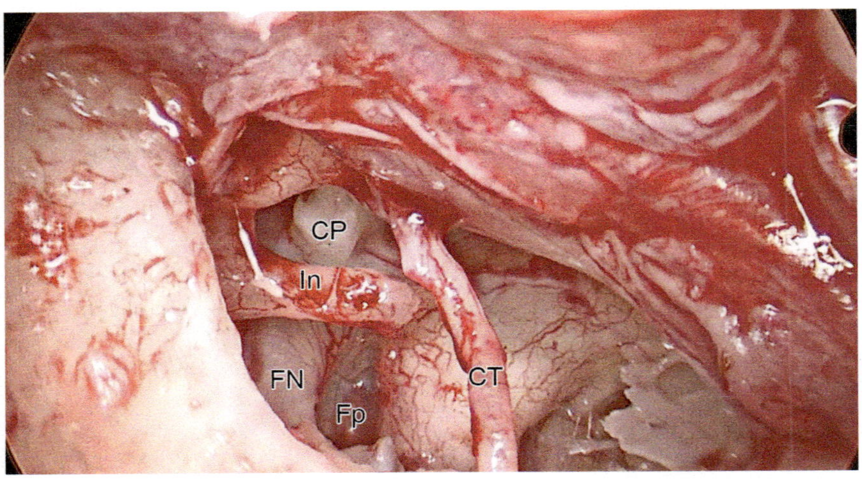

Fig. 32C: Inspection of stapes footplate (maginified view) and identification of landmarks.
(CP: cochleariform process; CT: chorda tympani; FN: facial nerve; Fp: stapes footplate; In: incus)

Creation of Fenestra

A control fenestra is then made over the *posterior third of the footplate* using a 0.3 mm perforator.

TIP

Prior to the next step, that is fenestration of the footplate, intravenous steroid (IV Hydrocortisone as per body weight) is administered to prevent vestibular shock that may occur due to sudden opening of the vestibule.

Thereafter, the fenestra is enlarged using perforators of 0.5, 0.7 mm successively.

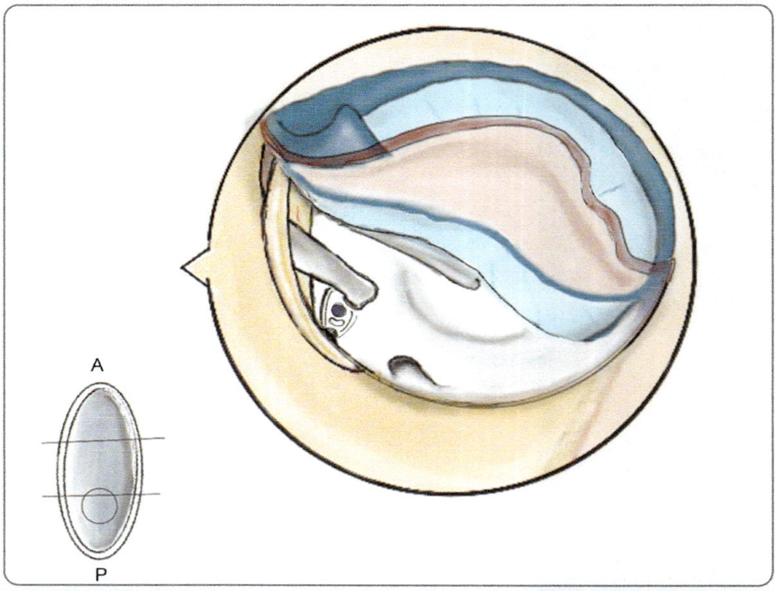

Fig. 33A: Creation of fenestra: Schematic depiction of the site of fenestration at posterior third of the footplate.

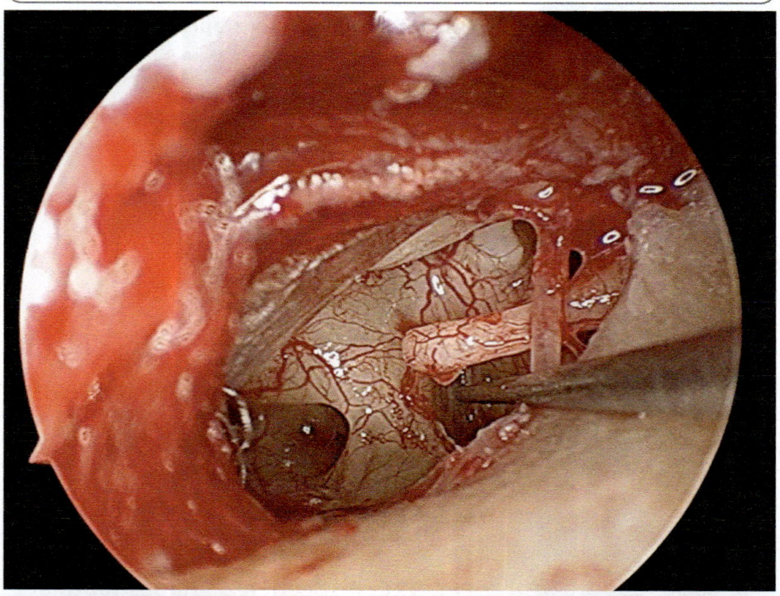

Fig. 33B: Creation of control fenestra using 0.3 mm perforator (left ear).

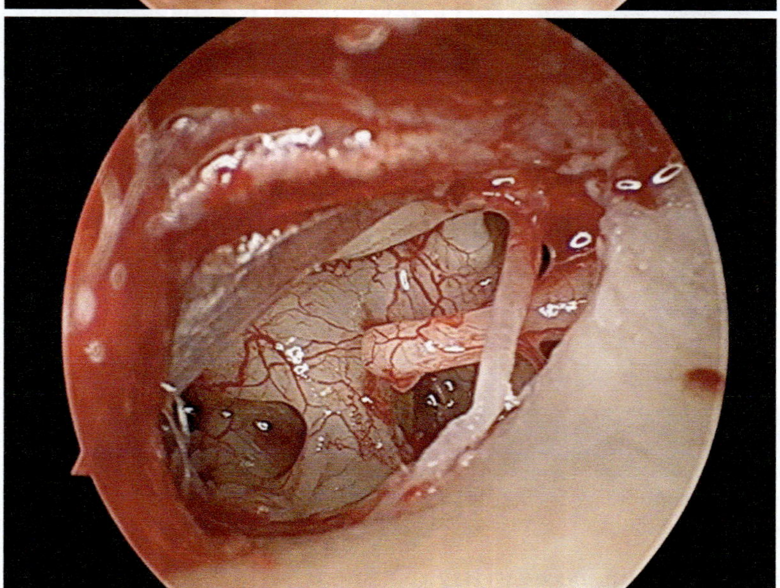

Fig. 33C: Creation of fenestra: Inspection of footplate after control fenestration for any gusher or footplate mobilization (left ear).

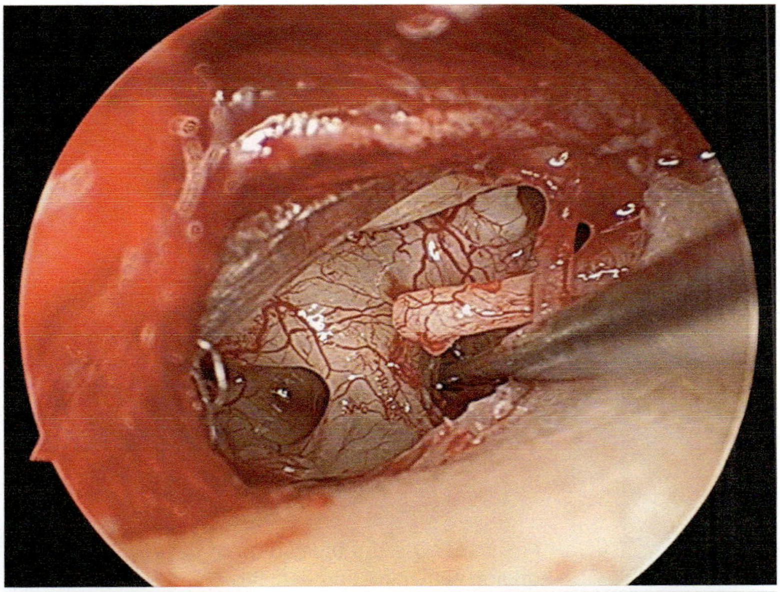

Fig. 33D: Creation of fenestra: Subsequent enlargement of the fenestra using perforators of increasing size (left ear).

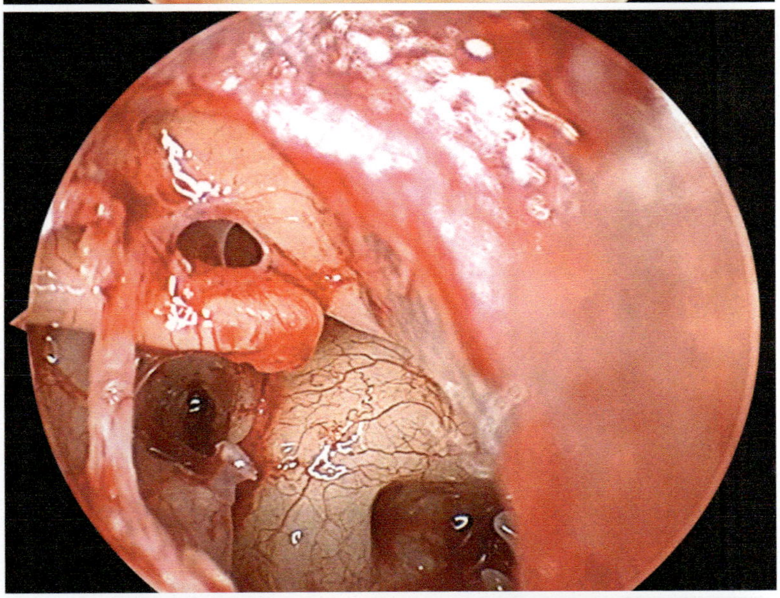

Fig. 33E: Creation of fenestra: Final size of fenestra (right ear).

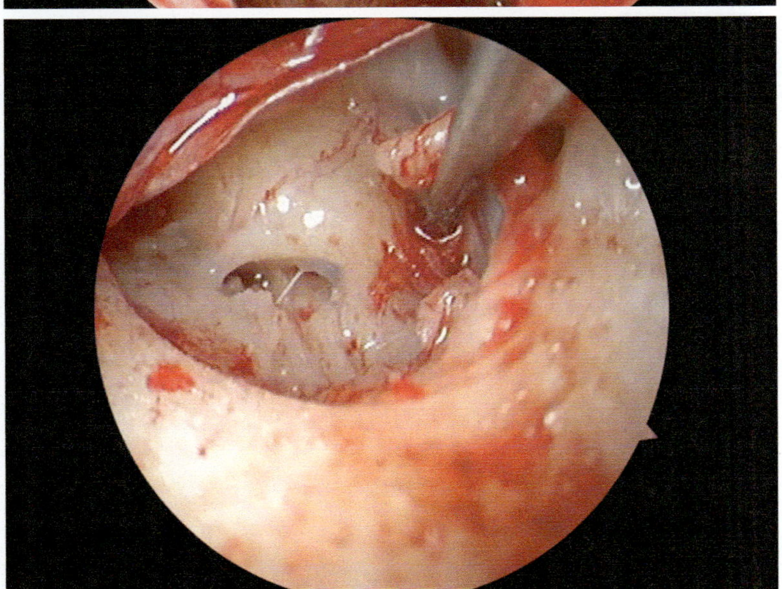

Fig. 34A: Hand burr being used to blue-line the vestibule in thick footplate (left ear).

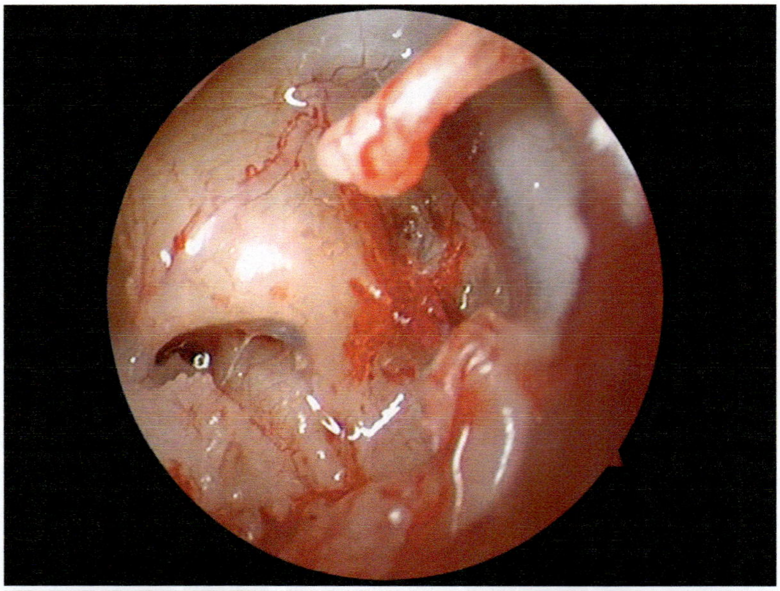

Fig. 34B: Note the blue lining of the vestibule after drilling with hand burr (left ear).

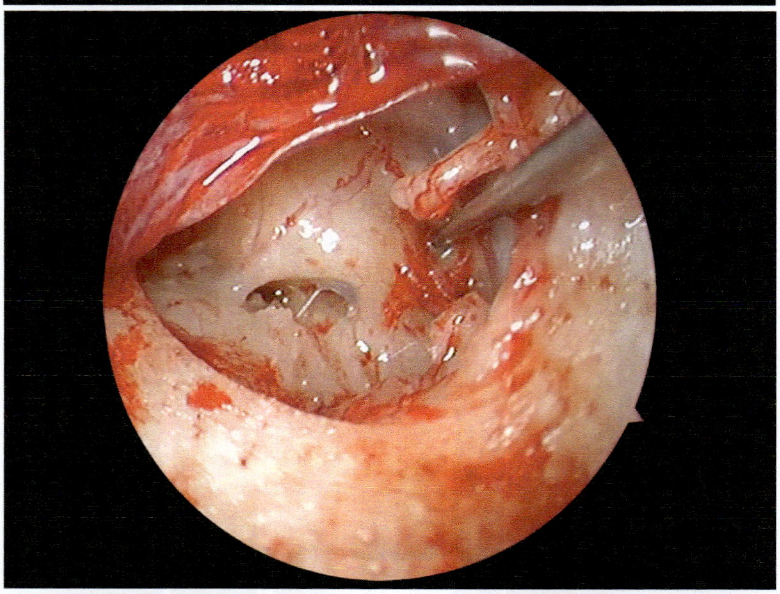

Fig. 34C: Subsequent use of perforator to create the fenestra of desired size (left ear).

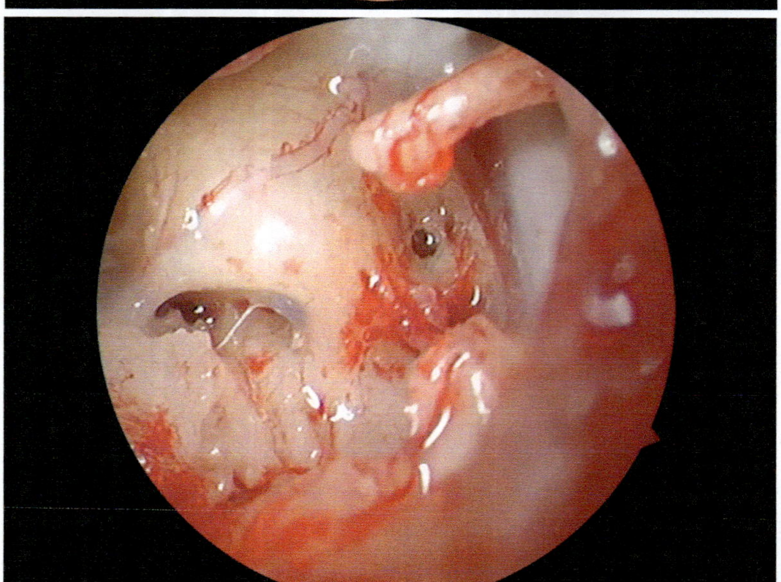

Fig. 34D: Final view after fenestration (left ear).

TIP

- In difficult situations with extremely hard footplate, 0.5 or 0.6 mm diamond burr with a skeeter *drill* should be used in a controlled manner to drill the footplate area to make it thinner (blue-lining of the vestibule is observed) followed by creation of a control fenestra using the perforator.

TIP

- Once the vestibule is opened, direct suctioning over the vestibule and use of adrenaline is to be strictly avoided.

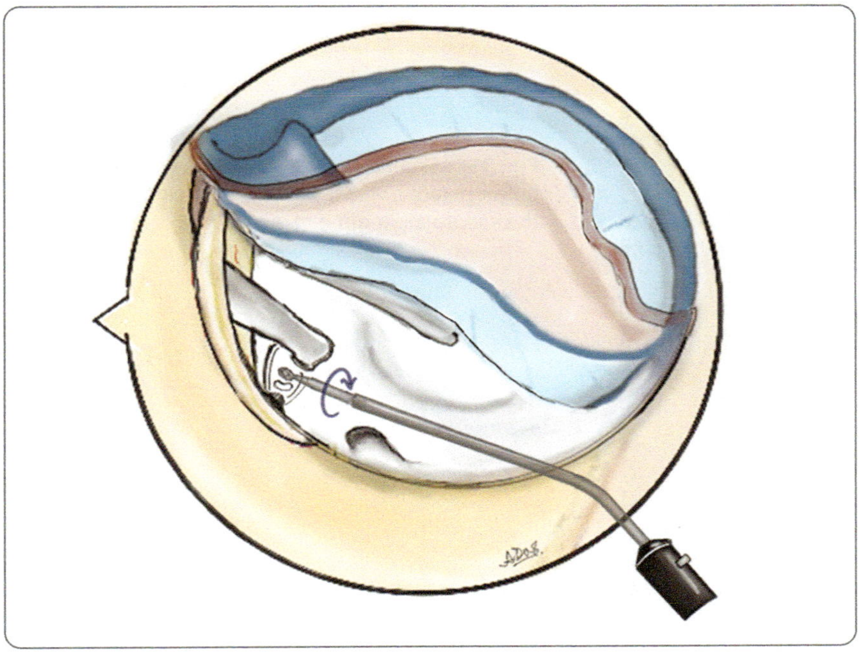

Fig. 35A: Skeeter drill being used to create fenestra: Schematic depiction.

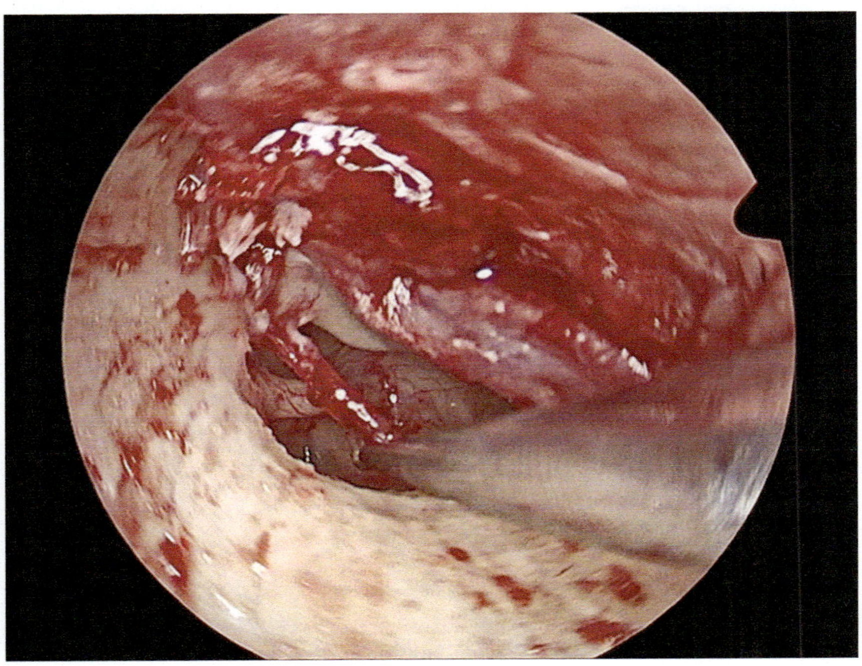

Fig. 35B: Skeeter drill being used to create fenestra (intraoperative view): Skeeter drill being introduced into middle ear (right ear).

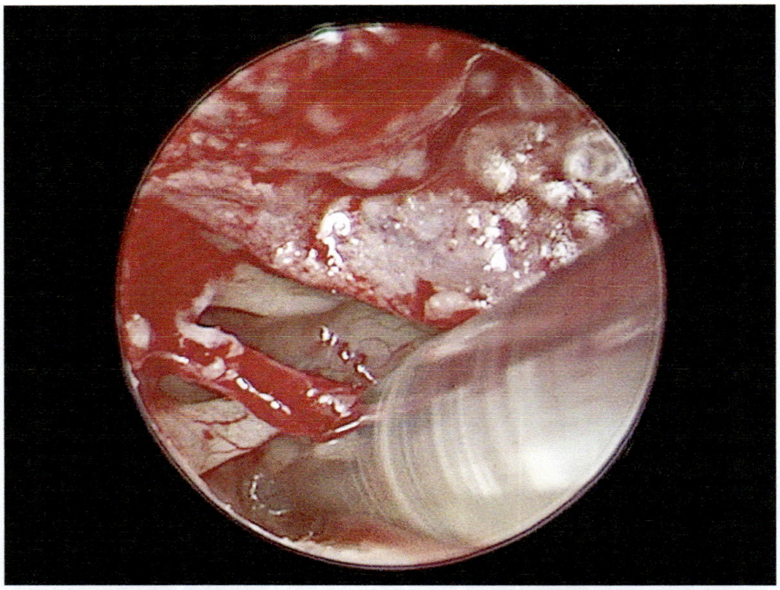

Fig. 35C: Skeeter drill being used to create fenestra (intraoperative view): Skeeter drill being used to drill thick footplate (right ear).

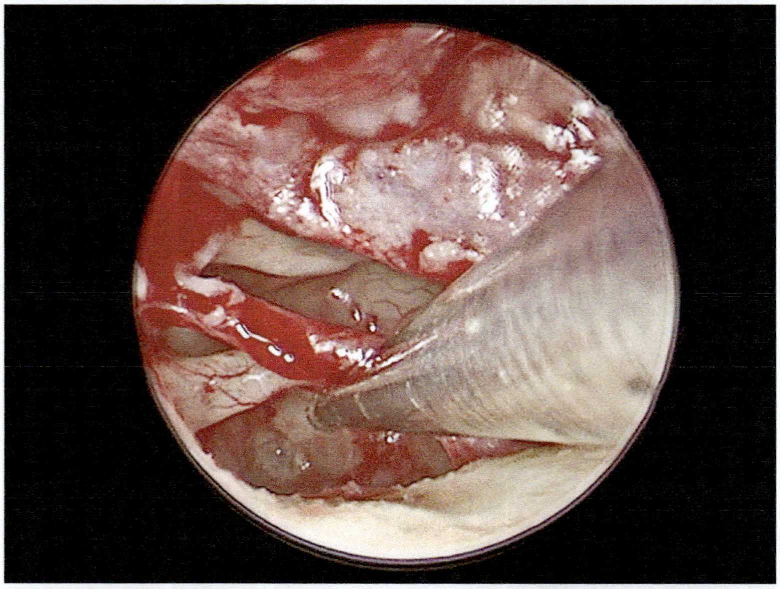

Fig. 35D: Skeeter drill being used to create fenestra (intraoperative view): First view of blue lining of vestibule (right ear).

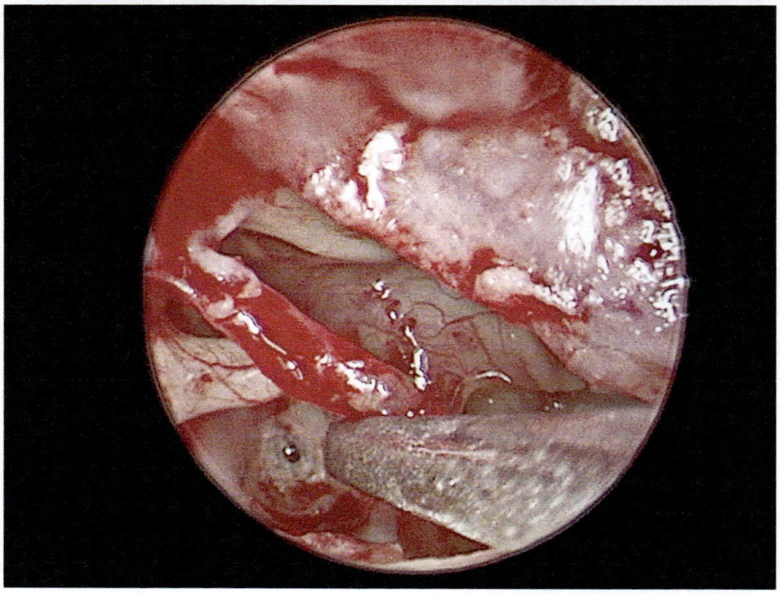

Fig. 35E: Skeeter drill being used to create fenestra (intraoperative view): Fenestra completed using perforator (right ear).

Preparation of Piston

PEARL **PREPARATION OF THE PISTON[4]**

The piston has to be adequately sized to ensure a proper fit:

- The length of the piston can be calculated as a = Distance from the under/medial surface of the long process of incus + b = Thickness of the footplate itself + c = 0.5 mm additional length inside the vestibule.
- The resultant length of the piston is the sum of the three and is measured using a Fisch measuring rod.
- Usually, the length has been found to be a (3.5 mm) + b (0.25 mm) + c (0.5 mm) = 4.25 mm.
- Once the piston length has been adequately sized, loop of the piston is widened by gently screwing motion using the shaft of a straight pick.
- Thereafter, the piston is grasped at its neck at an angulation of 30–40 degrees using a micro alligator forceps.

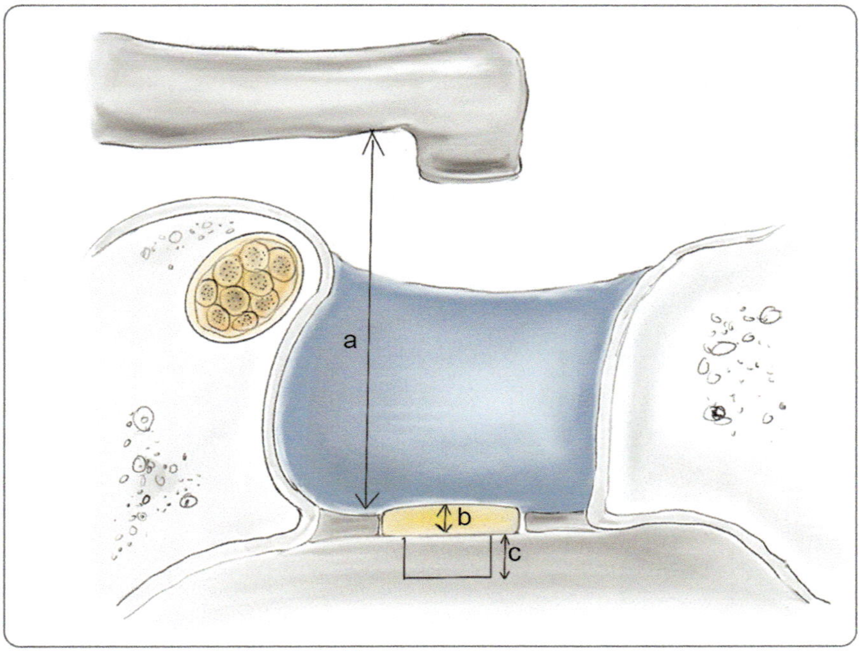

Fig. 36A: Calculation of length of piston: Schematic depiction (a—Distance from the under/medial surface of the long process of incus; b—Thickness of the footplate itself; c—0.5 mm additional length inside the vestibule).

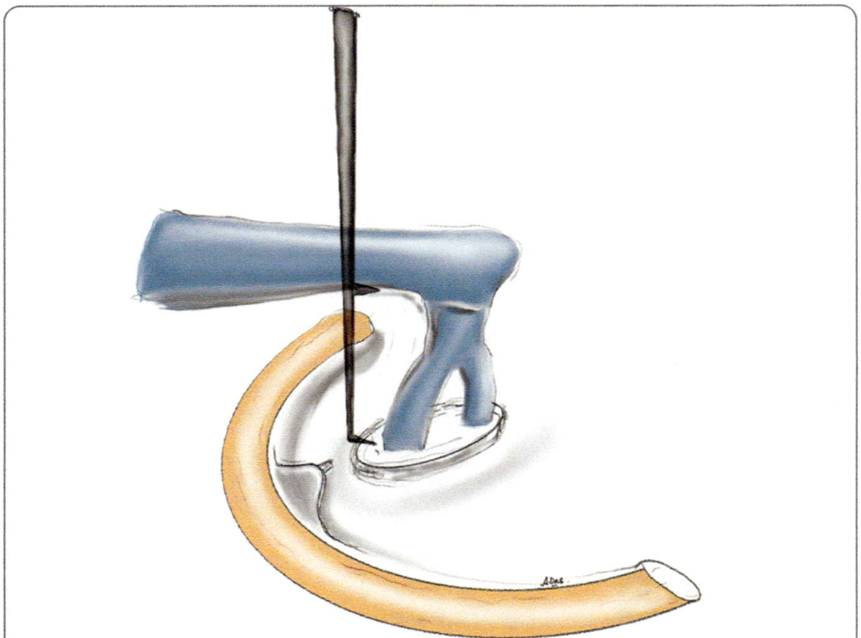

Fig. 36B: Calculation of length of piston by measurement of distance from the under/medial surface of the long process of incus to footplate: Schematic depiction (right ear).

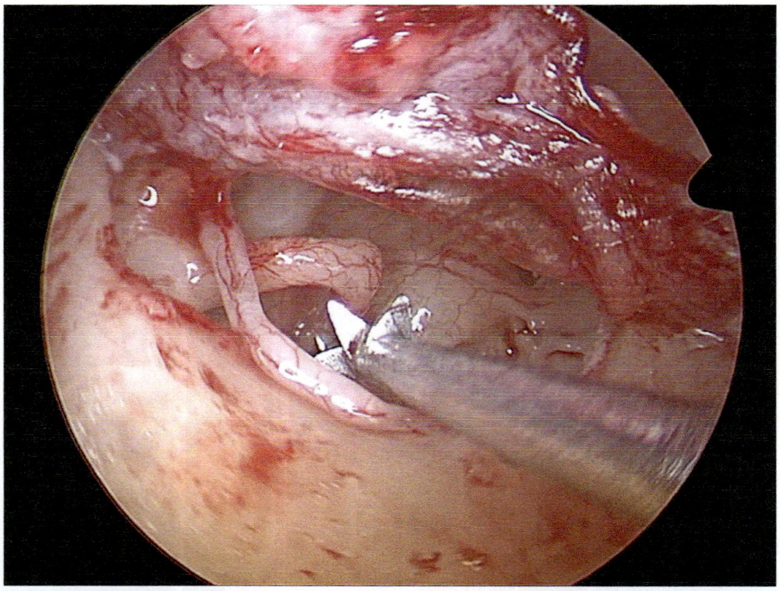

Fig. 36C: Calculation of length of piston using Fisch measuring rod: intraoperative view (right ear).

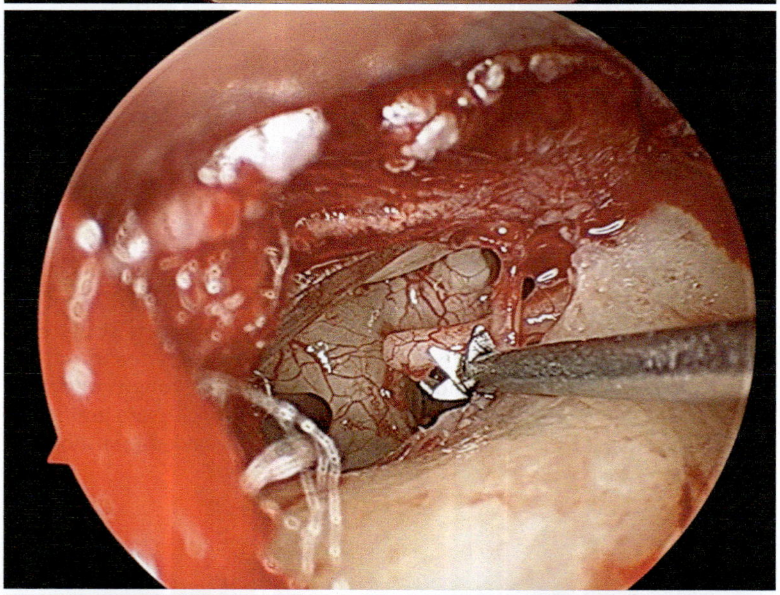

Fig. 36D: Calculation of length of piston using Fisch measuring rod: intraoperative view (left ear).

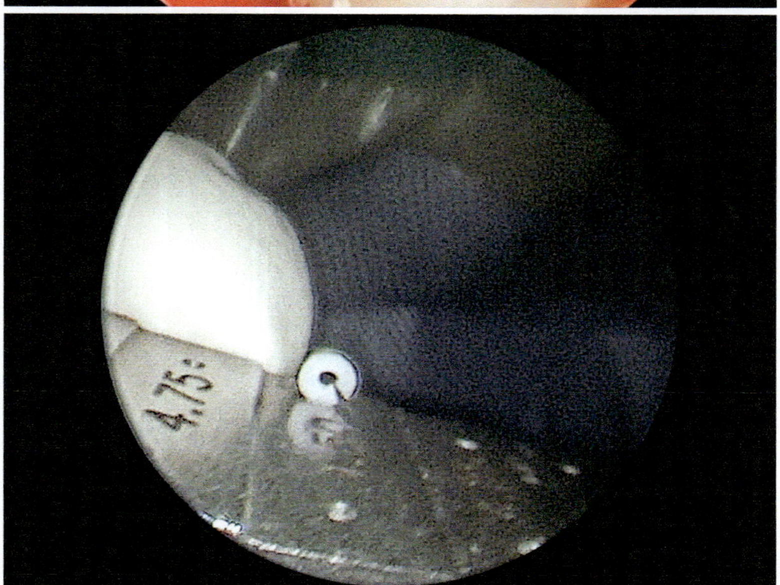

Fig. 37A: Placement of the piston in the measurement gauge.

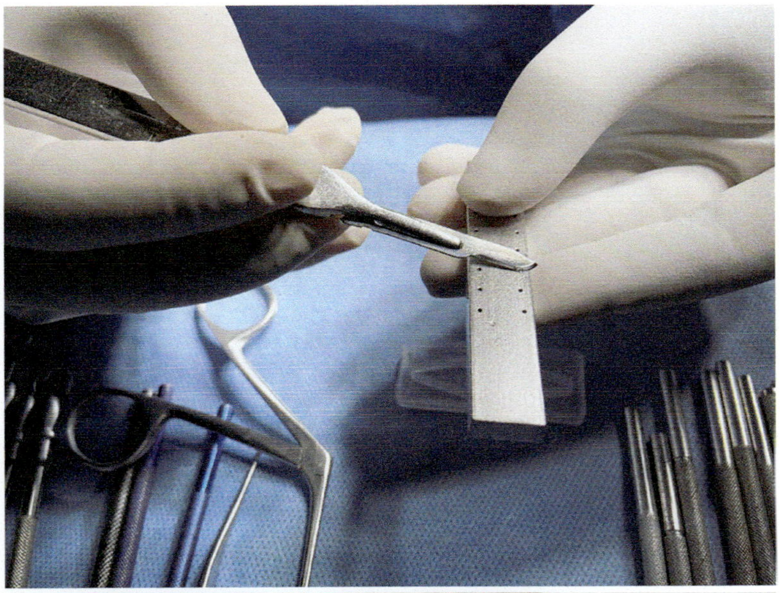

Fig. 37B: Trimming the piston.

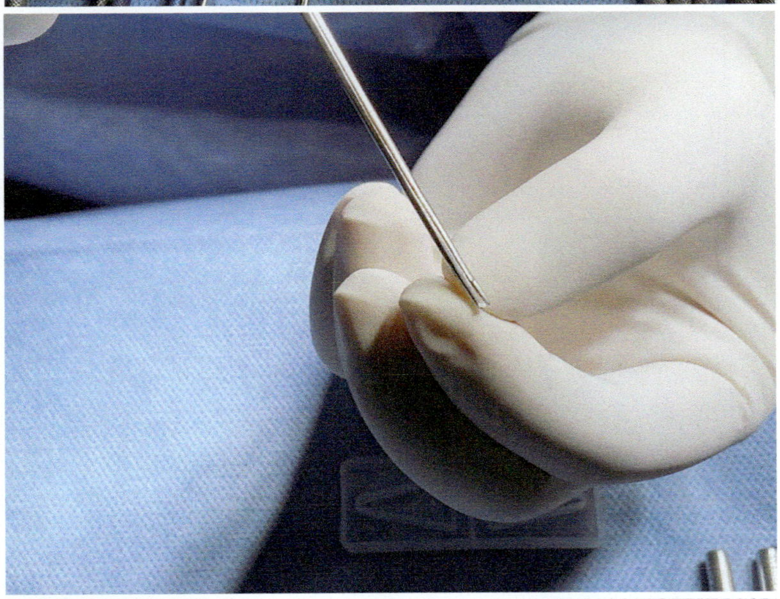

Fig. 37C: Once the loop of the piston has been widened by a pick, it is further opened using an alligator.

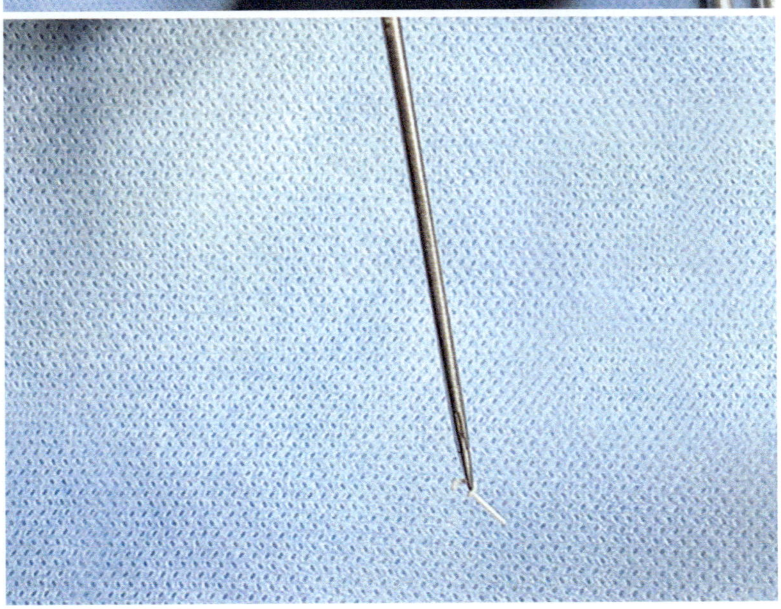

Fig. 37D: Method of holding the piston at its neck.

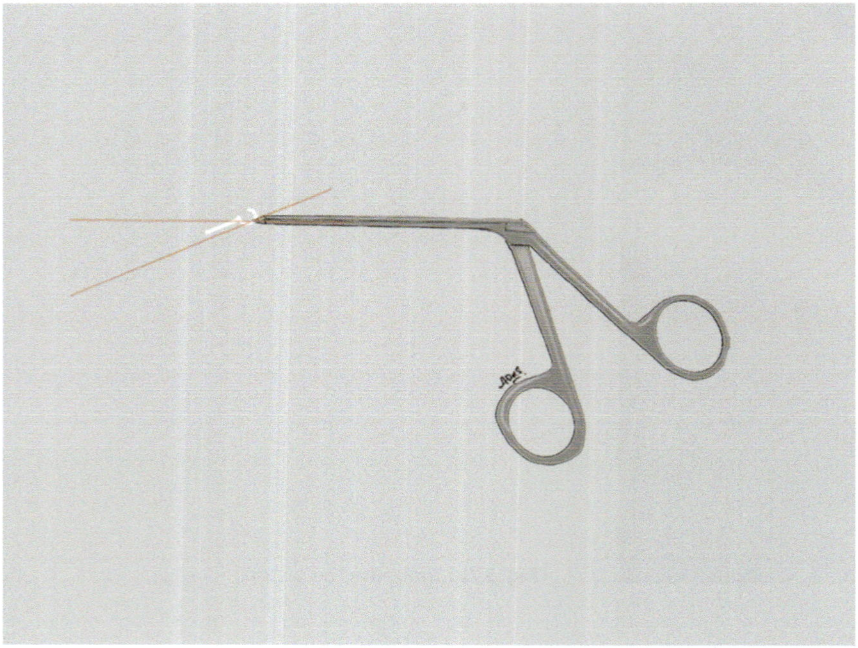

Fig. 37E: Schematic depiction of holding the piston.

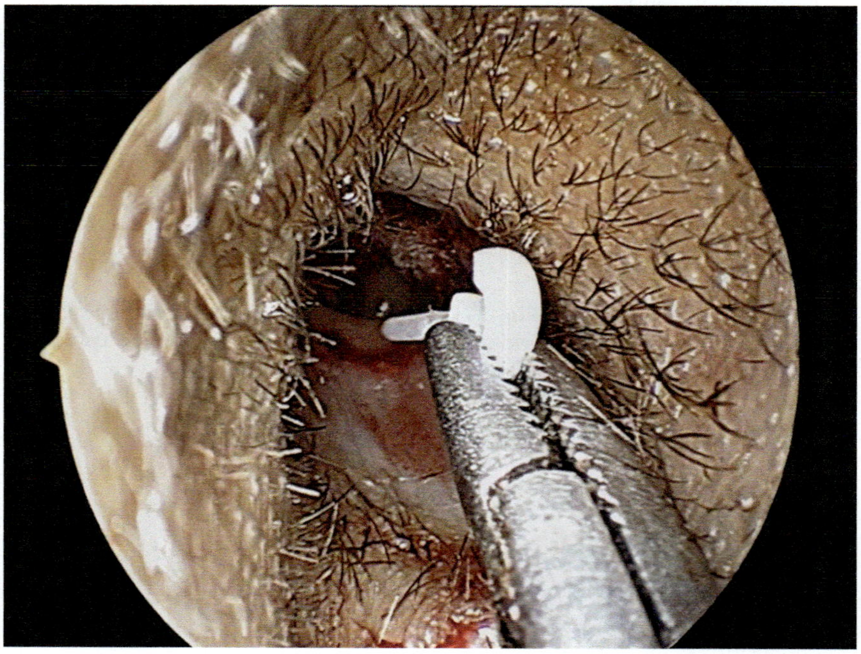

Fig. 37F: Method of insertion of the piston.

Piston Placement

We usually prefer a 0.5 mm Teflon stapes piston (Causse type) which is fitted adequately and crimped. Superior quality Teflon piston (Medtronic/Grace Medical) should be used to achieve best result.

- The distal end of the piston is first placed inside the vestibule, at the site of the fenestra
- The loop is then gently negotiated to fit the long process of incus using an angled (45°/90°) pick
- Depending on the fit, the piston can be further crimped to ensure optimal fit

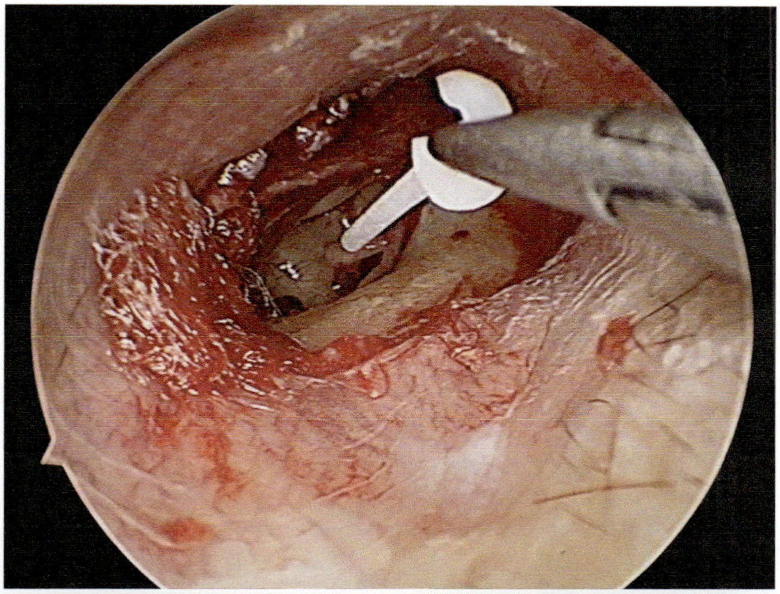

Fig. 38A: Placement of piston: Piston negotiated into middle ear (left ear).

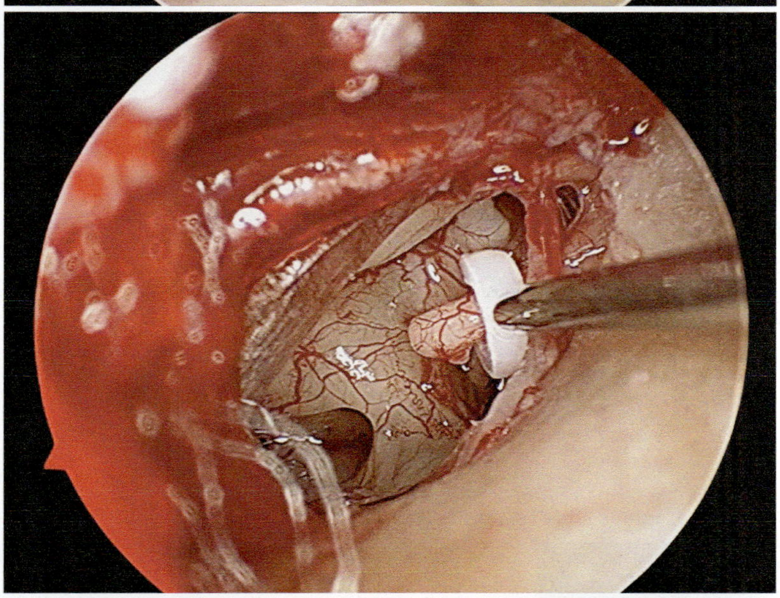

Fig. 38B: Placement of piston: Distal end of piston introduced into fenestra (left ear).

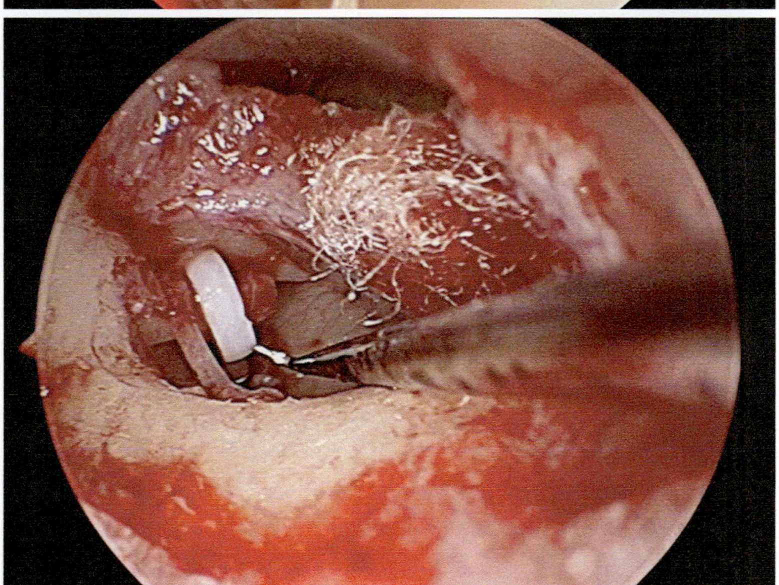

Fig. 38C: Placement of piston: Loop of piston negotiated to fit long process of incus with the help of pick (right ear).

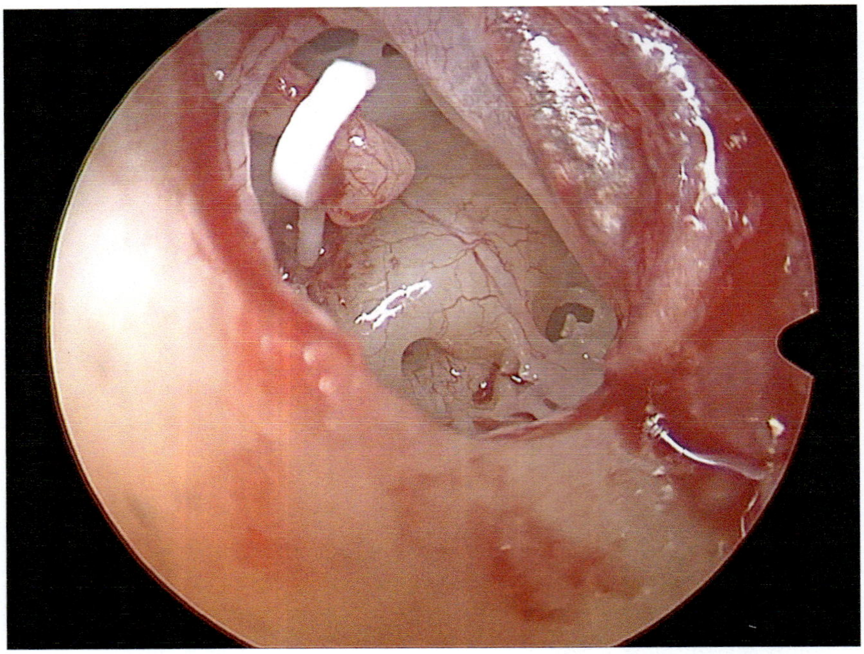

Fig. 38D: Placement of piston: Final view after proper placement (right ear).

TIP **TESTS FOR CORRECT PLACEMENT AND FIT OF STAPES PROSTHESIS**

- *"LIFT" test*: Gentle palpation of the incus to check the correct length of the prosthesis is called "Lift" test. In case the prosthesis is too short, it may get displaced out of the fenestra. In case of an excessively long prosthesis, movement of incus induces vertigo in patient. This indicates a long prosthesis which needs to be adequately shortened.
- *"BEND" test*: Anteroposterior movement of the shaft of the piston is used the check the fit of the stapes piston in the fenestra. An adequately fitted piston will not move on application of gentle pressure in the said direction whereas, a too-short prosthesis will get displaced out of the fenestra.

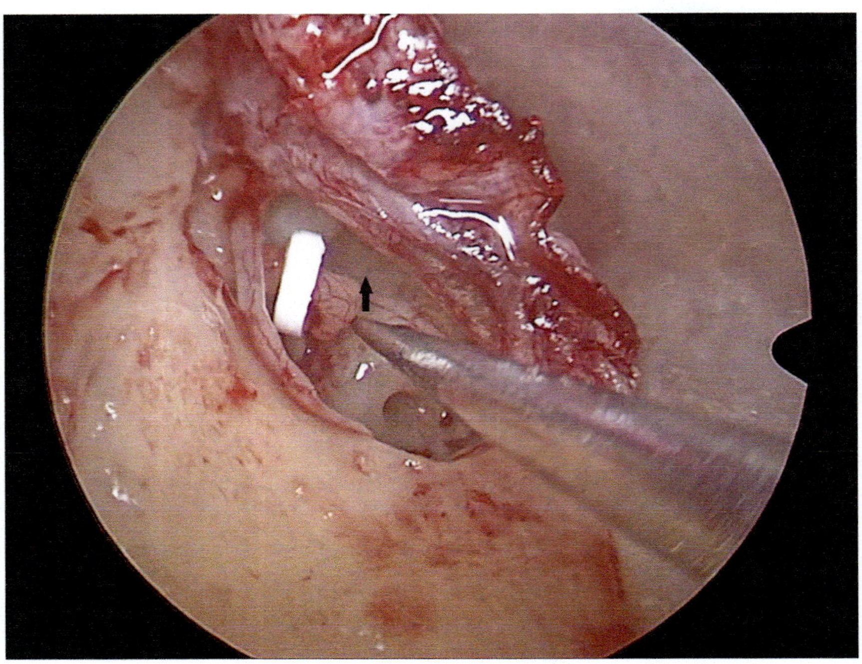

Fig. 39A: "Lift" test.

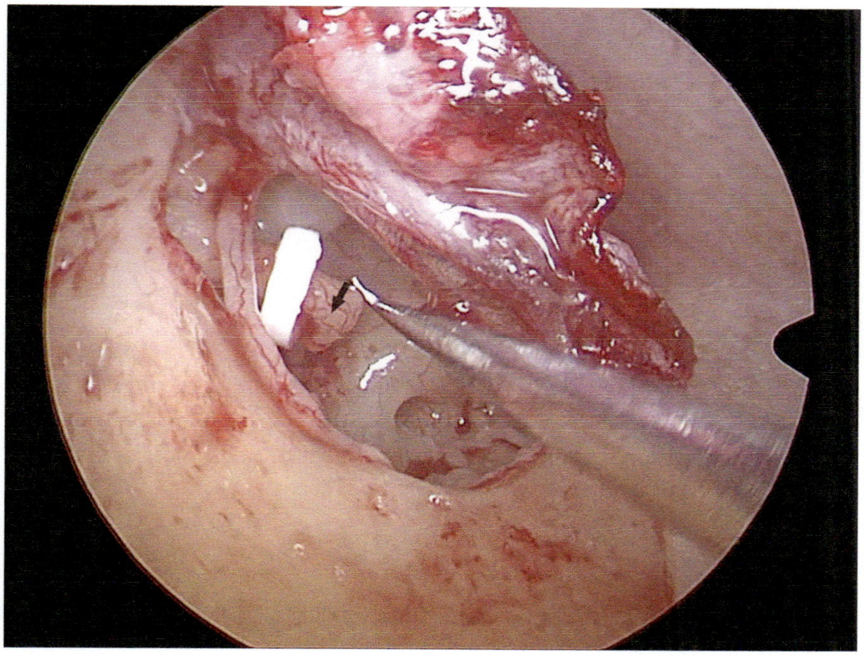

Fig. 39B: "Bend" test.

- Teflon piston is gently crimped with wire-crimper.
- Soft tissue seal obtained from a small postaural puncture wound is used to plug the fenestra.

TIP

A small stab wound is made in the postaural region and subcutaneous soft tissue is harvested. The collected tissue is directly transferred to its bed at the fenestra by a "no-touch" technique, that is, the soft tissue should not touch any surface of a used instrument or gloves or drapes in order to avoid postoperative granulation tissue formation.

- Tympanomeatal flap is repositioned back in its place
- Gelfoam is placed in the canal to stabilize the flap
- Routine postoperative medications are prescribed

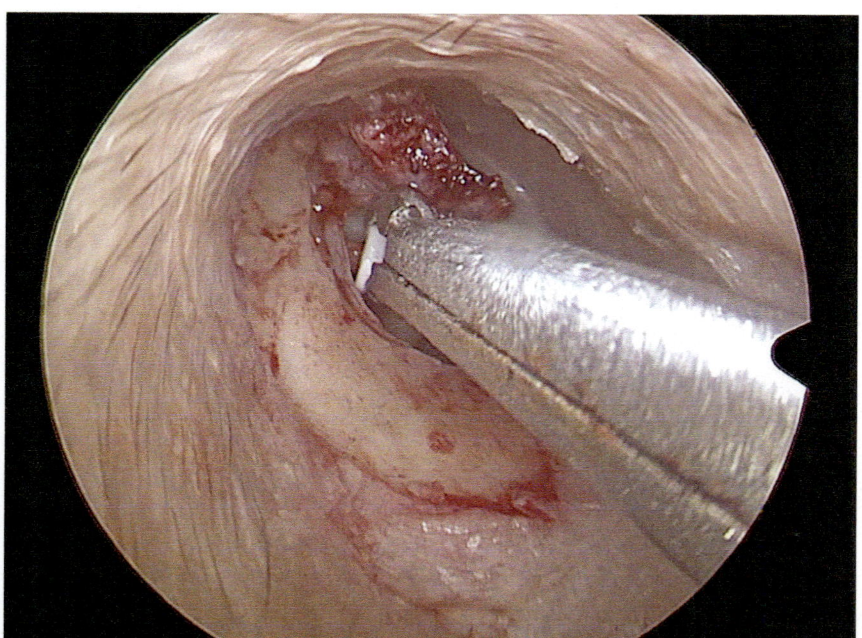

Fig. 40A: Piston being crimped with wire crimper.

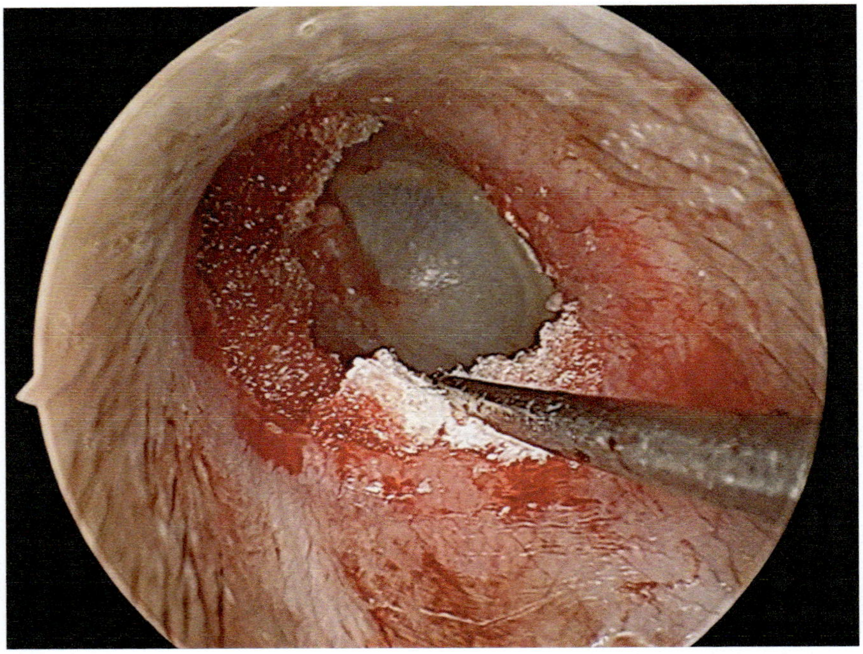

Fig. 40B: Tympanomeatal flap secured with gelfoam.

ENDOSCOPIC STAPEDECTOMY

- Majority of the cases operated by us endoscopically are stapedotomy as it is less invasive, carries lesser chance of inner ear damage with hearing results comparable with that of stapedectomy.
- Stapedectomy is reserved for select situations
- The initial steps till the removal of stapes suprastructure are the same as that for stapedotomy.

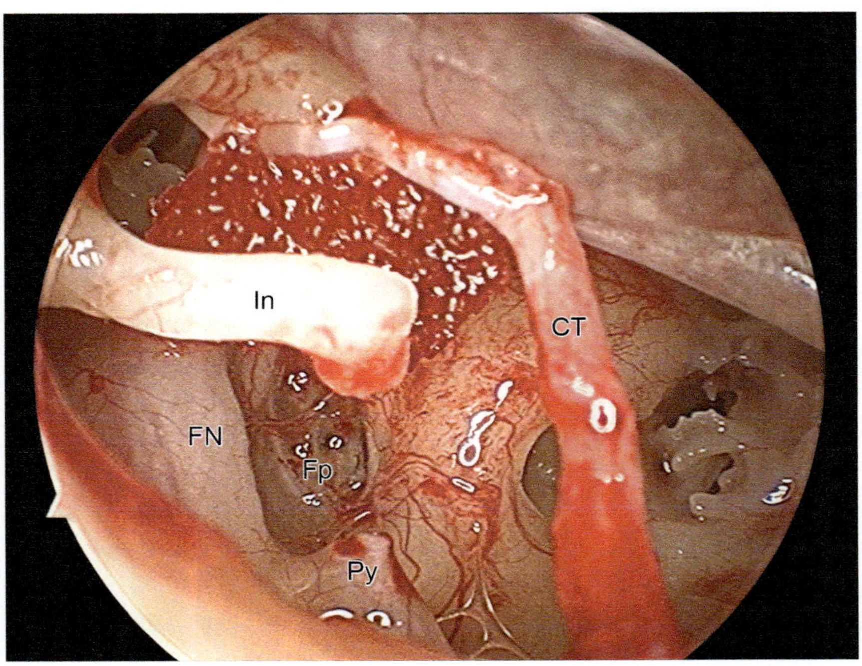

Fig. 41A: Floating footplate and landmarks around incudostapedial complex area (right ear).
(CT: chorda tympani nerve; FN: facial nerve; Fp: foot plate; In: incus; Py: pyramid)

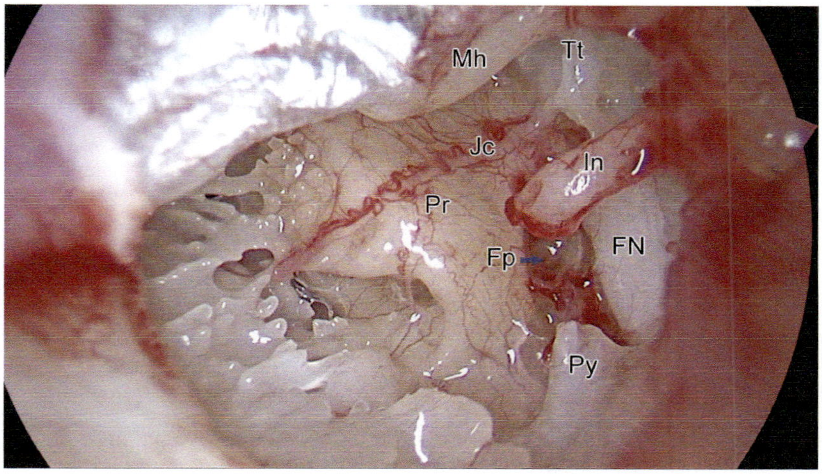

Fig. 41B: Floating footplate and landmarks around incudostapedial complex area (Left ear).
(FN: facial nerve; Fp: foot plate; In: incus; Mh: handle of malleus; Py: pyramid; Jc: Jacobson's nerve; Tt: tensor tympani tendon; Pr: promontory)

- **The footplate is retrieved with the help of a 2-mm angled pick.**

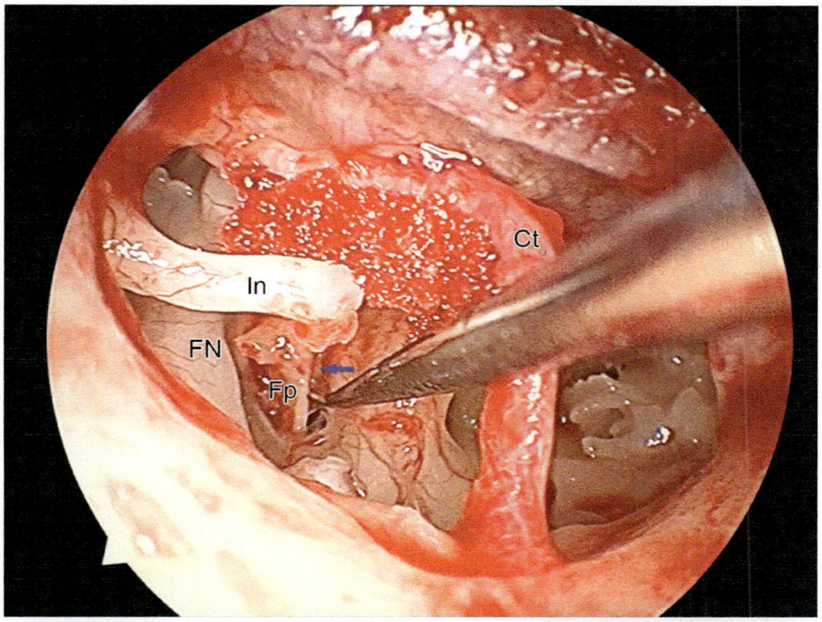

Fig. 42A: Footplate retrieved using a 2-mm angled pick (right ear).
(Ct: chorda tympani nerve; FN: facial nerve; Fp: foot plate; In: incus)

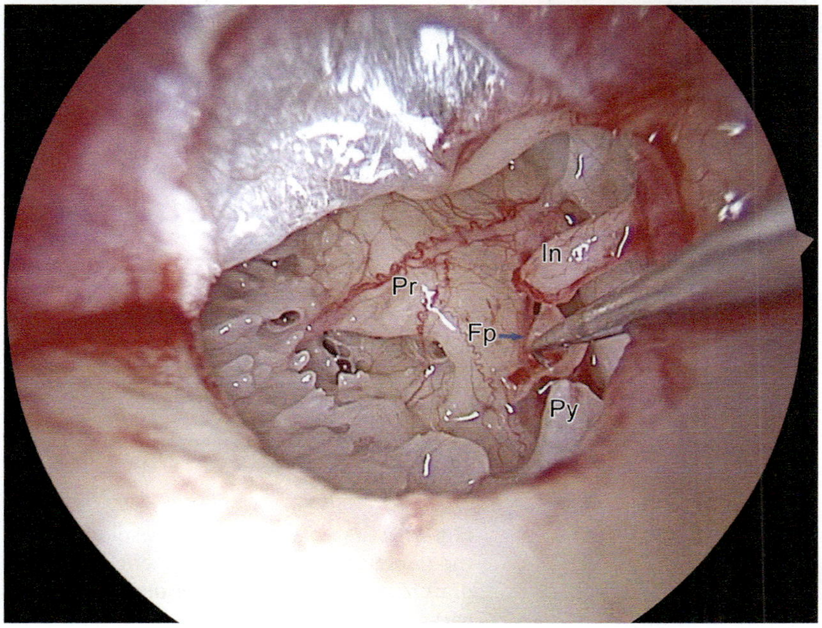

Fig. 42B: Footplate retrieved using a 2-mm angled pick (left ear).
(Fp: foot plate; In: incus; Pr: promontory; Py: pyramid)

TIP

In case a control fenestra has been made already, the footplate is fished out gently by engaging the 2-mm angled pick in the fenestra. In the absence of a control fenestra, the footplate is retrieved by engaging at the inferior border, close to the promontory.

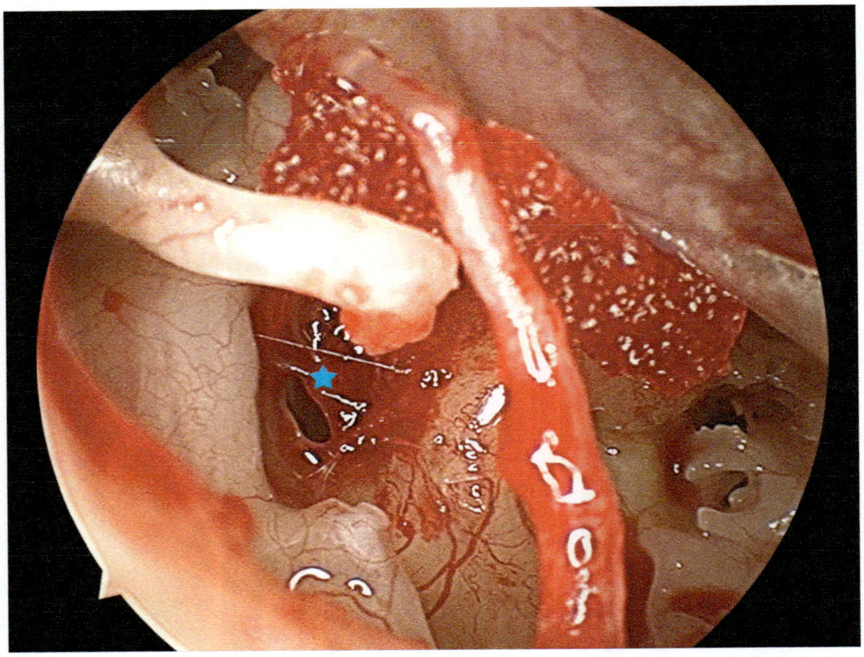

Fig. 43: Opening of the vestibule following removal of footplate (marked with *).

- *Grafting over the open vestibule:* We use crushed perichondrium, harvested from a small incision over the postaural region or vein graft to cover the vestibule.

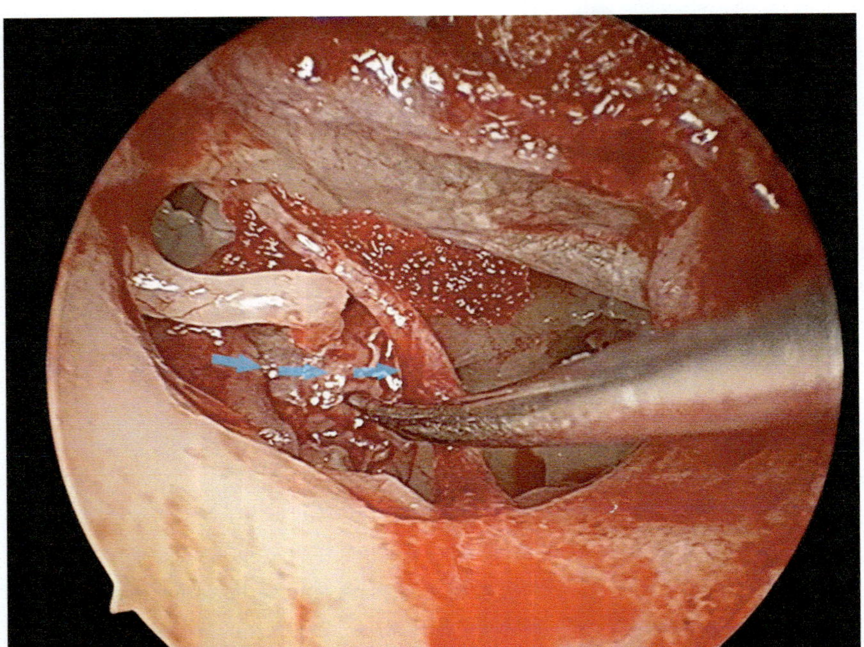

Fig. 44A: Graft placement over vestibule: Note the direction of placement of perichondrium graft from superior to inferior direction (right ear).

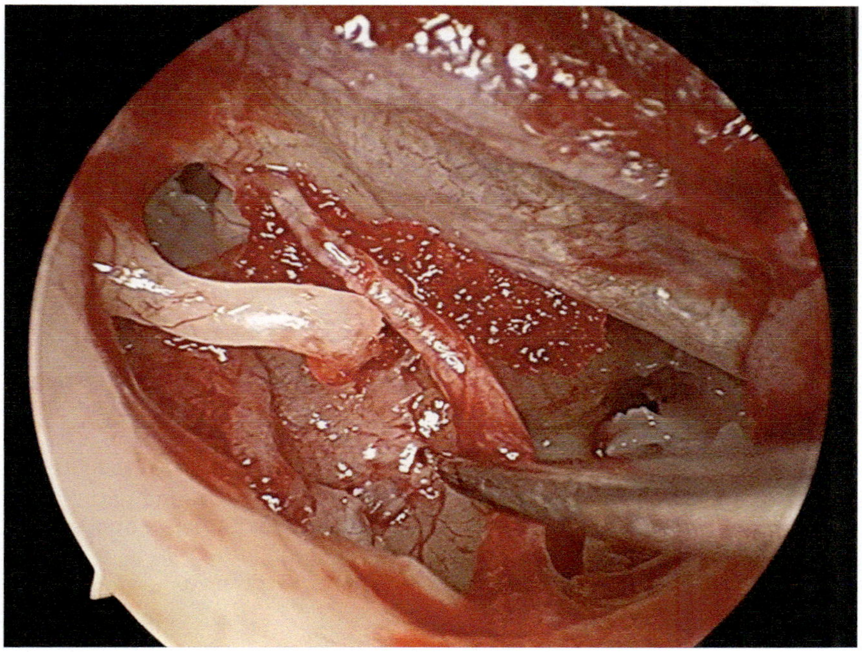

Fig. 44B: Graft placement over vestibule: Note the placement of perichondrium graft covering part of the horizontal segment of facial nerve above and promontory below (right ear).

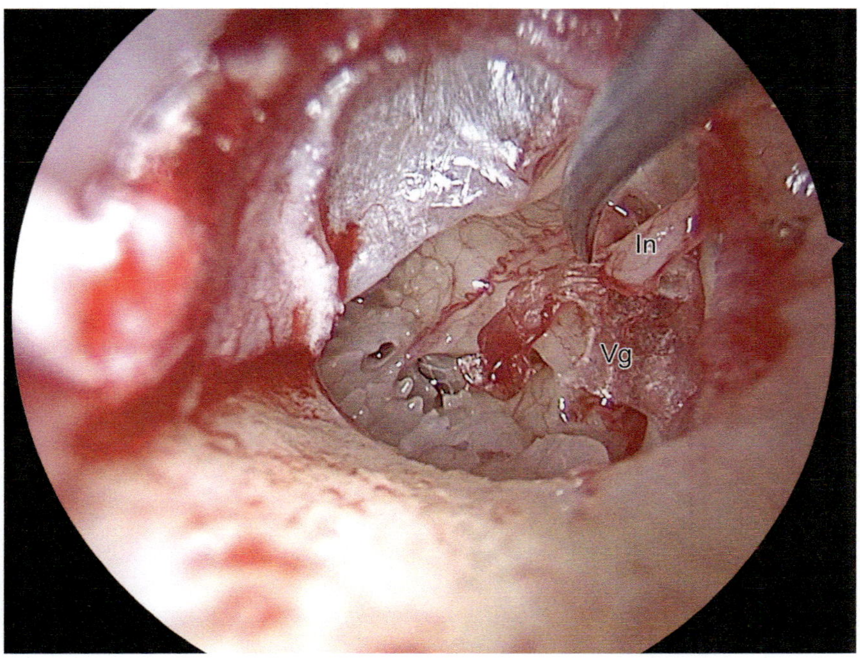

Fig. 44C: Graft placement over vestibule: Note the direction of placement of vein graft from superior to inferior direction (left ear). (Vg: vein graft; In: incus)

PEARL METHOD OF PLACEMENT OF GRAFT

The graft is laid from superiorly over the fallopian canal, then over the vestibule and extending inferiorly over the promontory. This technique of graft placement from superior to inferior region instead of doing so on the vestibule directly, makes it easier to lay the graft uniformly over the area. A small piece of gelfoam may be used to spread it out evenly over the said areas.

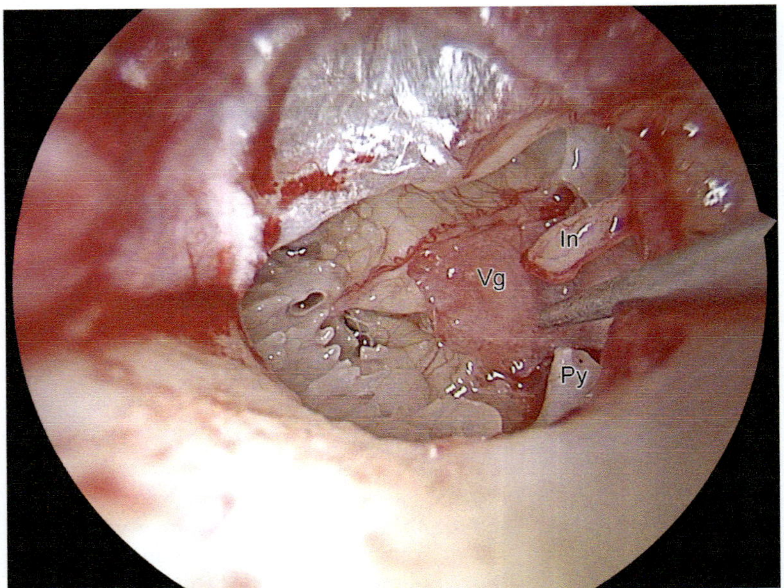

Fig. 44D: Graft placement over vestibule: Note the placement of vein graft covering part of the horizontal segment of facial nerve above and promontory below (left ear).
(Vg: vein graft; In: Incus; Py: pyramid)

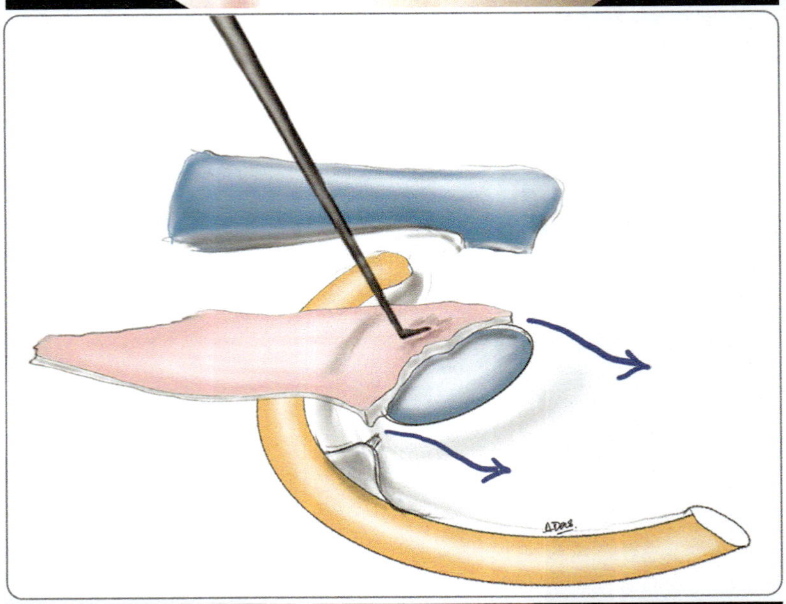

Fig. 45A: Schematic depiction of direction of grafting over open vestibule (superior to inferior).

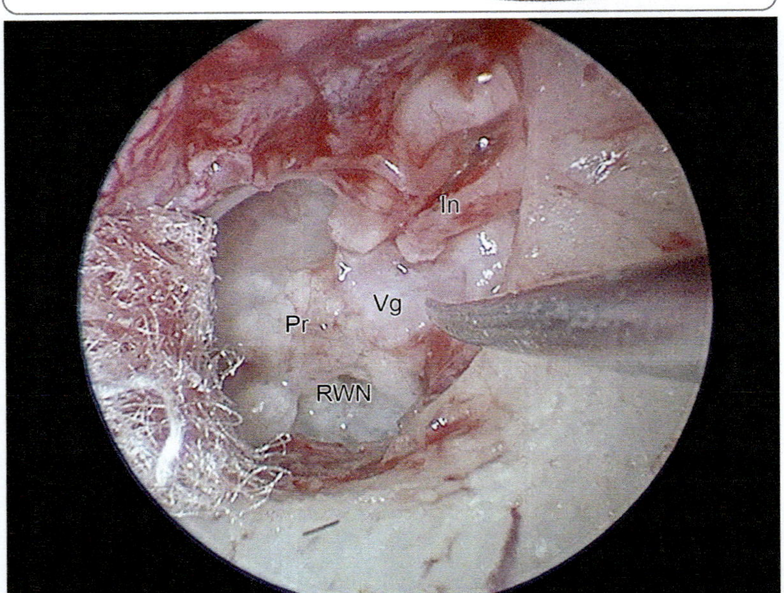

Fig. 45B: Vein graft placed over the vestibule.
(In: incus; Pr: promontory; Vg: vein graft; RWN: round window niche)

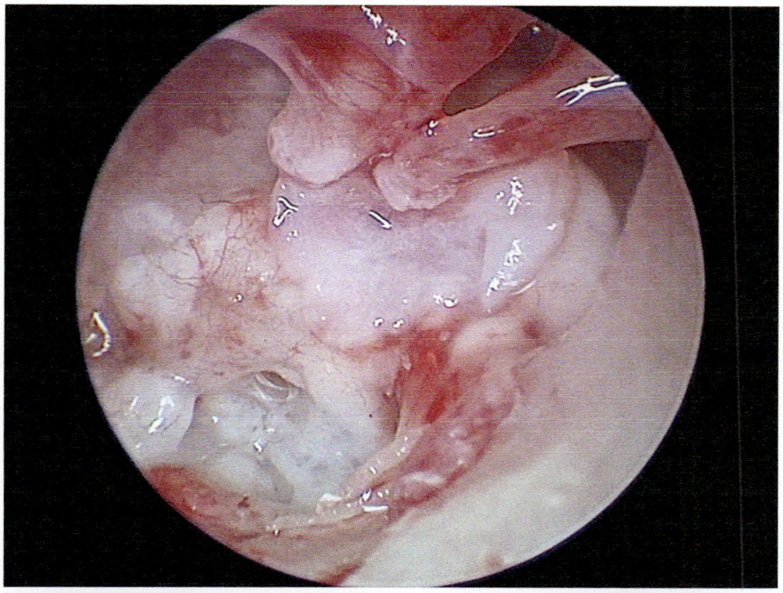

Fig. 45C: Vein graft placed over the vestibule.

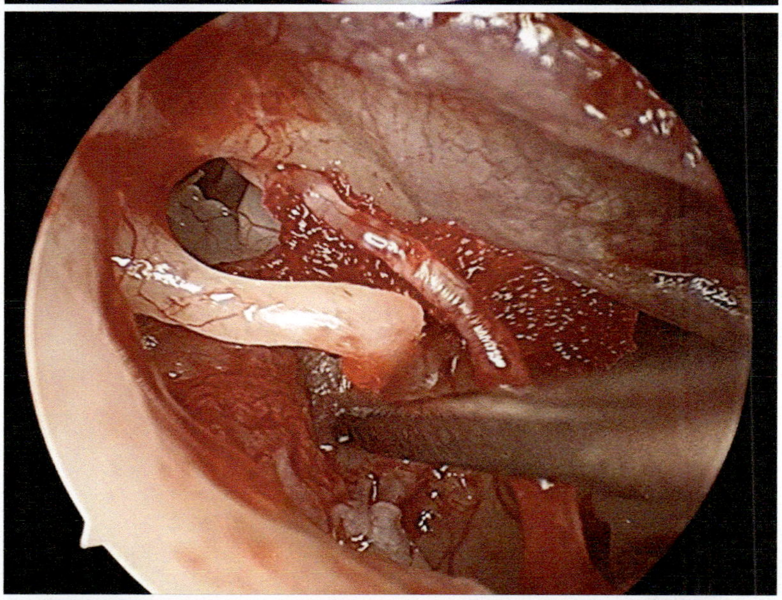

Fig. 46A: Preparation of the bed for placement of the piston over the graft (right ear).

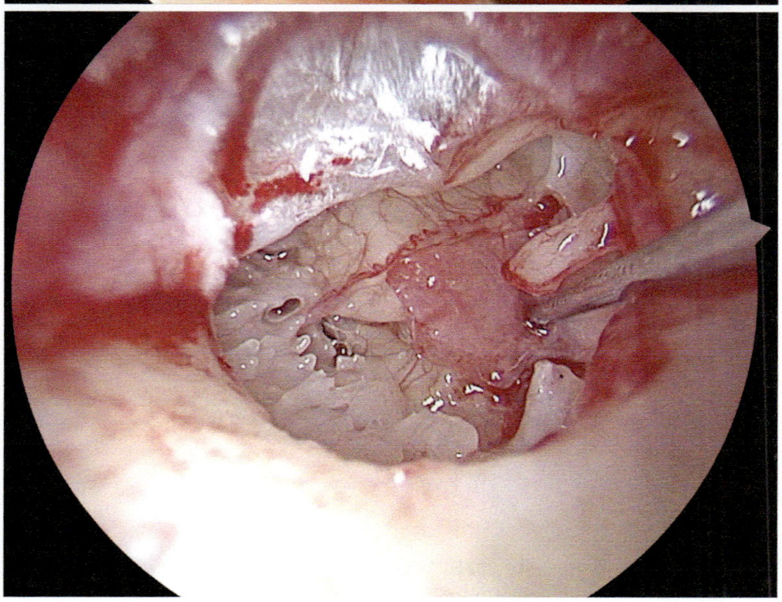

Fig. 46B: Preparation of the bed for placement of the piston over the graft (left ear).

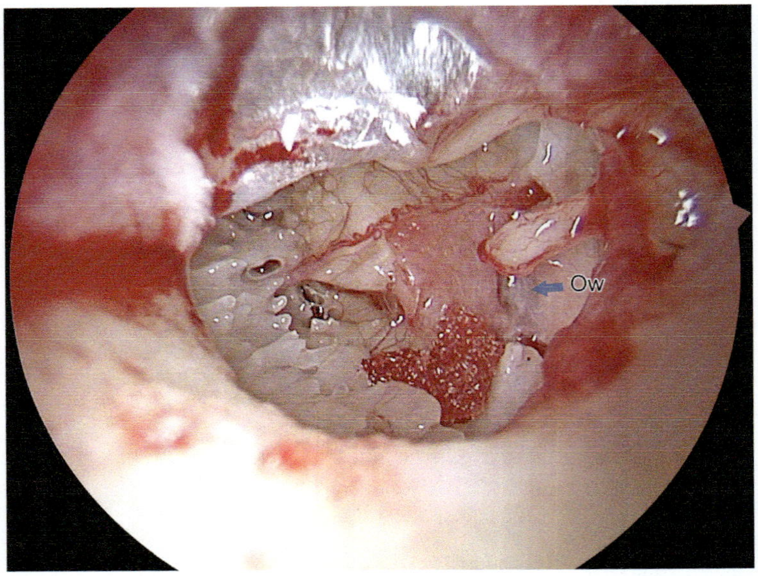

Fig. 46C: Blue lining of vestibule visible beneath the vein graft (left ear).
(Ow: oval window)

- Measurement of the piston length as in stapedotomy
- The piston is then placed at the center of the vestibule

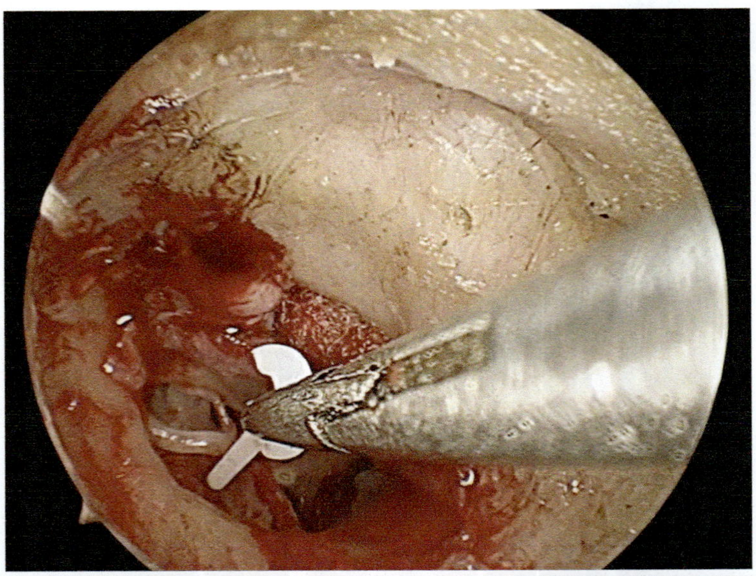

Fig. 47A: Piston being placed over the graft covering the vestibule (right ear).

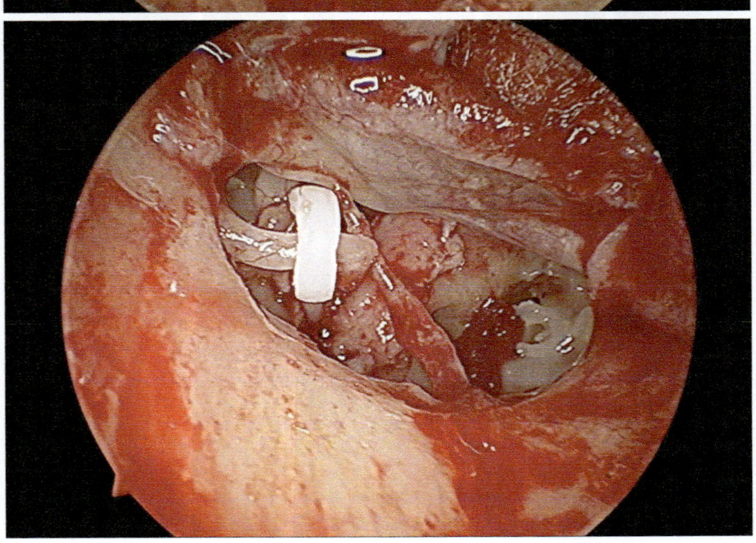

Fig. 47B: Final view of piston placed into vestibule over perichondrium graft (right ear).

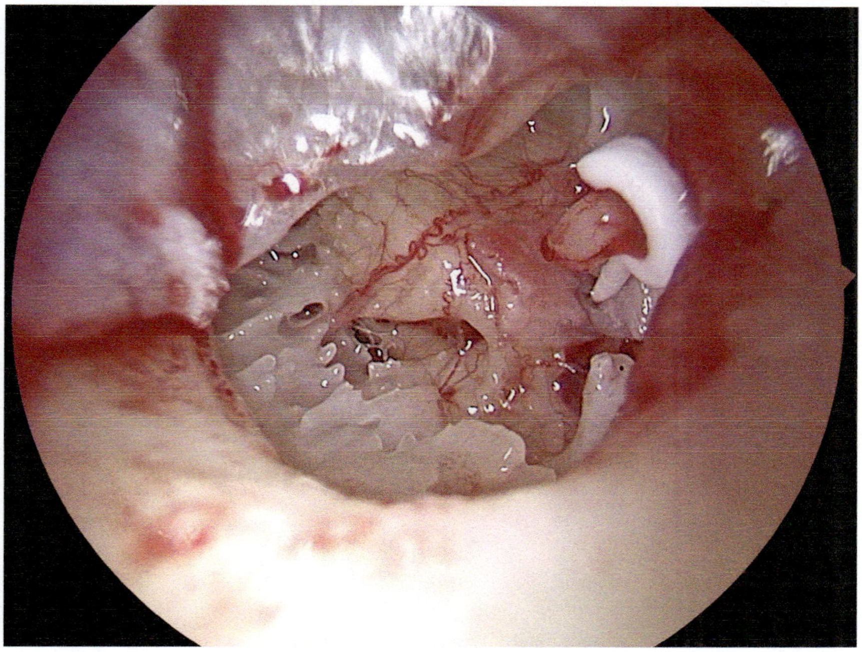

Fig. 47C: Final view of piston placed into vestibule over vein graft (left ear).

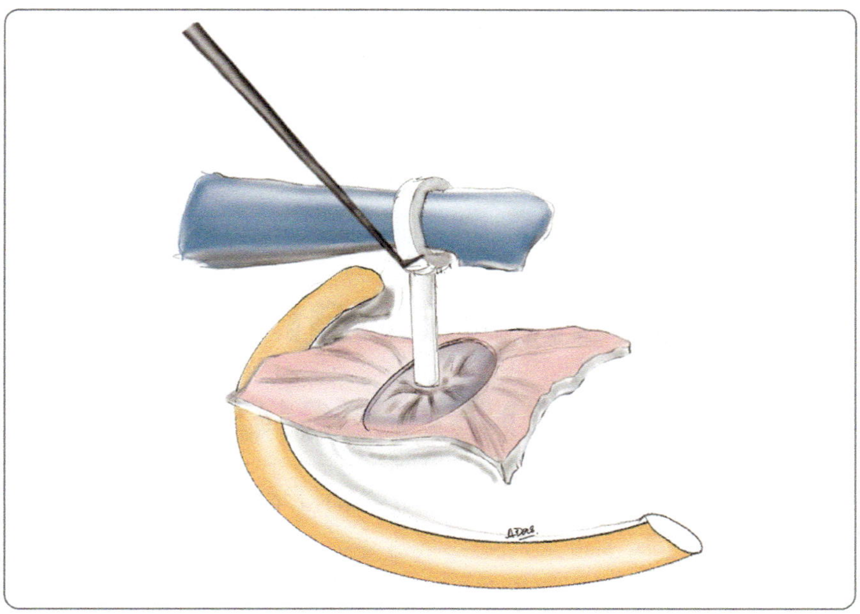

Fig. 48: Schematic representation of the final assembly of the piston over the graft covering the open vestibule.

- Tympanomeatal flap is repositioned back
- Gelfoam placed in the canal to stabilize the flap

REFERENCES

1. Chole RA, McKenna M. Pathophysiology of otosclerosis. Otol Neurotol. 2001;22(2):249-57.
2. Shea JJ. Symposium on the operation for mobilization of the stapes in otosclerosis. Laryngoscope. 1956;66:729-84.
3. Das A, Mitra S, Ghosh D, Sengupta A. Endoscopic Stapedotomy: Overcoming Limitations of Operating Microscope. Ear Nose Throat J. 2021;100(2):103-9.
4. Brackmann DE, Shelton C, Arriaga Moisés A. Avoidance and management of complications of otosclerosis surgery. Otolcgic surgery, 4th edition, 2006; pp. 260–1. Essay, Elsevier.

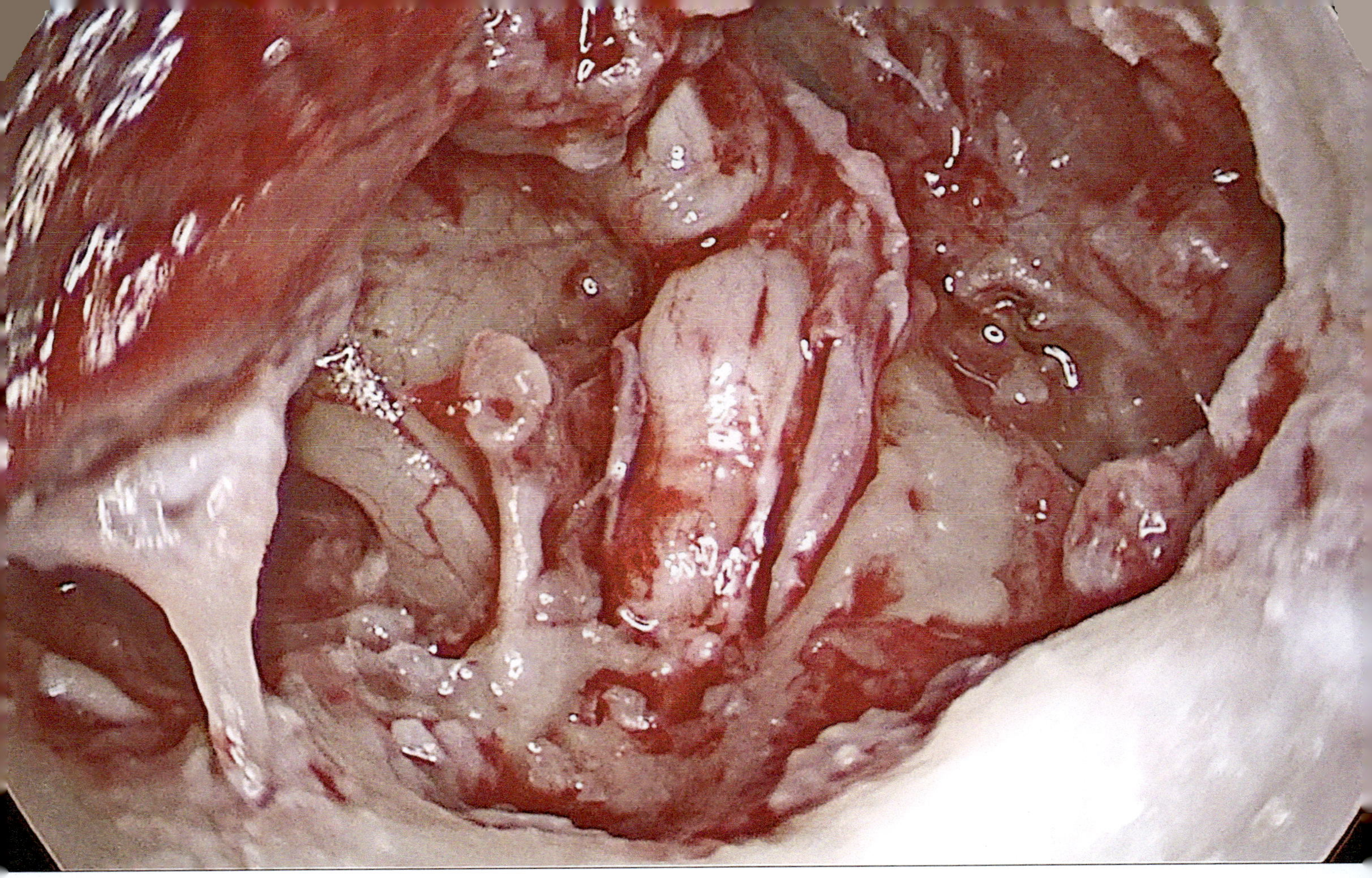

CHAPTER **14**

Endoscopic Transcanal Facial Nerve Decompression

Arindam Das, Sandipta Mitra

Chapter Outline

INTRODUCTION

Traumatic temporal bone fractures often present with facial nerve paralysis. Of the three types of temporal bone fractures—longitudinal, transverse and mixed type, facial nerve involvement is seen in up to 15–20% of longitudinal fractures and up to 50% of transverse fractures.[1,2] Temporal bone fractures have been recently classified into otic capsule-violating and otic capsule-sparing fractures. It has been seen that otic capsule-violating fractures carry five times higher incidence of facial nerve involvement than otic capsule-sparing fractures.[3] Overall incidence of grave long-term outcomes and complications are higher in otic capsule-violating fractures.

The severity of traumatic facial palsy encompasses a large number of pathophysiological conditions that may be:[4]

- Simple traction injury over an anatomically intact nerve
- Crush injury of the nerve fibers
- Partial nerve transection
- Complete nerve transection
- Loss of nerve segment

Apart from these, fractured bone fragments impinging on the nerve or intraneural hematoma may also jeopardize normal nerve conduction.

Facial nerve is a unique anatomical structure which passes through multiple planes of the temporal bone in a complex tortuous course. Hence, no single approach is adequate to address all segments of the nerve equally. Classically, the following approaches have been advocated for corresponding segments of facial nerve:

- Mastoidectomy for vertical/mastoid segment
- Transcanal atticotomy for horizontal/tympanic vsegment
- Middle cranial fossa approach for labyrinthine segment

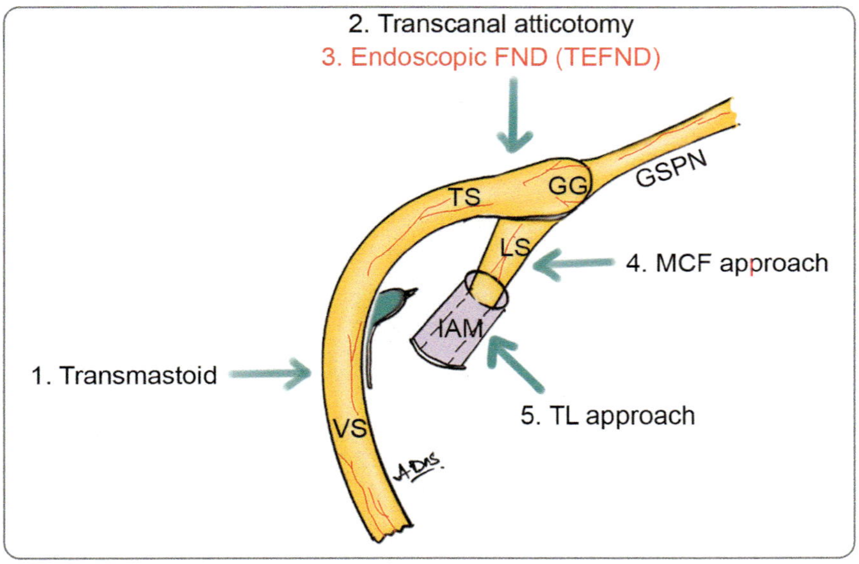

Fig. 1: Approaches to facial nerve decompression.
(TS: tympanic segment; GG: geniculate ganglion; GSPN: greater superficial petrosal nerve; IAM: internal acoustic meatus; LS: labyrinthine segment; MCF: middle cranial fossa approach; TL: translabyrinthine approach; VS: vertical segment; TEFND: transcanal endoscopic facial nerve decompression)

Endoscopic transcanal facial nerve decompression is a new surgical entity, only recently described in literature. It is a minimally invasive, functional surgery for addressing facial nerve injuries right from labyrinthine segment till second genu, proximal to processus pyramidalis.

However, the timing of the surgery is a matter of debate and lacks an internationally-accepted management protocol specific for traumatic facial palsy.

ENDOSCOPIC FACIAL NERVE DECOMPRESSION: CONCEPT OF SEGMENTAL DECOMPRESSION

- Endoscopic facial nerve decompression may be specified according to the site of affection
- Based on the site, endoscopic facial nerve decompression may be classified into:
  - *Type A*: Geniculate ganglion + Tympanic segment + Greater superficial petrosal nerve (most common)
  - *Type B*: Tympanic segment + Second genu (second most common)
  - *Type C*: Labyrinthine segment + Geniculate ganglion + Greater superficial petrosal nerve

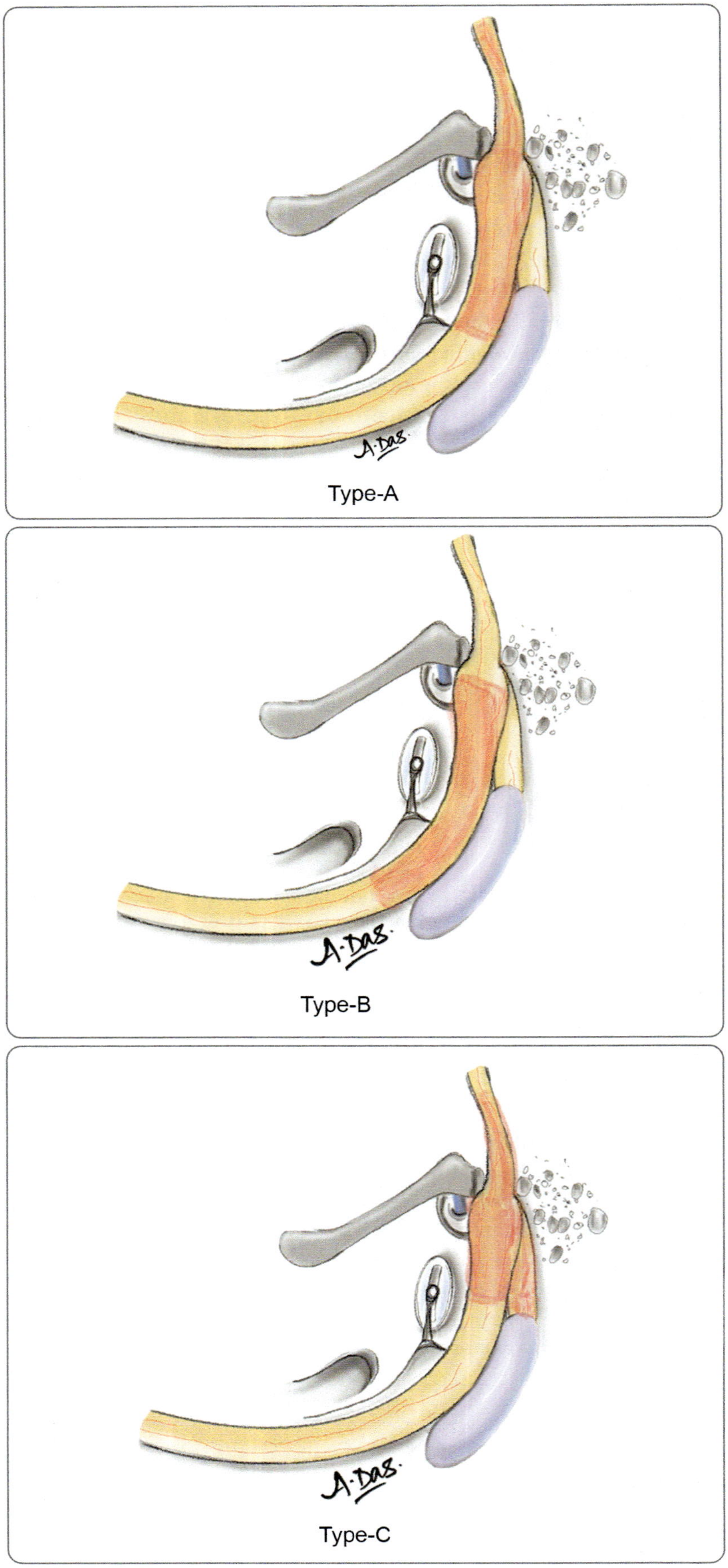

Fig. 2: Types of segmental facial nerve decompression (vide text).

RATIONALE OF ENDOSCOPIC TRANSCANAL FACIAL NERVE DECOMPRESSION

- Perigeniculate area is one of the most common sites affected in traumatic facial nerve paralysis.
- Conventionally, perigeniculate facial nerve injuries have been addressed by microscopic transcanal facial nerve decompression.
- However, this entails additional bone removal in the form of a complete atticotomy in order to attain adequate exposure of the site of injury.
- Endoscope via transcanal approach, offers a direct access to such a site of injury without the need for excess bone removal as in complete atticotomy.
- Site of injury and detection of multiple sites of involvement can be done early with the help of angled endoscope.
- A close-up magnified view helps to visualize the affected part of the nerve and compare the same with the adjacent normal segment (as close as the microvasculature supplying the nerve using Spectra-A and Spectra-B mode)
- Angled endoscopes help to visualize the greater superficial petrosal nerve

INDICATIONS OF ENDOSCOPIC TRANSCANAL FACIAL NERVE DECOMPRESSION

- Fractures traversing through perigeniculate area (area includes distal part of labyrinthine segment of facial nerve, geniculate ganglion, greater superficial petrosal nerve, first genu and proximal part of tympanic segment of facial nerve)
- House Brackmann Grade 4–6
- Time of presentation within 21 days of injury

CONTRAINDICATIONS OF ENDOSCOPIC TRANSCANAL FACIAL NERVE DECOMPRESSION

- Injuries involving vertical segment of facial nerve distal to processus pyramidalis
- Injuries involving multiple sites of the facial nerve (except subsites of perigeniculate area only)
- Narrow canal

TABLE 1: House-Brackmann grading system.

Grade	*Characteristics*
1	Normal facial muscle function and normal eye closure
2	On close inspection and slight facial muscle weakness noticeable. Complete eye closure with minimal effort
3	Obvious difference between two sides of face, but not disfiguring. Complete eye closure with maximal effort
4	Obvious facial muscle weakness and/or disfiguring asymmetry. Incomplete eye closure with maximal effort
5	Facial muscle motion barely perceptible. Incomplete eye closure with maximal effort
6	No facial muscle movement. Inability to close eye with maximal effort

Adapted from: House JW, Brackmann DE. Facial nerve grading system. Otolaryngol Head Neck Surg. 1985;93(2):146-7.

PREOPERATIVE CONSIDERATIONS

Primary survey, complete head, neck and neurological assessment.

Preoperative Investigations

- Topodiagnostic tests for facial nerve of special importance
    - *Schirmer's test*: Whatman 41 filter paper strips are placed in the lateral fornix of the lower eyelid to measure the basal lacrimal gland secretion. The test is *positive* in case of injury to the *first genu* or nerve segment *proximal* to it.
    - *Stapedial reflex*: Absent reflex indicates injury to vertical segment of facial nerve proximal to processus pyramidalis
- Computed tomography scan of temporomastoid region (fine 0.6 mm cuts) with 3D reconstruction
    - Gives clues about the trajectory of the fracture line traversing the temporal bone
    - The region around the geniculate ganglion fossa (GGF) is of critical importance
    - An enlarged GGF on temporal bone CT is an important indicator for the diagnosis of GGF fracture[4]
    - Helps to correlate intraoperative findings of edema, fibrosis, bony spicules impinging on the facial nerve in the perigeniculate area

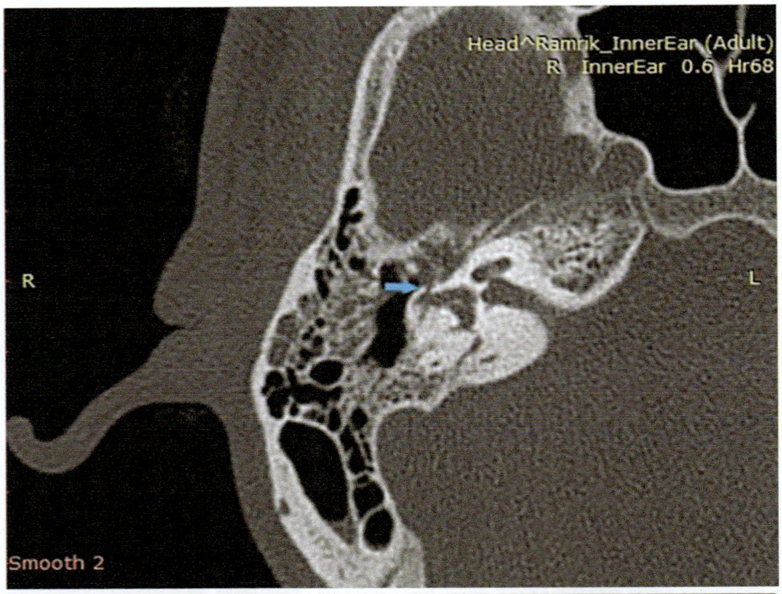

Fig. 3A: HRCT temporal bone in axial plane is showing fractured fragment (arrow).

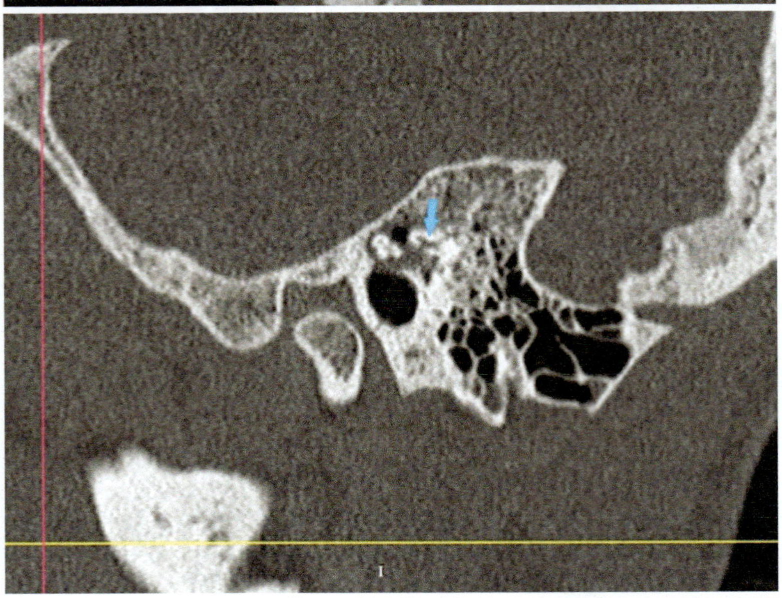

Fig. 3B: HRCT temporal bone in sagittal plane is showing fractured fragment (arrow).

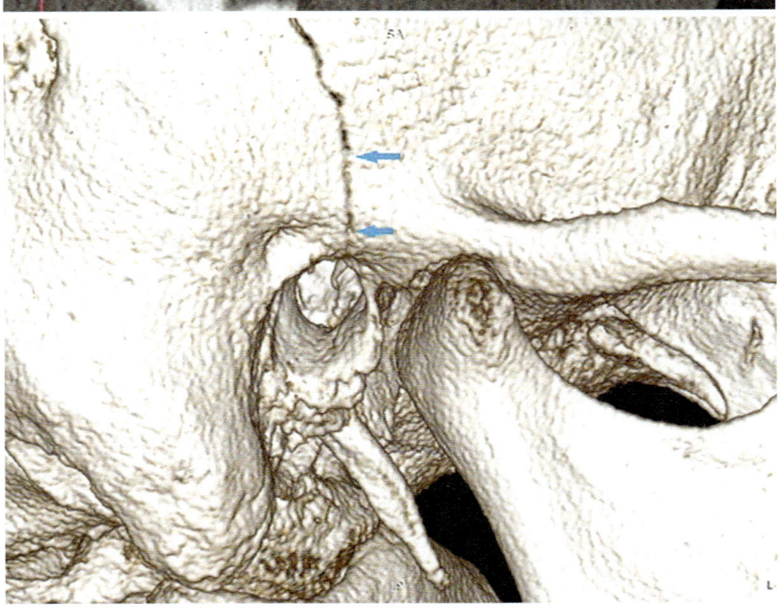

Fig. 3C: HRCT temporal bone is showing fracture line traversing squamous part of temporal bone into the external auditory canal (arrows).

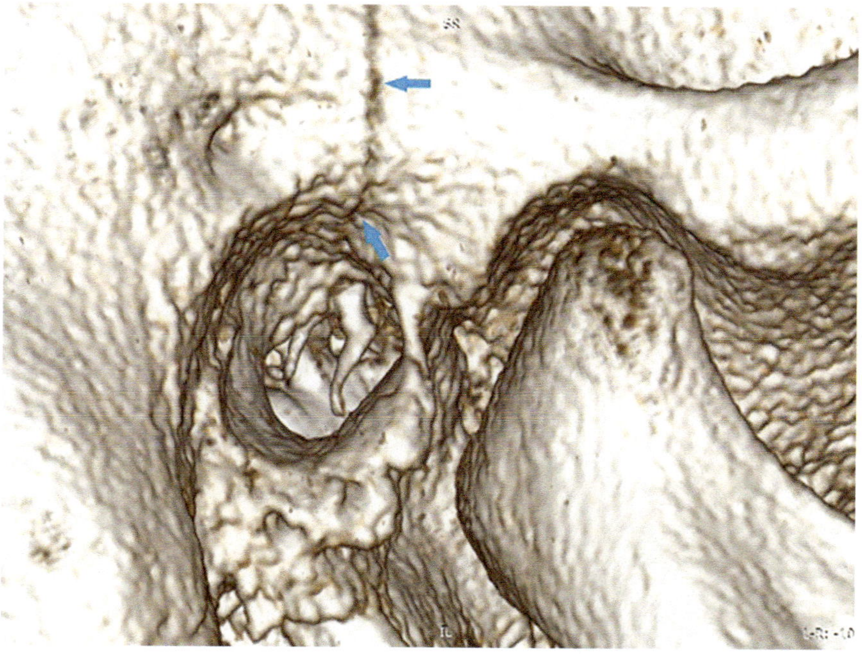

Fig. 3D: HRCT temporal bone is showing fracture line traversing squamous part of temporal bone into the external auditory canal (arrows)—Note the ossicles visible through the external auditory canal.

- Electrophysiological tests
    - Electroneuronography (ENoG) between 3 and 21 days of injury
    - More than 90% degeneration indicates poor prognosis and mandates surgical intervention
- Pure tone audiometry, tympanometry and SDS percentage
    - Patients with temporal bone trauma may suffer from ossicular chain disruption or otic capsule violation
    - Hence, a conductive or mixed hearing loss may be present and needs to be documented preoperatively in all cases
    - This additionally helps in planning of ossicular chain reconstruction and to explain postoperative hearing prognosis in cases of mixed hearing loss

STEPS OF SURGERY

1. *Anesthesia:* Hypotensive general anesthesia is preferred. Local four quadrant infiltration with 2% Lignocaine with Adrenaline (1:100,000).
2. *Tranexamic acid protocol* is followed to minimize intraoperative bleeding. Slow intravenous tranexamic acid bolus (10 mg/kg) half an hour before the start of surgery followed by infusion (5 mg/kg/hour). The infusion is prepared in normal saline. (Vide "Principles of Endoscopic Ear Surgery" chapter for further details)
3. *Endoscopy and observation of step deformity:* Fracture line in the external auditory canal may create a step-deformity that is palpated with ball point probe. Incision line is modified according to its location.

TIP

- Bleeding may occur at the line of incision due to post-traumatic granulation and neoangiogenesis.
- Monopolar ball point diathermy at low current setting is useful to control the bleeding.

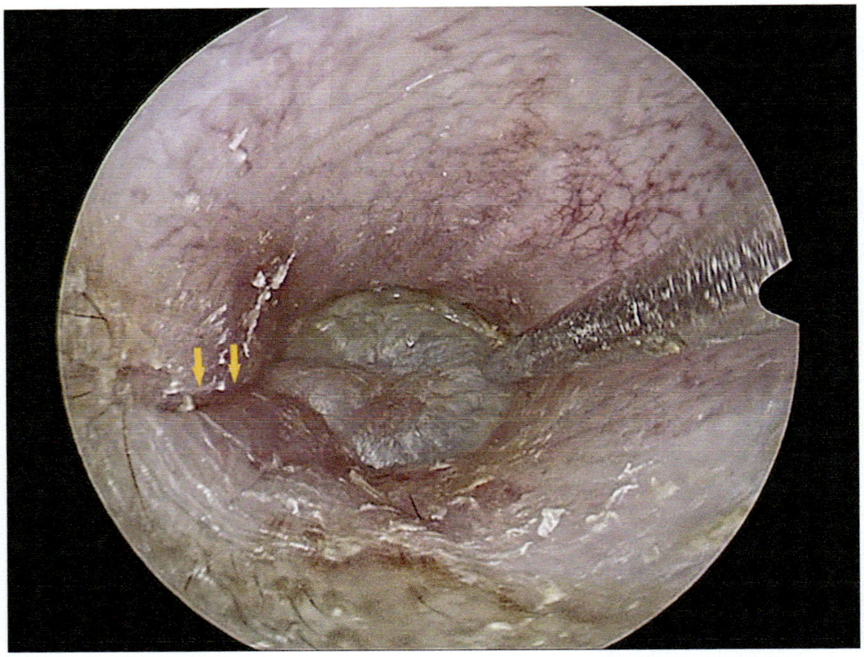

Fig. 4A: Endoscopy and observation of external auditory canal for step deformity.

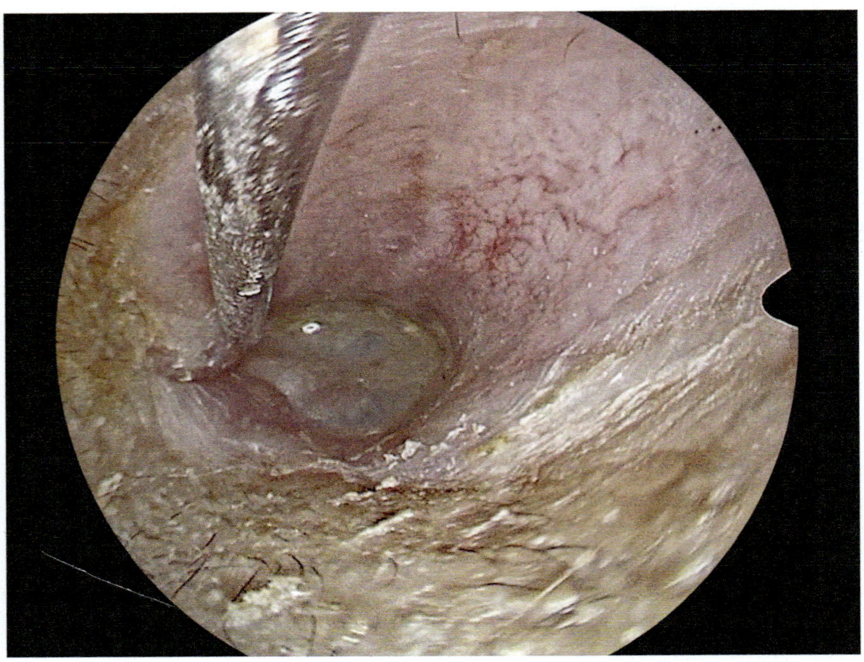

Fig. 4B: Palpation of the same as Figure 4A.

4. *Incision:* Same as for endoscopic transcanal atticotomy. Incision has three parts. A superior limb, an inferior limb and a horizontal limb connecting the two. The horizontal limb is fashioned at a distance of about 5–6 mm from the annulus with the help of a circular knife. The inferior limb is positioned at 6 o'clock clock position, 1 mm away from the inferior annulus and joins the lower border of the horizontal limb. The superior incision is placed keeping a width of 1 mm and is extended further anteriorly up to the Eustachian tube.

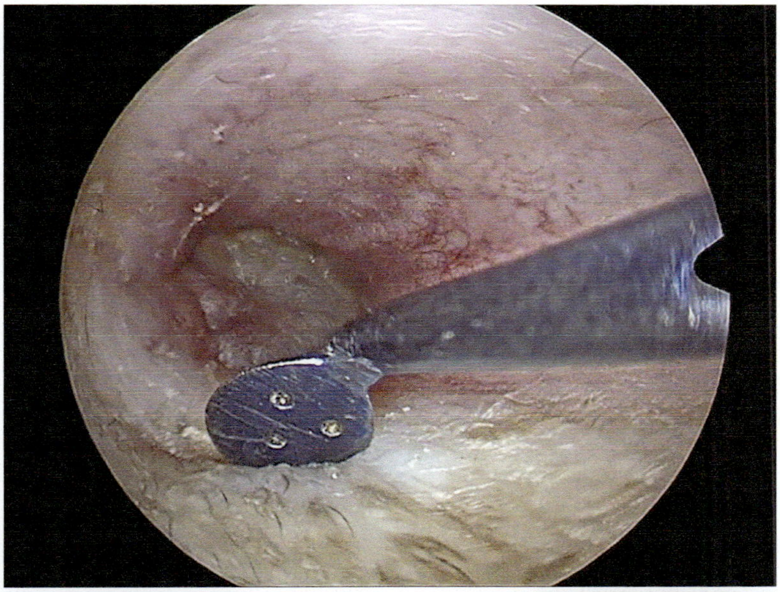

Fig. 5A: Incision: Marking of transcanal incision with round knife.

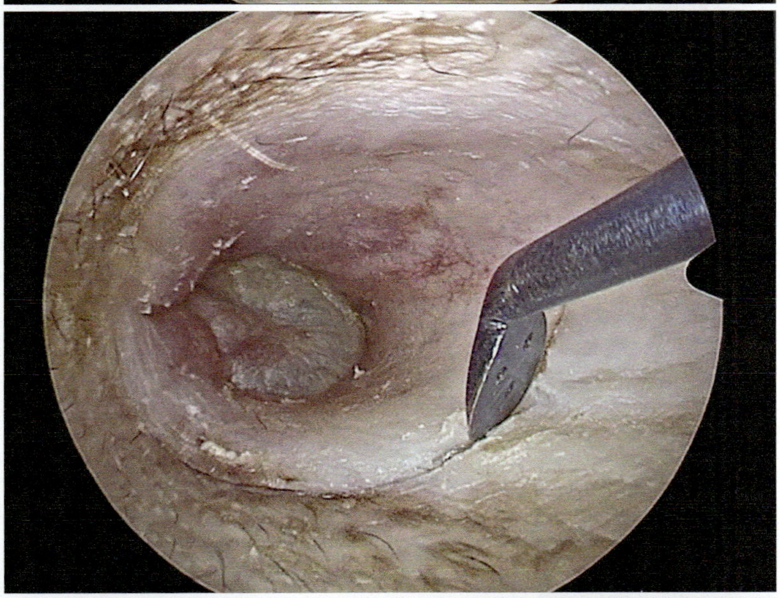

Fig. 5B: Incision: Horizontal limb of incision.

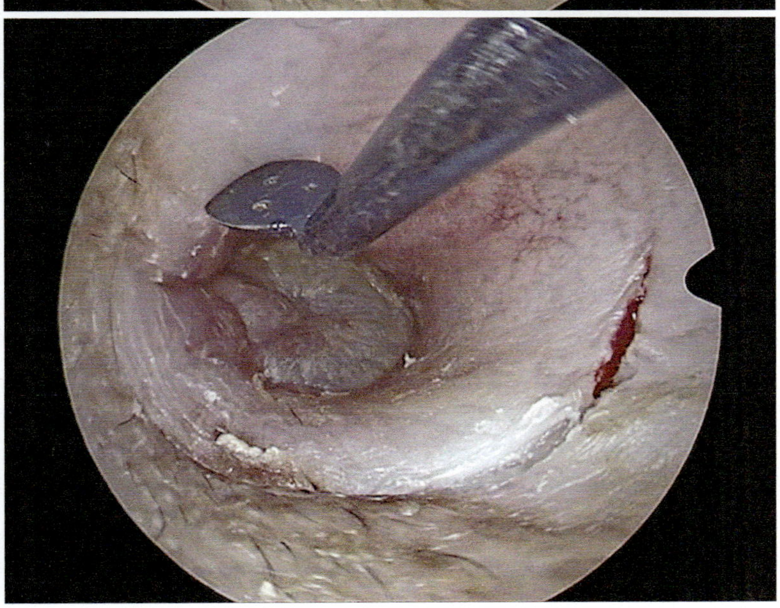

Fig. 5C: Incision: Superior limb.

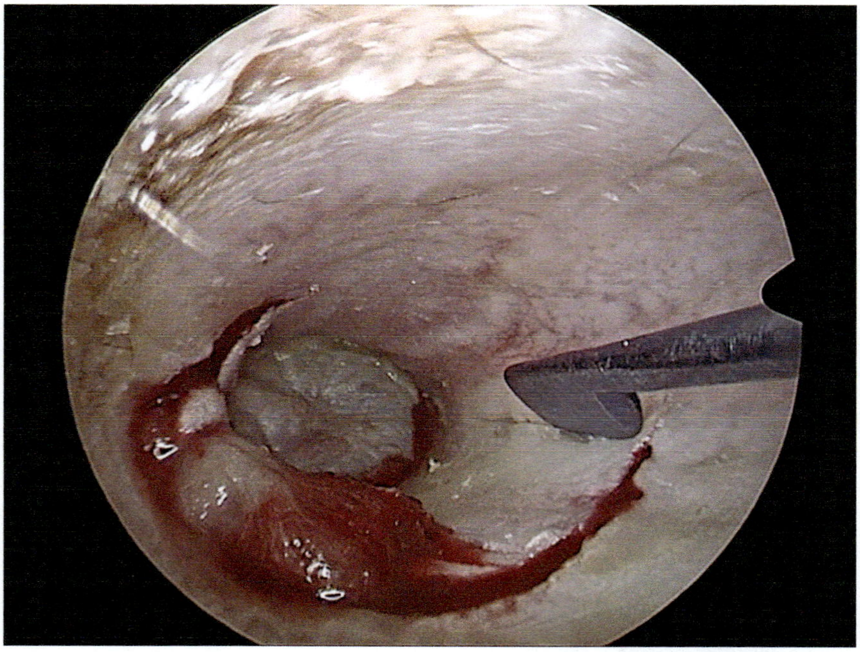

Fig. 5D: Incision: Inferior limb.

5. *Flap elevation:* Tympanomeatal flap is elevated up to annulus. After careful elevation of the flap, it is tucked inferiorly in the hypotympanum to protect it from the rotating burr tip.

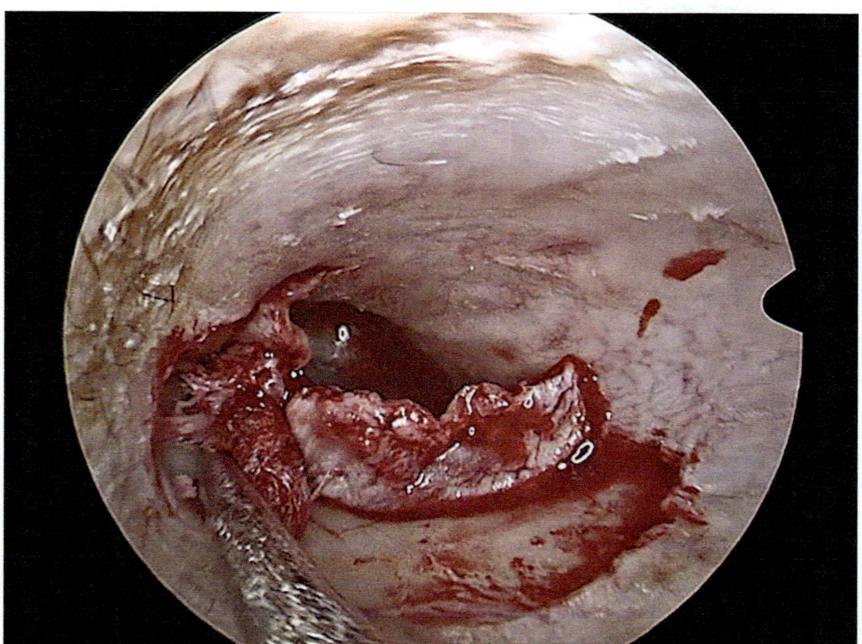

Fig. 6A: Flap elevation. Note the use of adrenaline-soaked cotton balls to maintain hemostasis and protection of flap.

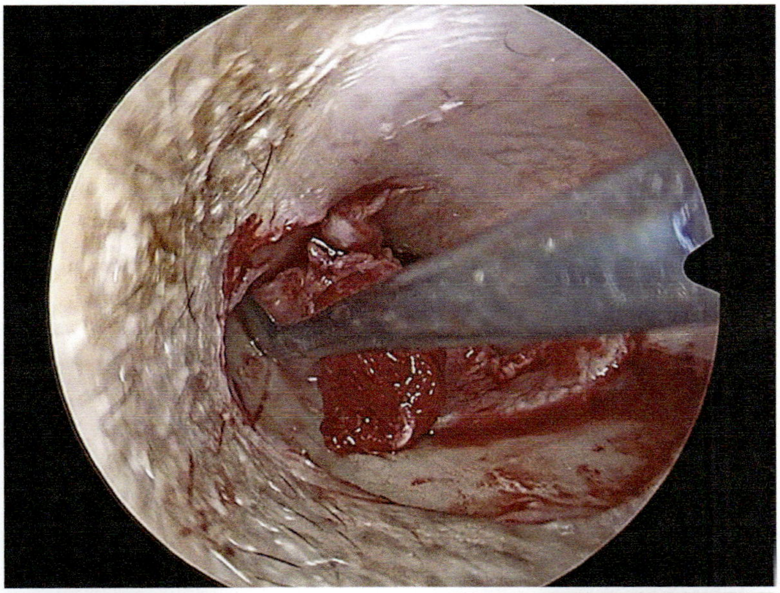

Fig. 6B: Superior flap elevation following fracture line.

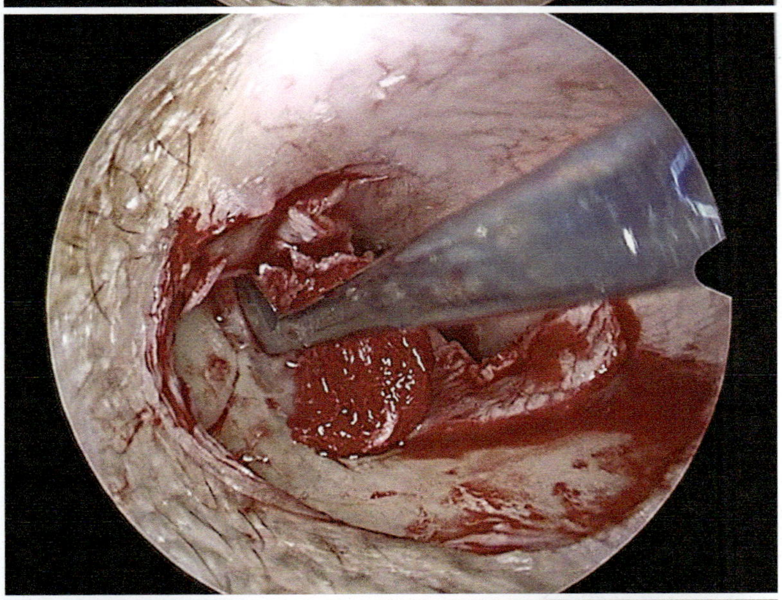

Fig. 6C: Exposure of fracture line following its trajectory.

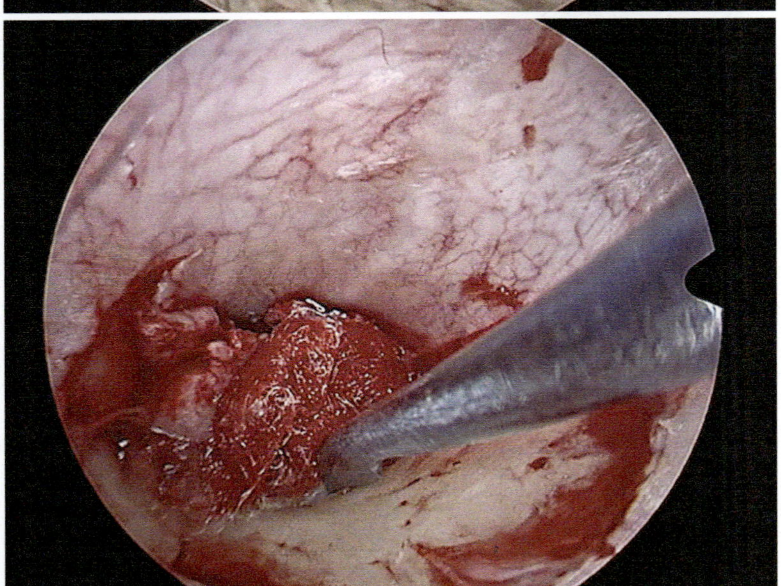

Fig. 6D: Annulus identification and elevation.

TIP

- Proper identification and elevation of the annulus is of prime importance as the tympanic membrane is often intact in these cases
- Sharp dissection may be required during annulus elevation as there is considerable amount of middle ear fibrosis owing to post-traumatic healing.

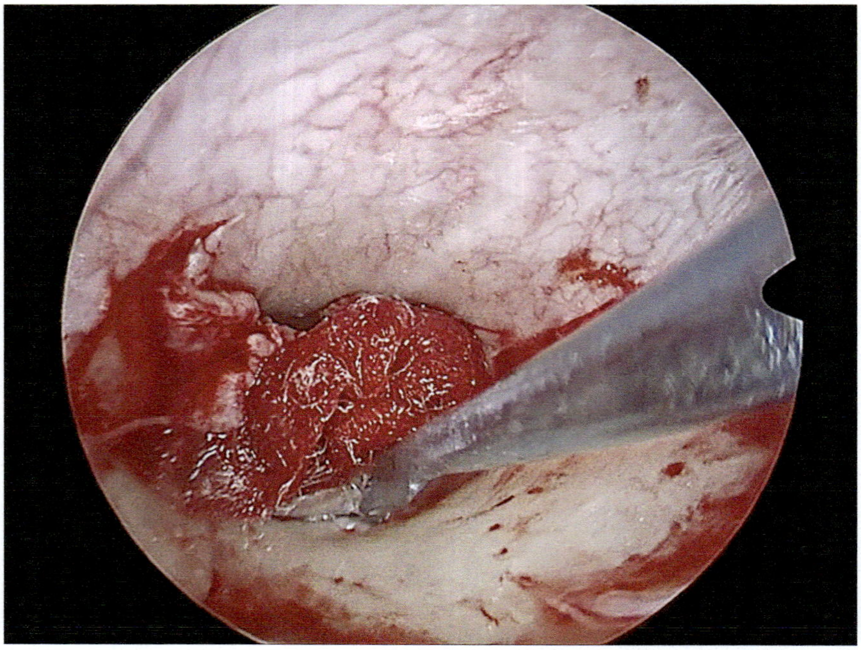

Fig. 7A: Sharp dissection to separate annulus from chorda tympani.

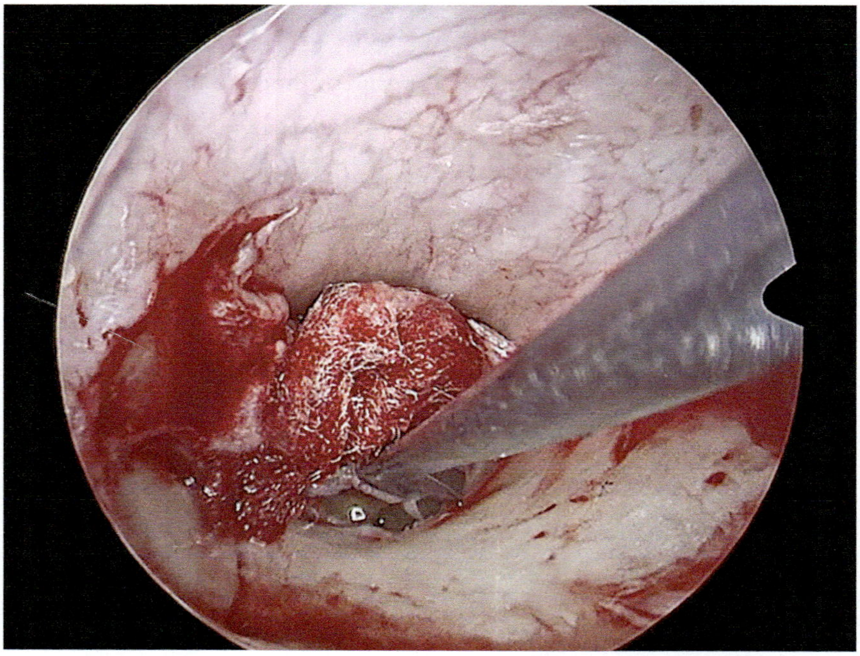

Fig. 7B: Annulus elevation to expose the middle ear.

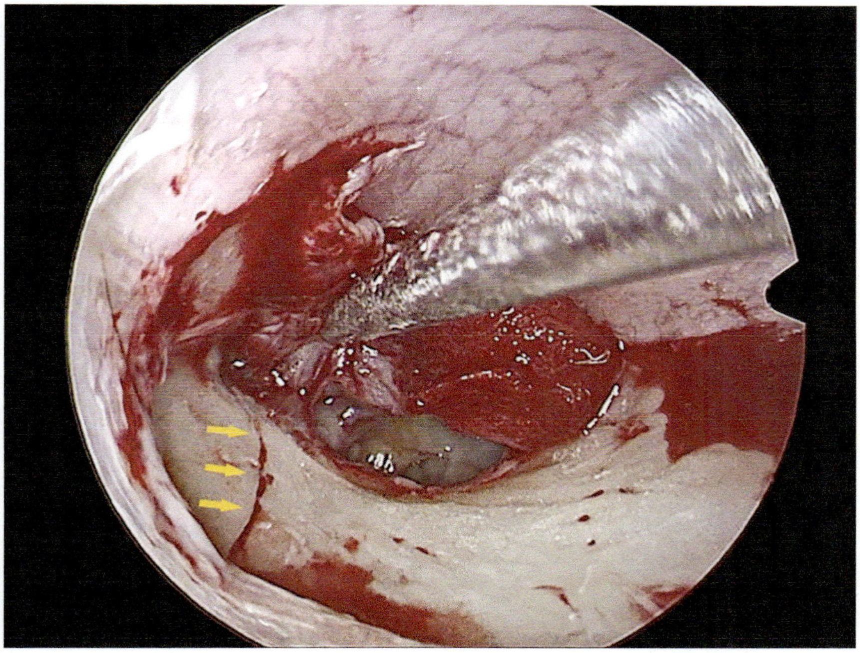

Fig. 7C: Flap elevation superiorly. Note the fracture line running along superior aspect of canal (yellow arrows).

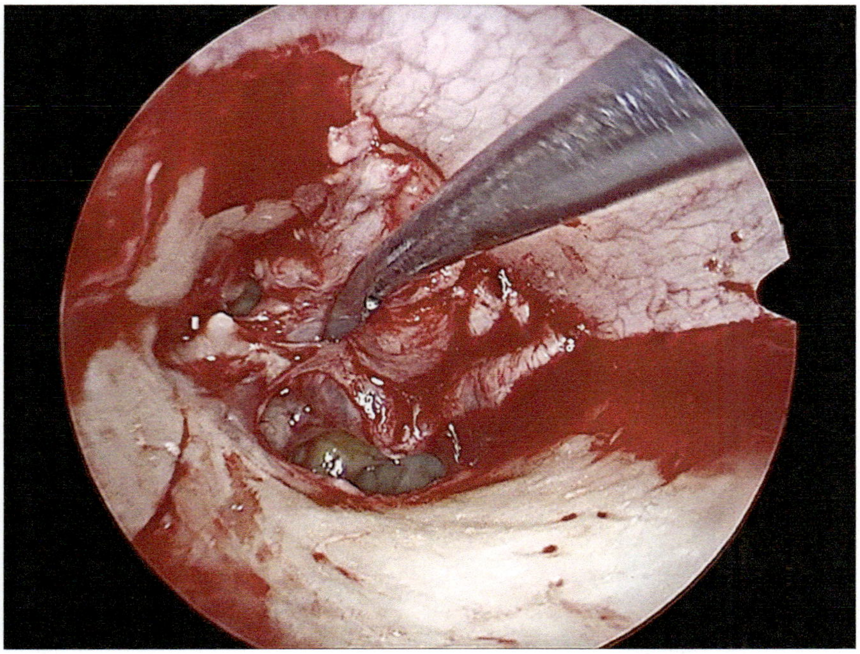

Fig. 7D: Anterior elevation of the flap from the malleus handle.

6. *Middle ear inspection and confirmation of diagnosis:* The following findings may be observed during exploration:
    - Organized hematoma, clots, hemosiderin (brownish-black) fluid
    - Middle ear fibrosis, bands around stapes superstructure
    - *Status of ossicular chain:* The ossicular assembly may be medialized or undergo anteroposterior dislocation
    - Involvement of greater superficial petrosal nerve (using a zero or 30-degree angled endoscope)
    - Displaced fractured fragments of bone indicating tentative site of facial nerve injury
    - Fibrosis around Eustachian tube opening

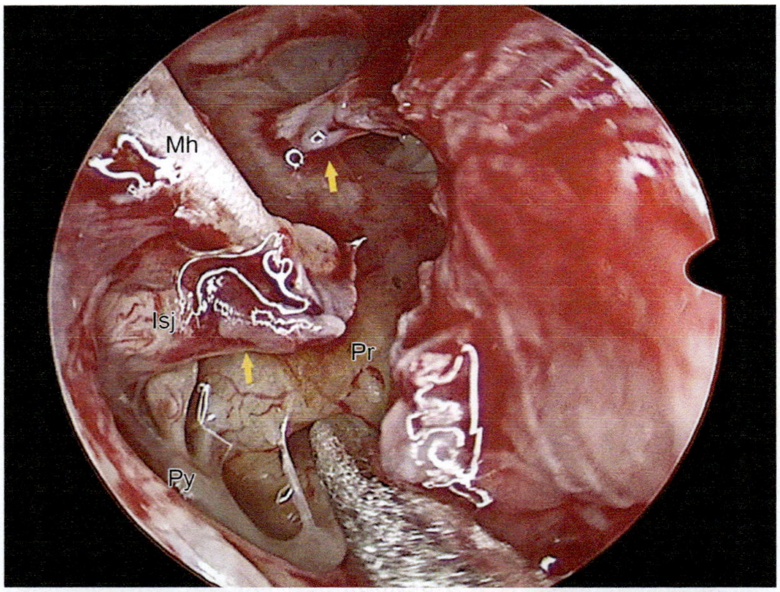

Fig. 8A: View of right middle ear. Yellow arrows—Fibrous bands.
(Isj: incudostapedial joint; Mh: malleus handle; Py: processus pyramidalis; Pr: promontory)

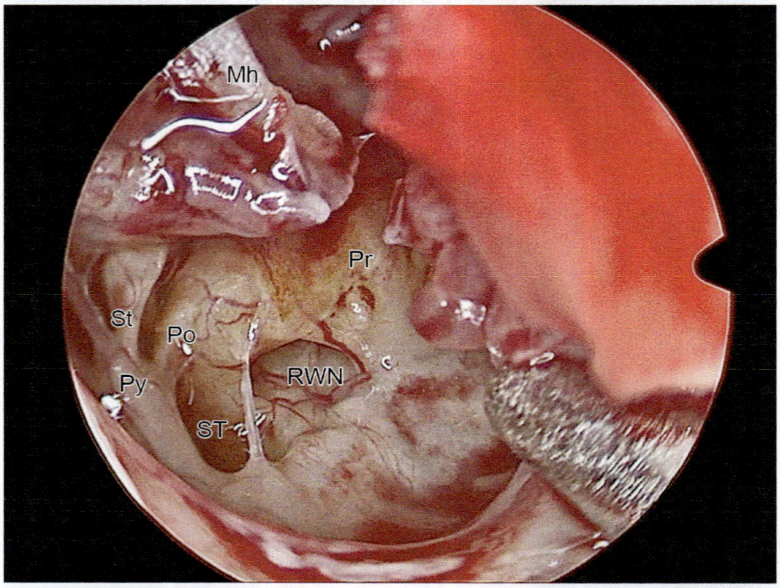

Fig. 8B: Panoramic view of middle ear and its landmarks.
(Mh: malleus handle; Py: processus pyramidalis; Pr: promontory; RWN: round window niche; ST: sinus tympani; Po: ponticulus.; St: stapedius tendon)

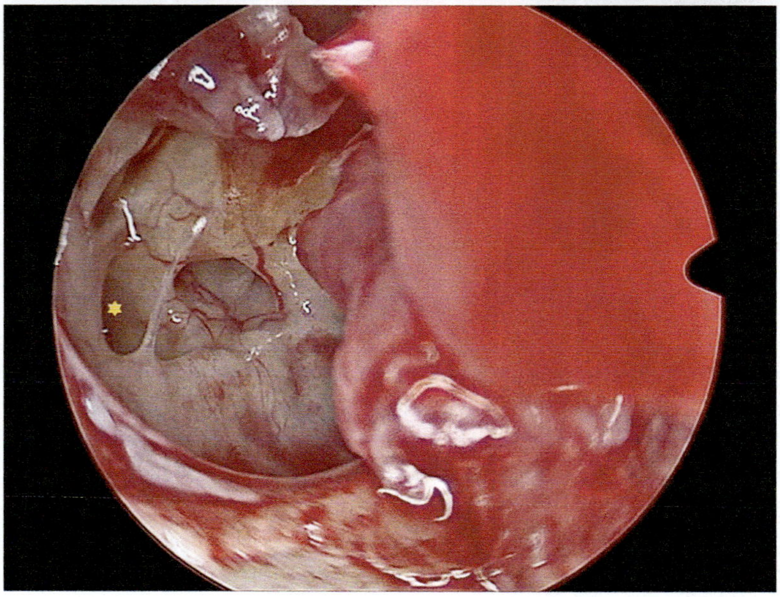

Fig. 8C: View of right middle ear. Asterisk—Sinus tympani.

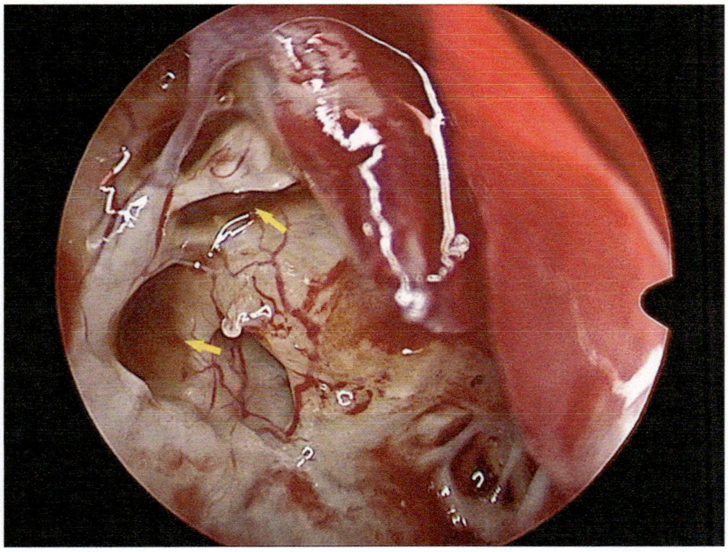

Fig. 8D: View of right middle ear. Yellow arrows—Hemosiderin (brownish-black) fluid.

7. *Endoscopic transcanal atticotomy:* Attic and the ossicular chain are exposed by performing a transcanal endoscopic atticotomy by drilling or curettage or Wilson bone punch or a suitable combination of them (Vide "Endoscopic Transcanal Atticotomy" chapter).

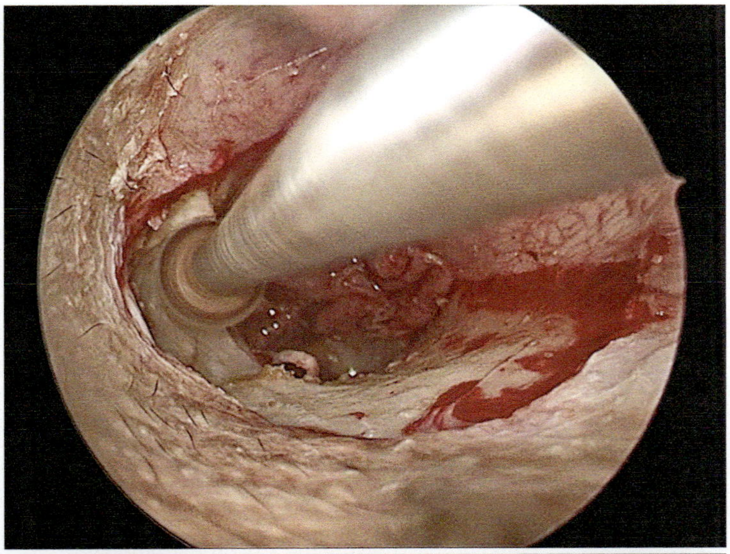

Fig. 9A: Endoscopic atticotomy. Drilling of lateral attic wall till it is thinned.

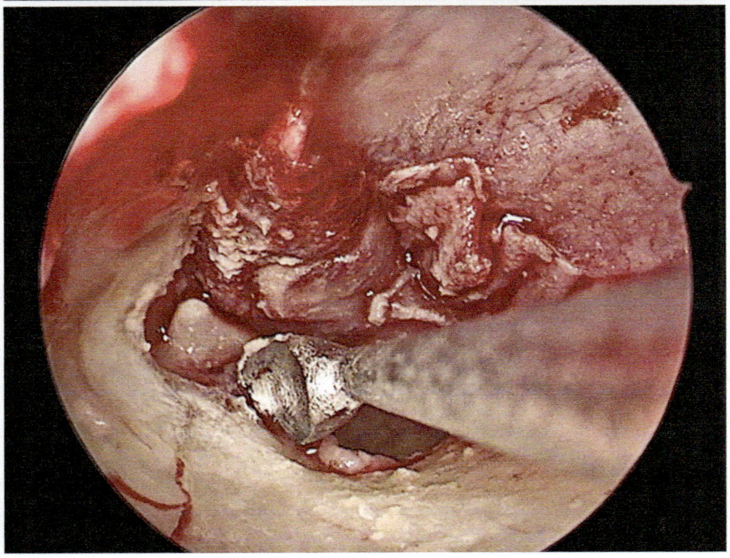

Fig. 9B: Endoscopic atticotomy. House curette used to remove posterosuperior canal wall.

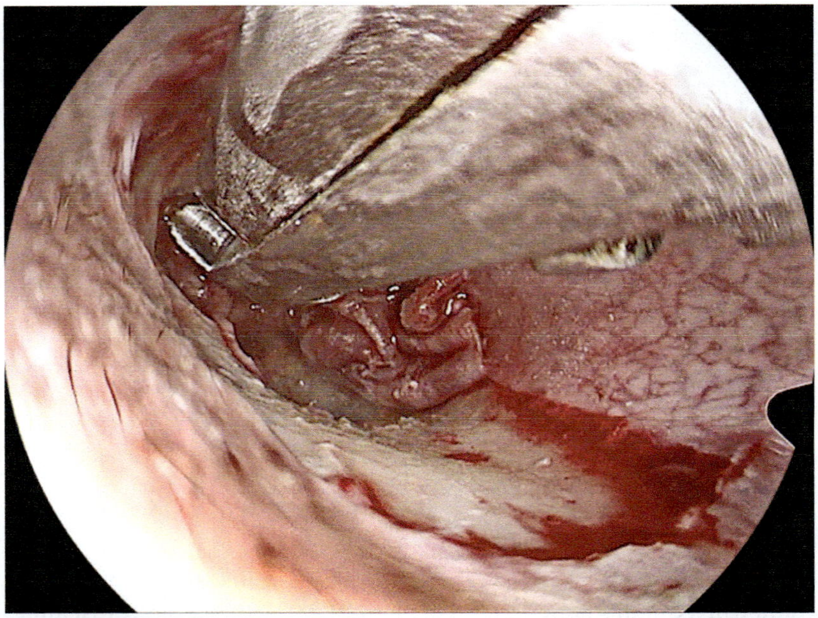

Fig. 9C: Endoscopic atticotomy. Wilson bone punch used to remove remaining bone of scutum.

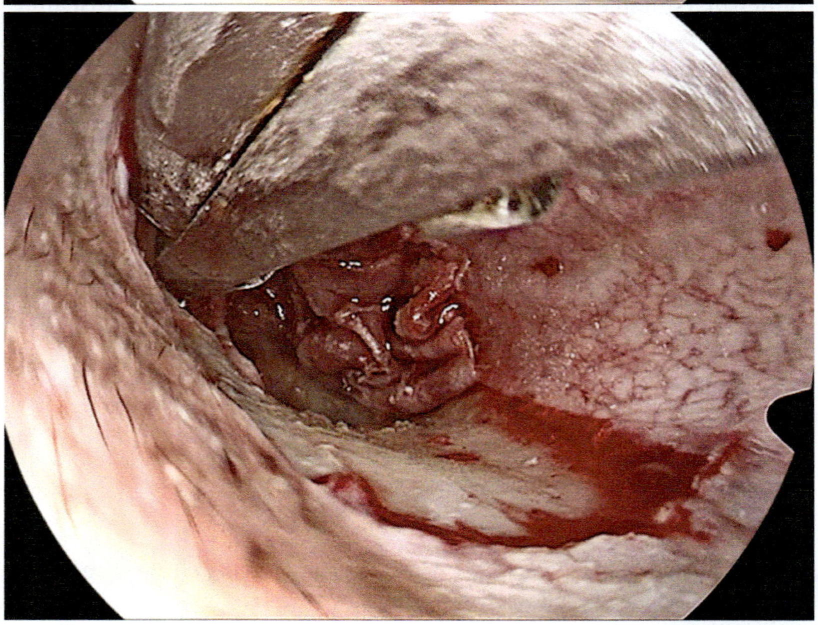

Fig. 9D: Endoscopic atticotomy. Wilson bone punch being used to enlarge the atticotomy window.

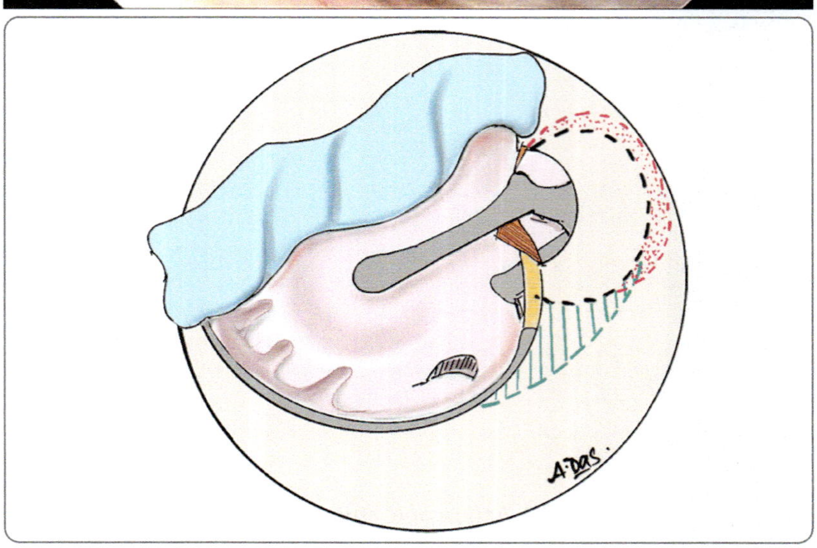

Fig. 9E: Dimensions of atticotomy window based on type on decompression; (black dotted line: Type A; green shaded area: Type B; red shaded area: Type C).

8. *Disarticulation of incudostapedial joint:* Incudostapedial joint is dislocated using a sharp pick in a posterior-to-anterior direction.

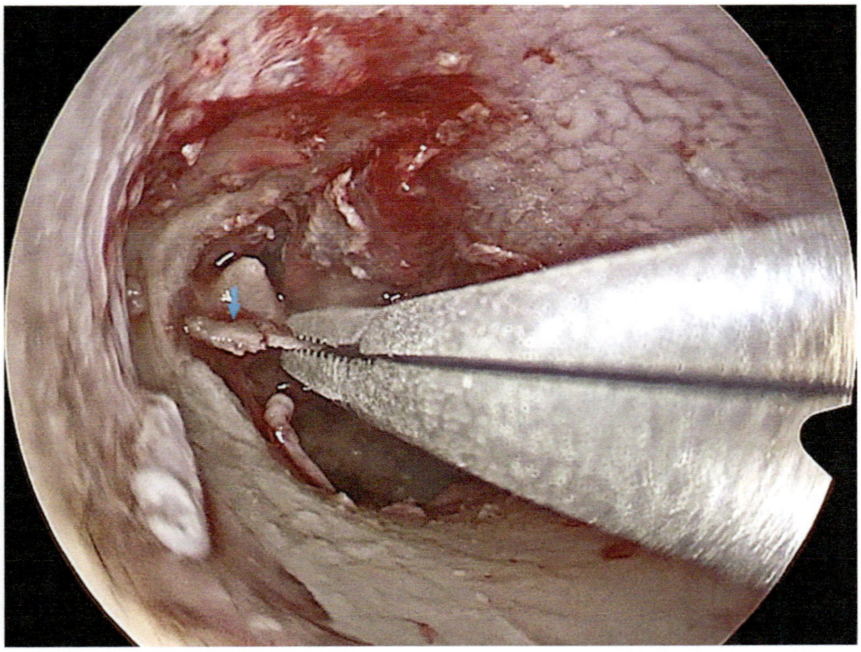

Fig. 10A: Last egg-shell piece of postero-superior canal wall bone taken out (arrow).

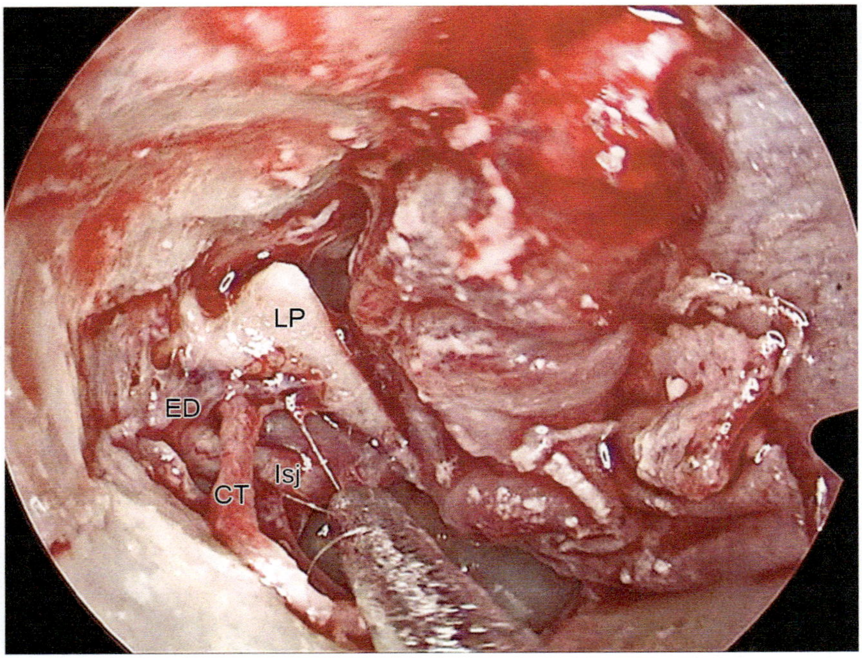

Fig. 10B: Exposure following atticotomy. (CT: chorda tympani; ED: epitympanic diaphragm; Isj: incudostapedial joint; LP: lateral process of malleus)

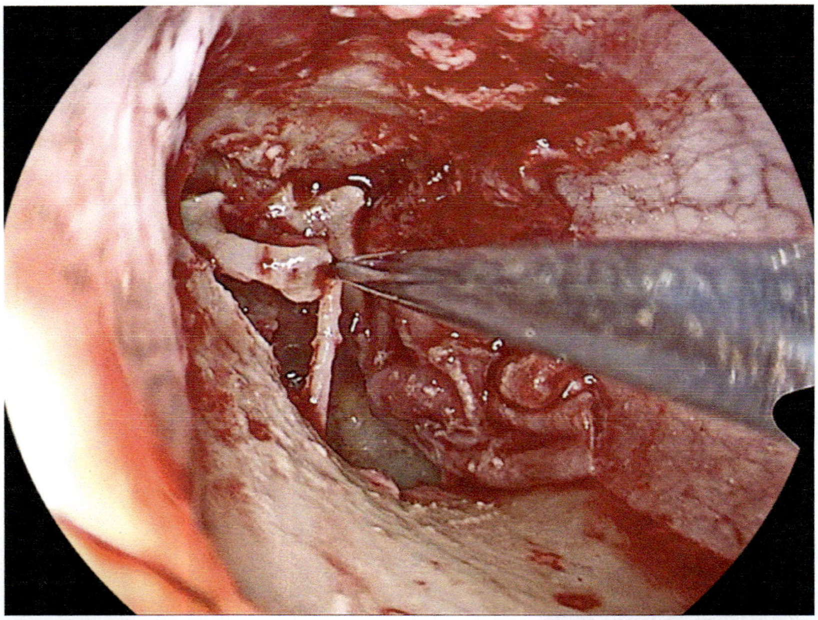

Fig. 10C: Disarticulation of incudostapedial joint.

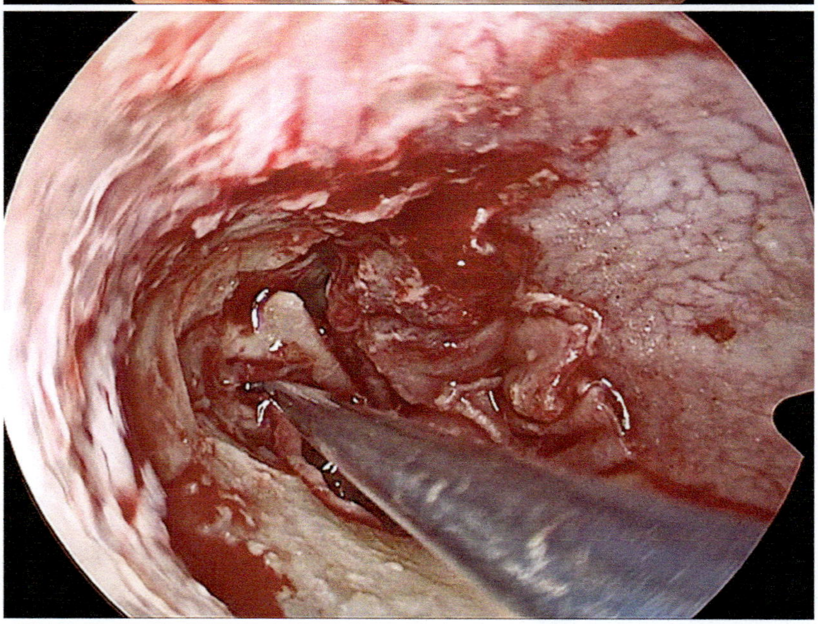

Fig. 10D: Disarticulation of incudomalleolar joint using 45 degree pick.

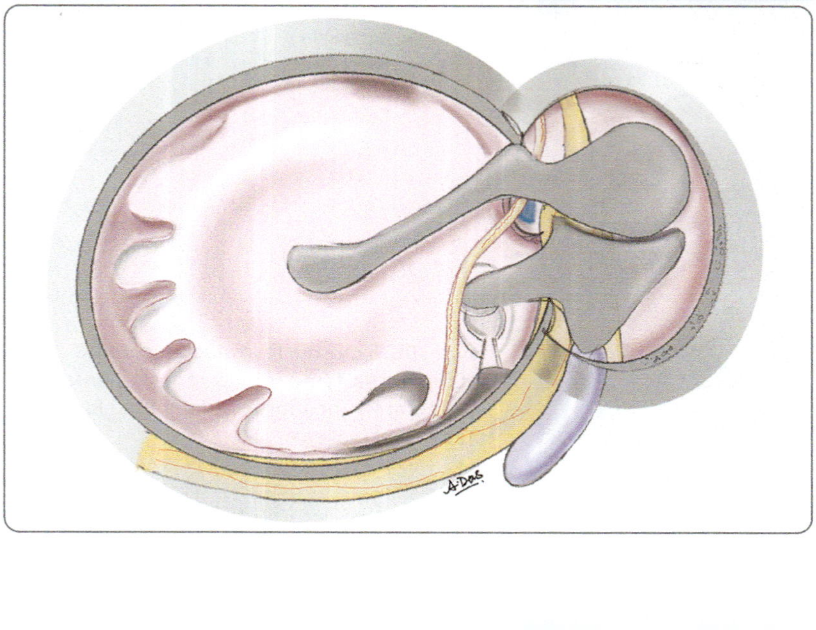

Fig. 10E: Pictorial depiction of working window following atticotomy.

9. *Disarticulation of incudomalleolar joint:* Similarly, the incudomalleolar joint is dislocated and incus is delivered out.

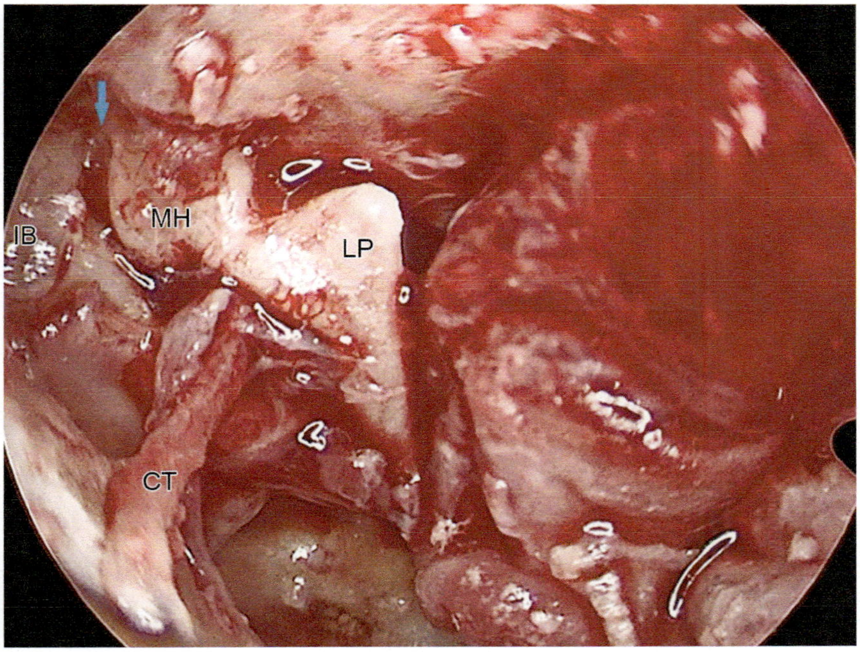

Fig. 11A: Identification of incudomalleolar joint (blue arrow).
(IB: incus buttress; MH: malleus head; LP: lateral process of malleus; CT: chorda tympani)

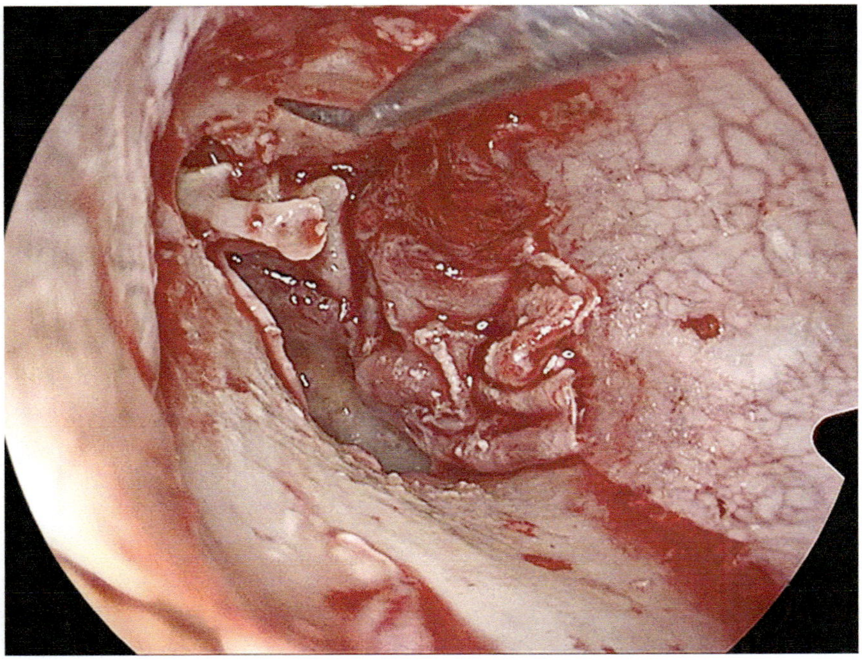

Fig. 11B: Extraction of incus through atticotomy window.

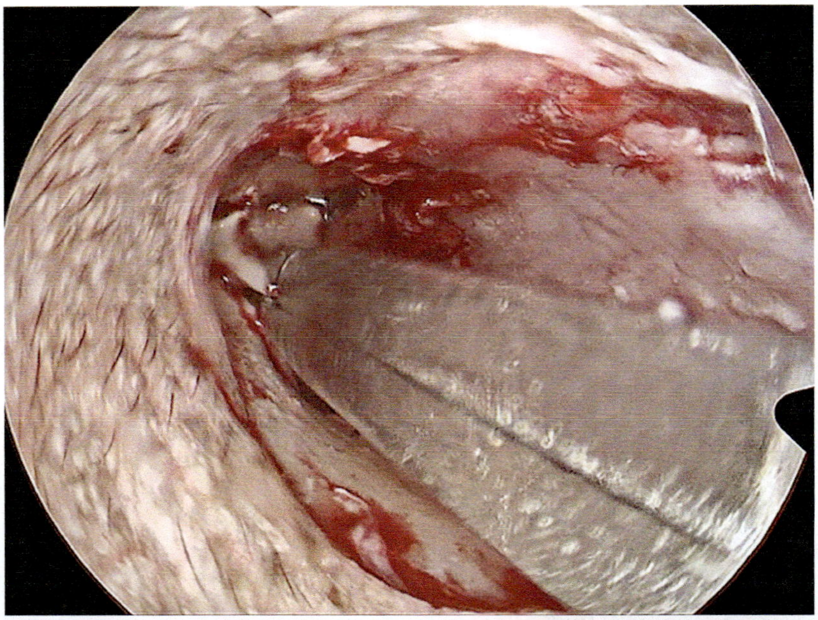

Fig. 11C: Incus being delivered out.

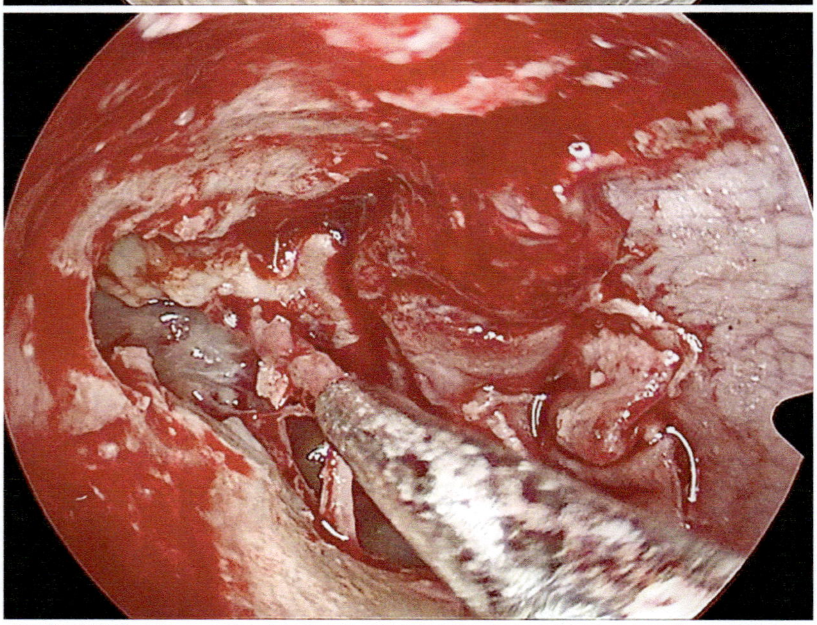

Fig. 11D: View of the epitympanum following removal of incus.

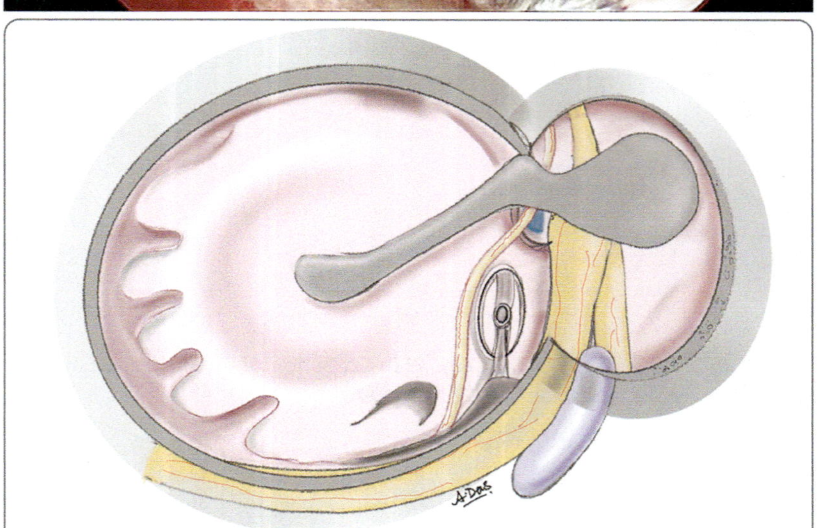

Fig. 11E: Pictorial depiction of exposure following incus removal.

10. *Nipping of malleus head:* Head of the malleus is nipped at its neck, using a malleus nipper, to expose the epitympanum.

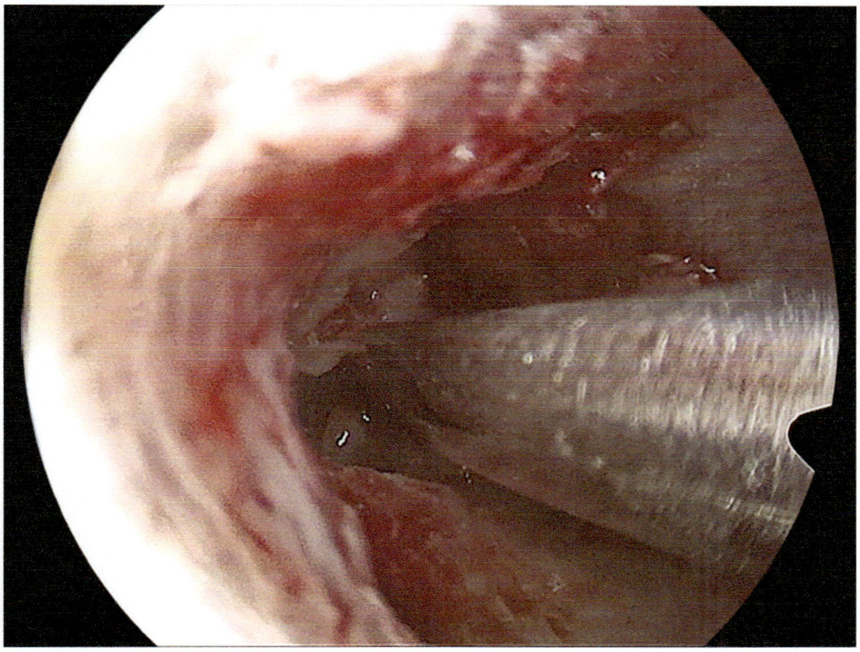

Fig. 12A: Nipping of malleus head. Engagement of the nipper at neck of malleus.

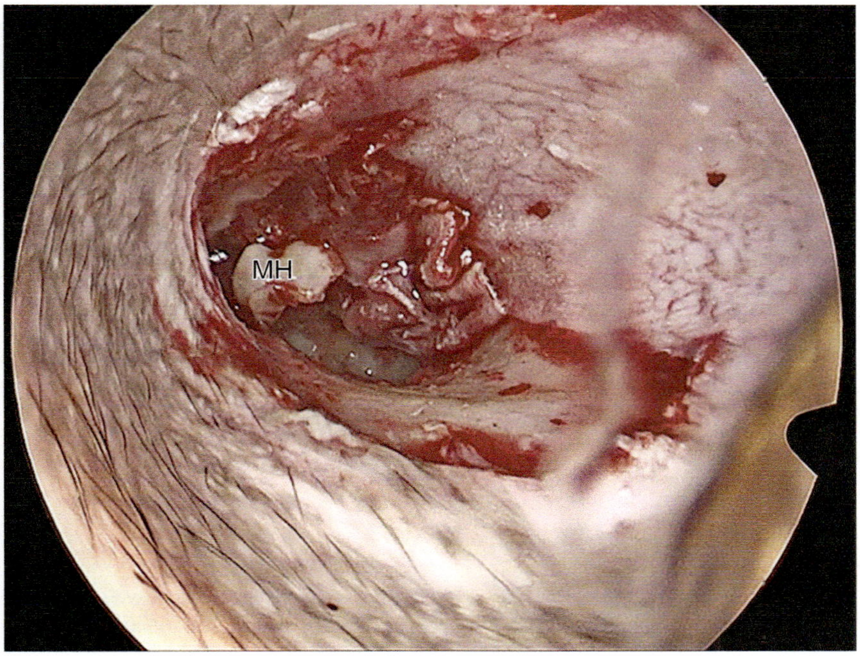

Fig. 12B: Nipping of malleus head: Malleus head being removed from epitympanum.
(MH: malleus head)

TIP

Final exposure should expose the full arc including anterior and posterior epitympanic spaces, lateral semicircular canal up to aditus, second genu, vertical segment up to pyramid. Limited canalplasty may be required to expose second genu. After complete exposure, tegmen tympani and lateral canal are inspected for signs of violation.

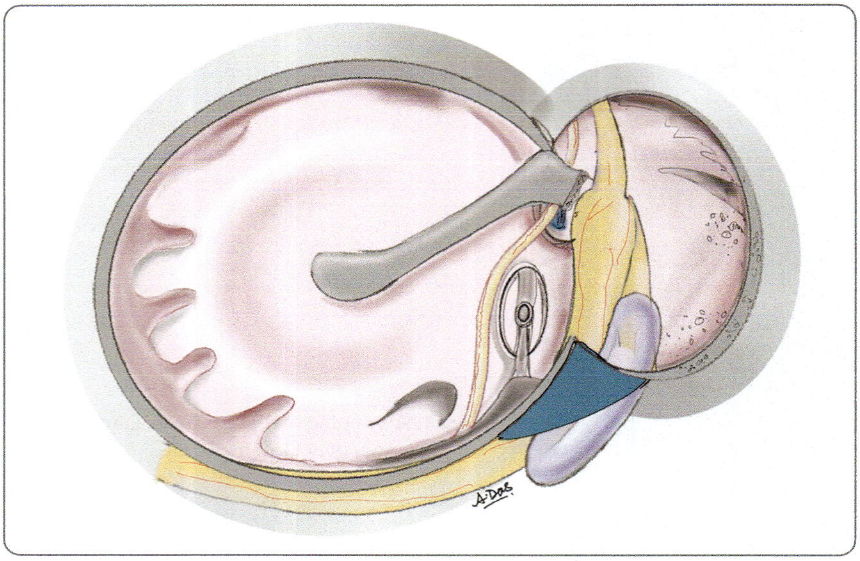

Fig. 13A: Before removal of canal wall bone to completely expose the second genu up to processus pyramidalis.

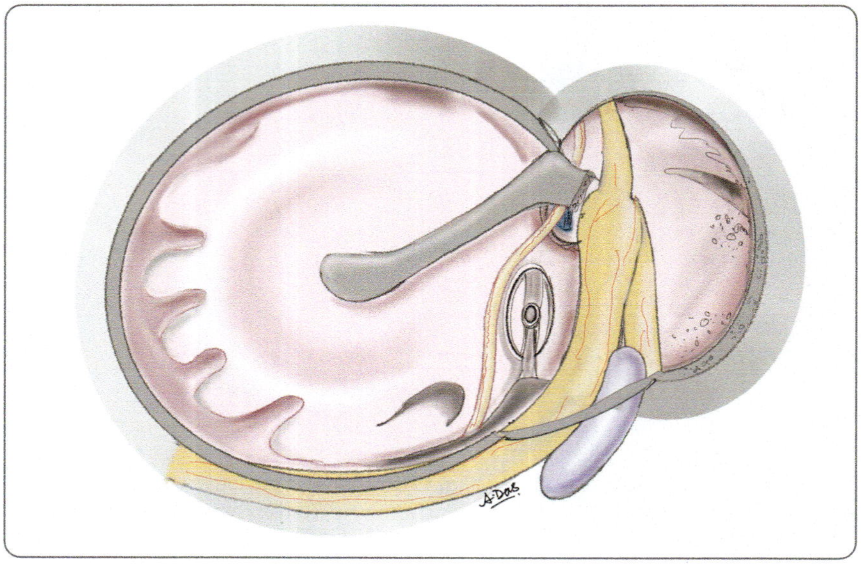

Fig. 13B: After removal of canal wall bone to completely expose the second genu up to processus pyramidalis.

11. *Dissection of organized tissue:* Affected part of the nerve is often found engulfed in granulation or fibrous tissue that forms as a part of healing. Intraneural hematoma may also be found imparting a dark color to the nerve instead of its normal pinkish hue.

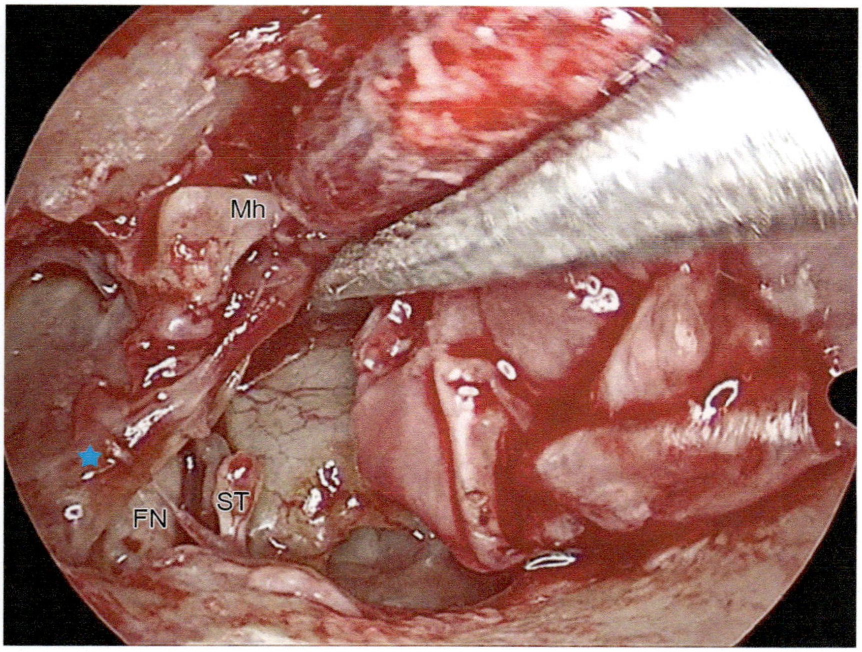

Fig. 14A: Dissection of organized tissues (blue star). Note the use of suction elevator to maintain the traction and countertraction for single-handed dissection.
(FN: facial nerve; Mh: malleus handle; ST: stapes)

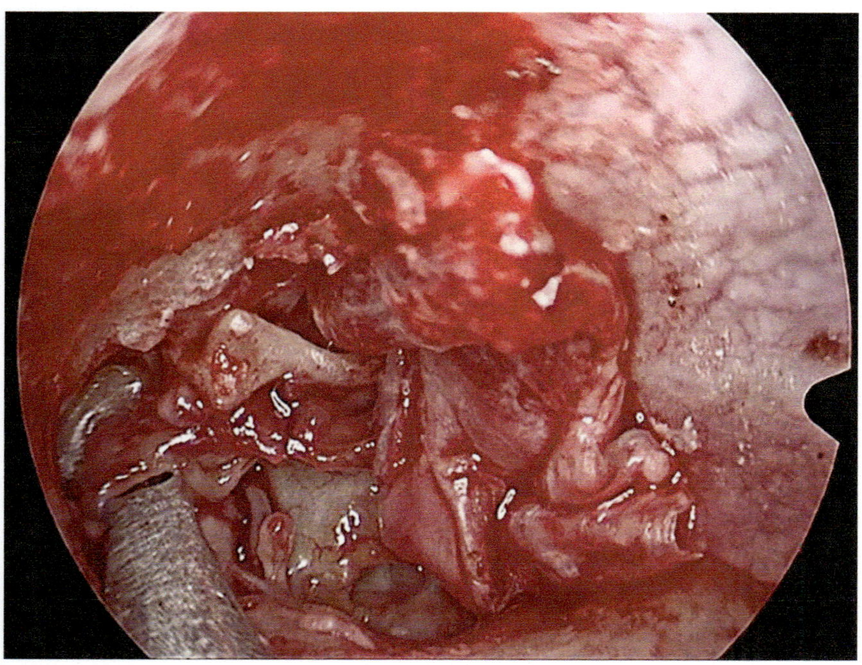

Fig. 14B: Dissection of organized tissues: Note the direction of suction elevator in posterior-to-anterior direction.

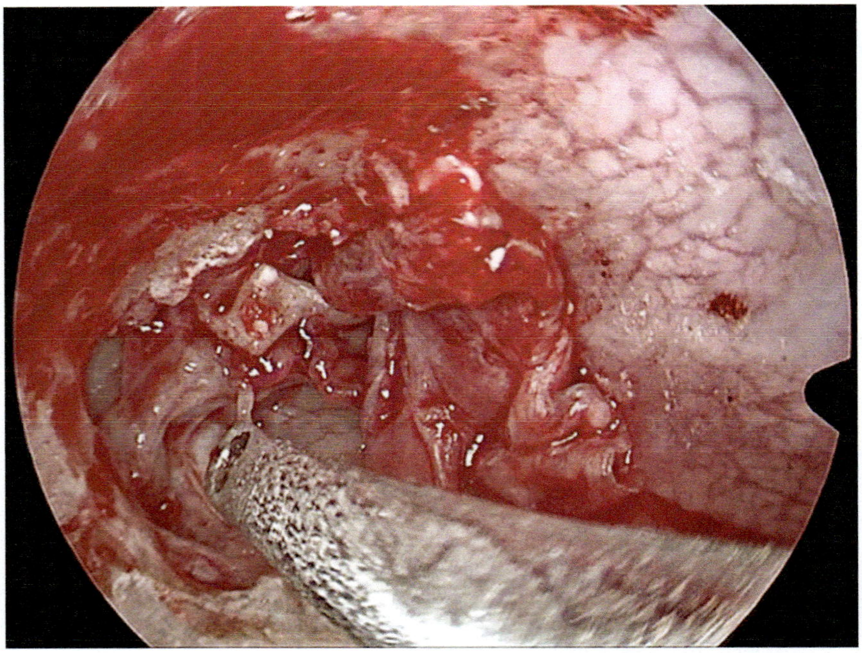

Fig. 14C: Dissection of organized tissues: Note the use of suction elevator to dissect the organized tissues of the facial nerve.

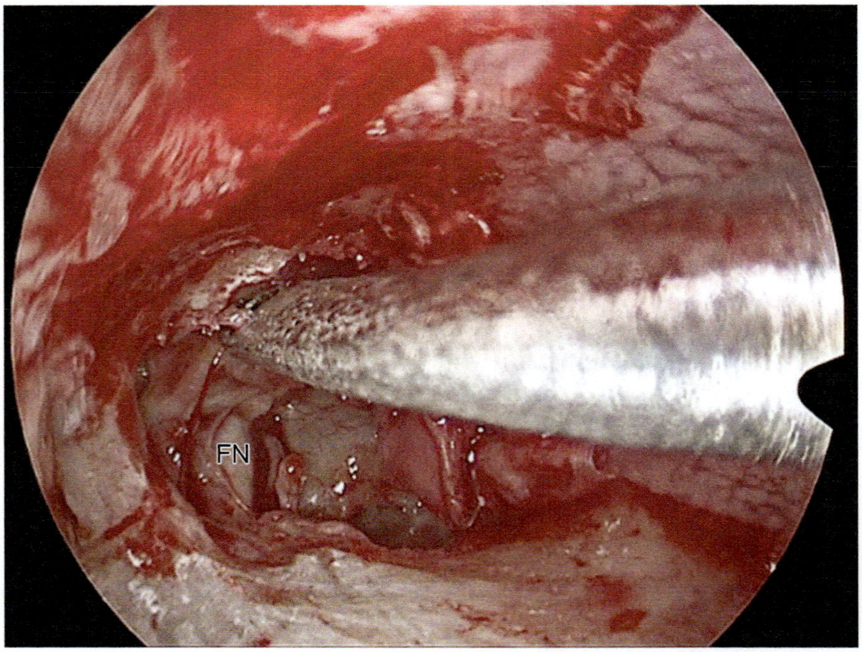

Fig. 14D: Dissection of organized tissues: Facial nerve exposed.
(FN: facial nerve)

PEARL

There may be considerable amount of bleeding from organized granulation tissue due to neoangiogenesis. Decongestion of the affected area with adrenaline-soaked cotton balls is helpful at this stage. Suction instruments are used at this stage to utilize traction–countertraction advantage of such instruments.

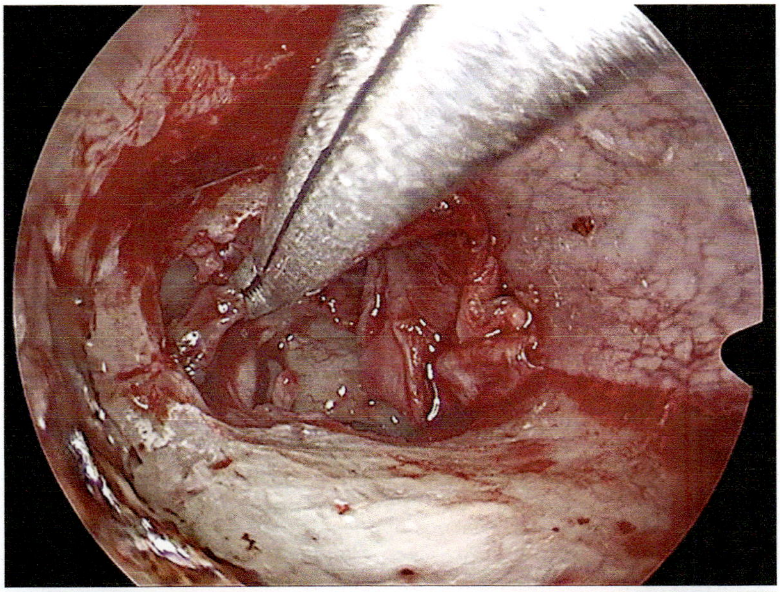

Fig. 15A: Separation of organized tissues from facial nerve using curved alligator forceps.

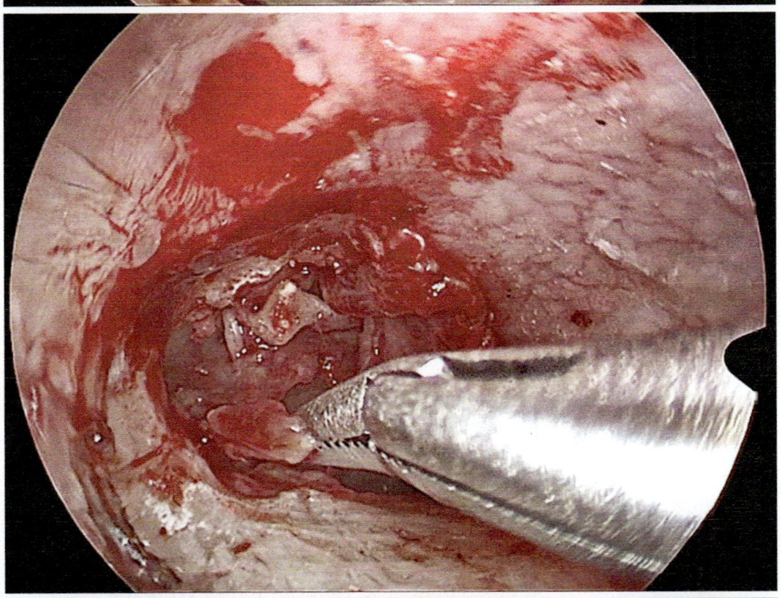

Fig. 15B: Removal of organized tissues over facial nerve using curved alligator forceps.

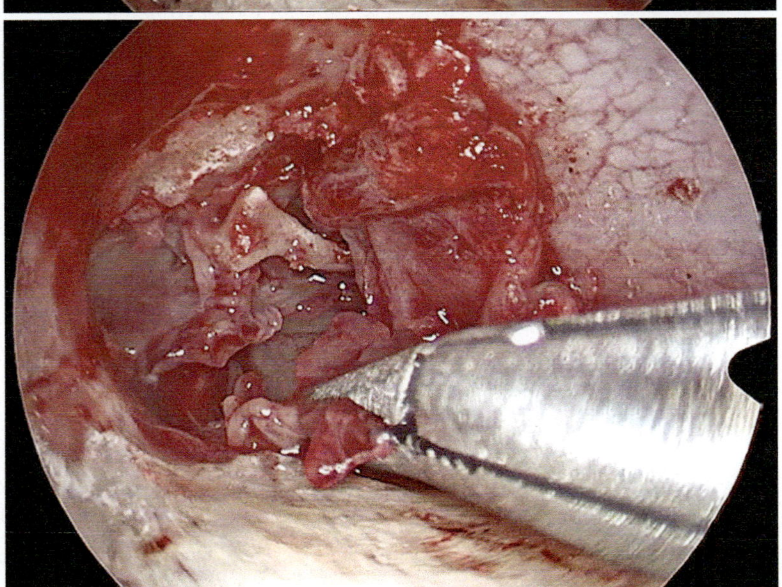

Fig. 15C: Clearance of organized tissues.

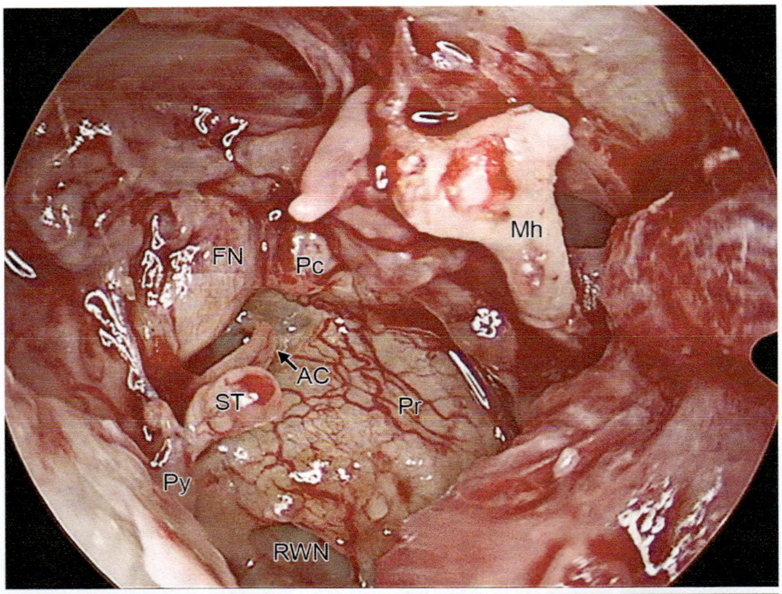

Fig. 15D: Exposure of nerve segment following clearance of organized tissues.
(AC: anterior crus of stapes; FN: facial nerve; Mh: malleus handle; Pc: processus cochleariformis; Py: processus pyramidalis; Pr: promontory; RWN: round window niche; ST: stapes)

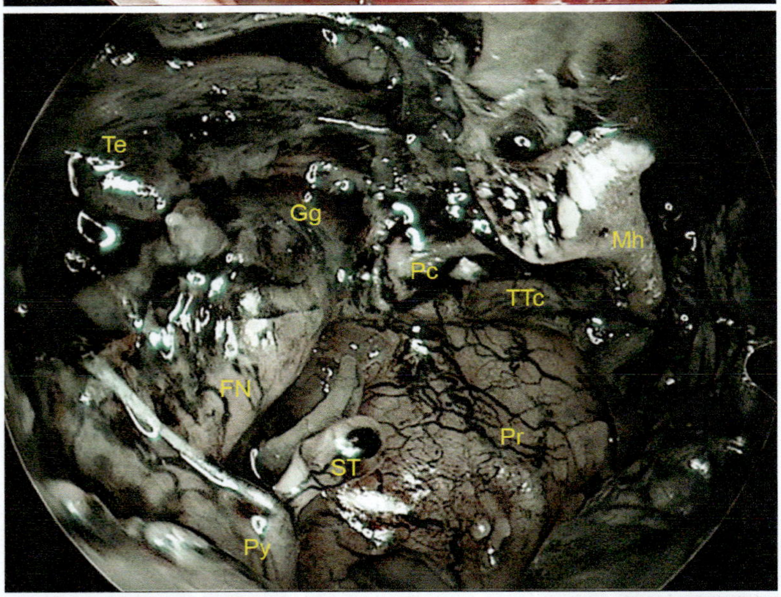

Fig. 16A: Spectra A mode view of exposed nerve segment. Note the color of the organized granulation tissues over the injured segment of the nerve.
(FN: facial nerve; Gg: geniculate ganglion; Mh: malleus handle; Pc: processus cochleariformis; Py: processus pyramidalis; Pr: promontory; ST: stapes; Te: tegmen plate; TTc: canal for tensor tympani)

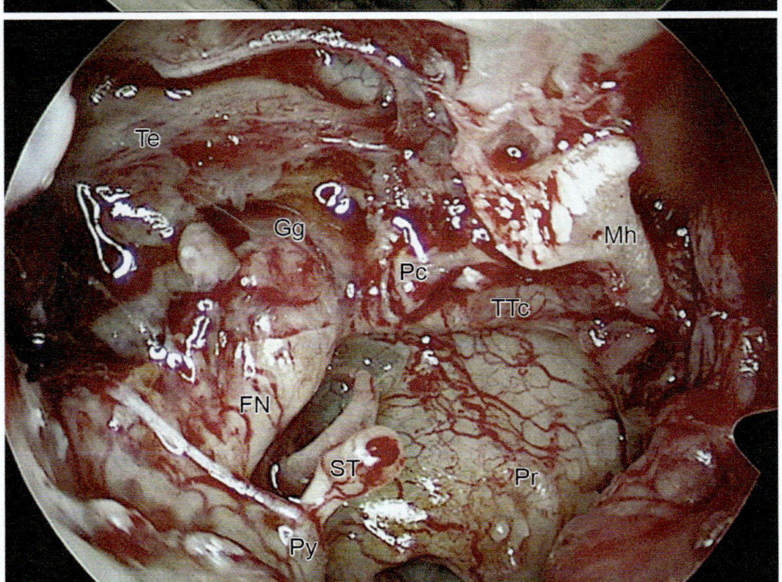

Fig. 16B: Spectra B mode view of exposed nerve segment. Note the color of the organized granulation tissues over the injured segment of the nerve.
(FN: facial nerve; Gg: geniculate ganglion; Mh: malleus handle; Pc: processus cochleariformis; Py: processus pyramidalis; Pr: Promontory; ST: Stapes; Te: Tegmen plate; TTc: Canal for tensor tympani)

12. *Dissection and exposure of facial nerve:*

- The following layers of tissues are expected at the site of injury (from outside-inward):
  - Mucosa with inflammatory tissues (as a part of healing process)
  - Fallopian canal bone
  - Facial nerve
- The plane of dissection is done between the mucosa and bone starting from a region away from the nerve, proceeding towards the injured segment of the nerve
- After dissection of mucosa, the area is packed with Adrenaline-soaked cotton balls and kept for a few minutes to control bleeding and increase field visibility
- Thickness of bone of the facial nerve is judged by palpation with a ball-point probe
- Bone of fallopian canal over the tympanic segment may be dehiscent in up to 50% of normal individuals
- The nerve is sharply dissected free from the organized tissues with the help of a pick or iris scissors
- Fractured fragments of bone of fallopian canal are often found impinged on the nerve. An angled alligator forceps or Bill's elevator is used to disimpact the bone chips from the underlying nerve.

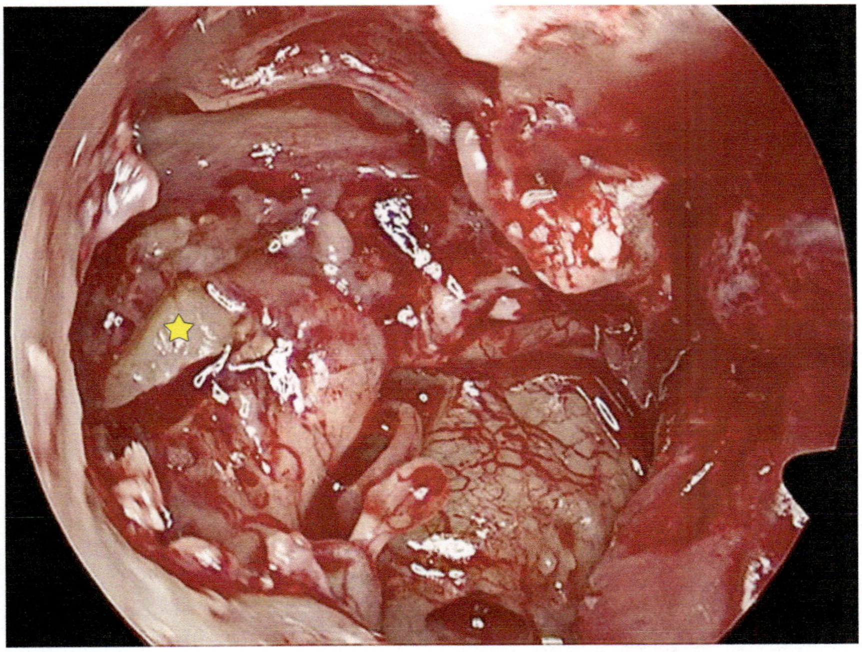

Fig. 17A: Bone chip impacted over horizontal segment of facial nerve (yellow star).

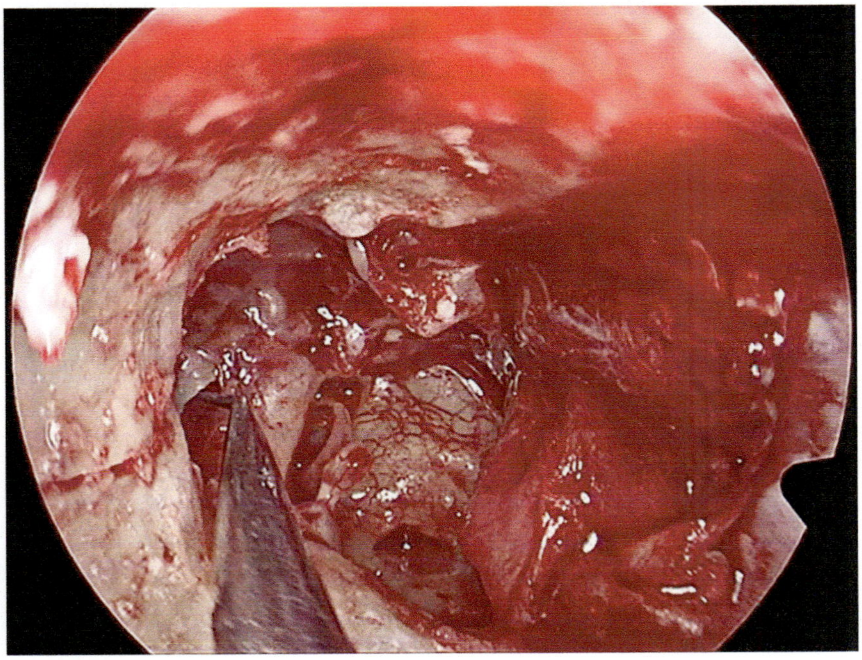

Fig. 17B: Bone chip being elevated off the facial nerve using angled pick.

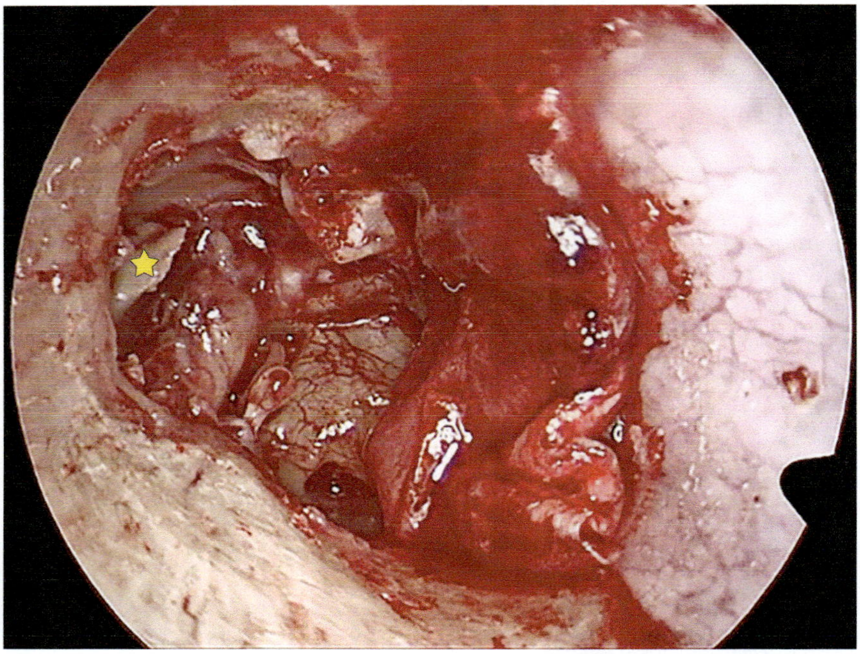

Fig. 17C: Disimpacted bone chip (yellow star).

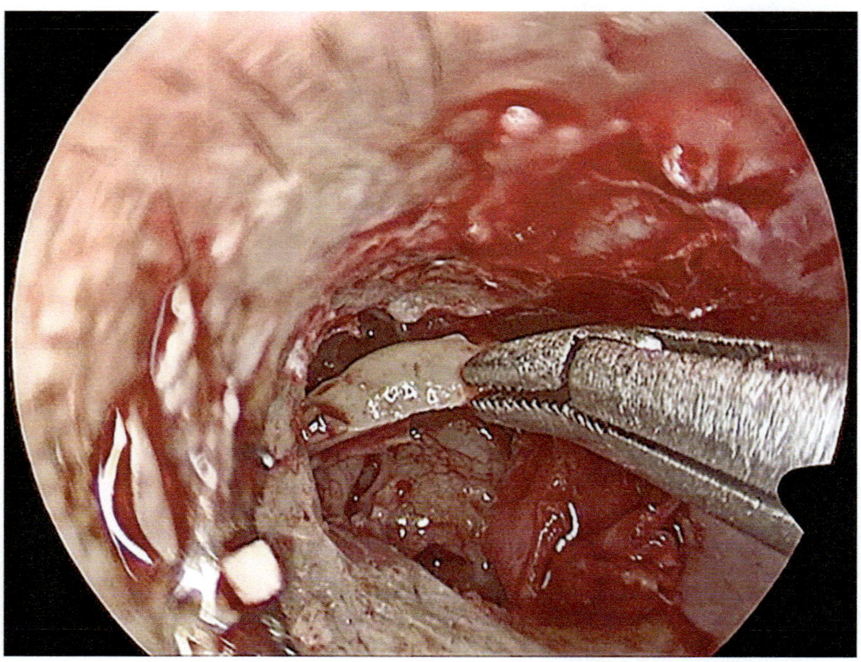

Fig. 17D: Disimpacted bone chip being taken out using an alligator forceps.

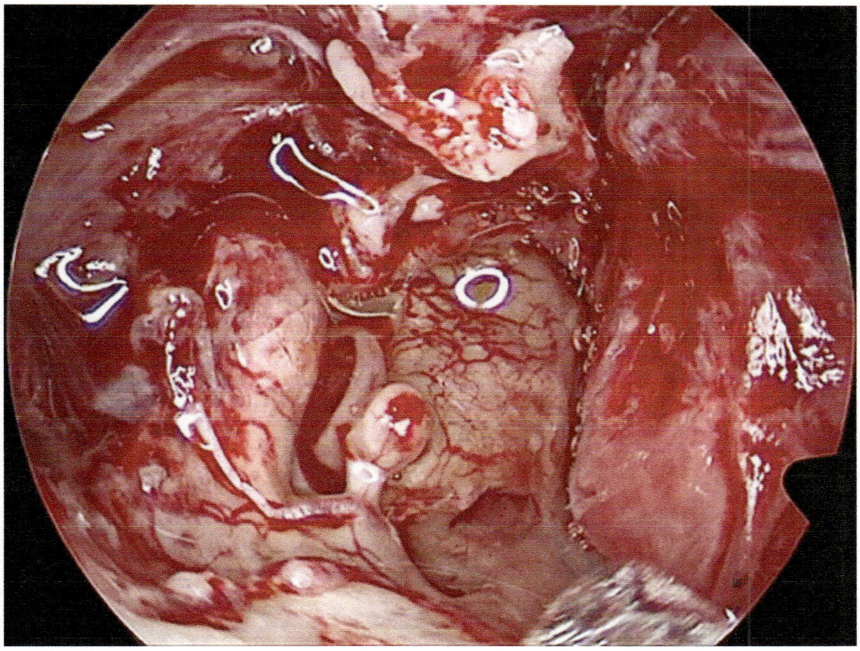

Fig. 17E: Nerve segment exposed after disimpaction.

13. *Fallopian canal drill:* The nerve is decompressed up to one centimeter proximal and distal to the area of affection.

TIP **RULES OF DRILLING OVER THE FALLOPIAN CANAL**

- Diamond burr larger than the caliber of the nerve trunk
- Direction of drilling parallel to the nerve
- Without exerting pressure over the nerve
- Continuous irrigation to be used while drilling
- Drilling continued till an egg-shell of bone is intact over the nerve

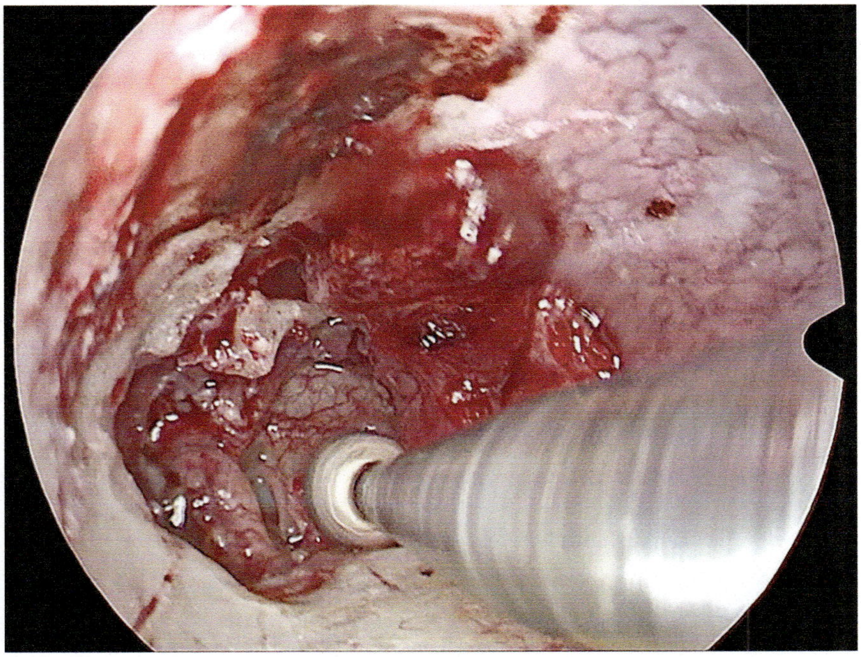

Fig. 18A: Canalplasty using diamond burr.

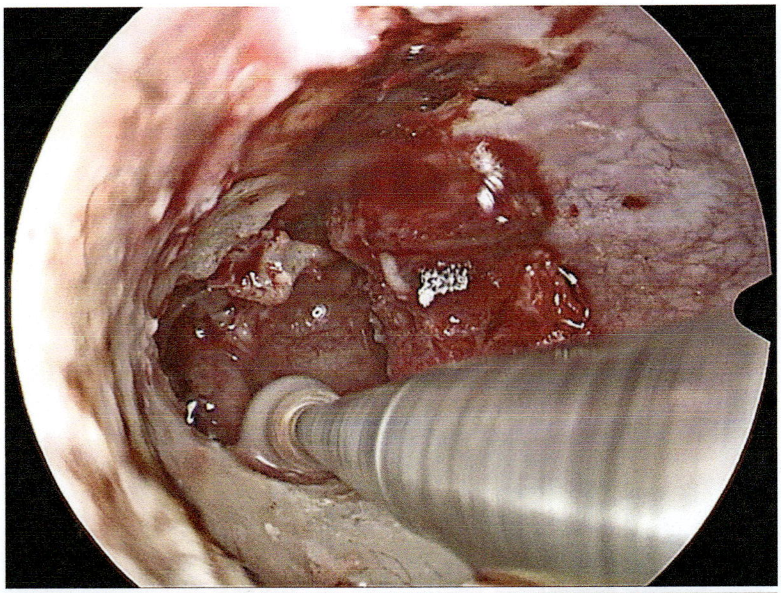

Fig. 18B: Fallopian canal drill. Complete exposure of nerve till second genu ensured.

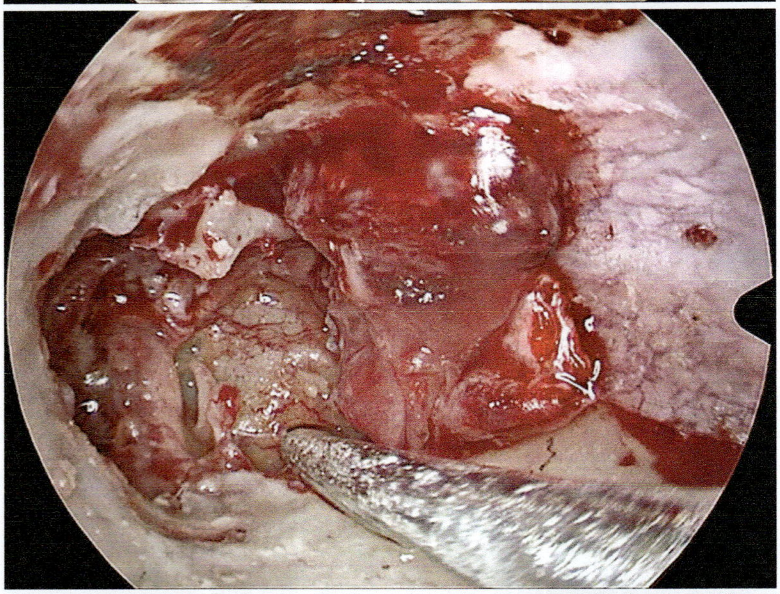

Fig. 18C: Fallopian canal drill. Visualization before commencement of further drilling.

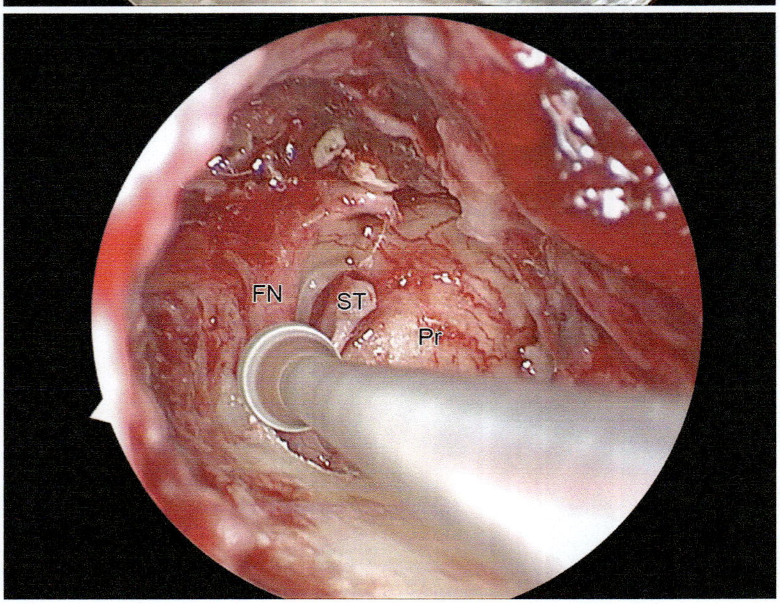

Fig. 18D: Fallopian canal drill. Drilling over tympanic segment of the fallopian canal.
(FN: facial nerve; Pr: promontory; ST: stapes)

14. *Egg shelling of fallopian canal bone:* Egg-shell bone is carefully lifted off the nerve sheath using a Bill's elevator.

TIP

One has to make sure that the egg-shell bone over the facial nerve has been exposed in its entire length before lifting off the bone fragments from the nerve.

PEARL

Bleeding is normally encountered during this process and is controlled using gelfoam soaked in adrenaline.

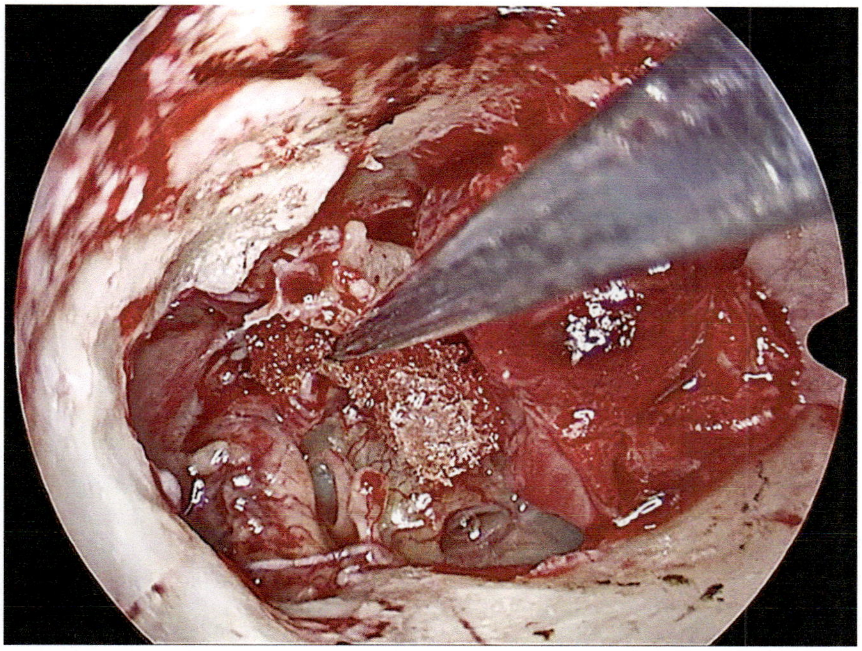

Fig. 19A: Remaining egg-shell bone over facial nerve.

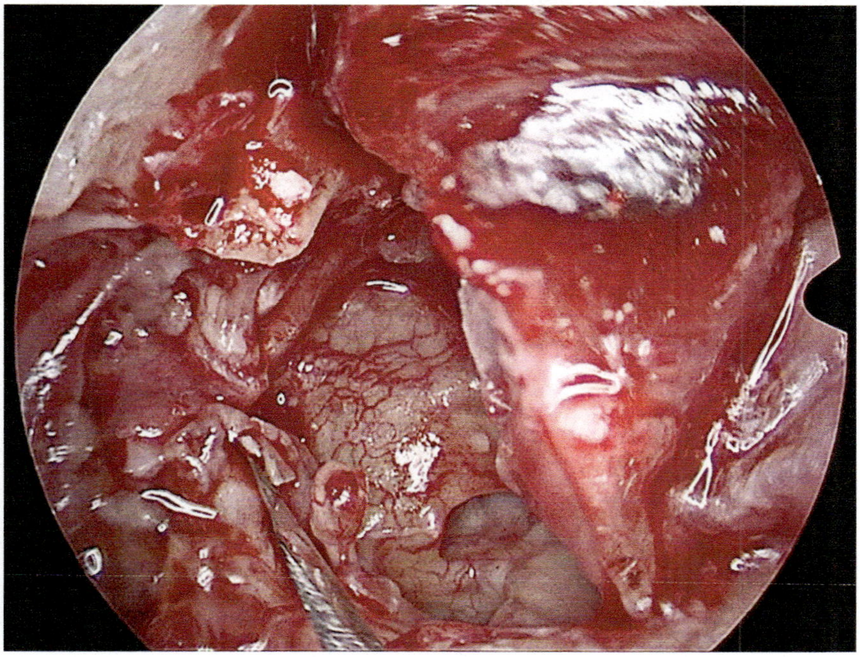

Fig. 19B: Egg-shell bone being removed using sharp sickle.

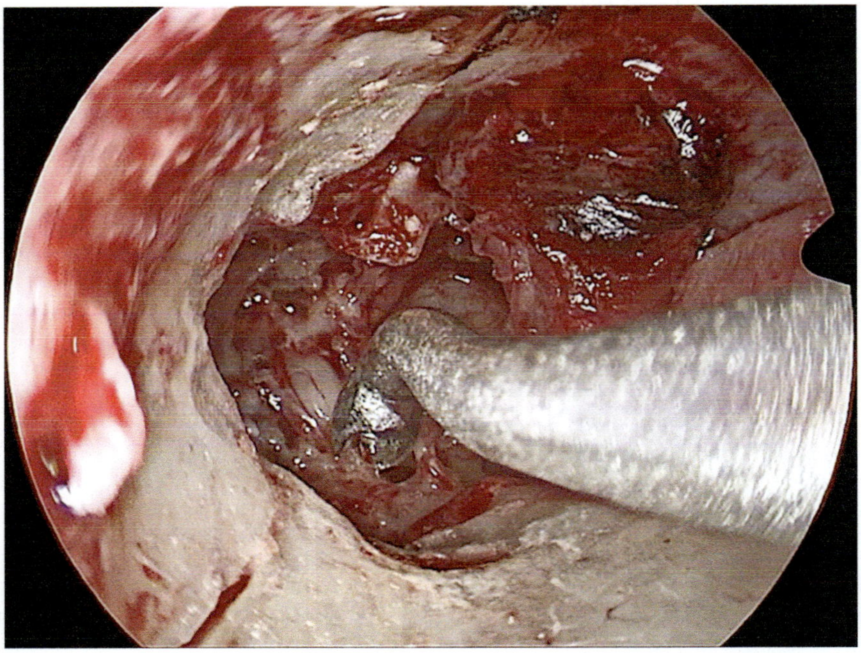

Fig. 19C: Thicker bone toward second genu being removed using a curved curette.

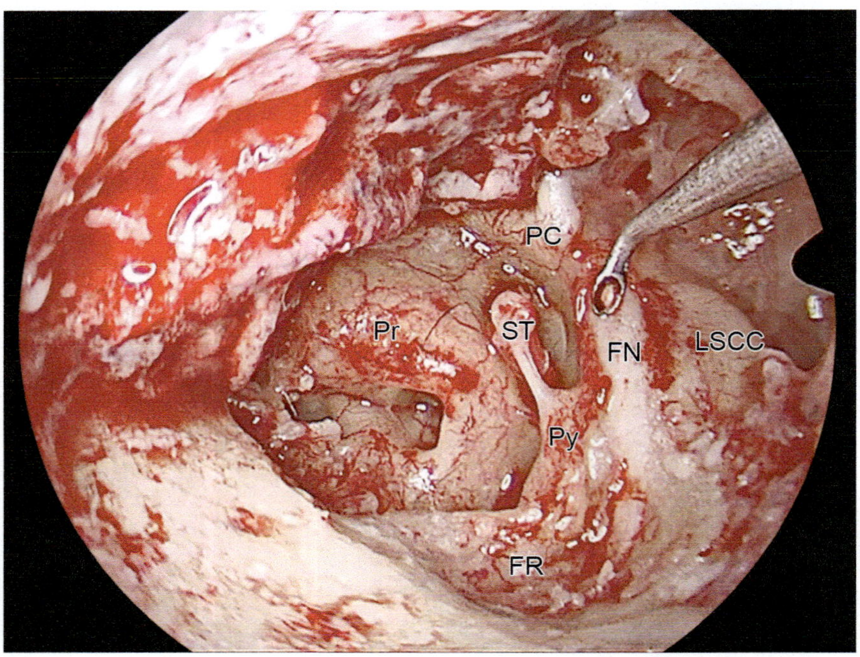

Fig. 19D: Exposure up to second genu. (FN: facial nerve; FR: facial recess; LSCC: lateral semicircular canal; PC: processus cochleariformis; Py: processus pyramidalis; Pr: promontory; ST: stapes)

15. *Incision over facial nerve sheath (neurolysis):*

- One should be familiar with the ultrastructure of the facial nerve before performing this crucial step of the surgery
- Facial nerve is composed of the following (from inside out):
  - Endoneurium
  - Perineurium
  - Epineurium

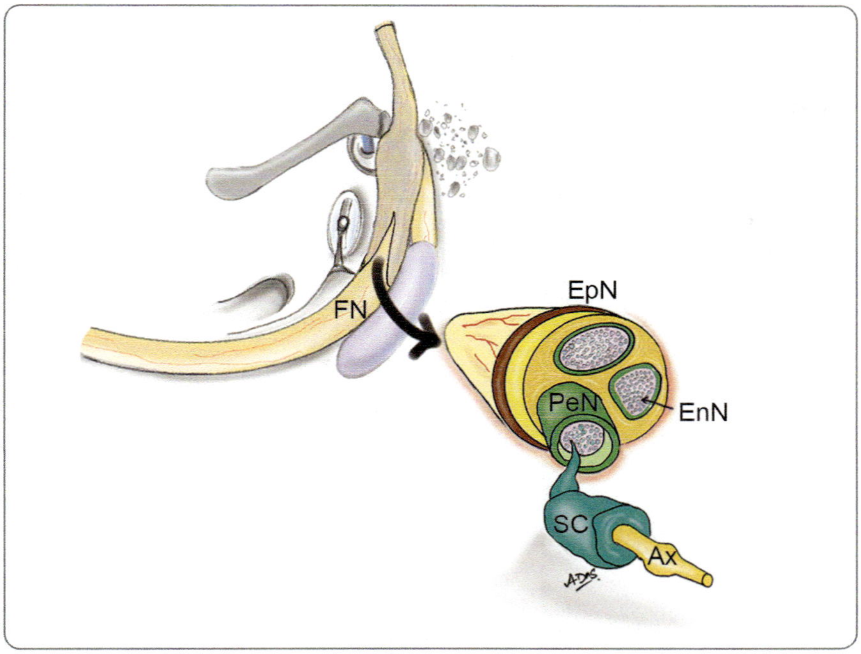

Fig. 20: Pictorial depiction of the layers of facial nerve and concept of nerve sheath incision. (It is the epineurium (EpN) that is incised during surgery.
(Ax: axon; EnN: endoneurium; EpN: epineurium; FN: facial nerve; PeN: perineurium; SC: Schwann cell)

- Facial nerve sheath, that is the epineurium, is incised sharply using a *tenotome/sharp sickle*
- The thickness of the facial nerve sheath varies from segment to segment; it is thicker in the mastoid/vertical segment, gradually gets thinner towards the geniculate ganglion and absent in the labyrinthine segment.

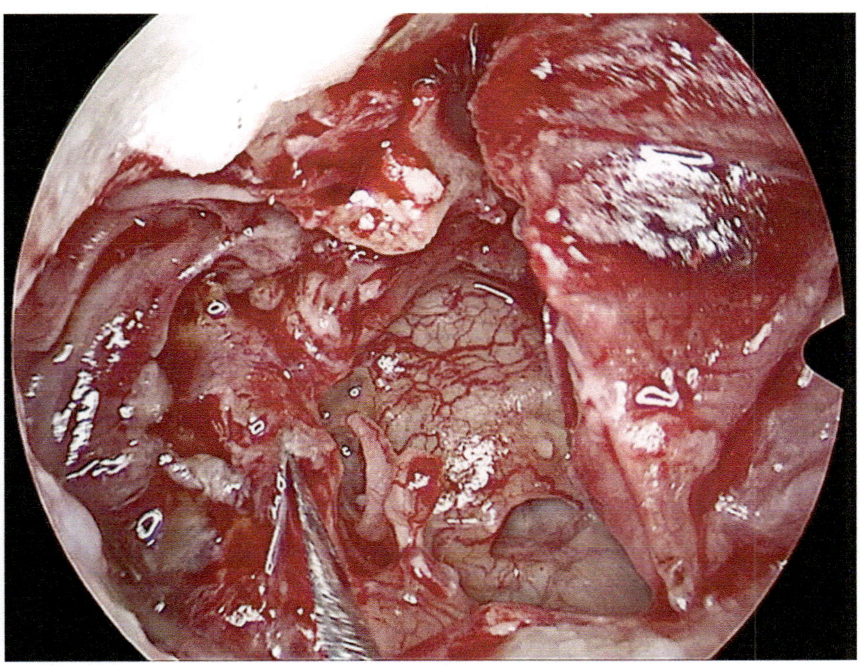

Fig. 21A: Engagement of the tenotome to excise the epineurium. Note the upward direction of the sharp tip of the instrument during the process.

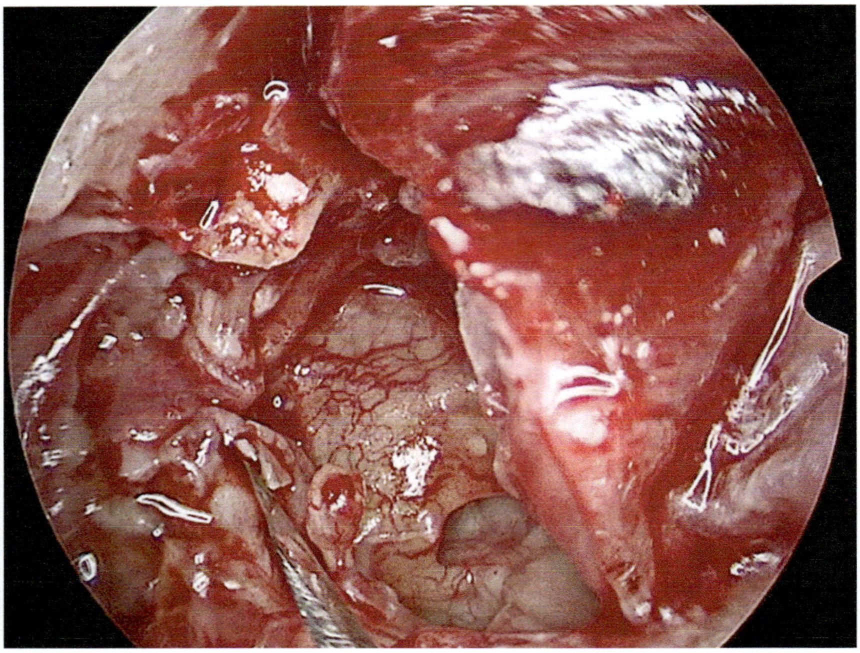

Fig. 21B: Incision of nerve sheath using tenotome. Note the upward direction of the sharp tip of the instrument during the process.

TIP

The sharp tip of the tenotome is to be directed upward, away from the nerve below. The decompressed nerve is allowed to bulge after the pressure of the edema or intraneural hematoma has been released.

PEARL

The decompressed nerve should finally be examined in its entire length before proceeding further.

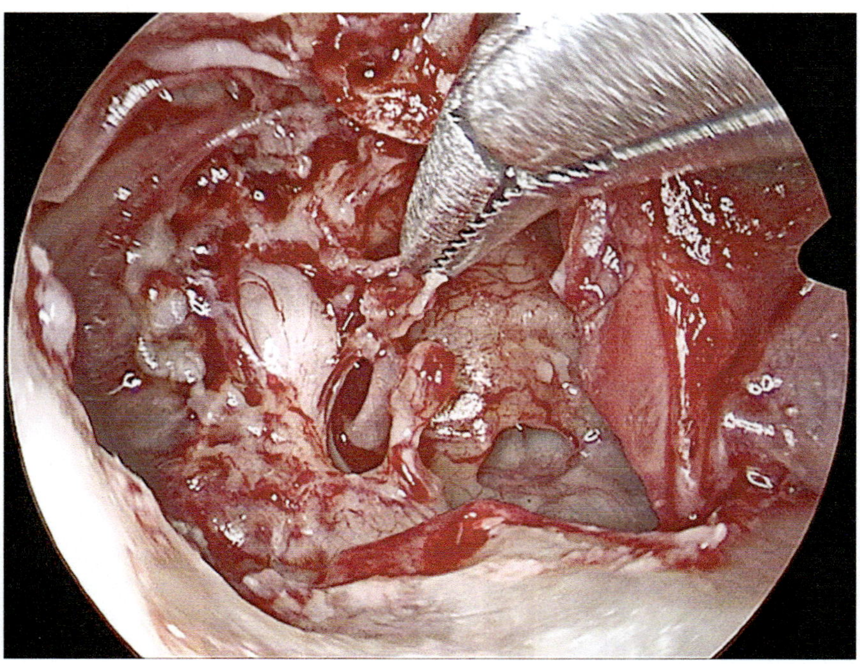

Fig. 22A: Separation of epineurium.

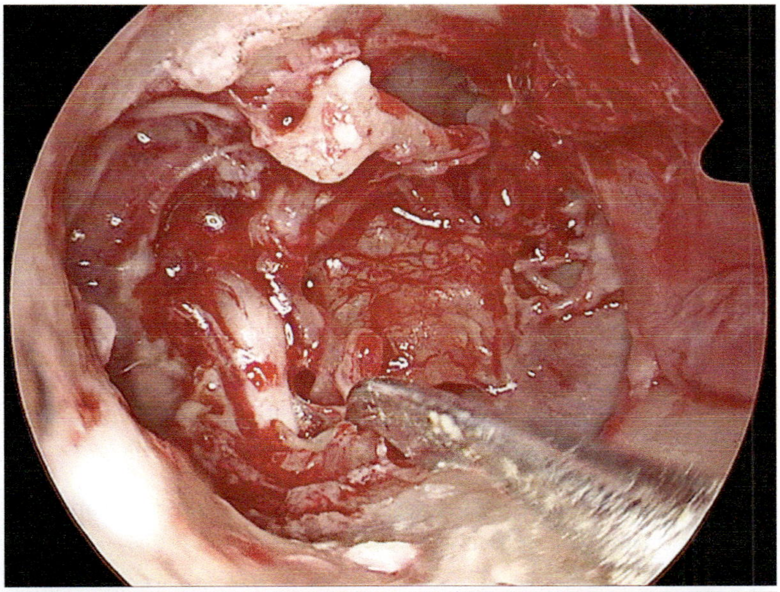

Fig. 22B: Tympanic segment decompressed.

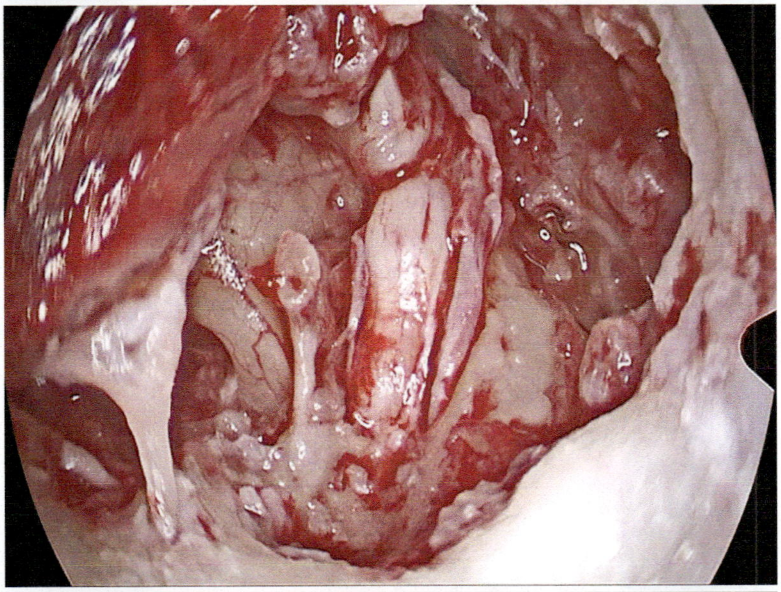

Fig. 22C: Note the bulging of the nerve following decompression.

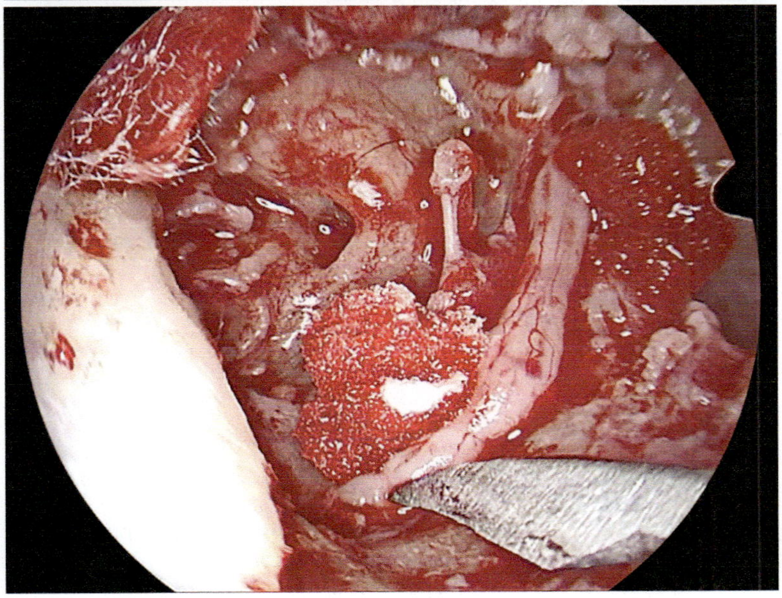

Fig. 22D: Incision of nerve sheath completed till second genu.

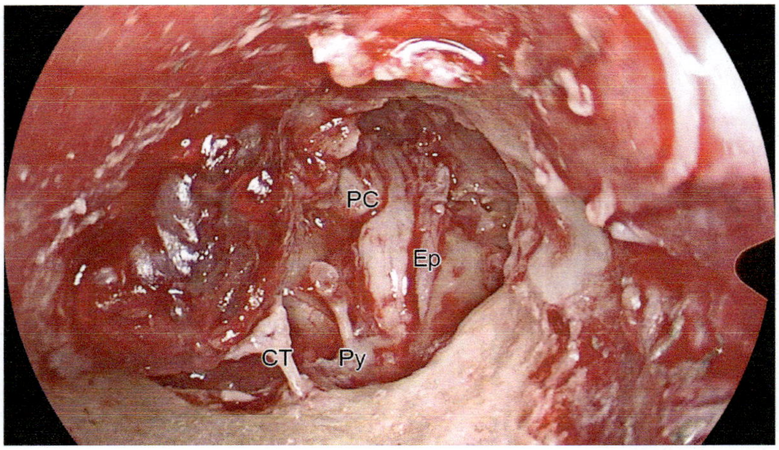

Fig. 22E: Type A decompression completed. (CT: chorda tympani; Ep: epineurium; PC: processus cochleariformis; Py: processus pyramidalis)

16. *Protecting the nerve from ossicular reconstruction assembly*: A strip of temporalis fascia graft is placed over the decompressed nerve in order to protect it from the subsequent ossicular reconstruction assembly.

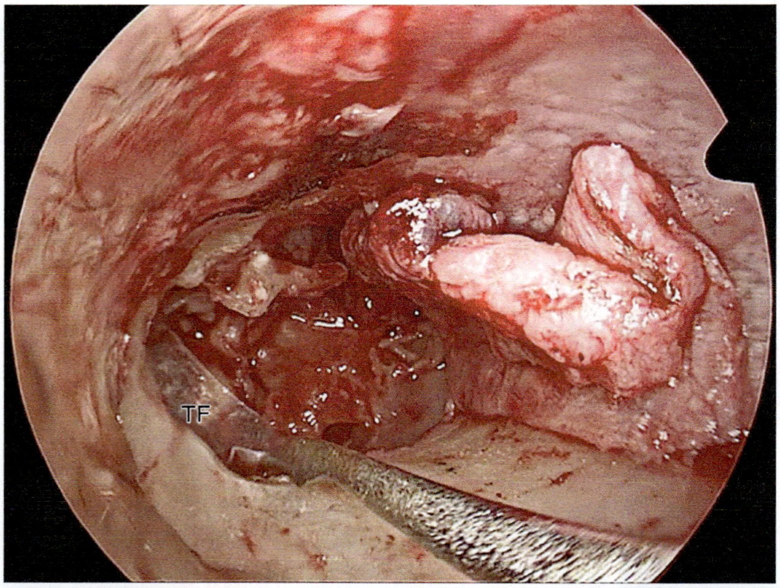

Fig. 23A: Strip of temporalis fascia being placed over decompressed nerve (right ear). (TF: temporalis fascia)

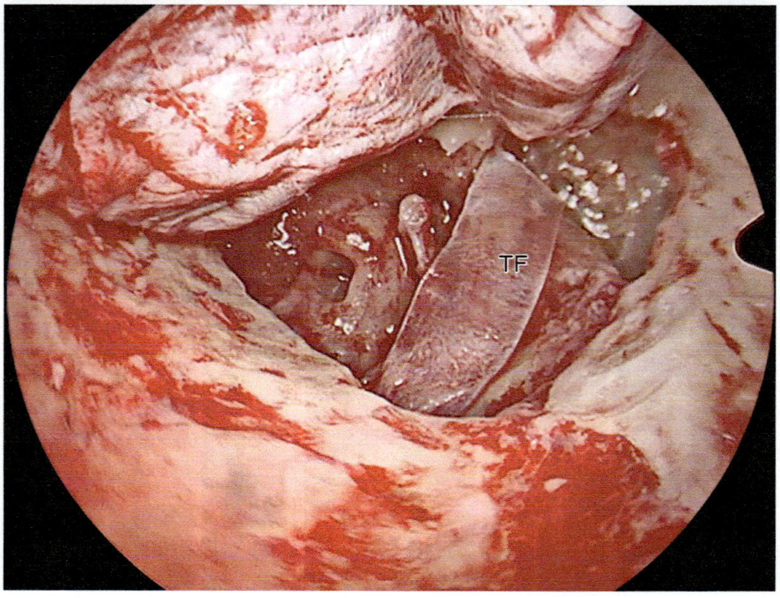

Fig. 23B: Strip of temporalis fascia being placed over decompressed nerve (left ear). (TF: temporalis fascia)

17. *Ossicular reconstruction:* The stapes superstructure is rarely disrupted in traumatic temporal bone fractures. Hence, in such situations, we prefer reconstruction with a partial ossicular replacement prosthesis (PORP). (Vide "Endoscopic Ossiculoplasty" chapter).

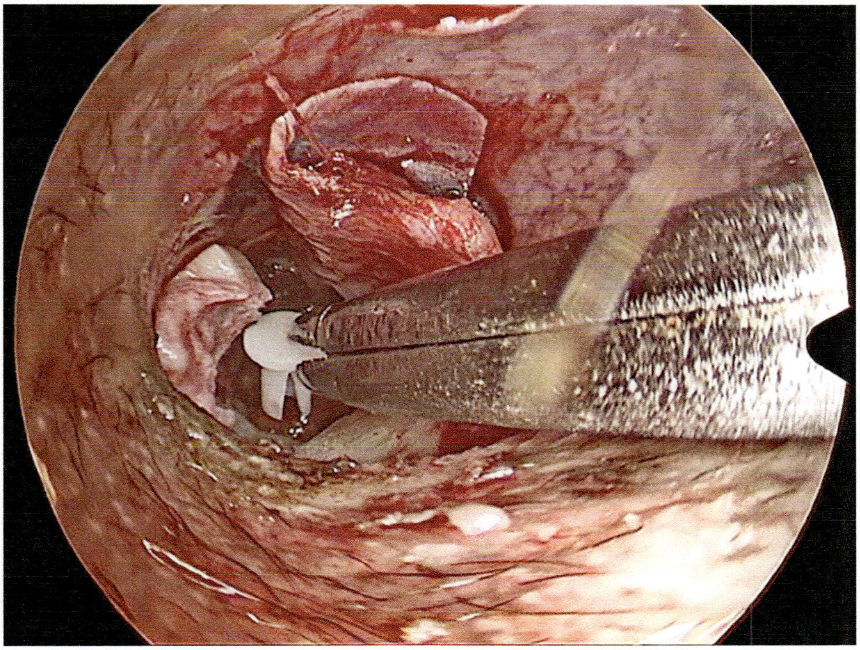

Fig. 24A: Ossicular chain reconstruction using partial ossicular replacement prosthesis (PORP). Note the posterosuperior canal wall already been reconstructed using cartilage.

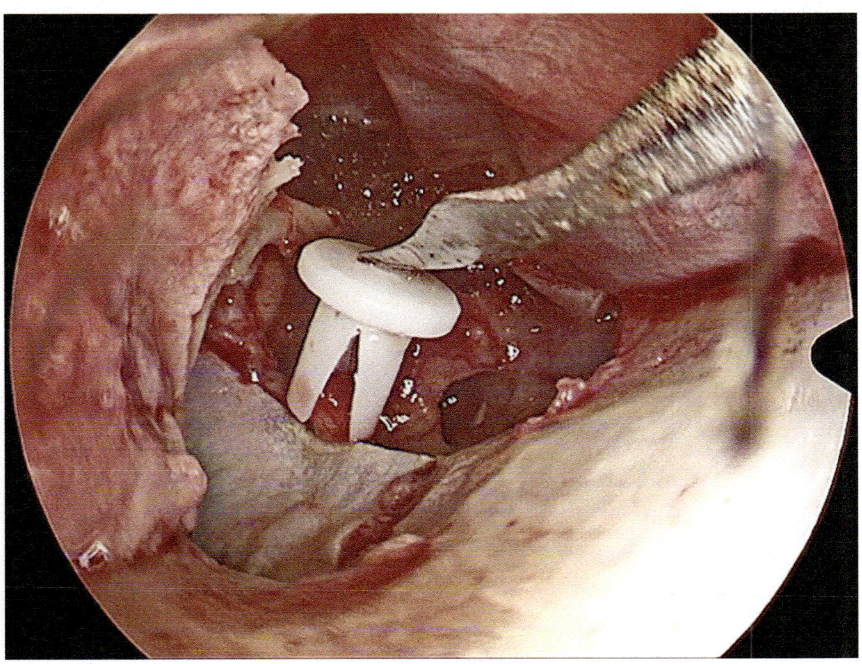

Fig. 24B: Ossicular chain replacement using partial ossicular reconstruction prosthesis (PORP). PORP being placed on stapes head.

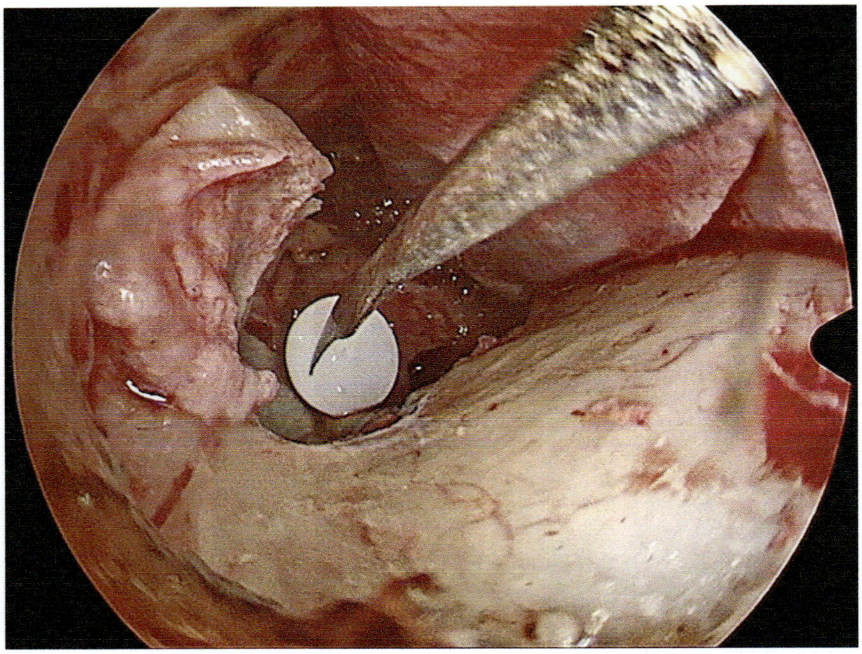

Fig. 24C: Ossicular chain reconstruction using partial ossicular replacement prosthesis (PORP). Vertical alignment of the PORP being checked.

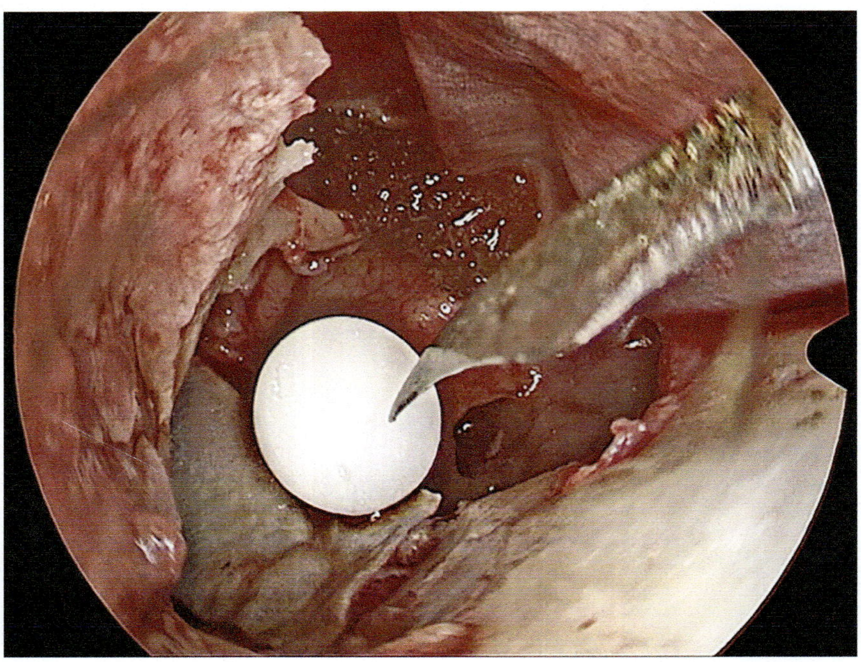

Fig. 24D: Ossicular chain reconstruction using partial ossicular replacement prosthesis (PORP). Demonstration of round window reflex.

18. *Temporalis fascia grafting*

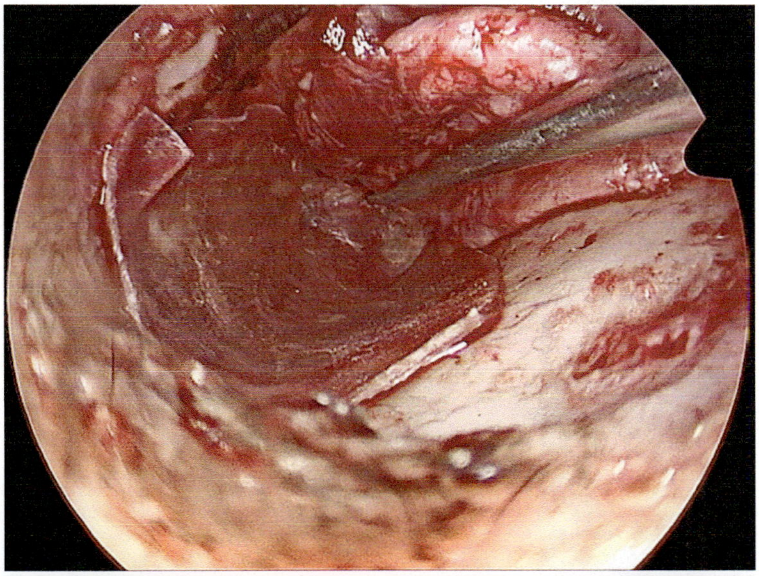

Fig. 25A: Temporalis fascia grafting.

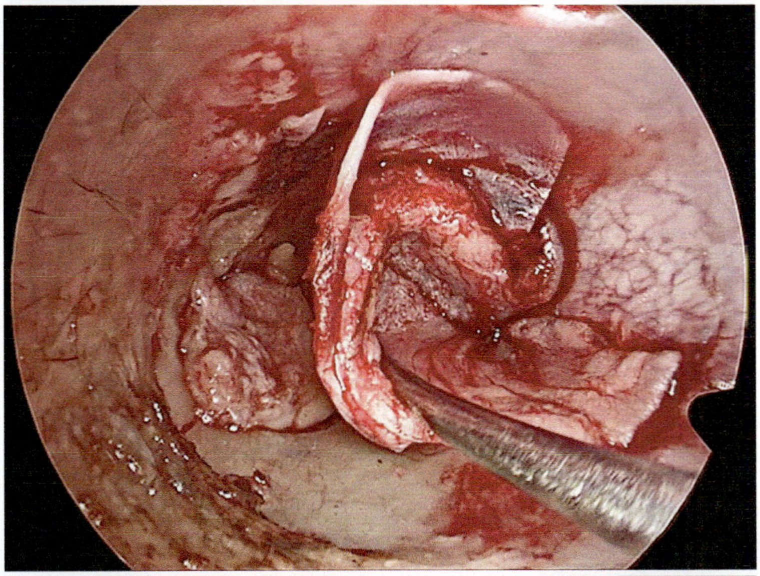

Fig. 25B: Repositioning of tympanomeatal flap.

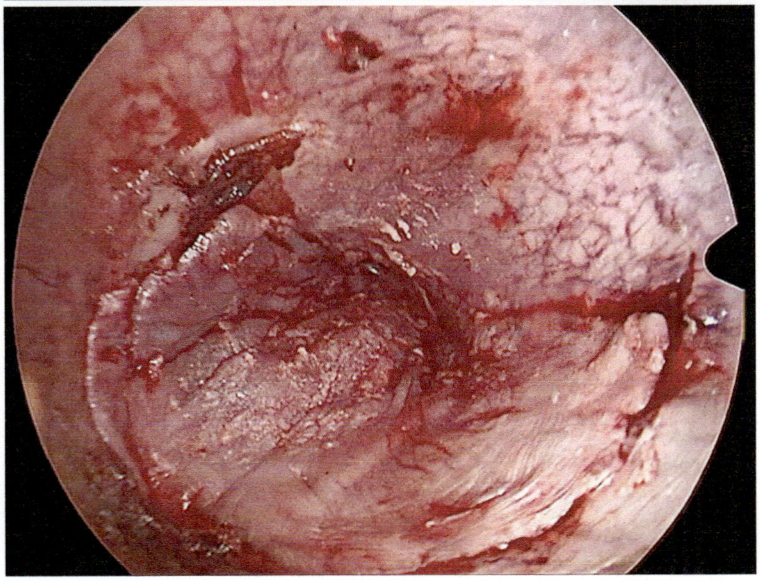

Fig. 25C: Note the edges of flap in alignment with the original site of incision.

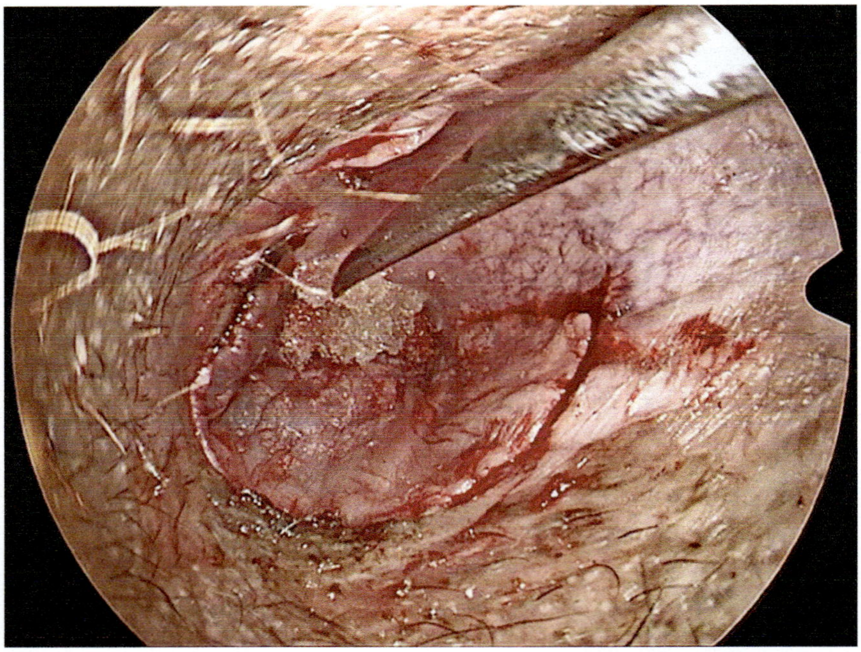

Fig. 25D: Gelfoam placement.

19. *Packing of middle ear and external auditory canal with gelfoam*

SPECIFIC POINTS RELATED SEGMENTAL DECOMPRESSION

Basic steps in terms of exposure remain the same for all the types.

- *Type A:* Steps to be followed as convention.
- *Type B:*
    - In order to decompress the distal segment of tympanic segment and mastoid segment proximal to processus pyramidalis, the posterosuperior canal wall bone needs to be removed
    - Canalplasty is done to remove this bone to ensure full exposure of the processus pyramidalis posterior to its base and ampullary end of lateral semicircular canal
    - Fallopian canal is thicker in this segment. It has to be drilled with a diamond burr.
    - Chorda tympani needs to be sacrificed sometimes to increase the exposure
    - Rotating burr should not touch the stapes or stapedius tendon to avoid sensorineural hearing loss

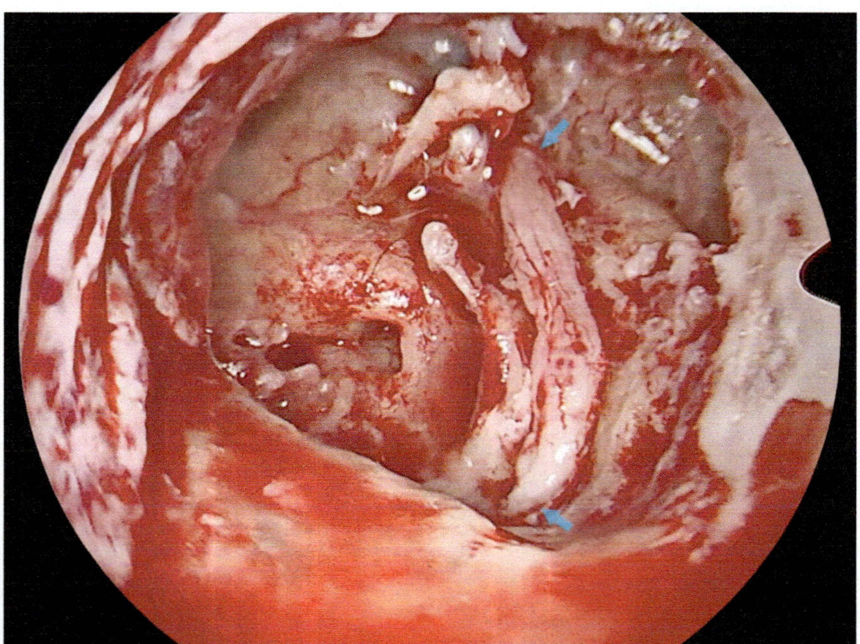

Fig. 26A: Type B decompression. Landmarks of type B decompression are first genu to second genu (blue arrows).

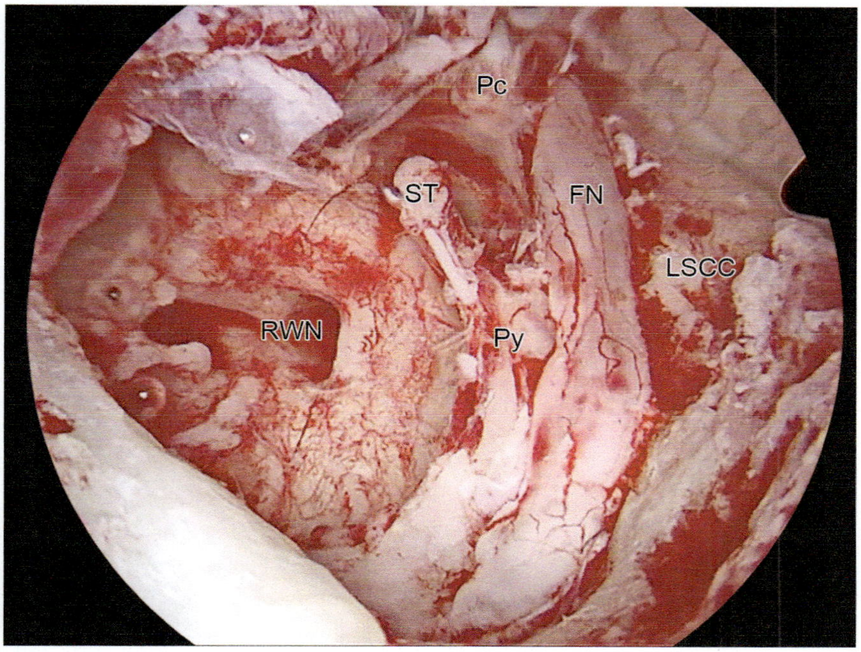

Fig. 26B: Type B decompression showing decompressed nerve segment and surrounding landmarks
(FN: facial nerve; LSCC: lateral semicircular canal; Pc: processus cochleariformis; Py: processus pyramidalis; RWN: round window niche; ST: stapes)

- *Type C:*
  - Exploration of labyrinthine segment is most challenging due to its difficult access
  - Endoscope gives a new perspective to address injuries in this region
  - Atticotomy should be wide enough so that instruments can reach up to tegmen
  - Supralabyrinthine cells are drilled using contra-angled handpiece or curetted with 0.8/1 mm curette
  - Geniculate crest is removed carefully without traumatizing the geniculate ganglion and tympanic segment
  - One must be extremely cautious not to injure the ampullary end of superior semicircular canal.

Exploration of Greater Superficial Petrosal Nerve

- Greater superficial petrosal nerve, is often not given much attention during facial nerve decompression
- However, owing to its important function of lacrimation, its dysfunction often leads to poor quality of life
- The nerve is often difficult to approach using the conventional microscopic transmastoid technique
- Endoscopes owing to their wide field of visualization and angulation, dissection in this region becomes much easier and safer without the need to remove excess bone
- Key points to be remembered during endoscopic GSPN decompression are:
  - Anterior epitympanic space should be widely exposed
  - Cog should be removed using a small curette

REFERENCES

1. Goodwin WJ Jr. Temporal bone fractures. Otolaryngol Clin North Am. 1983;16(3):651-9.
2. Patel A, Groppo E. Management of temporal bone trauma. Craniomaxillofac Trauma Reconstr. 2010;3(2):105-13.
3. Little SC, Kesser BW. Radiographic classification of temporal bone fractures: clinical predictability using a new system. Arch Otolaryngol Head Neck Surg. 2006;132(12):1300-4.
4. Lee LN, Lyford-Pike S, Boahene KD. Traumatic facial nerve injury. Otolaryngol Clin North Am. 2013;46(5):825-39.

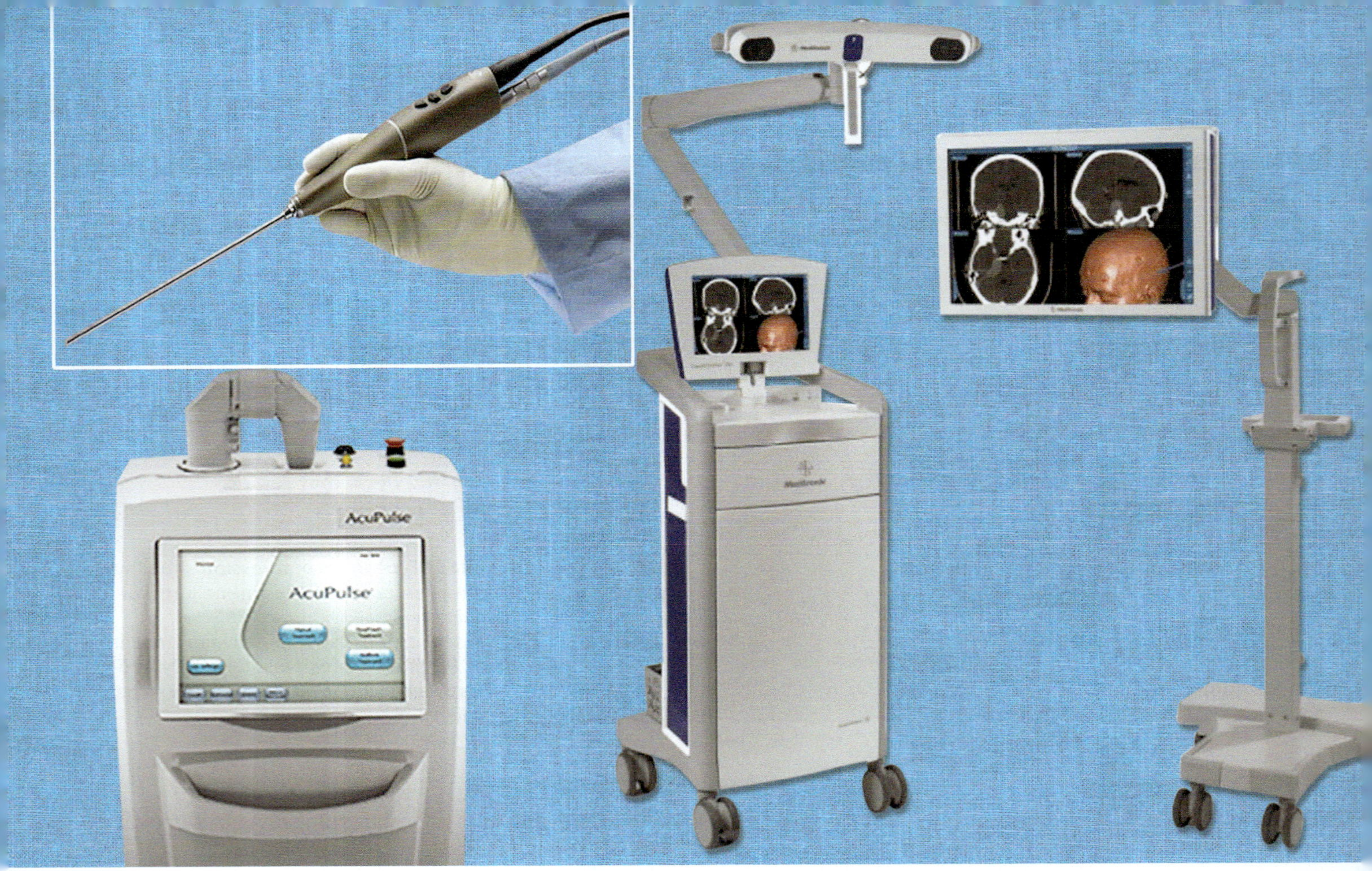

CHAPTER **15**

Recent Advances and Future of Transcanal Endoscopic Ear Surgery

Arindam Das, Sayan Hazra

Chapter Outline

INTRODUCTION

Operating microscope and Micromotor drill paved a new horizon in mastoid surgery, similarly transcanal endoscopic ear surgery (TEES) started to gain popularity with the advent of high-definition camera systems, endoscopes and host of armamentarium.

THREE-DIMENSIONAL HIGH-DEFINITION SYSTEM

Endoscopic ear surgery has often been criticized by otologists for its lack of depth perception. With the release of 4-mm high-definition three dimensional (3D) endoscopes, this shortcoming can be managed easily in the future. At present 0° and 30° angled 18 cm 3D scopes are available with digital and optical zoom comparable to the 2D system. The 3D effect is particularly suitable for convex or hollow structures such as the ear canal and middle ear cavity, thus providing better visualization of spatial relationships between key structures. The surgeon observes 3D stereoscopic images obtained from 3D scope, on a 26″ or 32″ monitor wearing 3D passive polarization glasses. 3D images can be converted back to 2D anytime if required in case surgeon feels uncomfortable by pressing a single switch. However, it is recommended to follow certain simple yet useful steps while operating on any 3D system to avoid such difficulties:

1. Initial few minutes of the surgery seem blurred and it takes time for the human eye to make adaptation with the polarization clip-on glasses.
2. Similarly, it will take few moments of adaptation again with change of position of the patient's head or that of the surgeon during the surgery.
3. The monitor is to be kept at distance of around 4 feet from the operating table at the surgeon's eye level, directly in view of the surgeon and assistant, thus providing a straight view and preventing any physical strain.
4. Background illumination of the theater is to be kept at a minimum to facilitate better visualization of the monitor, thus requiring lesser power from the light source as well as lesser glare on the screen.

Three-dimensional EES will prove to be an even better training and teaching tool in days to come.

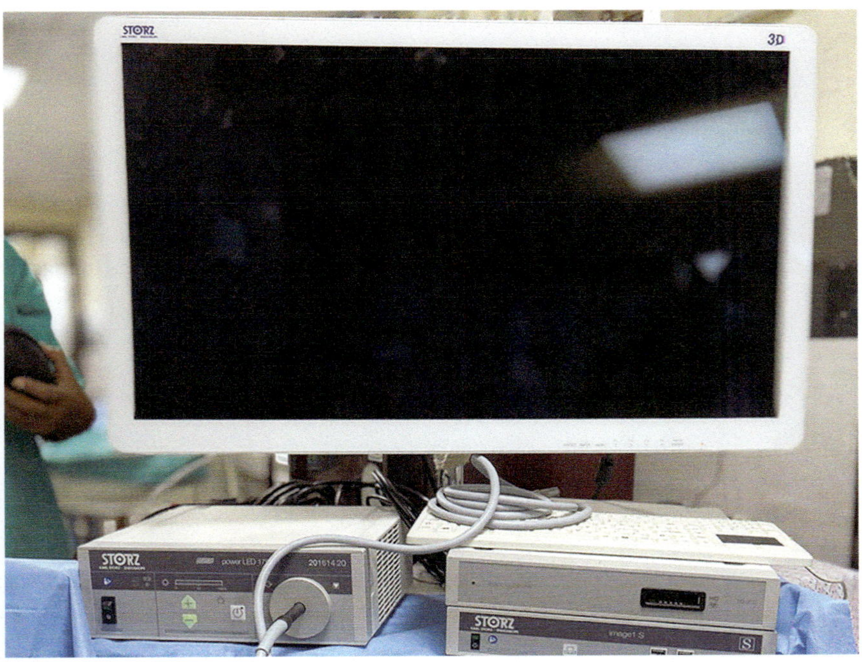

Fig. 1A: 32 inch 3D monitor with light source.

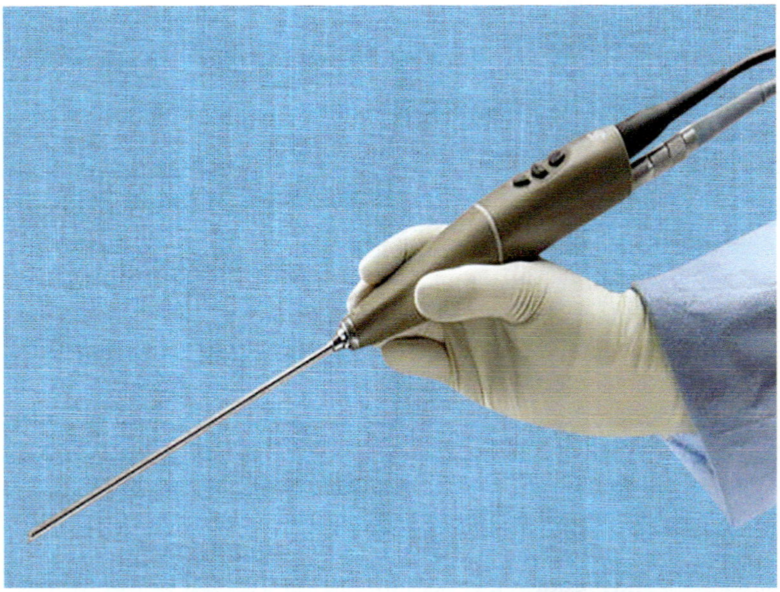

Fig. 1B: 3D endoscope.

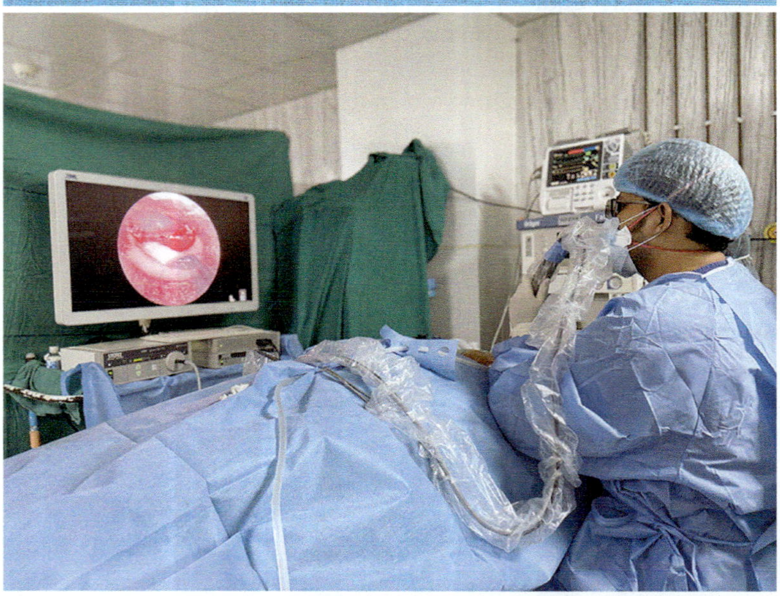

Fig. 1C: Depiction of position of surgeon and monitor.

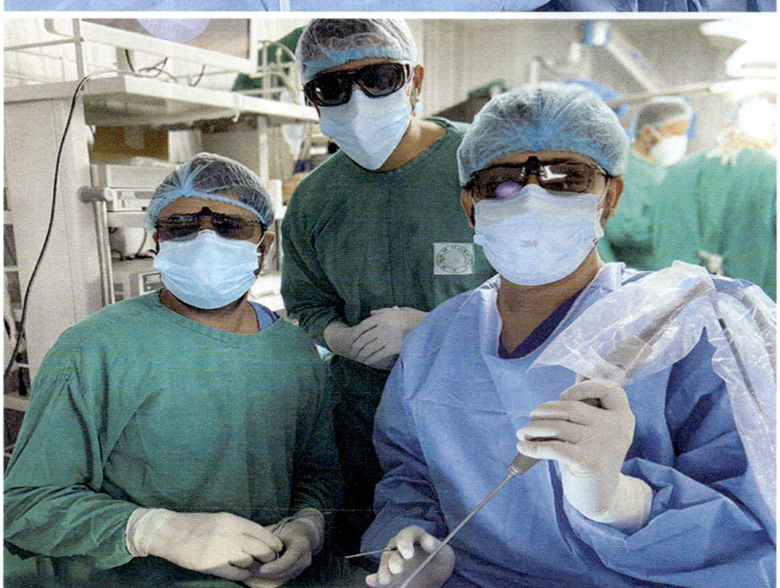

Fig. 1D: Surgeons wearing polarization glasses.

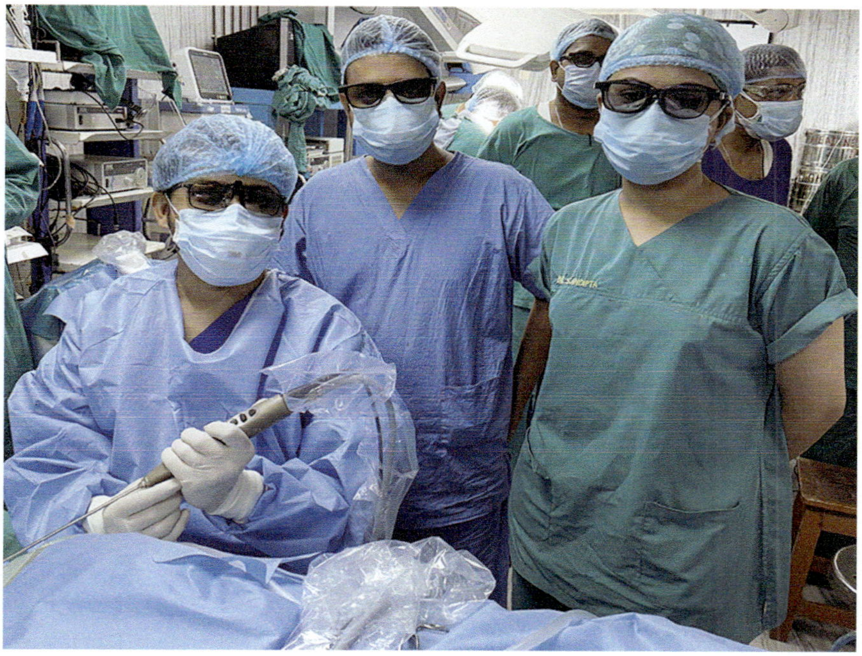

Fig. 1E: Surgeons (authors) wearing polarization glasses.

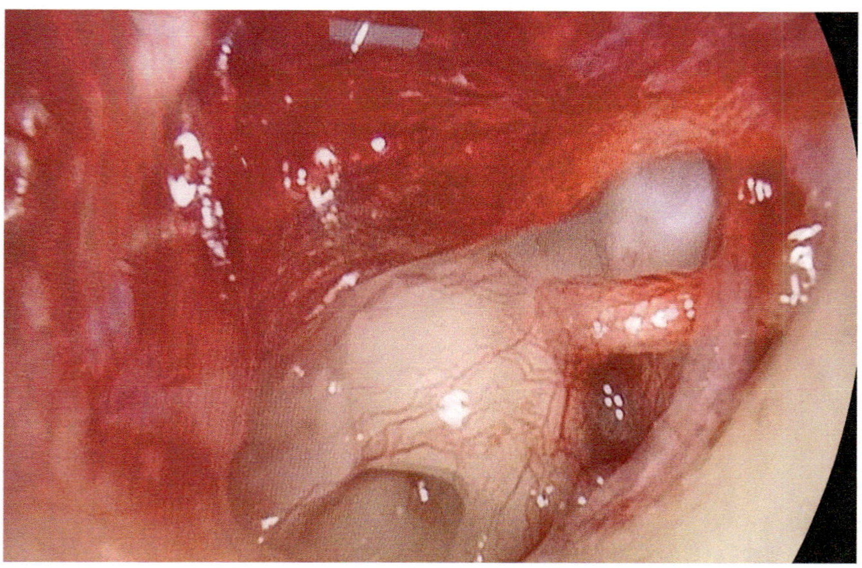

Fig. 2: 3D endoscopic view of left middle ear upon tympanotomy: As viewed on a 2D screen.

LASER

Lasers of different types (CO_2, Argon, Nd-YAG, etc.) are available, each with its own advantages of tissue penetration, precision and hemostatic properties. Flexible CO_2 laser with hand-held probe is a very useful tool during endoscopic ear surgery because of the precision and bloodless field it provides during extirpation of disease.

Lasers provide atraumatic surgery in relation to an intact ossicular chain. This unique property prevents any ossicular movement during stapes surgery or dissection of cholesteatoma.[1] Lasers have recently been used for myringotomy for its inherent bloodless sharp cutting property.[2] Use of Laser has been in vogue particularly for stapes surgery wherein it is used to cut the stapedius, evaporate the posterior crus and to make the fenestra on footplate with precision.

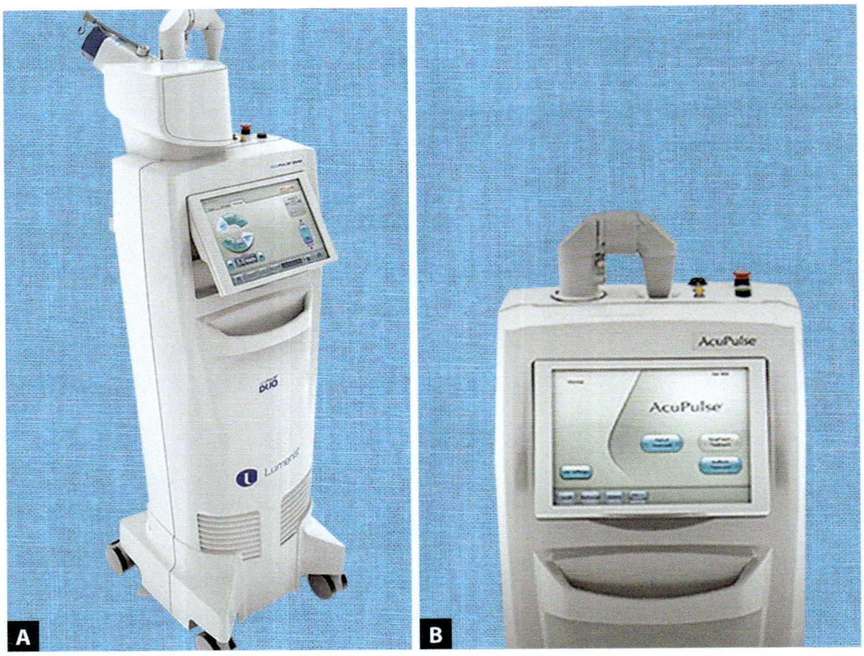

Fig. 3A and B: LASER machine used in transcanal endoscopic ear surgery (TEES).

Laser Probe in Endoscopic Ear Surgery

Flexible probe is needed since straight shot is not achievable without much bone removal. Handheld probes come in three varieties: (1) straight, (2) precurved and (3) malleable. The malleable ones are required in EES to negotiate beyond overhangs. Unlike microscopic Laser surgery where shots can be fired with micro-manipulator, Laser beam in EES needs to be fired close to structure. So, it is important to note that surgeon has to be aware while placing the probe and avoid touching nearby structures such as chorda which might get damaged by thermal damage of the probe tip. Similarly, while enlarging fenestra on foot-plate, standard perforators are to be used since beam size cannot be specified after the first firing due to unavailability of manipulator.

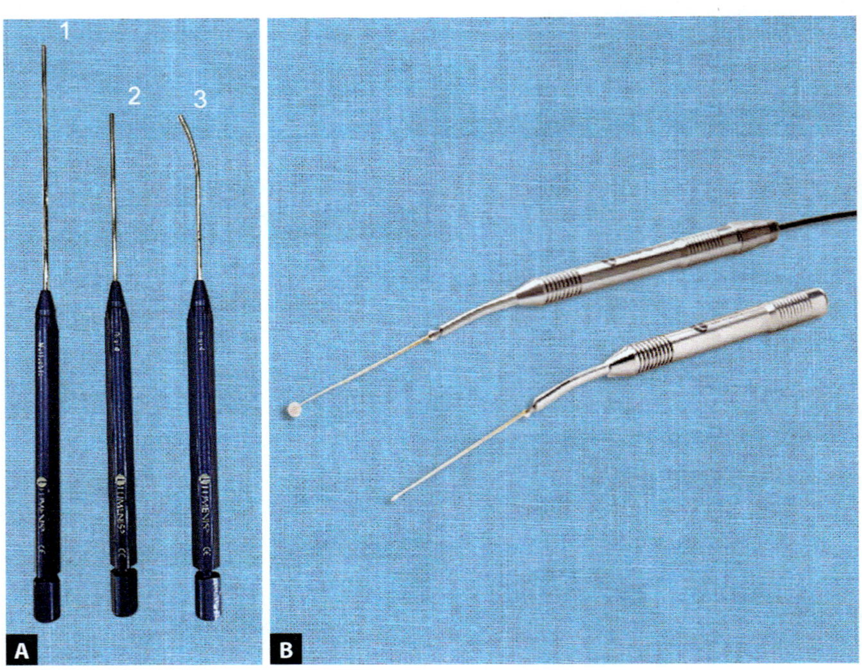

Fig. 4A and B: Handheld LASER probes, (1) malleable, (2) straight, (3) curved.

Safety protocol: In order to avoid injury to nearby vital structures while using Laser, saline soaked gel foams are placed over fallopian canal during entire procedure and footplate while working on stapedius and crura.

Laser specifications: The power of laser used ranges between 1 and 5 W with pulsed shooting.[3] Shooting time is generally 0.1 seconds for the tendon and between 0.05 and 0.1 seconds for the footplate. A minimum interval of 15–30 seconds is kept between every shooting on the footplate to allow the perilymph to cool. An average of 2–3 shots for the tendon, 4–7 shots for the crus, and single shot at footplate is used.

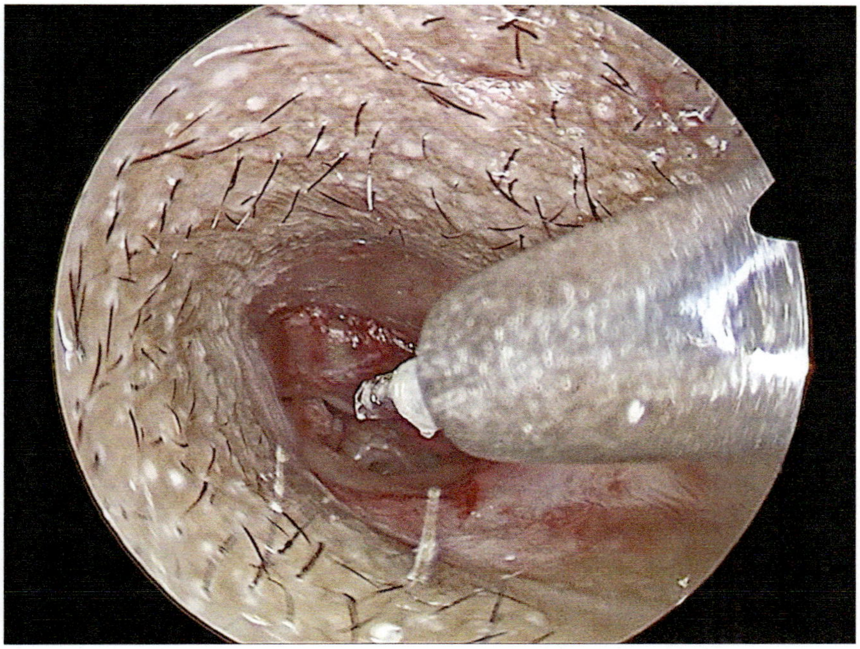

Fig. 5A: LASER probe being taken towards middle ear.

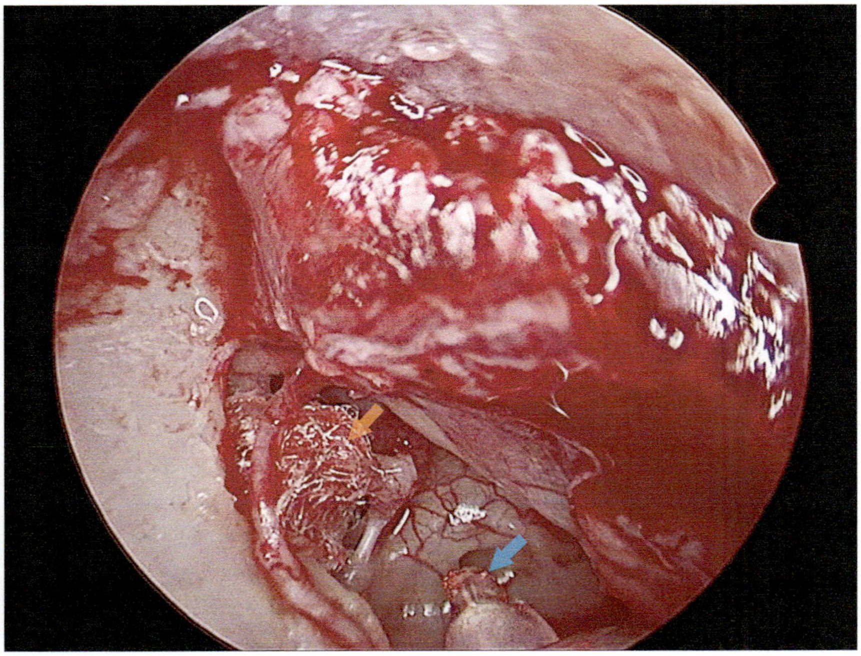

Fig. 5B: Orange arrow: Cottonoid to protect facial nerve, blue arrow: Laser Probe.

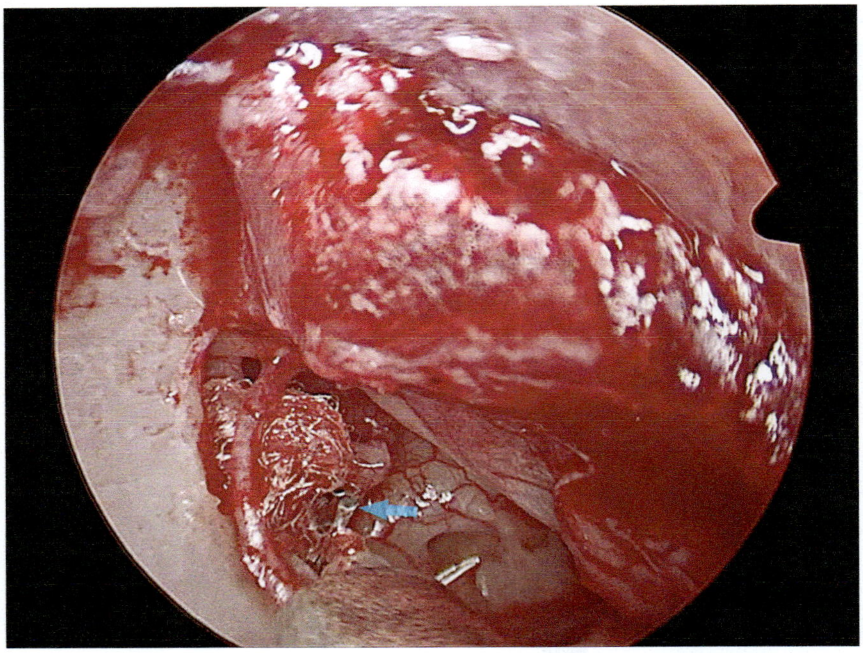

Fig. 5C: Blue arrow: Stapedius being vaporized.

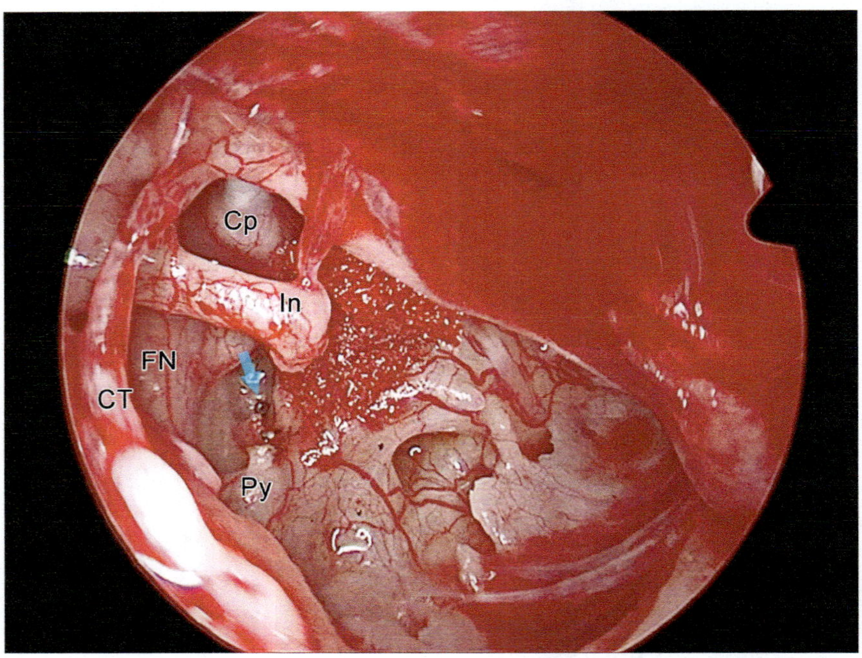

Fig. 5D: Blue arrow: Footplate fenestra created with regular perforator.
(Cp: processus cochleariformis; In: incus; FN: horizontal facial nerve; Py: pyramidalis process; CT: chorda tympani)

4K TECHNOLOGY AND NARROW-BAND IMAGING IN TEES

Development of high-definition visualization, such as 4K technology, which increases the magnification even further along with resolution, provides superior image sharpness and a much more detailed view of all anatomic and pathologic structures, which is particularly important when working around delicate and critical structures, thereby improving the safety and efficacy of the surgical procedure.

Use of narrow band imaging (NBI) has been in vogue in oncologic surgery. It uses a filter that allows different wavelengths of narrow band light (415 and 540 nm), in a sequential red-green-blue illumination, to pick up hypervascularity, which could indicate areas of dysplasia.

There has been interest in using this technology in non-cancer cases recently.[4]

Middle ear structures and disease process appear differently under the narrow band filter compared to ordinary LED or Halogen light. Tympanosclerosis and cholesteatoma being avascular in nature appear whiter than usual on NBI, whereas hypervascular structures, such as granulation tissue, are highlighted by the filter. This will facilitate better assessment of the extent of disease, and also ensure that small residual disease is not left behind at the time of operation.

The visualization modalities of the Storz Professional Image Enhancement System (SPIES), such as Clara, Chroma, and Spectra A and B, are available in both 2D and 3D systems. While Clara provides additional illumination for exploration of darker areas, the enhancement algorithms of Chroma, Spectra A and B facilitate the evaluation of the mucosal surface and the subepithelial vascularization. Their combination could be of particular interest in cholesteatoma surgery, as they may help in distinguishing cholesteatoma matrix from granulation tissue or normal mucosa. This property is utilized in facial nerve decompression surgery, wherein devitalized areas appear lighter and compression, hematoma, intraneural bleeding, neoangiogenesis appear hyperintense.

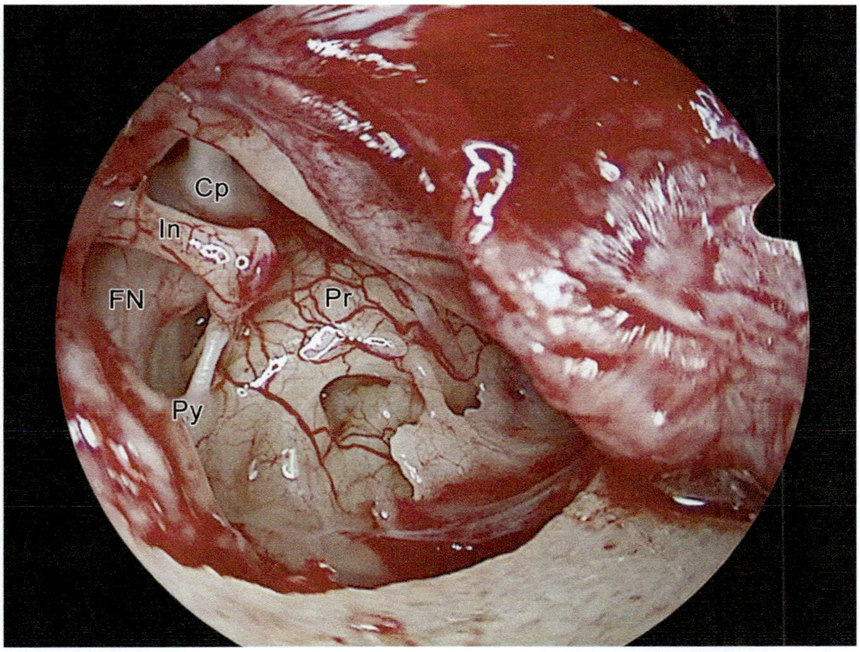

Fig. 6: Normal middle ear as seen in stapes surgery on Spectra B mode.
(Cp: processus cochleariformis; In: incus; FN: horizontal facial nerve; Py: pyramidalis process; Pr: promontory)

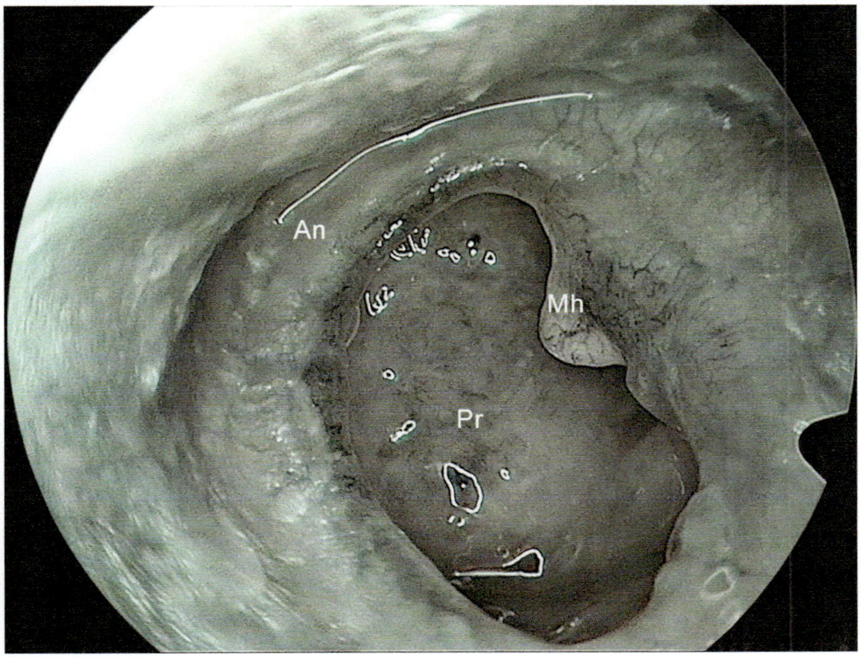

Fig. 7A: View of perforated tympanic membrane on Spectra A mode.
(An: annulus; Mh: malleus handle; Pr: promontory)

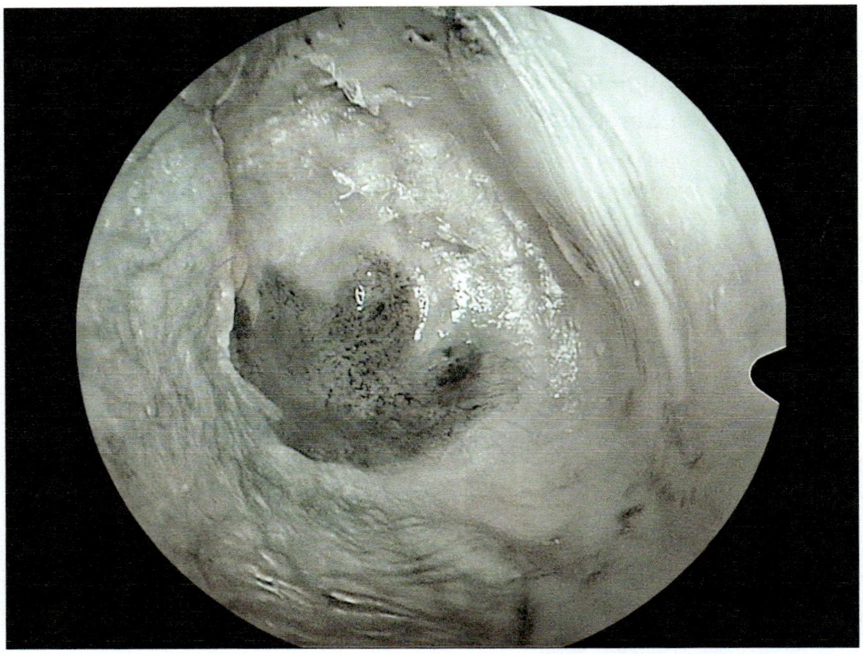

Fig. 7B: Granular myringitis with retracted membrane on spectra A mode.

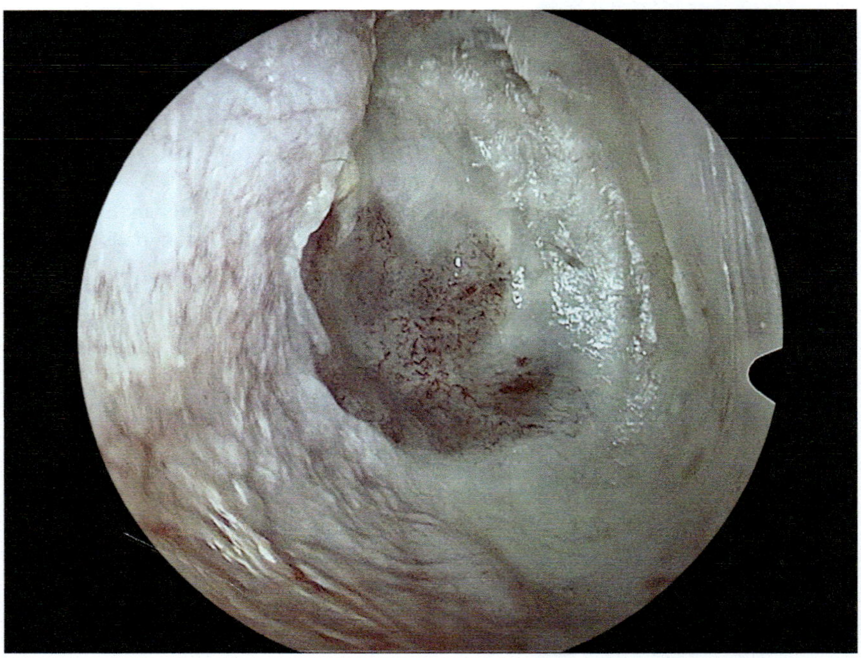

Fig. 7C: Granular myringitis with retracted membrane on spectra B mode.

The amalgamation of 4K magnification with NBI technology could improve the identification and dissection of middle ear pathologies, such as cholesteatoma, tympanosclerosis, carcinoma, etc., during middle ear surgery. The 4K magnification would allow a better visualization of the so-called hidden recesses such as sinus tympani, facial recess, and stapes foot plate while dissecting the disease.

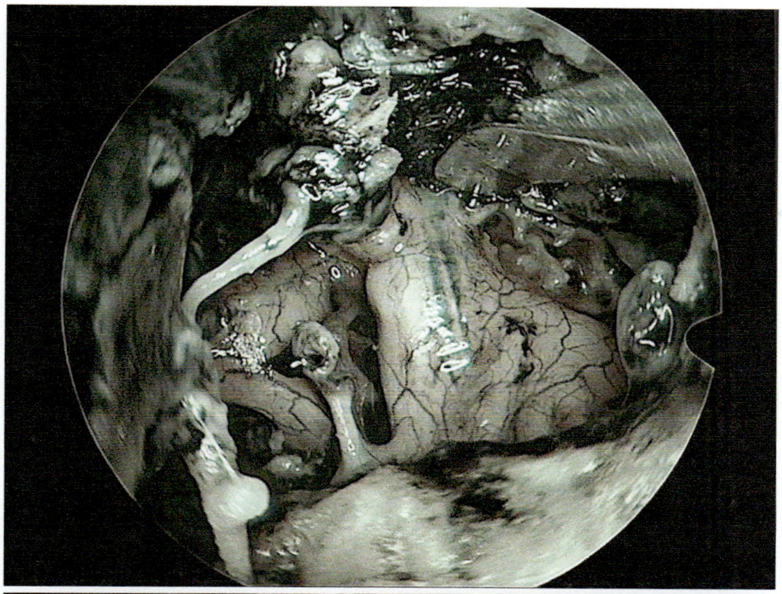

Fig. 8A: View of facial nerve decompression surgery on Spectra A mode (left ear).

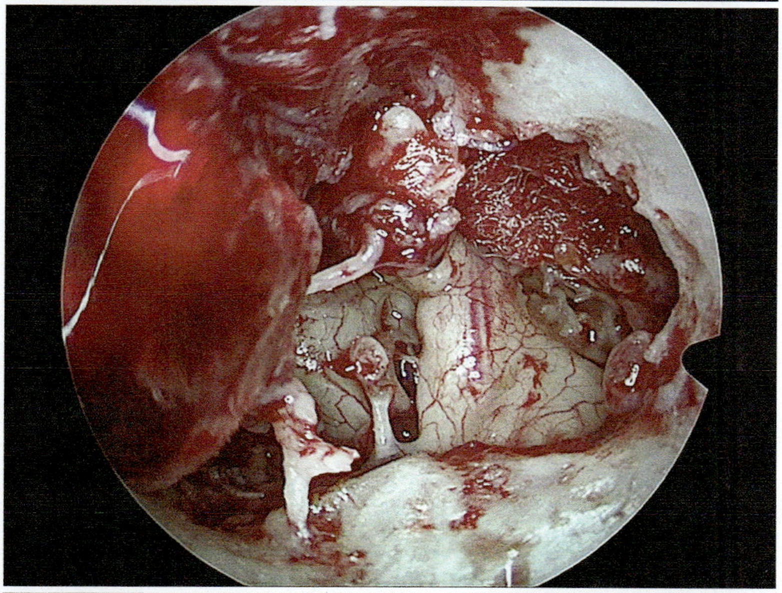

Fig. 8B: Corresponding views on Spectra B mode (left ear).

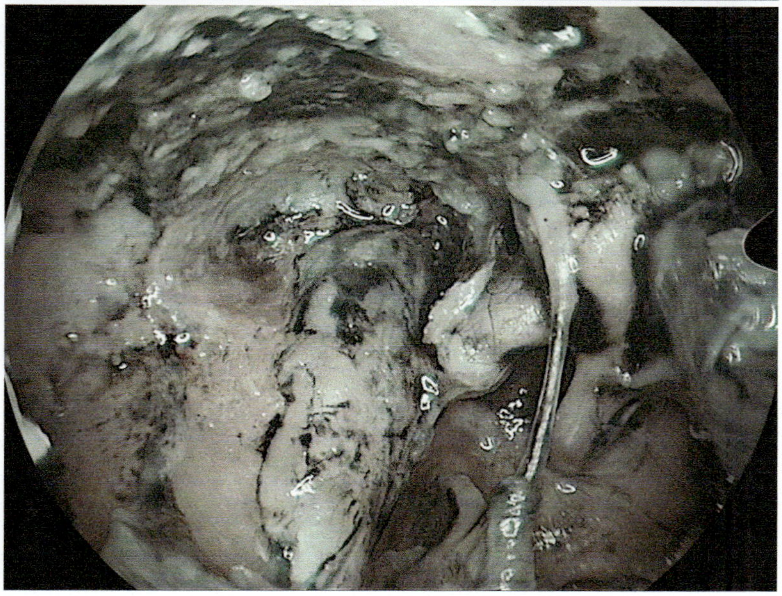

Fig. 8C: View of facial nerve decompression surgery on Spectra A mode (right ear).

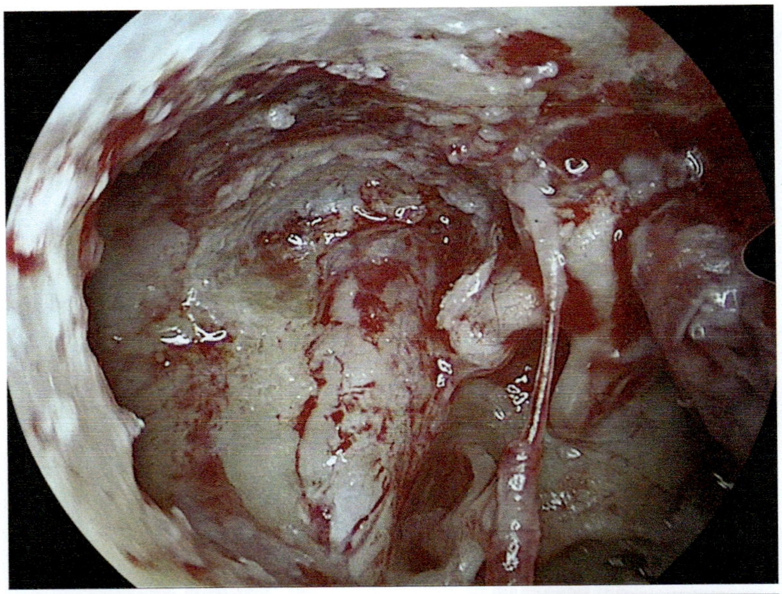

Fig. 8D: Corresponding views on Spectra B mode (right ear).

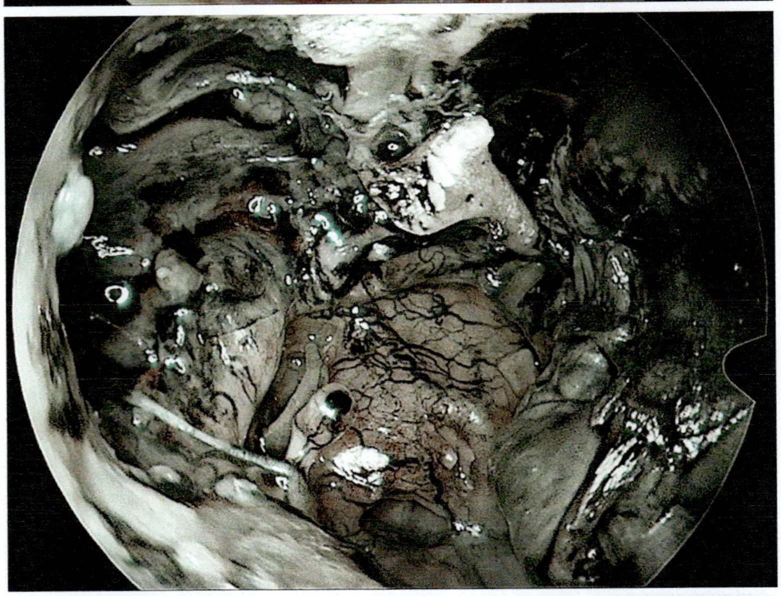

Fig. 8E: View of facial nerve decompression surgery on Spectra A mode (right ear).

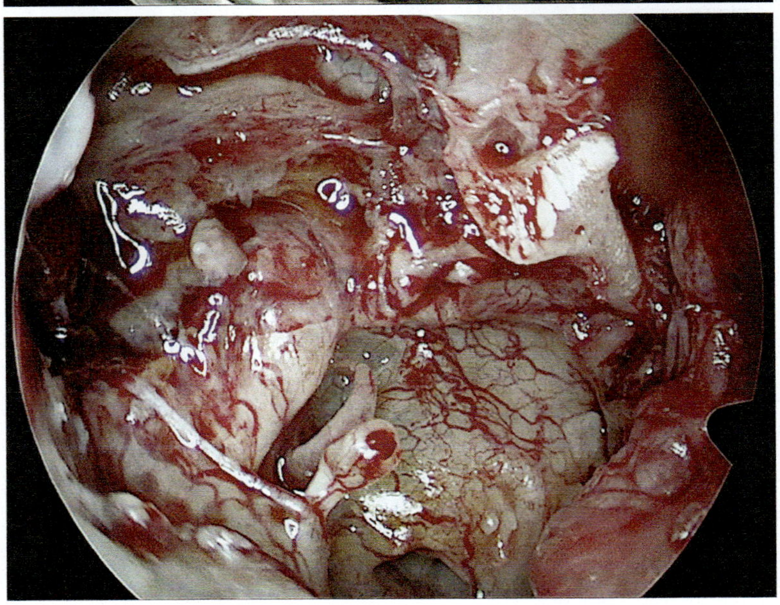

Fig. 8F: Corresponding views on Spectra B mode (right ear).

Piezosurgery

Piezoelectric surgery is another recently developed system by Mectron Medical Technology (Carasco, Genoa, Italy)[5] for cutting bone with microvibrations created by the piezoelectric effect which occurs when an electric current is passed through certain crystals and ceramics, causing them to oscillate at ultrasonic frequencies. The equipment consists of hand pieces, inserts, insert tips of various diameters, and peristaltic pumps that provide cooling during surgery by discharging a jet of physiologic saline solution.

The ultrasonic frequency of the device ranges from 24.7 to 29.5 kHz, and the amount of applied power ranges from 2.8 to 16 W. The cutting force can be programmed according to the density of the bone cut. The microvibrations created in the piezoelectric handpiece cause the inserts to vibrate linearly between 60 and 210 μm allowing a bone cut of only 0.3 to 0.6 mm width with no bone necrosis.

The piezoelectric surgery device is able to cut bone cleanly and quickly without causing necrosis or damage to nonmineralized tissue.[6] The system has the advantage of minimal damage to surrounding soft tissues, maximum surgical precision, and a blood-free surgical field, thus augmenting intraoperative visibility. Wide range of surgical inserts available makes it easy to use in endoscopic ear surgery. This property can be used in cholesteatoma surgery and skull base procedures wherein bone cuts are made without collateral damage to surrounding healthy tissues. EES being single handed surgery, this tool might come quite handy in days to come.

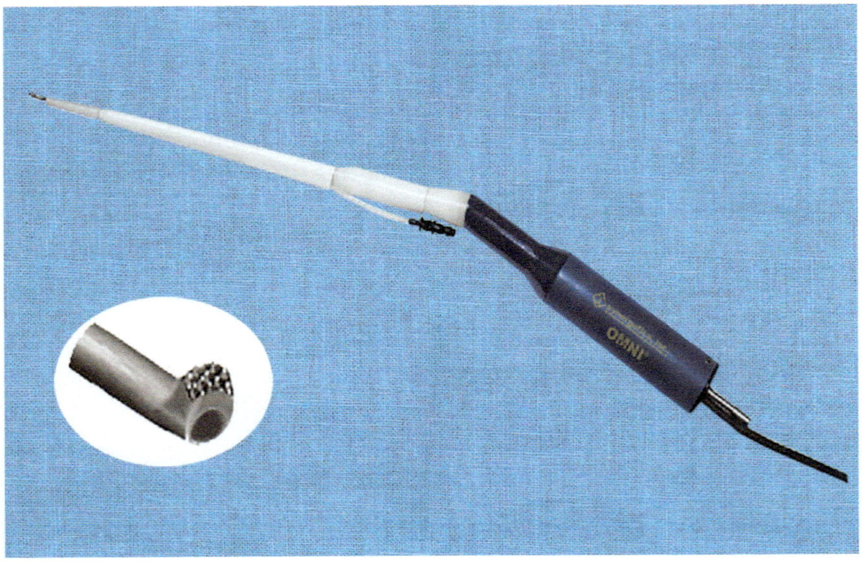

Fig. 9: Piezoelectric ultrasonic handpiece.

Neuronavigation and Intraoperative Doppler

Neuronavigation provides the surgical route map based on preoperative imaging of the patient. Since the realms of TEES has been increasing every day, it is pertinent to use image guidance systems to identify critical anatomical landmarks intraoperatively. These anatomic landmarks orient the surgeon during temporal bone drilling, to optimize access creation while minimizing bone removal and evading critical structures, such as the facial nerve, semicircular canals and sigmoid sinus. However, these landmarks are subject to high interindividual variability and chances of erosion by tumor, inflammation, or previous surgery.

Initially developed for neurosurgical procedures, these systems use computerized tracking devices to monitor the position of the endoscopes or instruments relative to the patient's anatomic landmarks. The system displays the location of the tip of a tracked drill, and other instruments, in real-time, on a navigation map of the patient's preoperative anatomy image.[7,8]

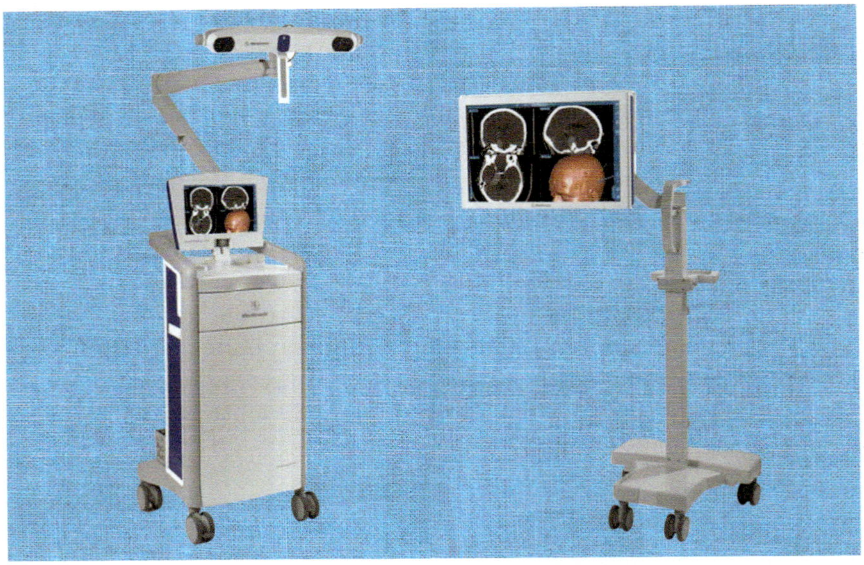

Fig. 10: Neuronavigation system.

With the development of new endoscopic surgical approaches to the inner ear, petrous apex and cerebello-pontine (CP) angle it is becoming ever more necessary to use special instruments in order to have the correct anatomical orientation during surgery. Neuronavigation provides helpful information to the surgeon while working deep in the skull base and the use of intraoperative Doppler ultrasound is helpful in detecting the appropriate position of the internal carotid artery during the endoscopic approach to inner ear lesions.

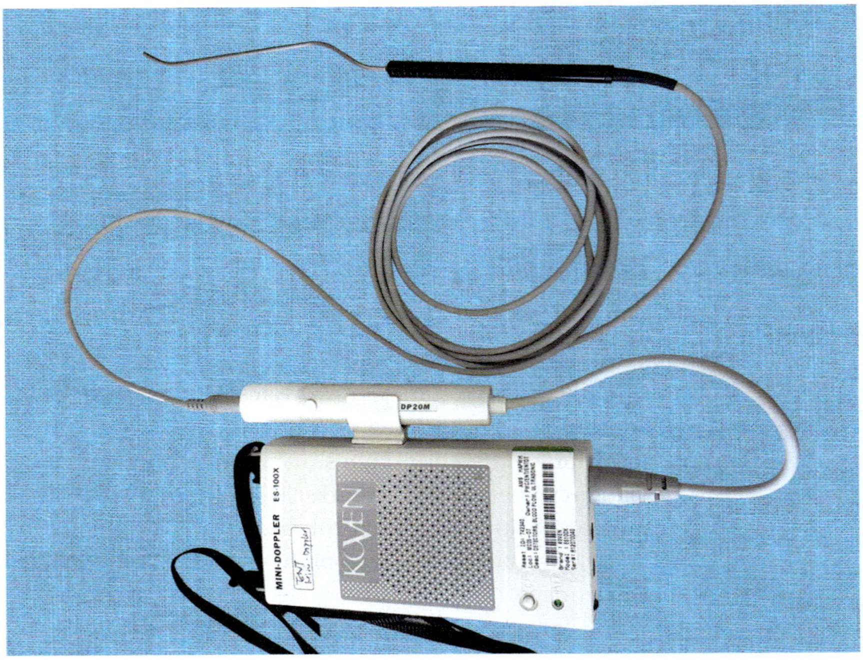

Fig. 11: Doppler ultrasound system with handheld probe.

Facial Nerve Monitor System

- Facial nerve monitor is a useful tool for intraoperative monitoring of facial nerve functional and anatomical integrity.
- Primarily used for—parotid and lateral skull base surgery.
- Needle electrode tips are inserted into ipsilateral orbicularis oculi and orbicularis oris along with a ground electrode. Myogenic potentials generated by giving electrical stimuli through a handheld probe are collected from electrodes on the muscles.

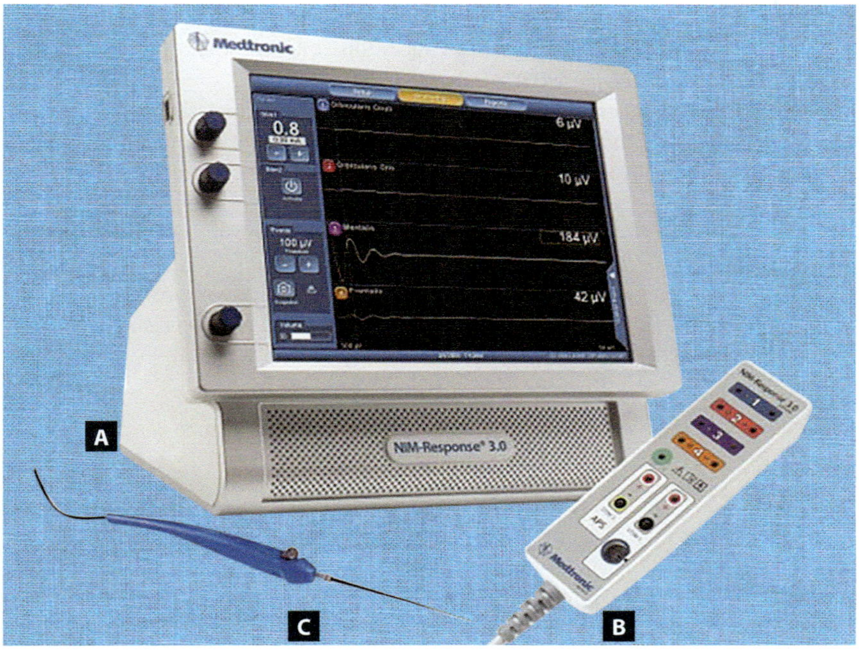

Fig. 12A to C: Intraoperative nerve monitoring systems. (A) Console; (B) Patient Interface; (C) Stimulator probe.

- Handheld probe is touched upon desired area to test the presence of facial nerve during middle ear dissection. Similarly, nerve integrity and functionality are tested by the probe in facial nerve decompression surgery.
- With recent widespread use of endoscopes in middle ear surgery it will prove to be an indispensable tool for procedures such as facial nerve decompression, epitympanic exploration, cochlear implantation and even routine mastoid surgery wherein precise knowledge of the location of facial nerve will prevent any inadvertent injury.

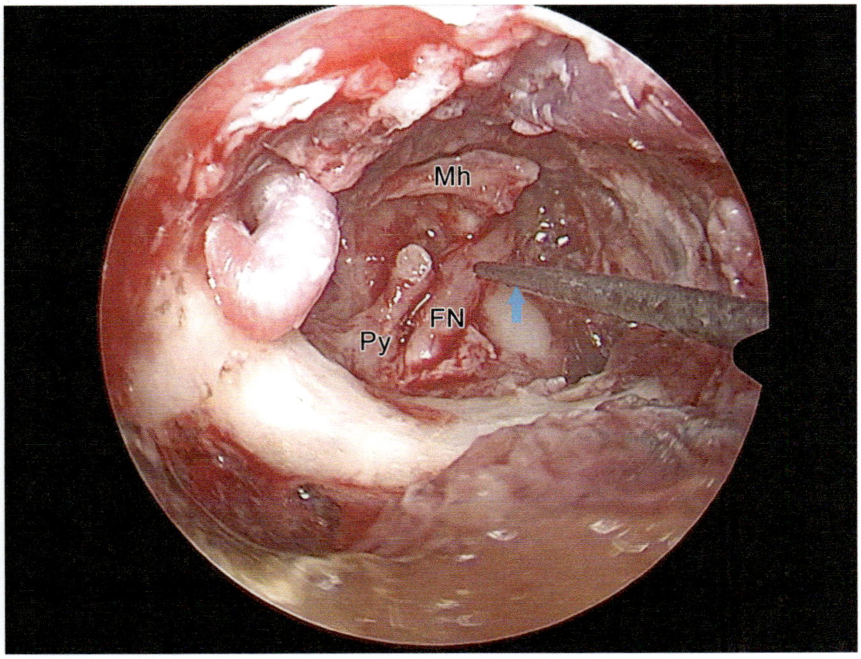

Fig. 13: Facial nerve integrity is being checked. (Py: processus pyramidalis; FN: facial nerve; Mh: malleus handle; Blue arrow—nerve stimulator probe)

In the last few years, the world has seen technical improvements and growing expertise in the handling of the endoscope allowing introduction of an exclusive endoscopic approach to the middle ear. Endoscopic instrumentation, techniques, and knowledge have been ever evolving, and in the future, endoscopic surgical techniques will gain even more importance in otologic surgery pertaining to lateral skull base, middle cranial fossa, and posterior fossa/CP angle pathologies. Who knows, in the coming years, use of automation, artificial intelligence, robotics, etc., might open up altogether different dimension to otology practice.

REFERENCES

1. Fyrmpas G, Tsetsos N, Katotomichelakis M, Rudic M. Lasers in endoscopic middle ear surgery: where do we stand today? Eur Arch Otorhinolaryngol. 2021;278(11):4169-77.
2. Silverstein H, Kuhn J, Choo D, Krespi YP, Rosenberg SI, Rowan P. Laser-assisted tympanostomy. Laryngoscope. 1996;106:1067-74.
3. Yetiser S. Flexible fiber optic carbon-dioxide laser assisted stapedotomy in otosclerosis. Int J Otolaryngol. 2016;2016:4958074.
4. Plaat B, Zwakenberg MA, Zwol JGV, Wedman J, van der Laan BFAM, Halmos GB, et al. Narrow-band imaging in transoral laser surgery for early glottic cancer in relation to clinical outcome. Head Neck. 2017;39(7):1343-8.
5. Piezosurgery medical manufactured by Mectron medical technology. Peizosurgery SRL, Via Portobello 12, 16039 Sestri Levante (GE), Italy.
6. Vercellotti T. Technological characteristics and clinical indications of piezoelectric bone surgery. Minerva Stomatol. 2004;53(5):207-14.
7. Stamm AC, Pignatari S, Sebusiani S. Image-guided endoscopic sinus and skull base surgery. Rev Bras Otorinolaringol. 2002;68:502-9.
8. Metson R, Cosenza M, Gliklish RE, Montgomery WW. The role of image-guidance systems for head and neck surgery. Arch Otolaryngol Head Neck Surg. 1999;125:1100-4.

Index

Page numbers followed by *f* refer to figure.

G

H

I

J

L

M

V

W

X